WORLD HEALTH ORGANIZATION

INTERNATIONAL AGENCY FOR RESEARCH ON CANCER

IARC Handbooks of Cancer Prevention

Carotenoids

Volume 2

This publication represents the views and expert opinions
of an IARC Working Group on the
Evaluation of Cancer-preventive Agents,
which met in Lyon,

10–16 December 1997

1998

Published by the International Agency for Research on Cancer,
150 cours Albert Thomas, F-69372 Lyon cedex 08, France

© International Agency for Research on Cancer, 1998

Distributed by Oxford University Press, Walton Street, Oxford, UK OX2 6DP (Fax: +44 1865 267782) and in
the USA by Oxford University Press, 2001 Evans Road, Carey, NC 27513, USA (Fax: +1 919 677 1303).
All IARC publications can also be ordered directly from IARC*Press*
(Fax: +33 4 72 73 83 02; E-mail: press@iarc.fr).

IARC Library Cataloguing in Publication Data

Carotenoids/
    IARC Working Group on the Evaluation of
    Cancer Preventive Agents (1997 : Lyon,
    France)

(IARC handbooks of cancer prevention ; 2)

1. Carotenoids – congresses. I. IARC Working Group on the Evaluation of Cancer
   Preventive Agents II Series

ISBN 92 832 3002 7   (NLM Classification: W1)
ISSN 1027-5622

International Agency For Research On Cancer

The International Agency for Research on Cancer (IARC) was established in 1965 by the World Health Assembly, as an independently financed organization within the framework of the World Health Organization. The headquarters of the Agency are in Lyon, France.

The Agency conducts a programme of research concentrating particularly on the epidemiology of cancer and the study of potential carcinogens in the human environment. Its field studies are supplemented by biological and chemical research carried out in the Agency's laboratories in Lyon and, through collaborative research agreements, in national research institutions in many countries. The Agency also conducts a programme for the education and training of personnel for cancer research.

The publications of the Agency contribute to the dissemination of authoritative information on different aspects of cancer research. A complete list is printed at the back of this book. Information about IARC publications, and how to order them, is also available via the Internet at: **http://www.iarc.fr/**

Note to the Reader

Anyone who is aware of published data that may influence any consideration in these *Handbooks* is encouraged to make the information available to the Unit of Chemoprevention, International Agency for Research on Cancer, 150 Cours Albert Thomas, 69372 Lyon Cedex 08, France

Although all efforts are made to prepare the *Handbooks* as accurately as possible, mistakes may occur. Readers are requested to communicate any errors to the Unit of Chemoprevention, so that corrections can be reported in future volumes.

Contents

List of Participants 1

Preamble 3

General Remarks 15

Carotenoids
1   **Chemical and physical characteristics of carotenoids** 23
1.1   Structure and nomenclature 23
1.2   General properties 27
       1.2.1 Relationships between structure, properties and biological activity 27
       1.2.2 Molecular size and shape 27
       1.2.3 Solubility 27
       1.2.4 Properties and molecular interactions of carotenoids *in vivo* 27
1.3   Properties of the conjugated polyene chain 28
       1.3.1 Light absorption and photochemical properties 28
       1.3.2 Chemical properties 28
1.4   Isolation and analysis 29
       1.4.1 General methods 29
       1.4.2 Identification 30
       1.4.3 Quantitative analysis 30
1.5   Data on individual compounds 30
       1.5.1 β-Carotene 30
       1.5.2 α-Carotene 31
       1.5.3 Lycopene 31
       1.5.4 Lutein 32
       1.5.5 Canthaxanthin 33
       1.5.6 Zeaxanthin 33
       1.5.7 β-Cryptoxanthin 34
       1.5.8 α-Cryptoxanthin 34
       1.5.9 Zeinoxanthin 35

2   **Occurrence, commercial sources, use and application, analysis and human exposure** 35
2.1   Carotenes 36
       2.1.1 β-Carotene 36
       2.1.2 α-Carotene 41
       2.1.3 Lycopene 43
2.2   Xanthophylls 44
       2.1.1 Lutein and zeaxanthin 44
       2.2.2 Cryptoxanthin 45
       2.2.3 Canthaxanthin 46

3   **Metabolism, klnetics and genetic variation** 46
3.1   Humans 47
        3.1.1   Intestinal digestion and absorption 47
        3.1.2   Transport in plasma 48
        3.1.3   Serum carotenoid concentrations 49
             3.1.3.1   Effects of β-carotene supplements 50
             3.1.3.2   Effects of tobacco smoking .51
             3.1.3.3   Effects of alcohol drinking 51
             3.1.3.4   Effects of other modulators .52
        3.1.4 Tissue carotenoid concentrations 52
             3.1.4.1   Effects of dietary intake 52
             3.1.4.2   Effects of supplemental intake 54
        3.1.5 Kinetics 54
        3.1.6 Metabolism 55
             3.1.6.1   β-Carotene 55
             3.1.6.2   β-Apocarotenoids 57
             3.1.6.3   Other carotenoids 57
        3.1.7   Genetic variation 58
3.2   Experimental models 58
        3.2.1   Non-human primates 58
        3.2.2   Preruminant calves and cows 59
        3.2.3   Ferrets 61
        3.2.4   Rats 62
        3.2.5   Other animal species 63
        3.2.6   Conclusion 64

4.   **Preventive effects** 64
4.1   Humans 64
        4.1.1   Studies of cancer occurrence 64
             4.1.1.1   Observational studies based on blood and other tissue measures of
                       carotenoids 64
             4.1.1.2   Observational studies based on dietary questionnaires 92
             4.1.1.3   Intervention trials 118
        4.1.2   Studies of intermediate end-points 130
             4.1.2.1   Observational studies of dietary and serum carotenoids 130
             4.1.2.2   Experimental studies of colorectal adenoma 131
             4.1.2.3   Experimental studies of cellular dysplasia and atypia 131
             4.1.2.4   Experimental studies of oral leukoplakia 132
             4.1.2.5   Experimental studies of cell proliferation 133
             4.1.2.6   Experimental studies of chromosomal damage 134
             4.1.2.7   Experimental studies of immunological end-points 135
             4.1.2.8   Summary 136
4.2   Experimental models 137
        4.2.1   Experimental animals 137
             4.2.1.1   β-Carotene 137
             4.2.1.2   β-Carotene with other potential inhibitors 179
             4.2.1.3   Canthaxanthin 191
             4.2.1.4   Canthaxanthin with other potential inhibitors 205
             4.2.1.5   Lycopene 207

	4.2.1.6	Lutein	211
	4.2.1.7	α-Carotene	212
	4.2.1.8	Fucoxanthin	215
	4.2.1.9	Astaxanthin	215
	4.2.1.10	Crocetin	216
	4.2.1.11	Mixtures of carotenoids	216
	4.2.1.12	Other end-points	219
4.2.2	Cells		220
	4.2.2.1	Mammalian cells *in vitro*	220
	4.2.2.2	Antimutagenicity in short-term tests	229
4.3	Mechanisms of cancer prevention		251
	4.3.1	Antioxidant properties	251
	4.3.2	Modulation of carcinogen metabolism	254
	4.3.3	Effects on cell transformation and differentiation	254
	4.3.4	Effects on cell-to-cell communication	254
	4.3.5	Inhibition of cell proliferation and oncogene expression	254
	4.3.6	Effects on immune function	254
	4.3.7	Inhibition of endogenous formation of carcinogens	254

5	**Other beneficial effects**	255
5.1	Photosensitivity disorders	255
5.2	Cardiovascular disease	255
5.3	Age-related macular degeneration and cataract	257
5.4	Other effects	259

6	**Carcinogenicity**	259
6.1	Humans	259
	6.1.1 ATBC study	259
	6.1.2 CARET	259
	6.1.3 Interpretation of trials suggesting carcinogenicity	260
6.2	Experimental animals	261
6.3	Mechanisms of carcinogenicity	262

7	**Other toxic effects**	263
7.1	Toxic and other adverse effects	263
	7.1.1	Humans	263
	7.1.2	Experimental animals	264
7.2	Reproductive and developmental effects	264
	7.2.1	Humans	264
	7.2.2	Experimental animals	265
7.3	Genetic and related effects	266
	7.3.1	Humans	265
	7.3.2	Experimental systems	266
		7.3.2.1	*In vitro*	266
		7.3.2.2	*In vivo*	270

8 **Summary of data** 270
8.1 Chemistry, occurrence and human exposure 270
8.2 Metabolism and kinetics 270
    8.2.1 Humans 270
    8.2.2 Experimental models 271
8.3 Cancer-preventive effects 271
    8.3.1 Humans 271
    8.3.2 Experimental systems 271
        8.3.2.1 Cancer-preventive activity 272
        8.3.2.2 Genetic and related effects 272
    8.3.3 Mechanisms of cancer prevention 275
8.4 Other beneficial effects 275
8.5 Carcinogenic effects 276
    8.5.1 Humans 276
    8.5.2 Experimental animals 276
8.6 Other toxic effects 276
    8.6.1 Humans 276
    8.6.2 Experimental systems 276

9 **Recommendations for research** 276

10 **Evaluation** 278
10.1 Cancer-preventive activity 278
    10.1.1 Humans 278
    10.1.2 Experimental animals 278
10.2 Overall evaluation 278

11 **References** 281

Appendix 1 The concept of activity profiles of mutagenicity 323

Appendix 2 Definitions of test codes 326

List of participants

Volume 2. Carotenoids

Lyon, 10–16 December 1997

J.A. Baron
7927 Rubin Bldg
Dartmouth-Hitchcock Medical Center
1 Medical Center Drive
Dartmouth Medical School
Lebanon, NH 03756
USA

J.S. Bertram
Cancer Research Center of Hawaii
University of Hawaii
1236 Lauhala St
Honolulu, HI 96813
USA

G. Britton
The University of Liverpool
Life Sciences Building
School of Biological Sciences
Crown Street
Liverpool L69 7ZB
United Kingdom

E. Buiatti
Centro di Documentazione per la Salute
Via Triachini 17
40100 Bologna
Italy

S. De Flora
Institute of Hygiene and Preventive Medicine
University of Genoa
Via A. Pastore 1
16132 Genoa
Italy

V.J. Feron
TNO-Nutrition and Food Research Institute
Toxicology Division
PO Box 360
3700 AJ Zeist
The Netherlands

M. Gerber
Centre de Recherche en Cancerologie
Centre Val d'Aurelle
Parc Euromedicine
34298 Montpellier Cedex 5
France

E.R. Greenberg
Norris Cotton Cancer Center
Dartmouth-Hitchcock Medical Center
1 Medical Center Drive
Lebanon, NH 03756
USA

R.J. Kavlock
Reproductive Toxicology Division (MD-71)
United States Environmental Protection Agency
NHEERL
Research Triangle Park, NC 27711
USA

P. Knekt
National Public Health Institute
Mannerheimintie 166
00300 Helsinki
Finland

W. Malone
Chemoprevention Branch
National Cancer Institute
Executive Plaza North
Suite 201
Bethesda, MD 20892
USA

S.T. Mayne
Department of Epidemiology and Public Health
School of Medicine
Yale University,
60 College Street
PO Box 208034
New Haven, CT 06520-8034
USA

H. Nishino
Department of Biochemistry
Kyoto Prefectural University of Medicine
Kawaramachi-Hirokoji
Kamigyo-ku
Kyoto 602
Japan

J.A. Olson
Iowa State University
Biochemistry and Biophysics Department
Ames, Iowa 50011
USA

H. Pfander
Department of Chemistry and Biochemistry
University of Bern
Freiestrasse 3
3012 Bern
Switzerland

W. Stahl
Institut für Physiologische Chemie I
Heinrich-Heine Universität
Postfach 10 37 51
4000 Dusseldorf
Germany

D.I. Thurnham
Howard Professor of Human Nutrition
University of Ulster
Coleraine County, Londonderry
BT52 1SA
United Kingdom

J. Virtamo
National Public Health Institute
Mannerheimintie 166
00300 Helsinki
Finland

R.G. Ziegler
Nutitional Epidemiology Branch
National Cancer Institute
Executive Plaza North 430
Bethesda, MD 20892
USA

Observers:

P. Astorg
INRA, Centre de Recherches de Dijon
Unité de Toxicologie Nutritionnelle
BP 1540
17 rue Sully
21034 Dijon Cedex
France

R. Goralczyk
F. Hoffmann-La Roche Ltd
Vitamins & Fine Chemicals
Human Nutrition and Health
Carotenoid Research Group
CH-4070 Basel
Switzerland

R.M. Salkeld
F. Hoffmann-La Roche Ltd
Vitamins & Fine Chemicals
Human Nutrition and Health
Vitamin Research Group
CH-4070 Basel
Switzerland

J.F. Steghens
Fédération de Biochimie
Höpital Edouard Herriot
69437 Lyon Cedex 03
France

Secretariat:

P. Boffetta
E. Heseltine *(Editor)*
R. Kaaks
V. Krutovskikh
C. Malaveille
A.B. Miller
H. Ohshima
B. Pignatelli
M. Plummer
M. Rautalahti
E. Riboli
R. Sankaranarayanan
H. Vainio *(Responsible Officer)*
J. Wilbourn
M.L. Zaidan Dagli

Technical Assistance:

M. Lézère
A. Meneghel
D. Mietton
S. Ruiz
J. Mitchell
S. Reynaud
J. Thévenoux

Unable to attend:
H.K. Biesalski, Universitat Hohenheim, Institut für Biologische Chemie, Institut 140, Fruwirthstr. 12, 70599 Stuttgart, Germany
G.S. Omenn, Executive Vice President for Medical Affairs, 608 Fleming Administration Building, Ann Arbor, Michigan 48109-1340, USA

Preamble to the *IARC Handbooks of Cancer Prevention*

The prevention of cancer is one of the key objectives of the International Agency for Research on Cancer (IARC). This may be achieved by avoiding exposures to known cancer-causing agents, by increasing host defences through immunization or chemoprevention or by modifying lifestyle. The aim of the *IARC Monographs* programme is to evaluate carcinogenic risks of human exposure to chemical, physical and biological agents, providing a scientific basis for national or international decisions on avoidance of exposures. The aim of the series of *IARC Handbooks of Cancer Prevention* is to evaluate scientific information on agents and interventions that may reduce the incidence of or mortality from cancer. This preamble is divided into two parts. The first addresses the general scope, objectives and structure of the *Handbooks*. The second describes the procedures for evaluating cancer-preventive agents.

Part One

Scope

Preventive strategies embrace chemical, immunological, dietary and behavioural interventions that may retard, block or reverse carcinogenic processes or reduce underlying risk factors. The term 'cancer prevention' is used to refer to interventions with pharmaceuticals, vitamins, minerals and other chemicals to reduce cancer incidence. The *IARC Handbooks* address the efficacy, safety and mechanisms of cancer-preventive strategies and the adequacy of the available data, including those on timing, dose, duration and indications for use.

Preventive strategies can be applied across a continuum of: (1) the general population; (2) subgroups with particular predisposing host or environmental risk factors, including genetic susceptibility to cancer; (3) persons with precancerous lesions; and (4) cancer patients at risk for second primary tumours. Use of the same strategies

or agents in the treatment of cancer patients to control the growth, metastasis and recurrence of tumours is considered to be patient management, not prevention, although data from clinical trials may be relevant when making a *Handbooks* evaluation.

Objective

The objective of the *Handbooks* programme is the preparation of critical reviews and evaluations of evidence for cancer-prevention and other relevant properties of a wide range of potential cancer-preventive agents and strategies by international working groups of experts. The resulting *Handbooks* may also indicate where additional research is needed.

The *Handbooks* may assist national and international authorities in devising programmes of health promotion and cancer prevention and in making benefit–risk assessments. The evaluations of IARC working groups are scientific judgements about the available evidence for cancer-preventive efficacy and safety. No recommendation is given with regard to national and international regulation or legislation, which are the responsibility of individual governments and/or other international authorities. No recommendations for specific research trials are made.

IARC Working Groups

Reviews and evaluations are formulated by international working groups of experts convened by the IARC. The tasks of each group are: (1) to ascertain that all appropriate data have been collected; (2) to select the data relevant for the evaluation on the basis of scientific merit; (3) to prepare accurate summaries of the data to enable the reader to follow the reasoning of the Working Group; (4) to evaluate the significance of the available data from human studies and experimental models on cancer-preventive activity, carcinogenicity and other beneficial and adverse effects; and (5) to evaluate data relevant to the understanding of mechanisms of action.

Working Group participants who contributed to the considerations and evaluations within a particular *Handbook* are listed, with their addresses, at the beginning of each publication. Each participant serves as an individual scientist and not as a representative of any organization, government or industry. In addition, scientists nominated by national and international agencies, industrial associations and consumer and/or environmental organizations may be invited as observers. IARC staff involved in the preparation of the *Handbooks* are listed.

Working procedures

Approximately 13 months before a working group meets, the topics of the *Handbook* are announced, and participants are selected by IARC staff in consultation with other experts. Subsequently, relevant clinical, experimental and human data are collected by the IARC from all available sources of published information. Representatives of producer or consumer associations may assist in the preparation of sections on production and use, as appropriate.

About eight months before the meeting, the material collected is sent to meeting participants to prepare sections for the first drafts of the *Handbooks*. These are then compiled by IARC staff and sent, before the meeting, to all participants of the Working Group for review. There is an opportunity to return the compiled specialized sections of the draft to the experts, inviting preliminary comments, before the complete first-draft document is distributed to all members of the Working Group.

Data for *Handbooks*

The Handbooks do not necessarily cite all of the literature on the agent or strategy being evaluated. Only those data considered by the Working Group to be relevant to making the evaluation are included. In principle, meeting abstracts and other reports that do not provide sufficient detail upon which to base an assessment of their quality are not considered.

With regard to data from toxicological, epidemiological and experimental studies and from clinical trials, only reports that have been published or accepted for publication in the openly available scientific literature are reviewed by the Working Group. In certain instances, government agency reports that have undergone peer review and are widely available are considered. Exceptions may be made on an ad-hoc basis to include unpublished reports that are in their final form and publicly available, if their inclusion is considered pertinent to making a final evaluation. In the sections on chemical and physical properties, on production, on use, on analysis and on human exposure, unpublished sources of information may be used.

Criteria for selection of topics for evaluation

Agents, classes of agents and interventions to be evaluated in the *Handbooks* are selected on the basis of one or more of the following criteria.

- The available evidence suggests potential for significantly reducing the incidence of cancers.
- There is a substantial body of human, experimental, clinical and/or mechanistic data suitable for evaluation.
- The agent is in widespread use and of putative protective value, but of uncertain efficacy and safety.
- The agent shows exceptional promise in experimental studies but has not been used in humans.
- The agent is available for further studies of human use.

Part Two

Evaluation of cancer-preventive agents

A wide range of findings must be taken into account before a particular agent can be recognized as preventing cancer. On the basis of experience from the *IARC Monographs* programme, a systematized approach to data presentation is adopted for *Handbooks* evaluations.

Outline of data presentation scheme for evaluating cancer-preventive agents

1. **Chemical and physical characteristics**

2. **Occurrence, production, use, analysis and human exposure**

   2.1   Occurrence
   2.2   Production
   2.3   Use
   2.4   Analysis
   2.5   Human exposure

3. **Metabolism, kinetics and genetic variation**

   3.1   Human studies
   3.2   Experimental models
   3.3   Genetic variation

4. **Cancer-preventive effects**

   4.1   Human studies
   4.2   Experimental models
          4.2.1   Experimental animals
          4.2.2   *In-vitro* models
   4.3   Mechanisms of cancer-prevention

5. **Other beneficial effects**

6. **Carcinogenicity**

   6.1   Humans
   6.2   Experimental animals

7. **Other toxic effects**

   7.1   Adverse effects
          7.1.1   Humans
          7.1.2   Experimental animals
   7.2   Genetic and related effects
          7.2.1   Humans
          7.2.2   Experimental models

8. **Summary of data**

   8.1   Chemistry, occurrence and human exposure
   8.2   Metabolism and kinetics
   8.3   Cancer-preventive effects
          8.3.1   Humans
          8.3.2   Experimental animals
          8.3.3   Mechanism of action
   8.4   Other beneficial effects
   8.5   Carcinogenicity
          8.5.1   Humans
          8.5.2   Experimental animals
   8.6   Toxic effects
          8.6.1   Humans
          8.6.2   Experimental animals

9. **Recommendations for research**

10. **Evaluation**

    10.1   Cancer-preventive activity
           10.1.1   Humans
           10.1.2   Experimental animals
    10.2   Overall evaluation

11. **References**

---

1.   Chemical and physical characteristics of the agent

The Chemical Abstracts Services Registry Number, the latest Chemical Abstracts Primary Name, the IUPAC Systematic Name and other definitive information (such as genus and species of plants) are given as appropriate. Information on chemical and physical properties and, in particular, data relevant to identification, occurrence and biological activity are included. A description of technical products of chemicals includes trade names, relevant specifications and available information on composition and impurities. Some of the trade names given may be those of mixtures in which the agent being evaluated is only one of the ingredients.

2.   Occurrence, production, use, analysis and human exposure

2.1   Occurrence

Information on the occurrence of an agent or mixture in the environment is obtained from data derived from the monitoring and surveillance of levels in occupational environments, air, water, soil, foods and animal and human tissues. When available, data on the generation, persistence and bio-accumulation of the agent are included. For mixtures, information is given about all agents present.

2.2 Production

The dates of first synthesis and of first commercial production of a chemical or mixture are provided; for agents that do not occur naturally, this information may allow a reasonable estimate to be made of the date before which no human use of, or exposure to, the agent could have occurred. The dates of first reported occurrence of an exposure are also provided. In addition, methods of synthesis used in past and present commercial production and methods of production that may give rise to different impurities are described.

2.3 Use

Data on production, international trade and uses and applications are obtained for representative regions. Some identified uses may not be current or major applications, and the coverage is not necessarily comprehensive. In the case of drugs, mention of their therapeutic applications does not necessarily represent current practice, nor does it imply judgement as to their therapeutic efficacy.

2.4 Analysis

An overview of current methods of analysis or detection is presented. Methods for monitoring human exposure are also given, when available.

2.5 Human exposure

Human uses of, or exposure to, the agent are described. If an agent is used as a prescribed or over-the-counter pharmaceutical product, then the type of person receiving the product in terms of health status, age, sex and medical condition being treated are described. For nonpharmaceutical agents, particularly those taken because of cultural traditions, the characteristics of use or exposure and the relevant populations are described. In all cases, quantitative data, such as dose-response

relationships, are considered to be of special importance.

3. Metabolism, kinetics and genetic variation

In evaluating the potential utility of a suspected cancer-preventive agent or strategy, a number of different properties, in addition to direct effects upon cancer incidence, are described and weighed. Furthermore, as many of the data leading to an evaluation are expected to come from studies in experimental animals, information that facilitates interspecies extrapolation is particularly important; this includes metabolic, kinetic and genetic data. Whenever possible, quantitative data, including information on dose, duration and potency, are considered.

Information is given on absorption, distribution (including placental transfer), metabolism and excretion in humans and experimental animals. Kinetic properties within the target species may affect the interpretation and extrapolation of dose-response relationships, such as blood concentrations, protein binding, tissue concentrations, plasma half-lives and elimination rates. Comparative information on the relationship between use or exposure and the dose that reaches the target site may be of particular importance for extrapolation between species. Studies that indicate the metabolic pathways and fate of the agent in humans and experimental animals are summarized, and data on humans and experimental animals are compared when possible. Observations are made on interindividual variations and relevant metabolic polymorphisms. Data indicating long-term accumulation in human tissues are included. Physiologically based pharmacokinetic models and their parameter values are relevant and are included whenever they are available. Information on the fate of the compound within tissues and cells (transport, role of cellular receptors, compartmentalization, binding to macromolecules) is given.

Genotyping will be used increasingly, not only to identify subpopulations at increased or decreased risk for cancers but also to characterize variation in the biotransformation of, and responses to, cancer-preventive and chemotherapeutic agents.

This subsection can include effects of the compound on gene expression, enzyme induction or inhibition, or pro-oxidant status, when such data are not described elsewhere. It covers data obtained in humans and experimental animals, with particular attention to effects of long-term use and exposure.

4. Cancer-preventive effects

4.1 Human studies

Types of studies considered. Human data are derived from experimental and non-experimental study designs and are focused on cancer, precancer or intermediate biological end-points. The experimental designs include randomized controlled trials and short-term experimental studies; non-experimental designs include cohort, case–control and cross-sectional studies.

Cohort and case–control studies relate individual use of, or exposure to, the agents under study to the occurrence or prevention of cancer in individuals and provide an estimate of relative risk (ratio of incidence or mortality in those exposed to incidence or mortality in those not exposed) as the main measure of association. Cohort and case–control studies follow an observational approach, in which the use of, or exposure to, the agent is not controlled by the investigator.

Intervention studies are experimental in design — that is, the use of, or exposure to, the agent is assigned by the investigator. The intervention study or clinical trial is the design that can provide the strongest and most direct evidence of a protective or preventive effect; however, for practical and ethical reasons, such studies are limited to observation of the effects among specifically defined study subjects of interventions of 10 years or fewer, which is relatively short when compared with the overall lifespan.

Intervention studies may be undertaken in individuals or communities and may or may not involve randomization to use or exposure. The differences between these designs is important in relation to analytical methods and interpretation of findings.

In addition, information can be obtained from reports of correlation (ecological) studies and case series; however, limitations inherent in these approaches usually mean that such studies carry limited weight in the evaluation of a preventive effect.

Quality of studies considered. The *Handbooks* are not intended to summarize all published studies. It is important that the Working Group consider the following aspects: (1) the relevance of the study; (2) the appropriateness of the design and analysis to the question being asked; (3) the adequacy and completeness of the presentation of the data; and (4) the degree to which chance, bias and confounding may have affected the results.

Studies that are judged to be inadequate or irrelevant to the evaluation are generally omitted. They may be mentioned briefly, particularly when the information is considered to be a useful supplement to that in other reports or when it is the only data available. Their inclusion does not imply acceptance of the adequacy of the study design, nor of the analysis and interpretation of the results, and their limitations are outlined.

Assessment of the cancer-preventive effect at different doses and durations. The Working Group gives special attention to quantitative assessment of the preventive effect of the agent under study, by assessing data from studies at different doses. The Working Group also addresses issues of timing and duration of use or exposure. Such quantitative assessment is important to clarify the circumstances under which a preventive effect can be achieved, as well as the dose at which a toxic effect has been shown.

Criteria for a cancer-preventive effect. After summarizing and assessing the individual studies, the Working Group makes a judgement concerning the evidence that the agent in question prevents cancer in humans. In making their judgement, the Working Group considers several criteria for each relevant cancer site.

Evidence of protection derived from intervention studies of good quality is particularly informative. Evidence of a substantial and significant reduction in risk, including a dose–response relationship, is more likely to indicate a real effect. Nevertheless, a small effect, or an effect without a dose–response relationship, does not imply lack of real benefit and may be important for public health if the cancer is common.

Evidence is frequently available from different types of studies and is evaluated as a whole. Findings that are replicated in several studies of the same design or using different approaches are more likely to provide evidence of a true protective effect than isolated observations from single studies.

The Working Group evaluates possible explanations for inconsistencies across studies, including differences in use of, or exposure to, the agent, differences in the underlying risk for cancer and metabolism and genetic differences in the population.

The results of studies judged to be of high quality are given more weight. Note is taken of both the applicability of preventive action to several cancers and of possible differences in activity, including contradictory findings, across cancer sites.

Data from human studies (as well as from experimental models) that suggest plausible mechanisms for a cancer-preventive effect are important in assessing the overall evidence.

The Working Group may also determine whether, on aggregate, the evidence from human studies is consistent with a lack of preventive effect.

4.2 Experimental models

4.2.1 Experimental animals

Animal models are an important component of research into cancer prevention. They provide a means of identifying effective compounds, of carrying out fundamental investigations into their mechanisms of action, of determining how they can be used optimally, of evaluating toxicity and, ultimately, of providing an information base for developing intervention trials in humans. Models that permit evaluation of the effects of

cancer-preventive agents on the occurrence of cancer in most major organ sites are available. Major groups of animal models include: those in which cancer is produced by the administration of chemical or physical carcinogens; those involving genetically engineered animals; and those in which tumours develop spontaneously. Most cancer-preventive agents investigated in such studies can be placed into one of three categories: compounds that prevent molecules from reaching or reacting with critical target sites (blocking agents); compounds that decrease the sensitivity of target tissues to carcinogenic stimuli; and compounds that prevent evolution of the neoplastic process (suppressing agents). There is increasing interest in the use of combinations of agents as a means of improving efficacy and minimizing toxicity. Animal models are useful in evaluating such combinations. The development of optimal strategies for human intervention trials can be facilitated by the use of animal models that mimic the neoplastic process in humans.

Specific factors to be considered in such experiments are: (1) the temporal requirements of administration of the cancer-preventive agents; (2) dose–response effects; (3) the site-specificity of cancer-preventive activity; and (4) the number and structural diversity of carcinogens whose activity can be reduced by the agent being evaluated. Other types of studies include experiments in which the end-point is not cancer but a defined preneoplastic lesion or tumour-related, intermediate biomarker. An important variable in the evaluation of the cancer-preventive response is the time and the duration of administration of the agent in relation to any carcinogenic treatment, or in transgenic or other experimental models in which no carcinogen is administered. Furthermore, concurrent administration of a cancer-preventive agent may result in a decreased incidence of tumours in a given organ and an increase in another organ of the same animal. Thus, in these experiments it is important that multiple organs be examined.

For all these studies, the nature and extent of impurities or contaminants present in the cancer-preventive agent or agents being evaluated are given when available. For experimental studies of mixtures, consideration is given to the possibility of changes in the physicochemical properties of the test substance during collection, storage, extraction, concentration and delivery. Chemical and toxicological interactions of the components of mixtures may result in nonlinear dose–response relationships.

As certain components of commonly used diets of experimental animals are themselves known to have cancer-preventive activity, particular consideration should be given to the interaction between the diet and the apparent effect of the agent being studied. Likewise, restriction of diet may be important. The appropriateness of the diet given relative to the composition of human diets may be commented on by the Working Group.

Qualitative aspects. An assessment of the experimental prevention of cancer involves several considerations of qualitative importance, including: (1) the experimental conditions under which the test was performed (route and schedule of exposure, species, strain, sex and age of animals studied, duration of the exposure, and duration of the study); (2) the consistency of the results, for example across species and target organ(s); (3) the stage or stages of the neoplastic process, from preneoplastic lesions and benign tumours to malignant neoplasms, studied and (4) the possible role of modifying factors.

Considerations of importance to the Working Group in the interpretation and evaluation of a particular study include: (1) how clearly the agent was defined and, in the case of mixtures, how adequately the sample composition was reported; (2) the composition of the diet and the stability of the agent in the diet; (3) whether the source, strain and quality of the animals was reported; (4) whether the dose and schedule of treatment with the known carcinogen were appropriate in assays of combined treatment; (5) whether the doses of the cancer-preventive agent were adequately monitored; (6) whether the agent(s) was absorbed, as shown by blood concentrations; (7) whether the survival of treated animals was similar to that of

controls; (8) whether the body and organ weights of treated animals were similar to those of controls; (9) whether there were adequate numbers of animals, of appropriate age, per group; (10) whether animals of each sex were used, if appropriate; (11) whether animals were allocated randomly to groups; (12) whether appropriate respective controls were used; (13) whether the duration of the experiment was adequate; (14) whether there was adequate statistical analysis; and (15) whether the data were adequately reported. If available, recent data on the incidence of specific tumours in historical controls, as well as in concurrent controls, are taken into account in the evaluation of tumour response. The observation of effects on the occurrence of lesions presumed to be preneoplastic or the emergence of benign or malignant tumours may in certain instances aid in assessing the mode of action of the presumed cancer-preventive agent. Particular attention is given to assessing the reversibility of these lesions and their predictive value in relation to cancer development.

Quantitative aspects. The probability that tumours will occur may depend on the species, sex, strain and age of the animals, the dose of carcinogen (if any), the dose of the agent and the route and duration of exposure. A decreased incidence and/or decreased multiplicity of neoplasms in adequately designed studies provides evidence of a cancer-preventive effect. A dose-related decrease in incidence and/or multiplicity further strengthens this association.

Statistical analysis. Major factors considered in the statistical analysis by the Working Group include the adequacy of the data for each treatment group: (1) the initial and final effective numbers of animals studied and the survival rate; (2) body weights; and (3) tumour incidence and multiplicity. The statistical methods used should be clearly stated and should be the generally accepted techniques refined for this purpose. In particular, the statistical methods should be appropriate for the characteristics of the expected data distribution and should account for interactions in multifactorial studies. Consideration is given as to whether the appropriate adjustments were made for differences in survival.

4.2.2 In-vitro models

Cell systems *in vitro* contribute to the early identification of potential cancer-preventive agents and to elucidation of mechanistic aspects. A number of assays in prokaryotic and eukaryotic systems are used for this purpose. Evaluation of the results of such assays includes consideration of: (1) the nature of the cell type used; (2) whether primary cell cultures or cell lines (tumorigenic or nontumorigenic) were studied; (3) the appropriateness of controls; (4) whether toxic effects were considered in the outcome; (5) whether the data were appropriately summated and analysed; (6) whether appropriate quality controls were used; (7) whether appropriate concentration ranges were used; (8) whether adequate numbers of independent measurements were made per group; and (9) the relevance of the end-points, including inhibition of mutagenesis, morphological transformation, anchorage-independent growth, cell–cell communication, calcium tolerance and differentiation.

4.3   Mechanisms of cancer prevention

Data on mechanisms can be derived from both human and experimental systems. For a rational implementation of cancer-preventive measures, it is essential not only to assess protective end-points but also to understand the mechanisms by which the agents exert their anticarcinogenic action. Information on the mechanisms of cancer-preventive agents can be inferred from relationships between chemical structure and biological activity, from analysis of interactions between agents and specific molecular targets, from studies of specific end-points *in vitro*, from studies of the inhibition of tumorigenesis *in vivo* and the efficacy of modulating intermediate biomarkers, and from human studies. Therefore, the Working Group takes account of mechanistic data in making the final evaluation of cancer-prevention.

Several classifications of mechanisms have been proposed, as have several systems for evaluating them. Cancer-preventive agents may act at several distinct levels. Their action may be: (1) extracellular, for example, inhibiting the uptake or endogenous formation of carcinogens, or forming complexes with, diluting and/or deactivating carcinogens; (2) intracellular, for example, trapping carcinogens in non-target cells, modifying transmembrane transport, modulating metabolism, blocking reactive molecules, inhibiting cell replication or modulating gene expression or DNA metabolism; or (3) at the level of the cell, tissue or organism, for example, affecting cell differentiation, intercellular communication, proteases, signal transduction, growth factors, cell adhesion molecules, angiogenesis, interactions with the extracellular matrix, hormonal status and the immune system.

Many cancer-preventive agents are known or suspected to act by several mechanisms, which may operate in a coordinated manner and allow them a broader spectrum of anticarcinogenic activity. Therefore, multiple mechanisms of action are taken into account in the evaluation of cancer-prevention.

Beneficial interactions, generally resulting from exposure to inhibitors that work through complementary mechanisms, are exploited in combined cancer-prevention. Because organisms are naturally exposed not only to mixtures of carcinogenic agents but also to mixtures of protective agents, it is also important to understand the mechanisms of interactions between inhibitors.

5.   Other beneficial effects

This section contains mainly background information on preventive activity; use is described in Section 2.3. An expanded description is given, when appropriate, of the efficacy of the agent in the maintenance of a normal healthy state and the treatment of particular diseases. Information on the mechanisms involved in these activities is described. Reviews, rather than individual studies, may be cited as references.

The physiological functions of agents such as vitamins and micronutrients can be described briefly, with reference to reviews. Data on the therapeutic effects of drugs approved for clinical use are summarized.

6.   Carcinogenicity

Some agents may have both carcinogenic and anti-carcinogenic activities. If the agent has been evaluated within the *IARC Monographs on the Evaluation of Carcinogenic Risks to Humans*, that evaluation is accepted, unless significant new data have appeared that may lead the Working Group to reconsider the evidence. When a re-evaluation is necessary or when no carcinogenic evaluation has been made, the procedures described in the Preamble to the *IARC Monographs on the Evaluation of Carcinogenic Risks to Humans* are adopted as guidelines.

7.   Other toxic effects

Toxic effects are of particular importance in the case of agents that may be used widely over long periods in healthy populations. Data are given on acute and chronic toxic effects, such as organ toxicity, increased cell proliferation, immunotoxicity and adverse endocrine effects. If the agent occurs naturally or has been in clinical use previously, the doses and durations used in cancer prevention trials are compared with intakes from the diet, in the case of vitamins, and previous clinical exposure, in the case of drugs already approved for human use. When extensive data are available, only summaries are presented; if adequate reviews are available, reference may be made to these. If there are no relevant reviews, the evaluation is made on the basis of the same criteria as are applied to epidemiological studies of cancer. Differences in response as a consequence of species, sex, age and genetic variability are presented when the information is available.

Data demonstrating the presence or absence of adverse effects in humans are included; equally, lack of data on specific adverse effects is stated clearly.

Findings in humans and experimental animals are presented sequentially under the headings 'Toxic and other adverse effects' and 'Genetic and related effects'.

The section 'Toxic and other adverse effects' includes information on immunotoxicity, neurotoxicity, cardiotoxicity, haematological effects and toxicity to other target organs. Specific case reports in humans and any previous clinical data are noted. Other biochemical effects thought to be relevant to adverse effects are mentioned. The reproductive and developmental effects described include effects on fertility, teratogenicity, fetotoxicity and embryotoxicity. Information from nonmammalian systems and *in vitro* are presented only if they have clear mechanistic significance.

The section 'Genetic and related effects' includes results from studies in mammalian and nonmammalian systems *in vivo* and *in vitro*. Information on whether DNA damage occurs via direct interaction with the agent or via indirect mechanisms (e.g. generation of free radicals) is included, as is information on other genetic effects such as mutation, recombination, chromosomal damage, aneuploidy, cell immortalization and transformation, and effects on cell–cell communication. The presence and toxicological significance of cellular receptors for the cancer-preventive agent are described.

The adequacy of epidemiological studies of toxic effects, including reproductive outcomes and genetic and related effects in humans, is evaluated by the same criteria as are applied to epidemiological studies of cancer. For each of these studies, the adequacy of the reporting of sample characterization is considered and, where necessary, commented upon. The available data are interpreted critically according to the end-points used. The doses and concentrations used are given, and, for experiments *in vitro*, mention is made of whether the presence of an exogenous metabolic system affected the observations. For studies *in vivo*, the route of administration and the formulation in which the agent was administered are included. The dosing regimens, including the duration of treatment, are also given. Genetic data are given as listings of test systems, data and references; bar graphs (activity profiles) and corresponding summary tables with detailed information on the preparation of genetic activity profiles are given in appendices. Genetic and other activity in humans and experimental mammals is regarded as being of greater relevance than that in other organisms. The *in-vitro* experiments providing these data must be carefully evaluated, since there are many trivial reasons why a response to one agent may be modified by the addition of another.

Structure–activity relationships that may be relevant to the evaluation of the toxicity of an agent are described.

Studies on the interaction of the suspected cancer-preventive agent with toxic and subtoxic doses of other substances are described, the objective being to determine whether there is inhibition or enhancement, additivity, synergism or potentiation of toxic effects over an extended dose range.

Biochemical investigations that may have a bearing on the mechanisms of toxicity and cancer-prevention are described. These are carefully evaluated for their relevance and the appropriateness of the results.

8. Summary of data

In this section, the relevant human and experimental data are summarized. Inadequate studies are generally not summarized; such studies, if cited, are identified in the preceding text.

8.1 Chemistry, occurrence and human exposure

Human exposure to an agent is summarized on the basis of elements that may include production, use, occurrence in the environment and determinations in human tissues and body fluids. Quantitative data are summarized when available.

8.2 Metabolism and kinetics

Data on metabolism and kinetics in humans and in experimental animals are given when these are considered relevant to the possible mechanisms of cancer-preventive, carcinogenic and toxic activity.

8.3 Cancer-preventive effects

8.3.1 Humans

The results of relevant studies are summarized, including case reports and correlation studies when considered important.

8.3.2 Experimental animals

Data relevant to an evaluation of cancer-preventive activity in experimental models are summarized. For each animal species and route of administration, it is stated whether a change in the incidence of neoplasms or preneoplastic lesions was observed, and the tumour sites are indicated. Negative findings are also summarized. Dose–response relationships and other quantitative data may be given when available.

8.3.3 Mechanism of action

Data relevant to the mechanisms of cancer-preventive activity are summarized.

8.4 Other beneficial effects

When beneficial effects other than cancer prevention have been identified, the relevant data are summarized.

8.5 Carcinogenicity

Normally, the agent will have been reviewed and evaluated within the *IARC Monographs* programme, and that summary is used with the inclusion of more recent data, if appropriate.

8.5.1 Humans

The results of epidemiological studies that are considered to be pertinent to an assessment of human carcinogenicity are summarized. When relevant, case reports and correlation studies are also summarized.

8.5.2 Experimental animals

Data relevant to an evaluation of carcinogenic effects in animal models are summarized. For each animal species and route of administration, it is stated whether a change in the incidence of neoplasms or preneoplastic lesions was observed, and the tumour sites are indicated. Negative findings are also summarized. Dose–response relationships and other quantitative data may be mentioned when available.

8.6 Toxic effects

Adverse effects in humans are summarized, together with data on general toxicological effects and cytotoxicity, receptor binding and hormonal and immunological effects. The results of investigations on the reproductive, genetic and related effects are summarized. Toxic effects are summarized for whole animals, cultured mammalian cells and non-mammalian systems. When available, data for humans and for animals are compared.

Structure–activity relationships are mentioned when relevant to toxicity.

9. Recommendations for research

During the evaluation process, it is likely that opportunities for further research will be identified. These are clearly stated, with the understanding that the areas are recommended for future investigation. It is made clear that these research opportunities are identified in general terms on the basis of the data currently available.

10. Evaluation

Evaluations of the strength of the evidence for cancer-preventive activity and carcinogenicity from studies in humans and experimental models are made, using standard terms. These terms may also be applied to other beneficial and adverse effects, when indicated. When appropriate, reference is made to specific organs and populations.

It is recognized that the criteria for these evaluations, described below, cannot encompass all factors that may be relevant to an evaluation of cancer-preventive activity. In considering all the relevant scientific data, the Working Group may assign the agent or other intervention to a higher or lower category than a strict interpretation of these criteria would indicate.

10.1 Cancer-preventive activity

These categories refer to the strength of the evidence that an agent prevents cancer. The evaluations may change as new information becomes available.

Evaluations are inevitably limited to the cancer sites, conditions and levels of exposure and length of observation covered by the available studies. An evaluation of degree of evidence, whether for a single agent or a mixture, is limited to the materials tested, as defined physically,

chemically or biologically. When the agents evaluated are considered by the Working Group to be sufficiently closely related, they may be grouped for the purpose of a single evaluation of degree of evidence.

Information on mechanisms of action is taken into account when evaluating the strength of evidence in humans and in experimental animals, as well as in assessing the consistency of results between studies in humans and experimental models.

10.1.1 Cancer-preventive activity in humans

The evidence relevant to prevention in humans is classified into one of the following four categories.

- *Sufficient evidence of cancer-preventive activity*
  The Working Group considers that a causal relationship has been established between use of the agent and the prevention of human cancer in studies in which chance, bias and confounding could be ruled out with reasonable confidence.
- *Limited evidence of cancer-preventive activity*
  The data suggest a reduced risk for cancer with use of the agent but are limited for making a definitive evaluation either because chance, bias or confounding could not be ruled out with reasonable confidence or because the data are restricted to intermediary biomarkers of uncertain validity in the putative pathway to cancer.
- *Inadequate evidence of cancer-preventive activity*
  The available studies are of insufficient quality, consistency or statistical power to permit a conclusion regarding a cancer-preventive effect of the agent, or no data on the prevention of cancer in humans are available.
- *Evidence suggesting lack of cancer-preventive activity*
  Several adequate studies of use or exposure are mutually consistent in not showing a preventive effect.

The strength of the evidence for any carcinogenic activity is assessed in parallel. Both cancer-preventive activity and carcinogenicity are identified and, when appropriate, tabulated by organ site. The evaluation also cites the population subgroups concerned, specifying age, sex, genetic or environmental predisposing risk factors and the presence of precancerous lesions.

10.1.2 Cancer-preventive activity in experimental animals

Evidence for prevention in experimental animals is classified into one of the following categories.

- *Sufficient evidence of cancer-preventive activity*
  The Working Group considers that a causal relationship has been established between the agent and a decreased incidence and/or multiplicity of neoplasms.
- *Limited evidence of cancer-preventive activity*
  The data suggest a preventive effect but are limited for making a definitive evaluation because, for example, the evidence of prevention is restricted to a single experiment, the agent decreases the incidence and/or multiplicity only of benign neoplasms or lesions of uncertain neoplastic potential or there is conflicting evidence.

- *Inadequate evidence of cancer-preventive activity*
  The studies cannot be interpreted as showing either the presence or absence of a preventive effect because of major qualitative or quantitative limitations (unresolved questions regarding the adequacy of the design, conduct or interpretation of the study), or no data on prevention in experimental animals are available.
- *Evidence suggesting lack of cancer-preventive activity*
  Adequate evidence from conclusive studies in several models shows that, within the limits of the tests used, the agent does not prevent cancer.

10.2 Overall evaluation

Finally, the body of evidence is considered as a whole, and summary statements are made that encompass the effects of the agents in humans with regard to cancer-preventive activity, carcinogenicity and other beneficial and adverse effects, as appropriate.

General Remarks

Experiments with animal models conducted in the 1960s and 1970s demonstrated that high doses of retinoids could inhibit carcinogenesis in several organs, including the respiratory tract. Many epidemiological studies carried out during the late 1970s and early 1980s showed negative associations between estimated intakes of vitamin A or β-carotene (provitamin A) and the risk for developing cancer at various sites. In well-nourished populations, however, no consistent relationships were found between cancer risk and plasma retinol concentrations. Following these observations, it was postulated that β-carotene itself, without transformation into retinol, might protect against cancer by its antioxidant capacity or by direct action or conversion to retinoid-like molecules. These suggestions captured the imaginations of many workers and stimulated much research (Peto et al., 1981). This monograph summarizes a great deal of that work and attempts to draw conclusions about the present and future trends in research.

Carotenoids

Of the various classes of pigments in nature, the carotenoids are among the most widespread and important and have attracted interest for a considerable time. In 1831, Wackenroder isolated carotene from carrots (*Daucus carota*), from which the class of compounds derives its name. In 1837, Berzelius gave the name 'xanthophylls' to the yellow pigments from autumn leaves. These reports mark the beginning of carotenoid research. Because of their ubiquitous occurrence, different functions and interesting properties, carotenoids are the subject of interdisciplinary research in many branches of science. The industrial production of carotenoids has also contributed much to knowledge in this field.

Early work on carotenoid chemistry is summarized in the book *Carotenoide* (Karrer & Jucker, 1948), which was followed by another, edited by Isler et al. (1971), who devised an economically feasible method for the industrial synthesis of carotenoids. Biochemical aspects have been covered in *The Biochemistry of the Carotenoids* (Goodwin, 1980, 1984), in *The Biochemistry of Natural Pigments* (Britton, 1983) and, more recently, in *Plant Pigments*, (Goodwin, 1988). The technical and nutritional applications of carotenoids have been treated in a book edited by Bauernfeind (1981). Recently, a new series, *Carotenoids* (Britton et al., 1995a,b), was started which will cover the entire field. Advances in all areas of research on carotenoids are covered in the published proceedings of the *International Symposia on Carotenoids* (Weedon, 1976; Goodwin, 1979; Britton & Goodwin, 1982; Davies & Rau, 1985; Krinsky et al., 1989; Britton, 1991, 1994, 1997).

β-Carotene is one of the agents being evaluated in the framework of the US National Cancer Institute chemoprevention plan. This programme includes a number of in-vitro and in-vivo preclinical studies and phase-I, phase-II and phase-III clinical chemoprevention trials (Kelloff & Boone, 1994).

Carotenoids occur in all three domains of life, i.e. eubacteria, archeobacteria and eukaryotes. More than 600 naturally occurring carotenoids are known today (Pfander et al., 1987; Kull & Pfander, 1995). Algae are a rich source of carotenoids, and more than 100 such compounds have been isolated from these organisms and characterized (Haugan et al., 1995). The most important source of carotenoids for humans is plants, in which the brilliant colours of the carotenoids are often masked by chlorophyll, e.g. in green leaves. The carotenoids are responsible for the beautiful colours of many fruits (citrus fruits, tomatoes, paprika, rose hips) and flowers (*Eschscholtzia, Narcissus*), as well as the colours of many birds (flamingo, cock of the rock, ibis, canary), insects (ladybird) and marine animals (crustaceans, salmon). Normally, carotenoids occur in low concentrations; nevertheless, total carotenoid production in nature has been estimated to be about 108 tonnes per year (Isler et al., 1967). Analysis of serum and human breast milk has shown that about 20 carotenoids derived from fruits and vegetables may be absorbed and metabolized by humans (Khachik et al., 1997).

Carotenoids produced industrially by synthesis or from natural extracts are widely used in feed to colour egg yolk, chickens, shrimp and farm-raised salmon or to colour food products such as margarine and cheese. Various methods have been developed for incorporation of carotenoids into foods: a microcrystalline dispersion in an edible fat is used to colour margarine, and β-carotene in the form of a microdispersion in a hydrophilic protective colloid is used in fruit juices.

Besides the β-carotenes, which are of commercial interest, many other naturally occurring carotenoids have been synthesized. The main emphasis has been on the synthesis of carotenoids in optically active forms, as it is these that are found in nature and are useful as reference standards for analytical work.

Given the large number of natural carotenoids, a detailed systematic nomenclature has been developed (Section 1). This handbook deals specifically with those compounds found predominantly in human blood and tissues and with which the most extensive studies of cancer prevention have been undertaken. The term 'carotenoid' covers all of these compounds; the term 'carotene' is restricted to the hydrocarbons, that is, compounds containing only hydrogen and carbon, and carotenoids containing oxygen functions are known as 'xanthophylls'. The provitamin A carotenoids are β-carotene and other compounds that contain one unsubstituted β ring, e.g. α-carotene and β-cryptoxanthin.

Because of their long system of conjugated double bonds, any carotenoid can theoretically exist not only in the all-*trans* (all-E) form but also in alternative forms with different geometrical arrangements of one or more of the double bonds, i.e. as *cis* (Z) isomers. Interconversion between the geometrical isomers occurs readily. The geometrical isomers have different physical and chemical properties, which must lead to differences in their bioavailability and biological activity. For all purposes of this handbook, $E = trans$ and $Z = cis$, and the terms *trans* and *cis* are used consistently.

The form in which a carotenoid is ingested is also important. Supplements can consist of formulations of pure, often crystalline material as a suspension in oil or in a stabilized, water-dispersible form. In natural foods, the structural matrix and molecular environment of a carotenoid are major determinants of its bioavailability. The isomeric composition of samples of a particular carotenoid from different sources may also vary. All β-carotene samples, for example, consist of mixtures of geometrical isomers, but the isomeric compositions are not always the same. Thus, β-carotene obtained from the alga *Dunaliella* can contain up to 50% *cis* isomers, whereas in most natural sources the level of *cis* isomers present is small (usually no more than 5–10%).

The many biological properties and functions of the carotenoids establish the importance of this class of compounds (Krinsky, 1994). During photosynthesis, direct excitation of carotenoids by light results in an excited singlet state; subsequent transfer of this excitation energy to chlorophyll initiates photosynthesis. The involvement of carotenoids can effectively extend the wavelength of light available to an organism for photosynthesis. Carotenoids are also important for photo protection of cells and tissues (Section 1).

In humans and in animals that require vitamin A for normal growth and development, the most important source is the ingestion and metabolism of carotenoids that can be converted to vitamin A. An adequate supply of vitamin A is not critical in affluent societies but may still be a severe problem in countries of the Third World. According to an estimate of WHO (Underwood & Arthur, 1996), 250 000–500 000 children go blind every year due to xerophthalmia, a disease caused by a deficiency of vitamin A, or die as a consequence of infectious diseases.

Oxidative processes may damage macromolecules such as proteins, lipids and DNA bases. Such damage may affect the proper functioning of cells and contribute to the development of cancer and of cardiovascular and other degenerative disease. Oxidative processes are also a necessary part of essential biological functions in cells, however, including those involved in intracellular signal transduction and control of cell proliferation or apoptosis. Thus, the health of an organism depends on a balance between oxidants and antioxidants.

The ability of carotenoids to act as antioxidants *in vitro* is well established; what is currently of great interest is whether they also behave as antioxidants *in vivo*, e.g. in low-density lipoproteins and in the membranes of cells susceptible to carcinogenesis. Other possible anti-carcinogenic effects of carotenoids could derive from their influence on immune functioning or induction/suppression of enzymes involved in xenobiotic detoxification, such as cytochrome P450, and the postulated growth regulation mediated by gap-junctional communication. Some carotenoids are metabolized to retinol or further to other retinoids, and may also induce biological effects mediated by retinoic acid receptors.

Issues in research on carotenoids and human cancer

A variety of investigative approaches has been used in the extensive body of research on the effect of carotenoids on carcinogenesis. Findings from in-vitro systems, animal models, human epidemiological studies and human clinical trials are discussed in Sections 4 and 6. Application of all of the disciplines involved in such studies will be needed to understand the possible effects of carotenoids in the prevention of cancer. When findings from various research fields point in a common direction, inference is relatively straight-forward. Associations seen in observational epidemiological studies may be clarified by clinical trials. The underlying mechanisms may be better understood from studies in animal models and *in vitro*.

The diverse data may, however, be difficult to integrate, as each research domain suggests different mechanisms or even different effects. Such discrepancies emphasize the limitations of each of the research methods, which may not provide relevant information for cancer prevention as currently conducted. Studies *in vitro* and in animal models rely on biological models of carcinogenesis, which may not correspond to the human situation with regard to cancer. For example, in-vitro systems isolated from tissue and blood proteins and protected from counter-regulatory physiological responses may suggest mechanisms that do not occur in humans. Animal models of cancer often involve specific carcinogens and a dosage schedule that is much more rapid than those to which humans are usually exposed. In addition, the physiology of organs can differ between humans and animals, further complicating extrapolation of results.

Many species have been used to study the relationship between exposure to carotenoids and cancer. Each species has advantages and limitations with regard to the human situation. For example, the absorption and transport of carotenoids in rodents differ markedly from those in humans, although the metabolism and functions of carotenoids in rodents and humans are similar. These issues must be considered carefully when extrapolating the results obtained in any given species to humans.

Epidemiology is also subject to several potential limitations. Estimates of dietary intake of carotenoids derived from questionnaires, food composition tables or biomarkers of nutritional exposure may be of only limited validity because questionnaires tend to reflect recent intake rather than intake at the time of cancer induction. Further, until recently, dietary databases did not contain data on the content of specific carotenes in food items. Confounding is a second major issue in nutritional epidemiology. Specific food constituents tend to be clustered by food group; e.g. vegetables and fruits are the main sources not only of carotenoids but also of other substances that have been postulated to protect against cancer. Since other nutrients may have cancer-protective properties, they themselves may underlie an apparent inverse association between carotenoid intake and cancer risk. Conceivably, an apparent protective effect of a high intake of carotenoids could be due to associated dietary factors, such as low fat intake and non-dietary lifestyle factors such as exercise, avoidance of cigarette smoking and leanness. Associations with intermediate end-points, increasingly used in nutritional epidemiology, may not parallel those with cancer itself. Indeed, it has been difficult even to define the criteria whereby an end-point is a valid intermediate marker of cancer.

Randomized intervention trials avoid the problems of measuring exposure and of confounding which bedevil observational studies; however, the evidence from clinical trials is restricted to the doses given, the duration and the stage of the natural history of the cancer under study. When possible chemopreventive agents such as the carotenoids are being tested, the agent being administered and the way in which it is administered may also differ in important ways from the situation in which carotenoids are obtained from foods. Thus, observational studies on nutrient–disease relationships and intervention studies in which an isolated nutrient is given do not necessarily examine the same questions.

Objectives of this handbook

The Working Group has critically evaluated work relevant to the potential role of carotenoids and cancer prevention carried out during the last two decades. An enormous volume of experimental research on the anti-cancer effects of β-carotene and other dietary and non-dietary carotenoids resulted from the enthusiasm that followed the original observation of an inverse association between dietary β-carotene and cancer risk. The hypothesis did not only affect experimental studies but resulted in expansion of interest in the whole field of carotenoids. It stimulated improvements in analytical techniques to measure the small concentrations of carotenoids in serum, and this in turn facilitated more detailed research on metabolism, genetic variation and the kinetics of carotenoid turnover in tissues. This handbook also describes and evaluates the outcomes of the large intervention trials that were conducted in the wake of the enthusiasm for the hypothesis and were made possible by the availability of β-carotene supplements. The outcome of that work is evaluated, and the direction that research is currently taking and areas where more research is still needed are defined.

References

Bauernfeind, J.C., ed. (1981) *Carotenoids as Colorants and Vitamin A Precursors. Technological and Nutritional Applications*, New York, Academic Press

Britton, G., ed. (1983) *The Biochemistry of Natural Pigments,* Cambridge, Cambridge University Press

Britton, G., ed. (1991) Proceedings of the 9th International Symposium on Carotenoids, Kyoto, Japan, 1990. *Pure Appl. Chem.,* **63**, 1–176

Britton, G., ed. (1994) Proceedings of the 10th International Symposium on Carotenoids, Trondheim, Norway, 1993. *Pure Appl. Chem.,* **66**, 931–1076

Britton, G., ed. (1997) Proceedings of the 11th International Symposium on Carotenoids, Leiden, The Netherlands, 1996. *Pure Appl. Chem.,* **69**, 2027–2173

Britton, G. & Goodwin, T.W., eds (1982) *Carotenoid Chemistry and Biochemistry*, Oxford, Pergamon Press

Britton, G., Liaaen-Jensen, S. & Pfander, H., eds (1995a) *Carotenoids,* Vol. 1A, *Isolation and Analysis,* Basel, Birkhäuser Verlag

Britton, G., Liaaen-Jensen, S. & Pfander, H., eds (1995b) *Carotenoids,* Vol. 1B, *Spectroscopy,* Basel, Birkhäuser Verlag

Davies, B.H. & Rau, W., eds (1985) Proceedings of the 7th International Symposium on Carotenoids, Munich, Germany, 1984. *Pure Appl. Chem.,* **57**, 639–821

Goodwin, T.W., ed. (1979) Proceedings of the 5th International Symposium on Carotenoids, Madison, USA, 1978. *Pure Appl. Chem.,* **51**, 435–657

Goodwin, T.W. (1980) Carotenoids in higher plants. In: Goodwin, T.W., ed., *The Biochemistry of the Carotenoids*, 2nd Ed, Vol. 1, *Plants,* London, Chapman & Hall, pp. 143–203

Goodwin, T.W., ed. (1984) *The Biochemistry of the Carotenoids*, 2nd Ed., Vol. 2, *Animals*, London, Chapman & Hall

Goodwin, T.W., ed. (1988) *Plant Pigments*, London, Academic Press

Isler, O., Ruegg, R. & Schwieter, U. (1967) Carotenoids as food colourants. *Pure Appl. Chem.,* **14**, 245–263

Isler, O., Gutmann, H. & Solms U., eds (1971) *Carotenoids*, Basel, Birkhäuser Verlag

Karrer, P. & Jucker, E., eds (1948) *Carotinoide,* Basel, Birkhäuser Verlag

Kelloff, G.J. & Boone, C.W., eds (1994) Cancer chemopreventive agents: Drug development status and future prospects. *J. Cell. Biochem.,* **Suppl. 20**, 110–140

Khachik, F., Spangler, C.J., Smith, J.C., Canfield, L.M., Steck, A. & Pfander, H. (1997) Identification, quantification, and relative concentrations of carotenoids and their metabolites in human milk and serum. *Anal. Chem.,* **69**, 1873–1881

Krinsky, N.I. (1994) The biological properties of carotenoids. *Pure Appl. Chem.*, **66**, 1003–1010

Krinsky, N.I., Mathews-Roth, M.M. & Taylor, R.F., eds (1989) *Carotenoids: Chemistry and Biology*, New York, Plenum Press

Kull, D. & Pfander, H. (1995) Appendix: List of new carotenoids. In: Britton, G., Liaaen-Jensen, S. & Pfander, H., eds, *Carotenoids*, Vol. 1A, *Isolation and Analysis*, Basel, Birkhäuser Verlag, Basel, pp. 295–317

Peto, R., Doll, R., Buckley, J.D. & Sporn, M.B. (1981) Can dietary beta-carotene materially reduce human cancer rates? *Nature*, **290**, 201–208

Pfander, H., Gerspacher, M., Rychener, M. & Schwabe, R. (1987) *Key to Carotenoids by Otto Straub*, 2nd Ed., Basel, Birkhäuser Verlag

Underwood, B.A. & Arthur, P. (1996) The contribution of vitamin A to public health. *FASEB J.* **10**, 1040–1048

Weedon, B.C.L., ed. (1976) Proceedings of the 4th International Symposium on Carotenoids, Bern, Switzerland, 1975. *Pure Appl. Chem.*, **47**, 97–243

Carotenoids

Carotenoids

Carotenoids

1. Chemistry

1.1 Structure and nomenclature

Carotenoids are a class of hydrocarbons (carotenes) and their oxygenated derivatives (xanthophylls). They consist of eight isoprenoid units joined in such a manner that their arrangement is reversed at the centre of the molecule, so that the two central methyl groups are in a 1,6-positional relationship and the remaining non-terminal methyl groups are in a 1,5-positional relationship. All carotenoids may be derived formally from the acyclic $C_{40}H_{56}$ structure, illustrated in Figure 1, with a long central chain of conjugated double bonds, by hydrogenation, dehydrogenation, cyclization or oxidation, or any combination of these processes. The class also includes compounds that arise from certain rearrangements or degradations of the carbon skeleton, provided that the two central methyl groups are retained. Retinoids, including retinol, all-*trans*-retinoic acid and 9-*cis*-retinoic acid (Fig. 2), are therefore not included in the class of carotenoids.

Rules for the nomenclature of carotenoids (semi-systematic names) have been published by the International Union of Pure and Applied Chemistry (IUPAC) and the IUPAC-International Union of Biochemistry Commissions on Biochemical Nomenclature (1975; Weedon & Moss, 1995). Trivial names are usually used for the most common carotenoids; however, when trivial names are used in a publication, it is recommended that the semi-systematic name be given, in parentheses or in a footnote, at the first mention. All specific names are based on the stem name 'carotene', which corresponds to the structure and numbering illustrated in Figure 3. The name of a specific compound is constructed by adding as prefixes two Greek letters that specify the two C_9 end groups (Fig. 4); these prefixes are cited in alphabetical order.

The oxygenated carotenoids (xanthophylls) are named according to the usual rules of organic chemistry. The functional groups most frequently observed are hydroxy, methoxy, carboxy, oxo and epoxy. Chirality and geometric configuration are designated conventionally as *R*/*S* or *E*/*Z*, respectively. In this handbook, the terms *trans* and *cis* are used for *E* and *Z*, respectively. Important, characteristic carotenoids (Fig. 5) are lycopene (φ,φ-carotene), β-carotene (β,β-carotene), α-carotene [(6'*R*)-β,ε-carotene], β-cryptoxanthin [(3*R*)-β,β-caroten-3-ol], zeaxanthin ((3*R*,3'*R*)-β,β-carotene-3,3'-diol), lutein (previously named 'xanthophyll' (3*R*,3'*R*,6'*R*)-β,ε-carotene-3,3'-diol), neoxanthin [(3*S*,5*R*,6*R*,3'*S*,5'*R*,6'*S*)-5',6'-epoxy-6,7-didehydro-5,6,5',6'-tetrahydro-β,β-carotene-3,5,3'-triol], violaxanthin [(3*S*,5*R*,6*S*,3'*S*,5'*R*,6'*S*)-5,6:5',6'-diepoxy-5,6,5',6'-tetrahydro-β,β-carotene-3,3'-diol], fucoxanthin [(3*S*,5*R*,6*S*,-3'*S*,5'*R*,6'*R*)-5,6-epoxy-3,3',5'-trihydroxy-6',7'-didehydro-5,6,7,8,5',6'-hexahydro-β,β-caroten-8-one 3'-acetate], canthaxanthin (β,β-carotene-4,4'-dione) and astaxanthin [(3*S*,3'*S*)-3,3'-dihydroxy-β,β-carotene-4,4'-dione].

Derivatives in which the carbon skeleton has been shortened by the formal removal of fragments from one end of a carotenoid are named 'apocarotenoids', the position of the point of cleavage being indicated, e.g. β-apo-8'-carotenal (8'-apo-β-caroten-8'-al). Derivatives in which fragments have been formally removed from both ends of the molecule are called 'diapocarotenoids', an example being bixin, the main component of the natural colorant annatto. Other structural variations are those of the norcarotenoids, in which one or more carbon atoms have been eliminated from within the typical C_{40} skeleton. A prominent example is the C_{37} skeleton of peridinin [(3*S*,5*R*,6*R*,3'*S*,5'*R*,-6'*R*)-5,6-epoxy-3,5,3'-trihydroxy-6,7-didehydro-5,6,5',6'-tetrahydro-10,11,20-trinor-β,β-caroten-19',11'-olide 3 acetate], which is characteristic of diatoms.

The structures and trivial and semisystematic names of all known naturally occurring carotenoids are listed in *Key to Carotenoids* (Pfander, 1987) and in the Appendix of *Carotenoids*,

Figure 1. The basic carotenoid skeleton, constructed from eight isoprenoid units

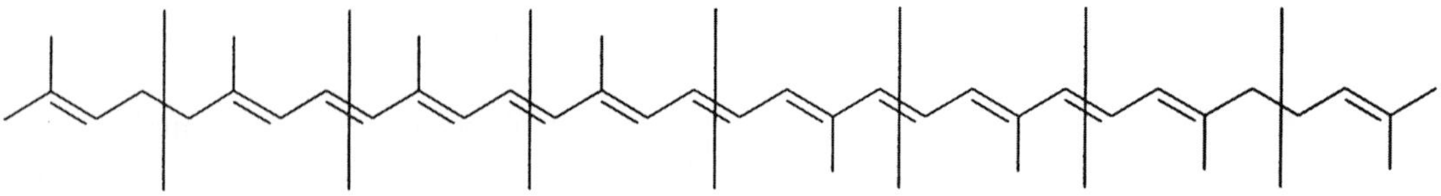

Figure 2. Structures of important retinoids

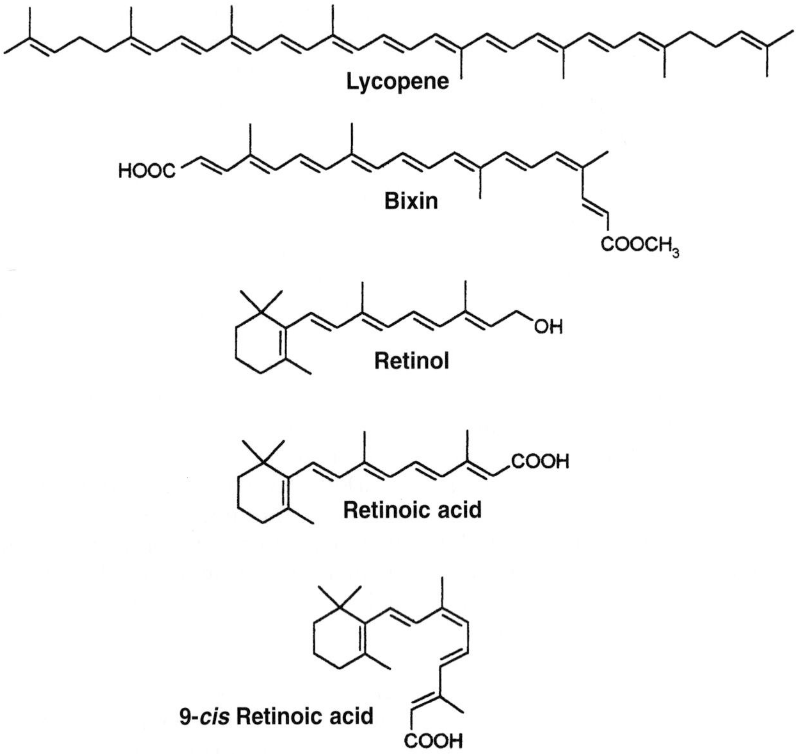

Lycopene

Bixin

COOCH$_3$

Retinol

Retinoic acid

9-*cis* Retinoic acid

COOH

Figure 3. Numbering scheme for carotenoids

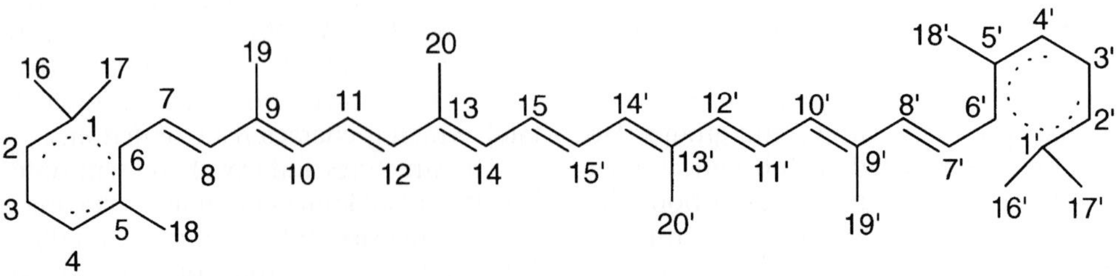

Figure 4. The seven end groups in carotenoids

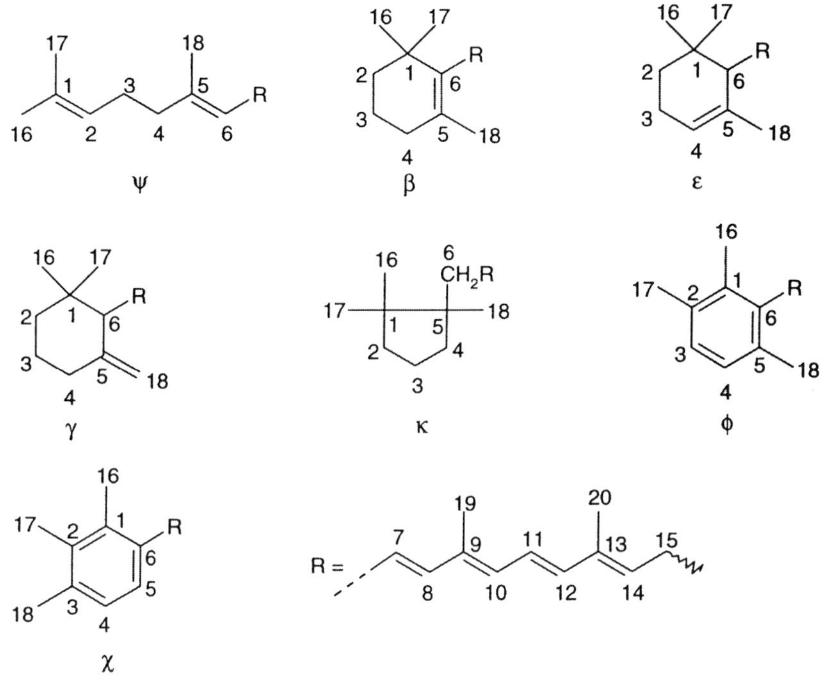

Volume 1A (Kull & Pfander, 1995), which also includes references for their spectroscopic and other properties. For many of the carotenoids listed, however, the structure (this term includes the stereochemistry) is still uncertain; in all these cases, reisolation followed by structural elucidation with modern spectroscopic methods (especially high-resolution nuclear magnetic resonance (NMR) spectroscopy) is absolutely necessary. About 370 of the naturally occurring carotenoids are chiral, bearing one to five asymmetric carbon atoms; most individual carotenoids occur in only one configuration in nature.

The *cis–trans* isomerism of the carbon–carbon double bonds is an important feature of the stereochemistry of carotenoids, because these geometric isomers may have different biological properties. The first comprehensive review of the *cis–trans* isomerism of carotenoids and vitamin A was published in 1962 (Zechmeister, 1962), and the literature in this field is extensive. Because of the number of double bonds, many geometric isomers (e.g.

1056 for lycopene and 272 for β-carotene) are theoretically possible. When in the *cis* configuration, the double bonds of the polyene chain can be considered as two groups: those with little steric hindrance (e.g. the central 15,15′ double bond and the double bonds that bear a methyl group, such as the 9,9′ and 13,13′ double bonds) and those with substantial steric hindrance (7,7′ and 11,11′ double bonds). Although isomers with sterically hindered *cis* double bonds are sometimes found, they are rare, and the number of *cis* isomers likely to be found is, in practice, reduced considerably, e.g. from a potential 1056 compounds to the actual number of 72 for lycopene.

Carotenoids usually occur in nature as all-*trans*-isomers, but exceptions are known, such as 9-*cis*-β-carotene in the alga *Dunaliella* and the 15-*cis*-phytoene isolated from carrots, tomatoes and other organisms. Some carotenoids readily undergo isomerization, and many *cis* isomers that are described in the literature as natural products may be artefacts. For experimental work, it must be kept in mind that geometric

Figure 5. Structures of important carotenoids

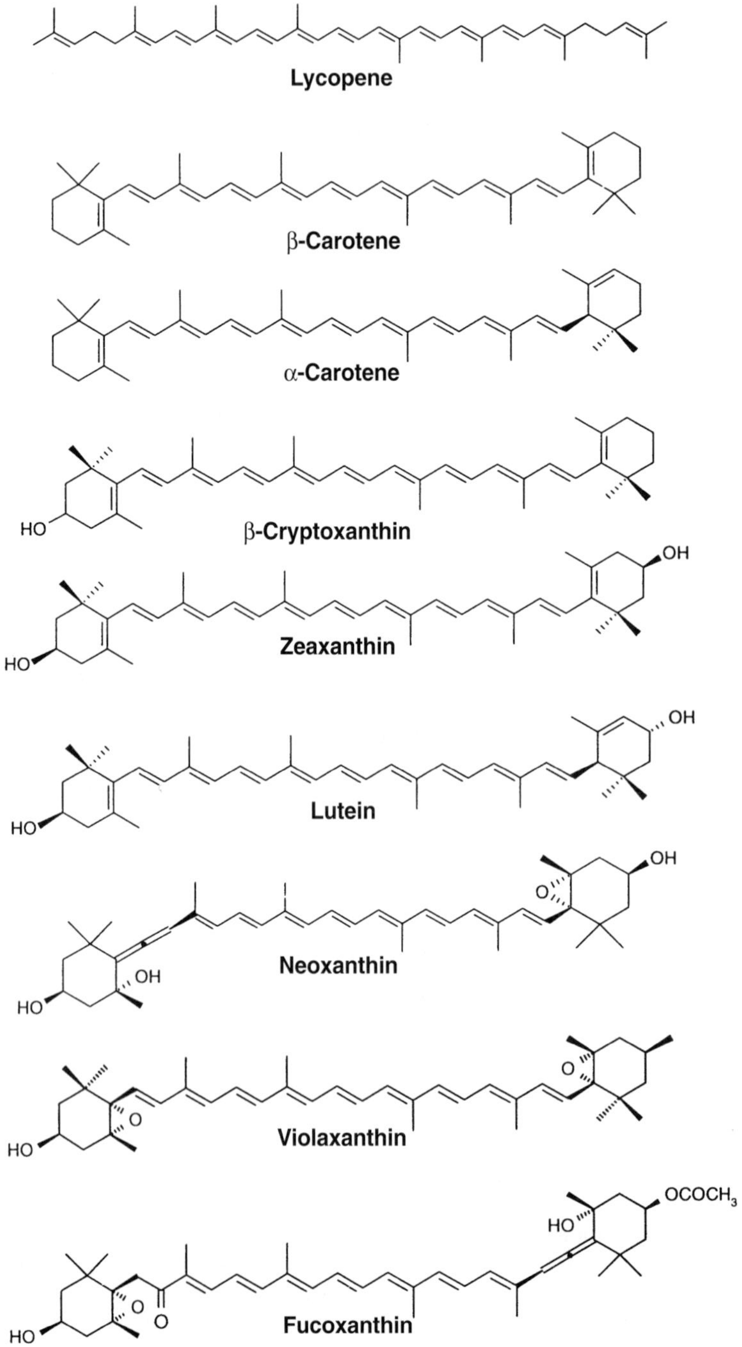

Lycopene

β-Carotene

α-Carotene

β-Cryptoxanthin

Zeaxanthin

Lutein

Neoxanthin

Violaxanthin

Fucoxanthin

isomerization may occur when a carotenoid is kept in solution. The percentage of *cis* isomers is usually low but is enhanced as the temperature rises above the ambient. Furthermore, the formation of *cis* isomers is increased by exposure to light.

This section consists of two parts. In the first part, the general properties of carotenoids as a group are considered. The information is derived largely from a recent review of the structures and properties of carotenoids in relation to function (Britton, 1995a). In the second part, information is given on the individual compounds covered in this handbook. Although those listed are the main carotenoids identified in human blood and tissues, more than 100 are likely to be ingested in the general human diet, some of them, notably astaxanthin, bixin, capsanthin, capsorubin and others, in significant amounts. Some main dietary carotenoids, especially the epoxides violaxanthin and neoxanthin which are major carotenoids in all green plants are not found in blood or tissues.

1.2 General properties

1.2.1 Relationships between structure, properties and biological activity

The natural functions and biological actions of carotenoids are determined by the physical and chemical properties of the molecules, which themselves are defined by the molecular structure. Carotenoids are largely rigid molecules, but some flexibility is associated with the end groups. The overall molecular geometry, i.e. the size and shape of the molecule and the presence of functional groups, determines the solubility and is the main feature that determines the ability of the carotenoid to fit into cellular and subcellular structures. The conjugated double-bond system also determines the chemical and photochemical properties that form the basis of its biological actions and functions. A third factor, the importance of which is often overlooked, is interaction between carotenoids and other molecules in their immediate vicinity, which can greatly alter the properties of carotenoids and thus affect their functioning *in vivo*.

1.2.2 Molecular size and shape

All coloured carotenoids in the all-*trans* configuration have an extended system of conjugated carbon–carbon double bonds and are consequently linear. The *cis* isomers are not linear, and their shape differs substantially from that of the all-*trans* form, so their ability to fit into subcellular structures may differ greatly from that of the all-*trans* form. The size and shape of the end groups also affects their fit. Acyclic compounds such as lycopene are essentially long, linear molecules with flexible end groups. When cyclic end groups are present, the molecule is shorter; the effective bulk of cyclic end groups is greater and depends on the preferred conformation, as determined by steric factors and the presence of substituent groups. Structural changes that appear to be minor can result in significant alterations in shape.

1.2.3 Solubility

Virtually all carotenoids that are obtained from a normal human diet, and certainly those found in blood and body tissues, are extremely hydrophobic molecules which form aggregates or adhere nonspecifically to structural surfaces. The exceptions include the norcarotenoid carboxylic acid nor-bixin, which is present in preparations of annatto, and the glycosyl esters found in saffron. *In vivo*, free (i.e. not aggregated) carotenoids are therefore expected to be restricted to hydrophobic (lipophilic) environments.

1.2.4 Properties and molecular interactions of carotenoids *in vivo*

Almost all of the information about the properties of carotenoids is derived from studies of the molecules in simple organic solutions. *In vivo*, however, carotenoids are part of a much more complex system and are in close proximity to other components such as lipids and proteins, frequently in ordered structures. The overall size, shape and hydrophobicity of a carotenoid are thus major determinants of its ability to fit into subcellular structures. As noted above, the structural details that define individual carotenoids also determine the precise orientation and the nature of any molecular interactions with the surroundings.

Carotenoids are commonly located in membranes, where they may be an integral part of the ordered membrane structure. The positioning of the carotenoid in the membrane is strongly dependent on structure, and differences are seen between carotenes and xanthophylls. The polar end groups of the xanthophylls interact with the polar, outer part of the membrane and allow the carotenoid to span the lipid bilayer (Gruszecki & Sielewiesiuk, 1990). Carotenes, with no polar end groups, are restricted to the hydrophobic inner core of the bilayer. Interactions between carotenoids and proteins are also of physiological importance, and the carotenoid is usually stabilized by such associations, which can significantly alter its physical and chemical properties.

Interactions between carotenoid molecules themselves can also affect their properties. The highly hydrophobic carotenoids show a strong tendency to aggregate and crystallize in aqueous media. This aggregation especially affects the light absorption and chemical reactivity of carotenoids and their effective size and solubility. This effect is particularly significant for the release of carotenoids from food matrices and their emulsification and absorption. In natural foods, carotenoids may be present in a micro-crystalline form, e.g. lycopene in tomatoes, and their solubilization when in this form (or as crystalline supplements) can be very inefficient. This property clearly has important consequences for their bioavailability. *cis* Isomers generally have a lesser tendency to crystallize than all-*trans* isomers, so that the *cis* isomers may be more readily solubilized, absorbed and transported.

1.3 Properties of the conjugated polyene chain

1.3.1 Light absorption and photochemical properties

The characteristic strong absorption of light in the visible region is attributed to a transition from the electronic ground state to the second singlet excited state. As the main absorption bands lie in the 400–500-nm region, the carotenoids are strongly coloured yellow, orange or red. The ultraviolet (UV)–visible absorption spectrum provides the first criterion for identifying a carotenoid and is also the basis for quantitative analysis.

Direct formation of the carotenoid triplet state from the excited singlet state is not favoured. Nevertheless, its formation by triplet–triplet energy transfer from other triplet state molecules, e.g. photosensitizers, can be very efficient because the triplet-state energy of carotenoids that contain more than seven conjugated double bonds is low. Transfer of energy from triplet species to carotenoids is usually very efficient and prevents the alternative energy transfer to oxygen, which would generate the highly reactive and destructive singlet oxygen. Carotenoids can also accept excitation energy from singlet oxygen, if any should be formed. The triplet carotenoid has too little energy to generate other species by energy transfer, and the excitation energy is dissipated harmlessly to the surroundings.

1.3.2 Chemical properties

Chemical reactions involving carotenoid end groups are important in classical chemistry for characterization and derivatization. The conjugated polyene chain is a reactive, electron-rich system that is susceptible to attack by electrophilic reagents, is responsible for the instability of carotenoids towards oxidation and is the most important part of the molecule in relation to free-radical chemistry.

Carotenoids are rapidly destroyed by oxidation, especially by free radicals such as the hydroxy radical and various peroxy radicals. The important fundamental chemistry of carotenoid radicals and of the reactions of carotenoids with oxidizing free radicals is not well understood. Carotenoid radicals may be charged or neutral and are very short-lived species. In principle, removal of one electron from the carotenoid molecule by oxidation gives the radical cation $Car^{+\bullet}$, whereas the addition of one electron by reduction generates the radical anion $Car^{-\bullet}$ (Simic, 1992). These charged radicals can be detected by their distinctive spectroscopic properties, with intense absorption in the near infrared region. The abstraction of a hydrogen atom from a saturated carbon atom in a position allylic to the polyene chain, by homolytic cleavage, would generate a neutral radical $Car^{\bullet}$. In all these radicals, delocalization of the unpaired electron over the conjugated polyene chromophore has a stabilizing effect and allows subsequent reactions to take place in many parts of the molecule. The same is true for carotenoid–adduct radicals which could be generated by the addition of a radical species such as a peroxy radical ROO• or the hydroxy radical HO• to the polyene chain.

The reactions between carotenoids (usually β-carotene) and peroxy radicals have been studied in organic solutions and in phospholipid liposomes. The reaction is usually attributed to direct addition of the peroxy radical to one of the suitable positions in the polyene chain of the carotenoid to give a resonance-stabilized, carbon-centred radical, e.g. ROO-Car•. At relatively low oxygen concentrations, a further peroxy radical could be added, to give a product that is not a free radical, e.g. ROO-Car-OOR. This process would consume peroxy radicals, and the carotenoid would act as an antioxidant. At higher oxygen concentrations, however, a carotenoid peroxy radical could be formed, e.g. Car-OO• or ROO-Car-OO•, and this could then act as a pro-oxidant, promoting hydrogen abstraction and peroxidation of unsaturated lipid and hence exacerbating damage (Burton & Ingold, 1984; Palozza & Krinsky, 1992a; Liebler, 1993). An alternative possibility is that the peroxy radical could abstract a hydrogen atom from a saturated CH_2 group allylic to the main polyene chromophore in a reaction analogous to the abstraction of hydrogen from an unsaturated lipid. Again, this could be followed by addition of a peroxy radical to generate a non-radical product, i.e. an antioxidant action, or of oxygen to generate a carotenoid–peroxy radical which would have prooxidant properties.

Series of apocarotenoids of different chain length have been reported to be products of chemical and free-radical oxidation of carotenoids and could be produced in tissues by nonspecific chemical or enzymic reactions or by specific excentric cleavage of carotenoids in the intestine.

All carotenoids react rapidly with oxidizing agents and free radicals, although the reactivity depends on the length of the polyene chromophore and on the nature of the end groups. Calculations show that the electron density is not uniform along the whole polyene chain but is greater towards the ends; there may therefore be preferred sites for reactions with electrophilic or free-radical species.

In discussing the mechanism by which β-carotene could act as an antioxidant or prooxidant, Truscott (1996) described interactions between radicals of β-carotene, vitamin E and vitamin C and concluded that β-carotene may quench or repair the vitamin E radical and vitamin C the β-carotene radical cation. This hypothesis highlights the need to consider possible interactions between carotenoids and other factors, in addition to the chemistry of the carotenoids themselves.

1.4 Isolation and analysis

Methods for the isolation and purification of carotenoids from natural sources are widely available and are described in detail, with worked examples, by Britton *et al.* (1995a), including many procedures for the high-performance liquid chromatography (HPLC) of carotenoids in blood, body tissues and foods. Details are also available of procedures for the analysis of the main carotenoids in blood plasma (Schüep *et al.*, 1995) and of geometrical isomers of β-carotene (Schierle *et al.*, 1995). More complex methods for the analysis of the many minor carotenoids present in blood have also been described (Khachik *et al.*, 1997). The use of spectroscopic methods for the analysis and characterization of carotenoids is discussed by Britton *et al.* (1995b). HPLC procedures are now available for the separation of mixtures of geometric isomers; however, very few isomers have been fully characterized and the position(s) of the *cis* double bond(s) established. A compound cannot be identified as a particular *cis* isomer without comparison with authentic (usually synthetic) standards. Therefore, in most published reports, use only of the general description '*cis* isomers' is justified.

1.4.1 General methods

As carotenoids are less stable than many other groups of substances, precautions and special procedures must be used to minimize the risk of degradation and formation of artefacts. In particular, exposure to oxygen, heat, light, acid and, in some cases, bases must be avoided whenever possible (Schiedt & Liaaen-Jensen, 1995). All operations should be carried out in an inert atmosphere (nitrogen or argon), at low temperature (room temperature, about 20 °C), in the dark or diffuse light, under acid-free conditions and with freshly purified, peroxide-free solvents. After carotenoids have been extracted from tissues, even when they are pure and in the crystalline state, they are susceptible to oxidation and may be broken down rapidly if samples are stored in the presence of even traces of oxygen; solids must be stored under vacuum or an inert gas (nitrogen or argon). Carotenoids are also susceptible to oxidative damage *in vivo* if they are exposed to oxidizing species or to the free radicals that may be generated.

The usual indication of carotenoid breakdown is bleaching, i.e. loss of colour, due to breakage of the chromophore. A variety of breakdown products have been detected, most often apocarotenoids of various chain lengths produced by cleavage of any of the double bonds in the polyene chain (Palozza & Krinsky, 1992b; Liebler, 1993). Similar products are derived from the chemical reaction between carotenoids and singlet oxygen or other oxidizing agents. The products of oxidative breakdown or similar oxidation products formed by metabolism of carotenoids may have biological activity.

Geometrical (*cis–trans*) isomerization occurs readily when carotenoids are exposed to factors such as light or heat and even occurs slowly in isolated, purified samples. Plasma or tissue samples should be stored at –70 °C or less to minimize degradative reactions or isomerization. Even carotenoid samples that are nominally all-*trans* usually contain small amounts of various *cis* isomers.

1.4.2 Identification
The following criteria must be fulfilled for identification of a carotenoid as a known compound (Schiedt & Liaaen-Jensen, 1995): (i) The UV–visible absorption spectrum (λ_{max} and fine structure) in at least two solvents must be consistent with the chromophore and identical to that of an authentic sample. (ii) The chromatographic properties must be identical to those of an authentic sample in two systems, preferably

thin-layer chromatography and HPLC, and co-chromatography with an authentic sample should be demonstrated. If possible a mass spectrum should be obtained which allows at least confirmation of the molecular mass.

Full elucidation of the structure requires a fully assigned NMR spectrum and, for chiral compounds, comparison of a circular dichroism spectrum with that of an authentic reference sample. A first criterion for identification is the UV–visible spectrum, which is characteristic of the chromophore of the molecule but generally gives no information about functional groups, except carbonyl groups conjugated with the polyene system. Not only the position of the λ_{max} but also the overall shape or fine structure of the spectrum convey information. A discussion of the relationship between chromophore and spectrum, with tabulated lists of λ_{max} values for natural carotenoids in several solvents, is given by Britton (1995b).

1.4.3 Quantitative analysis
The UV–visible spectrum also provides the basis for quantitative analysis of carotenoids. Tables of values for $A^{1\%}$ (usually in the order of 2500) and ε_{mol} (usually about 100 000) are also given by Britton (1995b).

1.5 Data on individual compounds
1.5.1 β-Carotene

IUPAC name
β,β-Carotene

Chemical Abstracts Services Registry Number
7235-40-7 (9Z, 13312-52-2; 13Z, 6811-73-0; 15Z, 19361-58-1)

Structure

Molecular formula
$C_{40}H_{56}$

Relative molecular mass
536

Melting-point
183 °C (from benzene–petroleum)

UV–visible spectrum
λ_{max} 425, 450, 477 nm (hexane, petroleum); 429, 452, 478 nm (acetone); 435, 462, 487 nm (benzene). $A^{1\%}$, 2592; ε_{mol}, 138 900 (450 nm, petroleum); $A^{1\%}$, 2337; ε_{mol}, 125 300 (462 nm benzene) (Britton, 1995b)

Mass spectrometry
M+ 536; major fragment ion at m/z 444 (M-92)

^{1}H-NMR (Englert, 1995)

^{13}C-NMR (Englert, 1995)

Infrared
(Bernhard & Grosjean, 1995)
Isolation
From green and other plant tissues (Britton, 1995c)

Natural sources
All green fruit and vegetables, carrots, many orange and yellow fruit

Geometrical isomers
(9-*cis*), (13-*cis*), (15-*cis*). Resolved by HPLC on Vydac 218TP54 C_{18} RP column (Schierle *et al.*, 1995), Vydac 201TP54 C_{18}RP column (Emenhiser *et al.*, 1995) or C_{30}RP column (Emenhiser *et al.*, 1995).

1.5.2 α-*Carotene*

IUPAC name
(6′R)-β,ε-Carotene

Chemical Abstracts Services Registry Number
7488-99-5

Structure

Molecular formula
$C_{40}H_{56}$

Relative molecular mass
536

Melting-point
187 °C (from petroleum or benzene–methanol)

UV–visible spectrum
λ_{max} 422, 445, 473 nm (hexane, petroleum); 424, 448, 476 nm (acetone); 432, 456, 485 nm (benzene). $A^{1\%}$, 2710; ε_{mol}, 145 300 (445 nm, hexane) (Britton, 1995b)

Mass spectrometry
M+ 536; major fragment ions at m/z 480 (M-56), 444 (M-92), 413 (M-123)

^{1}H-NMR
(Englert, 1995)
^{13}C-NMR
(Englert, 1995)

Infrared
(Bernhard & Grosjean, 1995)

Isolation
From green and other plant tissues (Britton, 1995c)

Sources
Carrots; some green fruit and vegetables; some yellow–orange fruit. Usually found with larger amounts of β-carotene

1.5.3 *Lycopene*

IUPAC name
ψ,ψ-Carotene

Chemical Abstracts Service Registry Number
502-68-5 (9Z, 64727-64-6; 13Z, 13018-46-7;
15Z, 59092-07-8)

Structure

Molecular formula
$C_{40}H_{56}$

Relative molecular mass
536

Melting-point
174 °C (from hexane or petroleum)

UV–visible spectrum
λ_{max} 444, 470, 502 nm (petroleum); 448, 474,
505 nm (acetone), 455, 487, 522 nm (benzene).
$A^{1\%}$, 3450; ε_{mol}, 184 900 (470 nm, petroleum);
$A^{1\%}$, 3370; ε_{mol}, 180 600 (487 nm, benzene)
(Britton, 1995b)

Mass spectrometry
M^+ 536; main fragment ions at m/z 467 (M-69),
444 (M-92), 430 (M-106)

^1H-NMR
(Englert, 1995)

^{13}C-NMR
(Englert, 1995)

Infrared
(Bernhard & Grosjean, 1995)

Isolation
From tomato (Britton, 1995c)

Sources
Tomato and tomato products; small amounts in
some fruits, e.g. watermelon

Geometrical isomers
Natural lycopene is mainly all-*trans*, accompa-
nied by 5Z, 9Z, 13Z and other isomers, which
are separated by HPLC on C_{30} RP columns
(Hengartner *et al.*, 1992; Emenhiser *et al.*,
1995). Prolycopene (7,9,7′,9′-tetra*cis*) occurs
naturally in tangerine, tomato and some other
fruit, e.g. passion fruit.

Comments
Poorly soluble in most solvents and natural
oils; crystallizes readily; very unstable in the
presence of oxygen

1.5.4 Lutein

IUPAC name
(3R,3′R,6′R)-β,ε-Carotene-3,3′-diol

Chemical Abstracts Services Registry Number
127-40-2

Structure

Molecular formula
$C_{40}H_{56}O_2$

Relative molecular mass
568

Melting-point
193 °C (from methanol)

UV–visible spectrum
λ_{max} 422, 445, 474 nm (ethanol); 432, 458, 487
nm (benzene). $A^{1\%}$, 2250; ε_{mol}, 144 800 (445 nm,
ethanol); $A^{1\%}$, 2236; ε_{mol}, 127 000 (458 nm, benzene) (Britton, 1995b)

Mass spectrometry
M^+ 568; major fragment ions at m/z 550 (M-18),
476 (M-92), 458 (M-18-92), 430 (M-138)

¹H-NMR
(Berset & Pfander, 1985)

¹³C-NMR
End-group assignment (Englert, 1995)

Isolation
From green leaves (Britton, 1995c)

Sources
Main carotenoid in all green fruit and vegetables; also present in other yellow–orange fruit, e.g. pumpkin; major carotenoid in egg yolk

Geometrical isomers
For separation and characterization of *cis* isomers, see Berset and Pfander (1985).

1.5.5 Canthaxanthin

IUPAC name
β-Carotene-4,4'-dione

Chemical Abstracts Services Registry Number
514-78-3

Structure

Molecular formula
$C_{40}H_{52}O_2$

Relative molecular mass
564

Melting-point
213 °C (from dichloromethane–methanol)

UV–visible spectrum
λ_{max} 474 nm (ethanol); 484 nm (benzene); 466 nm (petroleum); no fine structure. $A^{1\%}$, 2200; ε_{mol}, 124 100 (466 nm, petroleum); $A^{1\%}$, 2092; ε_{mol}, 118 000 (484 nm, benzene) (Britton, 1995b)

Mass spectrometry
M⁺ 564; fragment ion at *m/z* 472 (M-92). No diagnostic fragment ions

¹H-NMR
(Englert, 1995)

¹³C-NMR
End-group assignment (Englert, 1995)

Infrared
(Bernhard & Grosjean, 1995)

Sources
Characteristic carotenoid in marine animals, especially crustaceans (with astaxanthin); main pigment in trout; not a major human dietary component.

1.5.6 Zeaxanthin

IUPAC name
(3R,3'R)-β,β-Carotene-3,3'-diol

Chemical Abstracts Services Registry Number
144-68-3, 29472-68-2

Structure

Molecular formula
$C_{40}H_{56}O_2$

Relative molecular mass
568

Melting-point
215 °C (from methanol)

UV–visible spectrum
λ_{max} 428, 450, 478 nm (ethanol); 430, 452, 479 nm (acetone); 440, 463, 491 nm (benzene). $A^{1\%}$, 2480; ε_{mol}, 140 900 (450 nm, ethanol); $A^{1\%}$, 2340; ε_{mol}, 132 900 (452 nm, acetone) (Britton, 1995b)

Mass spectrometry
M+ 568; fragment ions at m/z 550 (M-18, low intensity), 476 (M-92)

¹H-NMR
(Englert, 1995)

¹³C-NMR
(Englert, 1995)

Infrared
(Bernhard & Grosjean, 1995)

Sources
Main food source: maize; also present in small amounts in many green and other fruits and vegetables; commonly present in egg yolk; also produced in high concentrations in some bacteria

Geometric isomers
Separation and characterization of 9-*cis*, 13-*cis* and others given by Englert *et al.* (1992) and Emenhiser *et al.* (1995).

1.5.7   β-Cryptoxanthin

IUPAC name
(3R)-β,β-Caroten-3-ol

Chemical Abstracts Services Registry Number
472-70-8

Structure

Molecular formula
$C_{40}H_{56}O$

Relative molecular mass
552

Melting-point
169 °C (from benzene–methanol)

UV–visible spectrum
λ_{max} 428, 450, 478 nm (ethanol); 425, 449, 476 nm (petroleum); 435, 463, 489 nm (benzene). A¹%, 2386; ε_{mol}, 131 900 (449 nm, petroleum) (Britton, 1995b)

Mass spectrometry
M+ 552; fragment ions at m/z 534 (M-18, low intensity), 460 (M-92)

¹H-NMR
End-group assignment (Englert, 1995)

¹³C-NMR
End-group assignment (Englert, 1995)

Sources
Present, usually in small amounts, in yellow–orange fruits and in maize; best sources: orange, peach, papaya; not a major dietary component

1.5.8   α-Cryptoxanthin

IUPAC name
(3'R, 6'R)-β,ε-Caroten-3-ol
Chemical Abstracts Services Registry Number
24480-38-4

Structure

Molecular formula
$C_{40}H_{56}O$

Relative molecular mass
552

UV–visible spectrum
λ_{max} 423, 446, 473 nm (ethanol); 421, 445, 475

nm (hexane); 433, 459, 488 nm (benzene). $A^{1\%}$, 2636; ε_{mol}, 145 500 (hexane); $A^{1\%}$, 2355; ε_{mol}, 130 000 (459 nm, benzene) (Britton, 1995b)

Mass spectrometry
M^+ 552; fragment ions at *m/z* 534 (M-18, low intensity), 496 (M-56), 460 (M-92), 414 (M-138)

¹H-NMR
End-group assignment (Englert, 1995)

¹³C-NMR
End-group assignment (Englert, 1995)

Sources
No major source; likely to be a minor component in many fruit and vegetables; often measured as part of cryptoxanthin.

1.5.9 Zeinoxanthin

IUPAC name
(3R,6'R)-β,ε-Caroten-3'-ol

Chemical Abstracts Services Registry Number
472-69-5

Structure

Molecular formula
$C_{40}H_{56}O$

Relative molecular mass
552

UV–visible spectrum
As for α-cryptoxanthin

Mass spectrometry
M^+ 552; fragment ions at *m/z* 534 (M-18 high density), 496 (M-56), 460 (M-92), 442 (M-18-92), 429 (M-123)

¹H-NMR
End-group assignment (Englert, 1995)

¹³C-NMR
End-group assignment (Englert, 1995)

Sources
No major source; likely to be a minor component of many fruit and vegetables; often measured as part of cryptoxanthin

2. Occurrence, Commercial Sources, Use and Application, Analysis and Human Use and Exposure

The most abundant source of carotenoids is plant tissues, although they are also found in microorganisms, insects, birds, fish and other animals. Only plants and microorganisms, however, can synthesize carotenoids *de novo*. Nature produces about 100 million tonnes of carotenoid pigments per year (Isler *et al.*, 1967); most of this output is in the form of fucoxanthin and peridinin (characteristic pigments in marine algae and diatoms, respectively) and β-carotene, lutein, violaxanthin and neoxanthin (in green leaves) (Ong & Tee, 1992). Zeaxanthin also occurs widely but in smaller amounts in green leafy vegetables, while others like lycopene, capsanthin and bixin constitute the pigments in specific plants.

The distribution of carotenoids in various plant materials has been reviewed (Borenstein & Bunnell, 1966; Bauernfeind, 1972; Goodwin, 1976, 1980; Speek *et al.*, 1988). Most of the data reported before 1980 were obtained by open-column chromatography, which did not permit adequate separation of carotenoids. More accurate quantification of carotenoids in foods has been possible since the introduction of HPLC. Information on the carotenoid composition of biological materials reported below is thus derived from recent references, when possible. Although modern methods allow improved qualitative and quantitative descriptions of the carotenoid composition of foods, assessing dietary intake will always be fraught with difficulties, which include the variable composition of vegetables through the year (Heinonen *et al.*, 1989), differences between what is eaten and what might be sampled for analysis, difficulties in assessing what is eaten, influence of the fat content of the diet on absorption and the influence of cooking methods on bioavailability (Micozzi *et al.*, 1990; Khachik *et al.*, 1992a). It is generally considered that cooking vegetables improves the bioavailability of carotenoids, since it breaks down the cellulose structure of the plant cell (Khachik *et al.*, 1992a; de Pee & West, 1996). One report (Micozzi *et al.*, 1990) suggested that microwave cooking has a destructive effect and that much more xanthophylls were destroyed than hydrocarbons; however, later studies indicated that carotenoids were generally (with the exception of epoxy-carotenoids) resistant to heating by microwaving, boiling and stewing (Khachik *et al.*, 1992a).

Ever since the elucidation of the structure of β-carotene and other carotenoids, much effort has been devoted to the synthesis of carotenoids and other polyenes. The first synthesis of β-carotene was reported independently by Karrer and Eugster (1950), Inhoffen *et al.* (1950) and Milas *et al.* (1950). The method of Inhoffen *et al.* was later developed into an industrial process, and synthetic β-carotene has been produced commercially since 1954. Today, six synthetic carotenoids (Fig. 6) have become commercially important as colourants for food and feed: 8'-apo-β-caroten-8'-al (β-apo-8'-carotenal) (C_{30}), β-apo-8'-carotenoic acid ethyl ester (ethyl 8'-apo-β-caroten-8'-oate) (C_{30} skeleton), citranaxanthin (5',6'-dihydro-5'-apo-18'-nor-β-caroten-6'-one (C_{33}), β-carotene (C_{40}), canthaxanthin (C_{40}) and a mixture of the stereoisomers of astaxanthin ((3RS,3'RS)-3,3'-dihydroxy-β,β-carotene-4,4'-dione) (C_{40}).

Natural extracts and carotenoids isolated from them are also produced commercially, including β-carotene from the alga *Dunaliella* and from red palm oil, lycopene from tomatoes and lutein from marigold flowers. There may be considerable variation in the geometrical isomer composition of a carotenoid from different natural sources and between natural and synthetic products.

The commercial products are available as crystalline materials or in formulations such as solutions or suspensions in natural oils or stabilized, water-soluble beadlets. The physical state of the carotenoid may differ substantially in different preparations and from that in the natural microenvironment within a food matrix.

It is not intended in this review to describe all of the more than 100 carotenoids that occur in foods eaten by humans: only the specific carotenes, α-carotene, β-carotene and lycopene, and the xanthophylls, lutein, zeaxanthin, β-cryptoxanthin and canthaxanthin, are considered. α- and β-carotene, β-cryptoxanthin, lycopene and lutein are the main carotenoids in serum or plasma, and a relatively limited number of foods are the major contributors to these carotenoids in the diet. Table 1 shows both the uniformity and diversity of diets in western countries, with marked differences in the contributions made by different carotenoids. For example, carrots, citrus products and tomato products make major contributions to the dietary supplies of α-carotene, β-cryptoxanthin and lycopene, respectively; carrots and spinach are major dietary sources of β-carotene and lutein, respectively, but the greater diversity of foods that supply the latter components increases the differences between countries and reduces the contribution made by specific foods. This is especially so in the case of lutein. It must also be realized that specific food types affect the bioavaibility of carotenoids in blood, and caution should be exercised in using specific foods as proxies for the intake of specific carotenoids. Dietary preferences, cooking methods and many other factors (de Pee & West, 1996) have a major influence on the true contribution of specific foods to the carotenoid composition of plasma.

2.1 Carotenes
2.1.1 β-Carotene
2.1.1.1 Occurrence

In temperate and tropical countries, important food sources of β-carotene are green leafy vegetables, carrots, peas and beans; carrots are a major source of both β- and α-carotene in many countries in the world. Dairy products and margarines contribute to less than 1% of daily

Figure 6. Carotenoids produced by industrial synthesis

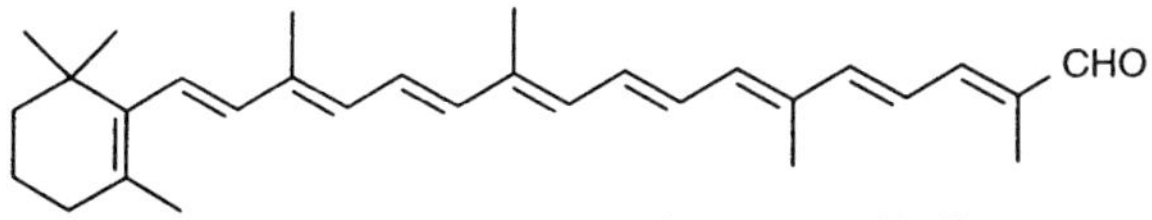

β-Apo-8'-carotenal (8'-apo-β-caroten-8'-al)

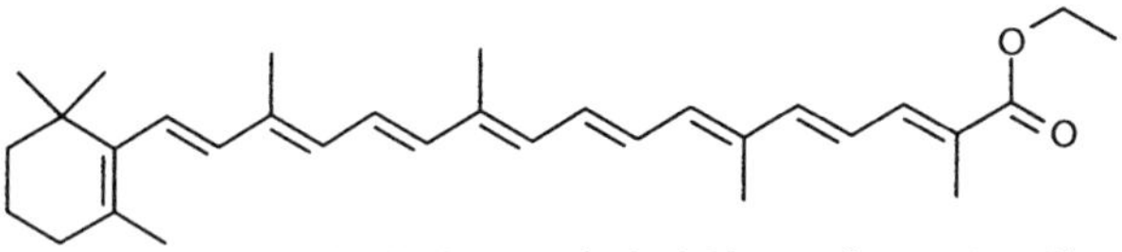

β-Apo-8'-carotenoic acid ethyl ester (ethyl 8'-apo-β-caroten-8'-oate)

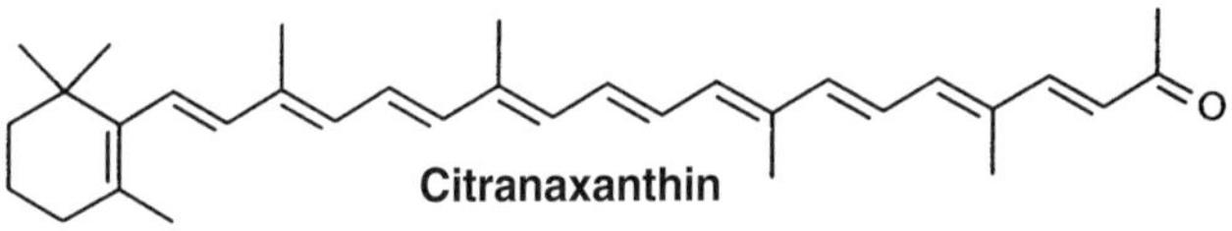

Citranaxanthin

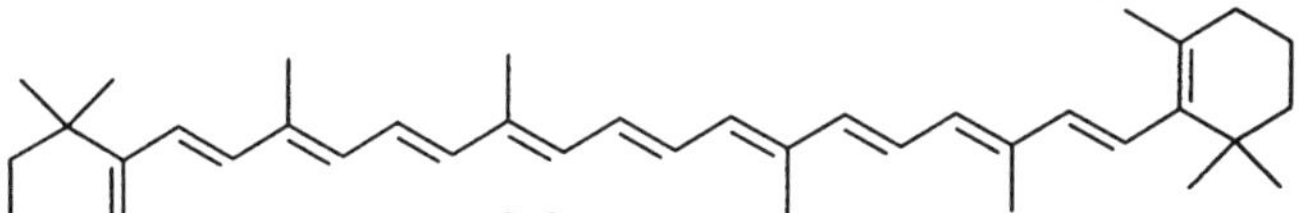

β-Carotene

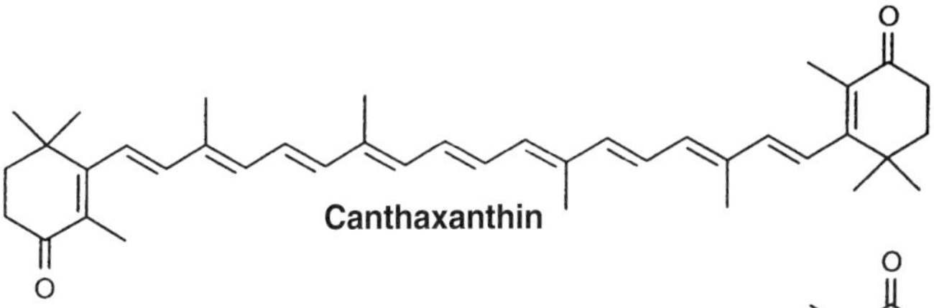

Canthaxanthin

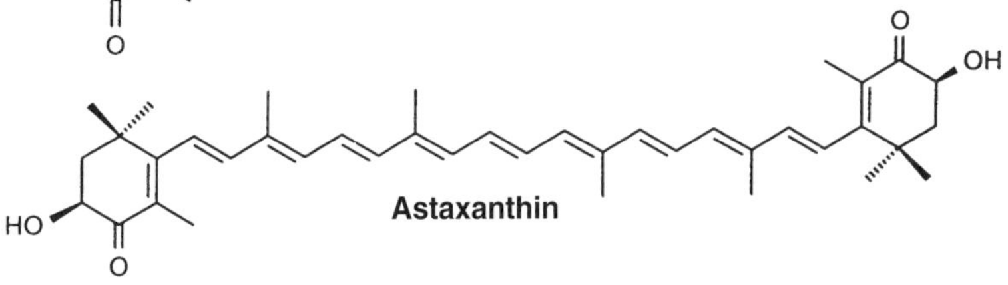

Astaxanthin

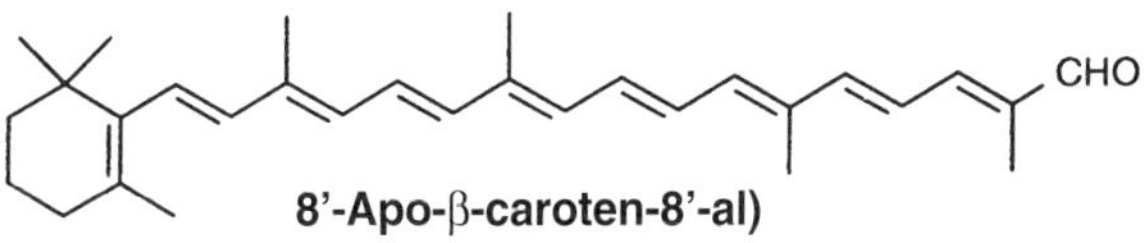

8'-Apo-β-caroten-8'-al)

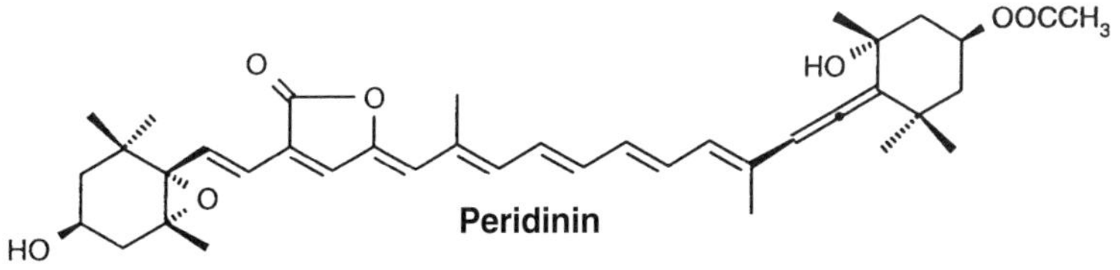

Peridinin

Table 1. Major food sources of carotenoids in five European (n = 80) and one US study (n = 1102)

Carotenoid	France Food	%	Ireland Food	%	Netherlands Food	%	Spain Food	%	United Kingdom Food	%	USA (women) Food	%
β-Carotene	Carrots	38	Carrots	60	Carrots	42	Carrots	24	Carrots	53	Carrots	25
	Spinach	14	Tomatoes and products	13	Spinach	14	Spinach	26	Soups	10	Cantaloupe melon	6
α-Carotene	Carrots	82	Carrots	90	Carrots	87	Carrots	60	Carrots	88	Carrots	51
	Oranges	6	Coleslaw	5	Oranges	5	Tangerines	17	Coleslaw	6	Soups	17
β-Cryptoxanthin	Orange juice	50	Oranges	42	Tangerines	41	Tangerines	53	Orange juice	45	Orange juice	38
	Oranges	30	Tangerines	28	Orange juice	33	Oranges	38	Oranges	26	Oranges	34
Lycopene	Fresh tomatoes	25	Tomatoes		Tomato soup	29	Tomatoes		Tomatoes		Tomatoes	
	Tinned tomatoes	16	Tinned	23	Fresh tomatoes	16	Puree	42	Fresh	21	Fresh puree/sauce	18
	Pizza	16	Soup	17	Pizza	16	Sauce	42	Tinned	20	Pasta	12
Lutein	Spinach	31	Peas	19	Spinach	30	Spinach	34	Peas	36	Spinach	14
	Mixed vegetables	6	Broccoli	16	Broccoli	10	Lettuce	16	Broccoli	8	Collard/ mustard/turnip grains	14
	Cucumber	6							Eggs	8		

From Chug-Ahuja et al. (1993)

Table 2. Concentrations of β-carotene and lutein in green leafy vegtables in Europe, Malaysia and North America

Country	Vegetable	β-Carotene (% of total)	Lutein (mg/100 g)	β-Carotene (mg/100 g)	Reference
Germany	Green pepper (capsicum)	24	7.99	5.49	Gross (1991)
Spain	Lettuce (leaf type)	33	0.34	0.17	Granado et al. (1992)
	Green pepper (raw)	38	0.34	0.21	
	Spinach (raw)	41	4.23	3.25	
	Green beans (raw)	29	0.36	0.17	
United Kingdom	Spinach (raw)	41	5.87	4.02	Hart & Scott (1995)
	Watercress (raw)	36	10.71	5.92	
	Broccoli (raw)	36	1.61	0.92	
	Savoy cabbage (outside leaves, raw)	45	14.46	11.84	
	Peas (frozen, raw)	21	1.63	0.43	
	Lettuce (leaf type)	55	1.61	1.98	
Malaysia	Chinese cabbage	75	0.96	3.02	Tee & Lim (1991)
	Coriander	70	1.34	3.17	
	Drumstick leaves	51	7.13	7.54	
	Lettuce	57	< 0.01	< 0.01	
	S. androgumus	29	29.91	13.35	
North America	Broccoli (raw)	32	2.83	2.33	Khachik et al. (1992a)
	Spinach (raw)	31	9.50	8.90	
	Green beans	31	0.59	0.47	

intake of β-carotene; however, the importance of this source is difficult to quantify, and the availability of β-carotene in these products is probably much higher than that in vegetables. In tropical countries, mangoes, papaya and red palm oil are also important sources of β-carotene.

In green leafy vegetables, β-carotene and lutein can account for more than 80% of all carotenoids (Khachik et al., 1992a; Ong & Tee, 1992; Hart & Scott, 1995). It has been suggested that green leafy vegetables contain approximately equal amounts of β-carotene and lutein (Heinonen et al., 1989), but the proportions of the two carotenoids vary widely (Table 2).

2.1.1.2 Commercial sources
Pure β-carotene is synthesized industrially and is the major carotenoid available commercial-

ly. In addition, extracts rich in β-carotene but also containing other carotenoids are produced industrially from palm oil, algae (Dunaliella) and fungi (Blakeslea trispora).

2.1.1.3 Use and application
The use of β-carotene (EC160a) as a colour in foodstuffs is authorized under European Parliament Directive 94/36/EC (Klepsch & Baltas, 1994). For the purposes of the Directive, 'colours' are substances that add or restore colour to food. The addition of β-carotene to unprocessed foods or to various unflavoured milk and cream products is not allowed; however, β-carotene is one of very few colourants that may be added to margarine, butter and some cheeses. β-Carotene is also used as a colourant in e.g. fruit juices, soft drinks and

corn flakes, but its contribution in these products to total intake is probably minor. β-Carotene, lycopene and lutein are also used more generally as food colourants (Klepsch & Baltas, 1994).

In the United States, β-carotene is classified as 'generally recognized as safe' by the Food and Drug Administration (Select Committee of GRAS Substances, 1979). β-Carotene has been used since 1975 in the United States to treat photosensitivity in adults with erythropoietic protoporphyria (see section 5.1), at doses of < 180 mg/d (Mathews-Roth *et al.*, 1977).

2.1.1.4 Analysis

The carotenoids have a characteristic absorption spectrum, and their concentrations can be calculated from specific extinction coefficients (see Section 1). It was reported that the collection of plasma in containers coated with ethylenediamine tetraacetic acid depressed the concentrations by 50% (Stacewicz-Sapuntzakis *et al.*, 1987); however, it has also been reported that the concentrations in serum and heparinized plasma are indistinguishable (Thurnham *et al.*, 1988a).

Carotenoids are separated by liquid chromatography, and numerous methods have been developed to separate carotenoids in the organic solvent after extraction from foods and blood samples. Although some 20 or more carotenoids are found regularly in blood (Thompson *et al.*, 1985; Khachik *et al.*, 1997), usually only the five best-known ones, i.e. β-carotene, α-carotene, lutein, lycopene and β-cryptoxanthin, are analysed (Nells & De Leenheer, 1983; Ito *et al.*, 1987; Thurnham *et al.*, 1988a; Cantilena & Nierenberg, 1989; Kaplan *et al.*, 1990; Krinsky *et al.*, 1990a; Nierenberg & Nann, 1992; Stahl *et al.*, 1993). A variety of internal standards can be used, including tocopherol acetate, tocopherol nicotinate, tocol, retinyl acetate, echinenone and β-apo-8'-carotenal. The choice of the internal standard depends on the chromatographic technique and whether a single or two-channel detector is used. Quantification of β-carotene by liquid chromatography is associated with a coefficient of variation of 5–10%.

The methods used for extraction from food (Tee & Lim, 1991; Khachik *et al.*, 1992a; Hart & Scott, 1995) differ from those used to extract blood samples, since the preparation of the initial extracts of foods is more complicated: the sample must be representative of the edible fraction, and it must be e.g. homogenized, possibly cooked or saponified. The last step obviates the use of esters as internal standards, and echinenone and β-apo-8'-carotenal are the most commonly used. The method of liquid chromatography used depends on the degree of resolution of the carotenoids in the extract required. A useful summary of the factors that affect the liquid chromatography of carotenoids is available (Craft, 1992).

2.1.1.5 Human use or exposure

The best known human use for β-carotene is to provide vitamin A (Bendich & Olson, 1989), but it can also be used therapeutically in some cases of erythropoietic protoporphyria (Mathews-Roth *et al.*, 1977). Other possible uses are still poorly defined.

Exposure to carotenoids in the diet is universal. They appear to be absorbed by duodenal mucosal cells through a mechanism involving passive diffusion, similar to that for cholesterol and the products of triglyceride lipolysis (Parker, 1996; see also section 3.1.6). In most industrialized countries, fruit and vegetables provide an average of 2–3 mg/d of provitamin A carotenoids, of which β-carotene is the principal component (Granado *et al.*, 1996), although the intake may be much higher in persons who regularly eat e.g. carrots (Gregory *et al.*, 1990; Scott *et al.*, 1996). The availability of carotenoids from food sources is limited, however, by the physical matrix in which they are ingested and their dissolution in dietary lipids in the gut (de Pee *et al.*, 1995; Parker, 1996). β-Carotene is found in most blood samples. The amount present in samples in developing countries is often low, probably reflecting diets low in carotene and/or fat and poor bioavailability of carotenes from vegetable sources (de Pee *et al.*, 1995). An unknown amount is converted to retinol as it crosses the gut and little is left to pass into the bloodstream as β-carotene *per se*. Thus, only about 10% of carotene was present as β-carotene in the blood of British adults (Thurnham & Flora, 1988); however, the concentration of plasma β-carotene in this survey was relatively low (median, 0.24 mmol/L in men, 0.32 μmol/L in women) in comparison with those in other parts of Europe, such as France (0.38 and 0.62 μmol/L; Howard et al., 1996), Germany (0.43 and 0.61 μmol/L; Heseker et al., 1991) and Northern Ireland (0.37 and 0.57 μmol/L; Howard et al., 1996). This discrepancy probably reflects the relatively low consumption of vegetables (120 g/d) and fruit (60 g/d) in Great Britain (Gregory et al., 1990) in comparison with the reported figure of 700 g/d in France (Drewnowski et al., 1997; see also Table 3).

Since the availability of fruit and vegetables is often seasonal, the dietary concentrations of carotenoids may fluctuate during the year. Furthermore, seasonal factors such as light and heat (Takagi et al., 1990) also affect the amounts of carotenoids in fruit and vegetables. The plasma concentrations of β-carotene frequently correlate with the dietary intake of carotenoids (Roidt et al., 1988; Stryker et al., 1988; Nierenberg et al., 1989; Ascherio et al., 1992; Cooney et al., 1995; Saintot et al., 1995) and vegetables (Drewnowski et al., 1997). Seasonal variations in the intake of β-carotene have been reported by some authors (Nathanail & Powers, 1992; Rautalahti et al., 1993; Olmedilla et al., 1994; Cooney et al., 1995) but not others (Thurnham & Flora, 1988; Cantilena et al., 1992), perhaps due to differences in the amounts consumed. Thus, when seasonal differences are not found, vegetable intake may be low (Gregory et al., 1990) or vary little during the year (Cantilena et al., 1992). The amount of β-carotene converted to retinol may also affect seasonal fluctuations in plasma β-carotene. Scott et al. (1996) found no difference in the dietary intake of β-carotene among women in four-day, weighed samples, yet their plasma β-carotene was significantly lower in winter and spring than at other times of the year. Low intakes of β-carotene may be inadequate to support the synthesis of vitamin A and increase plasma β-carotene, as is the case in many developing countries (Ascherio et al., 1992).

Another factor that affects the plasma concentrations of carotenoids is turnover. The half-lives of plasma β-carotene, α-carotene and β-cryptoxanthin are short (7–14 days) in comparison with those of lycopene (12–33 days) and lutein (33–61 days) (Micozzi et al., 1992; Rock et al., 1992). Plasma concentrations are probably maintained from deposits in adipose tissues, which in the case of β-carotene represent > 65% of the total body pool (Bendich & Olson, 1989; Kaplan et al., 1990).

The plasma concentrations of β-carotene in humans vary considerably, due not only to differences in dietary habits. After supplementation with 20 mg/d β-carotene, the concentrations in plasma were increased by an average of 10-fold, but the concentrations after two months were strongly correlated with the baseline values ($r = 0.64$, $p < 0.001$) (Albanes et al., 1992). As all subjects in this study had the same intake, individuals appear to differ substantially with regard to the absorption of β-carotene (Dimitrov et al., 1988). Similar findings were reported by O'Neill and Thurnham (1988) in persons receiving single doses of 32–40 mg of supplemental carotenoids.

Smoking also influences β-carotene concentrations, which are generally lower in smokers than nonsmokers (Thompson et al., 1985; Stryker et al., 1988; Thurnham, 1990; Albanes et al., 1991; Ascherio et al., 1992; Brady et al., 1996; Fukao et al., 1996). Smokers tend to consume fewer vegetables than nonsmokers (Ascherio et al., 1992; Margetts & Jackson, 1993; Brady et al., 1996), and it was suggested that diet alone accounts for the lower plasma carotenoid concentrations (Brady et al., 1996); even after correction for differences in intake, however, plasma β-carotene concentrations are 20–50% lower in smokers (Gregory et al., 1990; Thurnham, 1994). The effects of smoking is discussed in more detail in section 3.1.3.

2.1.2 α-Carotene
2.1.2.1 Occurrence
α-Carotene occurs in most vegetables and fruits but usually at concentrations much lower than those of β-carotene. Important natural sources of α-carotene are carrots (Bushway et al., 1986; Micozzi et al., 1992), red palm oil (Ong & Tee,

Table 3. Lutein and β-carotene concentrations (μmol/L) in plasma from men and women in studies in Europe, Japan and North America

Study	Lutein Men Mean (SD)	Lutein Men No.	Lutein Women Mean (SD)	Lutein Women No.	β-carotene Men Mean (SD)	β-carotene Men No.	β-carotene Women Mean (SD)	β-carotene Women No.	Reference
UK National Survey	0.34[a] (0.177)	429	0.34[a] (0.19)	443	0.29 (0.29)	871	0.37 (0.262)	892	Gregory et al. (1990)
Belfast, Northern Ireland	0.27 (0.13)	88	0.29 (0.14)	79	0.37 (0.25)	88	0.57 (0.37)	79	Howard et al. (1996)
Cambridge, UK (middle aged women only)			0.41 (0.14)	168			0.54 (0.27)	168	Scott et al. (1996)
Toulouse, France	0.56 (0.23)	100	0.61 (0.28)	106	0.38 (0.26)	100	0.63 (0.53)	106	Howard et al. (1996)
Montpellier, France	NR		NR		1.0 (0.40)	30	1.6 (0.60)	68	Saintot et al. (1994)
Madrid, Spain	0.20 (0.09)		0.24 (0.21)	54	0.22 (0.14)	57	0.37 (0.23)	54	Olmedilla et al. (1994)
German National Survey	NR	57	NR		0.43 (0.10–1.6)[b]	278	0.61 (0.16–2.2)[b]	367	Heseker et al. (1991)
Washington, USA (middle-aged persons)	0.31 (0.14)	55	0.34 (0.16)	55	0.29 (0.18)	55	0.41 (0.26)	55	Stacewicz-Sapuntzakis et al. (1987)
Nurses Study, USA	0.35 (0.10)	121	0.33 (0.11)	186	0.46 (0.29)	121	0.58 (0.37)		Ascherio et al. (1992)
Rural Japan (middle-aged persons)	NR		NR		0.55 (0.49)	356	1.15 (0.74)		Thurnham et al. (1997)
Rural Pakistan (infants)	0.17 (0.10)	101	0.17 (0.12)	90	ND		ND		

NR, not reported; ND, not detected
[a] Median (Thurnham & Flora, 1988)
[b] Median and range

1992) and mangoes (Cooney *et al.*, 1995). In these foods, not only is the proportion of α-carotene almost equal to that of β-carotene, but the concentrations of carotenoids are much higher than in other foods. As reports from The Gambia (Villard & Bates, 1987), Malaysia and Thailand (Tee & Lim, 1991), however, indicate that mangoes contain no α-carotene, there may be some interspecies variation. The concentration of α-carotene in most fruits is usually < 0.1 mg/100 g of edible fraction (Tee & Lim, 1991; Ong & Tee, 1992).

2.1.2.2   Commercial sources
α-Carotene is not synthesized commercially, but it is present in variable amounts in carotene extracts from various plants.

2.1.2.3   Analysis
Because of the structural similarities between α- and β-carotene, the two analytes tend to run close together when analysed by liquid chromatography. Nevertheless, they are usually easily separated. Most of the chromatographic methods used to separate β-carotene from other carotenoids can be used to separate α-carotene as well (see section 2.1.1.4).

2.1.2.4   Human use or exposure
Human use of and exposure to α-carotene are similar to those for β-carotene. It is found in most blood samples, although the concentrations are usually much lower than those of β-carotene (Thurnham & Flora, 1988), except when the diet contains a large proportion of carrots (Micozzi *et al.*, 1992), red palm oil (Adelekan *et al.*, 1989) or mangoes (Cooney *et al.*, 1995). α-Carotene is a provitamin A carotene since it retains one of the β rings intact; however, it is considered to have one-half of the biological potency of β-carotene as a source of retinol (Bauernfeind, 1972).

2.1.3   Lycopene
2.1.3.1   Occurrence
Lycopene is the predominant carotenoid in tomatoes; it also occurs at high concentrations (2–4.5 mg/100 g) in several deep-orange or reddish fruits such as papaya, watermelon and pink grapefruit (Ong & Tee, 1992). Preparations like tomato paste contain more than 10 times more lycopene (33–68 mg/100 g) than fresh tomatoes (about 4 mg/100 g) (Khachik *et al.*, 1992a; Tonucci *et al.*, 1995). A wide range of concentrations has been reported in different types of tomatoes, the pear-shaped variety being a particularly rich source (62 mg/100 g; Granado *et al.*, 1992).

2.1.3.2   Commercial sources
Lycopene is not synthesized commercially, but an extract of tomatoes which contains mainly lycopene is available.

2.1.3.3   Use and application
The use of lycopene (EC160d) as a colour is authorized by the European Parliament in many fruit preparations, meat and fish products, confectionery and drinks in which a red colour is desired and tomatoes are not a constituent; however, the addition of lycopene to tinned and bottled tomatoes and tomato-based sauces is not permitted (Klepsch & Baltas, 1994). The integrity of carotenoids is often preserved under quite demanding conditions, for example in tomato paste, which is typically prepared by dehydration at high temperature over an extended period under slight vacuum (Khachik *et al.*, 1992a). The deep red colour of the lycopene pigment therefore lends itself to widespread use as a colourant in many processed foods such as beans, fish, soups and sauces.

2.1.3.4   Analysis
In developed countries, lycopene is one of the main carotenoids in blood samples, and several methods for its analysis have been described (Thurnham *et al.*, 1988a; Cantilena & Nierenberg, 1989; Olmedilla *et al.*, 1990; Nierenberg & Nann, 1992; Stahl & Sies, 1992; Stahl *et al.*, 1993; Ritenbaugh *et al.*, 1996; Scott *et al.*, 1996). Isomers of lycopene have been detected in both biological samples (Stahl & Sies, 1992; Stahl *et al.*, 1993; Clinton *et al.*, 1996) and foods (Stahl & Sies, 1992; Clinton *et al.*, 1996), but foods usually contain mainly all-*trans*-lycopene while biological samples have a higher proportion of *cis* isomers (Clinton *et al.*, 1996). Most liquid chromatographic methods

do not provide baseline separation of the iso-mers, although separation of a set of 15 geo-metric isomers of lycopene identified by NMR has been reported (Hengartner *et al.*, 1992).

2.1.3.5 *Human use or exposure*

A threefold difference in dietary intakes of lycopene has been reported, from 1 mg/d in Spain (Granado *et al.*, 1996) to 2–3 mg/d in the United States (Chug-Ahuja *et al.*, 1993; Yong *et al.*, 1994). The concentrations of lycopene in blood samples also vary considerably between countries. The predominant source of lycopene in developed countries is tomatoes, which are consumed both as the fruit and as a constituent of many processed foods. Lycopene appears to be better absorbed from processed tomato prod-ucts than from the fresh fruit (Stahl & Sies, 1992; Gärtner *et al.*, 1997), perhaps because the *cis* isomers are absorbed better than all-*trans*-lycopene (Stahl & Sies, 1992). The latter accounts for 79–91% of all lycopene in tomatoes, tomato paste and tomato soup (Clinton *et al.*, 1996). Heating tomato juice with a small amount of oil has been reported to in-crease the formation of 9-*cis*-lycopene (Stahl & Sies, 1992). Khachik *et al.* (1992a), however, reported no difference in the chromatographic profile of raw and stewed tomatoes and tomato paste, but the *cis* isomers of lycopene formed during the processing of lycopene-containing foods may concentrate in the lipid fraction and be absorbed preferentially to all-*trans*-lycopene. This possibility is supported by reports of analyses of lycopene in biological samples, in which the *cis* isomers predominate. The proportion of *cis* isomers in serum ranged from 58 to 72% and that in prostate tissue from 79 to 88% (Clinton *et al.*, 1996).

The higher absorption of lycopene from processed foods may explain the higher serum concentrations of lycopene in blood from per-sons in developed countries such as France (Howard *et al.*, 1996), Great Britain (Gregory *et al.*, 1990), Northern Ireland (Howard *et al.*, 1996) and the United States (Ritenbaugh *et al.*, 1996) and the low concentrations or absence in blood from persons in developing countries such as China (Yang *et al.*, 1984), India (Das *et al.*, 1996), Pakistan (Thurnham *et al.*, 1997) and Thailand (Thurnham *et al.*, 1990). It has been reported that the plasma concentration of lycopene is better correlated with its dietary concentration than is that of β-carotene (Scott *et al.*, 1996). Unfortunately, the somewhat restricted distribution of sources of lycopene in the diet limits the usefulness of this carotenoid as a general marker of vegetable intake.

Smoking appeared to have no effect on serum lycopene concentrations in several stud-ies (Thompson *et al.*, 1985; Stryker *et al.*, 1988; Thurnham, 1994; Brady *et al.*, 1996), in con-trast to β-carotene. Lycopene also differs from β-carotene in showing no consistent difference in serum concentrations between the sexes (Stacewicz-Sapuntzakis *et al.*, 1987; Thurnham & Flora, 1988; Brady *et al.*, 1996). Furthermore, the concentrations of lycopene in serum appear to fall with age (Gregory *et al.*, 1990; Brady *et al.*, 1996), whereas this phenomenon has not been observed for other carotenoids. The plasma half-life is reported to be 12–33 days, which is longer than that of β-carotene (Rock *et al.*, 1992).

2.2 Xanthophylls
2.2.1 *Lutein and zeaxanthin*
2.2.1.1 *Occurrence*

As indicated earlier, lutein is one of the major carotenoids in green plants throughout the world (Khachik *et al.*, 1992a; Ong & Tee, 1992) and is the most prevalent carotenoid in blood samples (Thurnham *et al.*, 1997), although it is often not the most concentrated in plasma in industrialized countries (Thurnham & Flora, 1988; Micozzi *et al.*, 1992; Rock *et al.*, 1992; Brady *et al.*, 1996). Lutein is present in the serum of children with malnutrition or fat-absorption problems, even if no other carotenoid is detectable. The widespread occur-rence of lutein in both vegetables and fruit, coupled with the high concentrations in some green vegetables (Table 2), undoubtedly accounts for its almost universal appearance in blood (Table 3). Zeaxanthin is usually only a minor component of plasma, except when maize is a staple dietary cereal.

Particularly rich sources of lutein in western diets are broccoli and spinach (containing 3 and 10 mg/100 g, respectively; Khachik *et al.*, 1992a) and watercress (10.7 mg/100 g; Hart &

Scott, 1995). Tee and Lim (1991) reported concentrations of 20–30 mg/100 g in certain leafy vegetables in Malaysia. Zeaxanthin is far less abundant in foodstuffs than lutein, although it is found especially in yellow corn (Gross, 1991), spinach (Granado *et al.*, 1992) and sweet red peppers (Granado *et al.*, 1992).

2.2.1.2   Commercial sources
The main supply of lutein is derived by extraction from marigold flowers (*Tagetes* sp.; lutein esters) or from dried, powdered alfalfa (Isler *et al.*, 1967; Nonomura, 1990).

2.2.1.3   Use and application
Lutein (E161b) is permitted for use as a food colour in the European Community and may be used in a variety of products, including alcoholic and nonalcoholic drinks, preserved fruits and vegetables, confectionery, baked wares and decorations, milk products and cheeses, sauces and seasonings, fish, meat and fish products and nutritional supplements in amounts of 50–500 mg/kg (Klepsch & Baltas, 1994). Another major use for lutein is as an additive to chicken feed to colour egg yolks.

2.2.1.4   Analysis
Concentrations of lutein and zeaxanthin are determined by spectrophotometry (see Section 1). Several methods have been reported for their analysis in plasma (Thurnham *et al.*, 1988a; Olmedilla *et al.*, 1990; Craft, 1992; Nierenberg & Nann, 1992; Ritenbaugh *et al.*, 1996; Scott *et al.*, 1996). Although zeaxanthin and lutein can be fully resolved chromatographically, the procedure requires considerable time. As a consequence, simpler methods in which the two compounds are eluted together, because of their similar polarity, have generally been used in surveys. The dissection of human and monkey retinas for extraction of lutein and zeaxanthin has been describedin detail (Bone *et al.*, 1988; Handelman *et al.*, 1992).

2.2.1.5   Human use or exposure
About 1–2 mg/d of lutein are reportedly consumed in European and American countries (Chug-Ahuja *et al.*, 1993; Yong *et al.*, 1994; Granado *et al.*, 1996; Scott *et al.*, 1996). Lutein

must compete with the other carotenoids for entry into the mucosal cells lining the gut (Kostic *et al.*, 1995). Furthermore, the uptake of lutein into the triglyceride-rich lipoproteins is reported to be only 85% as efficient as that of β-carotene or lycopene when fed as an encapsulated supplement with a standard, low-carotene meal (O'Neill & Thurnham, 1998); however, long-term supplementation with a high dose of β-carotene did not affect the serum lutein concentration (Albanes *et al.*, 1997), and the concentrations of lutein in the serum in various population groups cover a wide range (Table 3).

Serum lutein can be used as a biomarker of vegetable intake (Thurnham *et al.*, 1997). Lutein is widely distributed in foods but is found predominantly in the leaves of green plants, which are eaten in almost all cultures. Although β-carotene is also present in green leaves in similar amounts to lutein and has also been proposed as a marker of intake (Drewnoski *et al.*, 1997), the concentrations in serum represent the amount left after the formation of retinol and retinoic acid in the gut. Plasma β-carotene also tends to be more labile than lutein, since β-carotene turns over more rapidly in blood, the half-lives being < 12 and 33–61 days, respectively (Rock *et al.*, 1992). The plasma concentrations of luteinare better correlated with estimate carotenoid intakes than for β-carotene (Scott *et al.*, 1996). The metabolism and distribution of lutein in tissues are discussed in Section 3.

2.2.2   Cryptoxanthin
2.2.2.1   Occurrence
Cryptoxanthin includes α-cryptoxanthin, β-cryptoxanthin and zeinoxanthin. Only β-cryptoxanthin is usually measured in blood plasma, because reference compounds are not readily available for the other cryptoxanthins. β-Cryptoxanthin is found mainly in fruits, in amounts ranging from 17 mg/100 g in jackfruit to 1.48 mg/100 g in papaya (Tee & Lim, 1991). Three fruits, papaya, starfruit and tree tomatoes, are reported to contain > 1 mg/100 g (Tee & Lim, 1991). Citrus fruit are a major source of β-cryptoxanthin in western countries, at concentrations of 80–1800 mg/100 g (Mangels *et al.*, 1993; Hart & Scott, 1995).

2.2.2.2 Commercial sources

β-Cryptoxanthin is not synthesized commercially. Extracts rich in β-cryptoxanthin are available in analytical quantities only.

2.2.2.3 Use and application

Cryptoxanthin is not listed in the EC Directorate for food colours.

2.2.2.4 Analysis

β-Cryptoxanthin is separated by HPLC and quantified by spectrophotometry (see Section 1). In some of the methods (Stacewicz-Sapuntzakis *et al.*, 1987; Thurnham *et al.*, 1988a), the peak of β-cryptoxanthin overlaps with that of α-tocopherol, but they are easily distinguished since they absorb at different wavelengths.

2.2.2.5 Human use or exposure

β-Cryptoxanthin is commonly found in plasma samples collected in western countries, the population means varying from 0.13 mmol/L in men in the United Kingdom (Thurnham & Flora, 1988) to 0.6 mmol/L in Spanish women (Olmedilla *et al.*, 1994). The plasma concentration of β-cryptoxanthin is usually lower than that of both β-carotene and lutein (Stacewicz-Sapuntzakis *et al.*, 1987; Thurnham & Flora, 1988; Cantilena *et al.*, 1992; Cooney *et al.*, 1995), unless oranges are particularly common in the diet, as reported from Spain (Olmedilla *et al.*, 1994). β-Cryptoxanthin has provitamin A activity. The plasma concentrations are usually higher in women than in men (Thurnham & Flora, 1988; Olmedilla *et al.*, 1994; Howard *et al.*, 1996). The half-life of β-cryptoxanthin in blood is < 12 days, similar to those of the other main provitamin A carotenoids (Rock *et al.*, 1992).

2.2.3 Canthaxanthin
2.2.3.1 Occurrence

Canthaxanthin is a red–orange pigment found in crustaceans, sea trout, algae, bacteria and some edible mushrooms. It is also present in the axion tissues of flamingos and other red-feathered birds (Hathcock *et al.*, 1990).

2.2.3.2 Commercial sources

β-Carotene is used as the starting material for the commercial synthesis of canthaxanthin.

2.2.3.3 Use and application

Canthaxanthin (EC161g) is approved for use as a food additive in the European Community but only for the colouring of Strasbourg sausages to a level of 15 mg/kg (Klepsch & Baltas, 1994). The predominant uses of canthaxanthin are in feed for laying hens, in order to colour egg yolks, in broiler production and in salmon and trout farming. Canthaxanthin has been marketed under a number of trade names as a tablet for 'tanning' the skin, in which deposition in subcutaneous tissues simulates the appearance of a tan, but this use has been discontinued in some countries. In Europe, capsules containing 10 mg β-carotene and 15 mg canthaxanthin are used at doses < 150 mg/d as a treatment for erythropoietic protoporphyria.

2.2.3.4 Analysis

Canthaxanthin can be measured by spectrophotometric methods (see Section 1). When the standard methods of reversed-phase liquid chromatography now adopted by many workers for the analysis of carotenoids in blood, tissue and food extracts are used, canthaxanthin elutes in the early part of the chromatogram, between lutein and β-crytoxanthin (Thurnham *et al.*, 1988a; van Vliet *et al.*, 1991). Canthaxanthin has also been reported to co-elute with β-apo-10′-carotenoid (van Vliet *et al.*, 1991). Canthaxanthin is unlikely to be a major component of plasma in North America or the United Kingdom, but no systematic study has been reported.

3. Metabolism, Kinetics and Genetic Variation

The metabolism of carotenoids has been studied since the early 1920s, when certain yellow plant pigments were found to stimulate the growth of vitamin A-deficient rats. Later in that decade, Thomas Moore showed that β-carotene, the most active of these plant pigments, was converted to vitamin A in rats *in vivo*. Until recently, carotenoids were considered in mammalian physiology only in terms of their provitamin A activity. The bioavailability and metabolism of carotenoids are significantly affected by dietary, physiological and matrix-associated factors (Erdman *et al.*, 1993; Olson, 1994; Wang, 1994; de Pee & West, 1996; Parker, 1996, 1997), including consumption of dietary fat together with the carotenoids, release of the bile acids necessary to form lipid micelles, the amount of carotenoids present in the diet, the dietary matrix and crystalline structure of the carotenoid in the matrix, processing and cooking, nutritional status (vitamin A and carotenoid concentrations), individual host-related factors such as disease states and genetic factors.

Most of the early studies of carotenoid metabolism focused on β-carotene. More recently, other carotenoids, such as lutein, canthaxanthin, lycopene, 4,4'-dimethoxy-β-carotene, ethyl β-apo-8'-carotenoate, and β-apo-8'-carotenal, have been studied both in humans and in experimental animals. The metabolism of carotenoids has been reviewed extensively (Erdman *et al.*, 1993; Olson, 1994; Wang, 1994; de Pee & West, 1996; Parker, 1996; Furr & Clark, 1997; Parker, 1997). Although there is little information on carotenoids other than β-carotene, it is clear that the absorption and metabolism of different carotenoids varies markedly. They may also mutually influence their bioavailability, as has been demonstrated for β-carotene, lutein and zeaxanthin (High & Day, 1951; Micozzi *et al.*, 1992; Kostic *et al.*, 1995; Gärtner *et al.*, 1996).

3.1 Humans

3.1.1 Intestinal digestion and absorption

Dietary carotenoids in foods exist in two major forms: as true solutions in oil, as in red palm oil, or as parts of the matrices of vegetables and fruit. The matrix is usually complex, consisting of fibre, digestible polysaccharides and proteins. Because carotenoids are often not fully disrupted during food preparation or during their passage through the intestine, their bioavailability can vary from < 10%, such as in largely intact raw carrots, to > 50% in oily solutions or in synthetic, gelatin-based, commercial preparations (Olson, 1994; Parker, 1996; Furr & Clark, 1997). Methods for evaluating the extent of absorption have been reviewed (Bowen *et al.*, 1993; Parker, 1997). Hydrocarbon carotenoids, like β-carotene and lycopene, are solubilized in the lipid core of micelles in the gut lumen or alternatively form small clathrate complexes with conjugated bile acids, of which deoxycholate and cholate are the most effective (Olson, 1994). Xanthophyll esters must be hydrolysed before absorption. As in membranes, xanthophylls and carotenes associate differently with micelles (Furr & Clark, 1997): hydrocarbon carotenoids tend to associate with the lipophilic core of membranes and micelles. The absorption process does not seem to involve special epithelial transporters.

The factors that lower the bioavailability of carotenoids, apart from incomplete release from food matrices, include the presence of fibre, particularly pectins, in the diet; lack of fat in the diet; the presence of undigested lipids, including fat substitutes; inadequate bile flow; various clinical conditions involving lipid malabsorption and reduced gastric acidity (Olson, 1994; Parker, 1996; Furr & Clark, 1997). The absorption and conversion efficiency of carotenoids in humans and animals decreases as the amount ingested increases (Brubacher & Weiser, 1985; Furr & Clark, 1997).

Carotenoids appear to be absorbed by duodenal mucosal cells by a mechanism involving passive diffusion, similar to that for cholesterol and the products of triglyceride lipolysis (Parker, 1996). One of the earliest human experiments to investigate the events that occur during intestinal absorption of β-carotene was reported in 1966 (Goodman *et al.*, 1966a). Tritiated β-carotene (plus 47 or 91 μg unlabelled β-carotene) dissolved in 2 ml olive oil and emulsified in 50 ml skimmed milk was fed to two patients in whom polyethylene cannulae had been inserted in the thoracic duct in the neck. Radiolabel was absorbed into the lymph 3–10 h after feeding; about 20% of the label was recovered, of which 70–80% was in the chylomicrons, and 60–70% was present as vitamin A esters, indicating that the human intestine has an extremely limited ability to absorb unchanged dietary β-carotene into the lymph.

When carotenoids are present in substantial amounts, they can interfere with each other's absorption. The action is not mutually competitive, however, since β-carotene inhibits canthaxanthin and lutein absorption, whereas the latter have lesser or no effects on β-carotene absorption (White *et al.*, 1994; Kostic *et al.*, 1995). The mechanism of this interaction has not been defined. Vitamin E and carotenoids also interact, since vitamin E supplements tend to lower plasma carotenoid concentrations, although small amounts of vitamin E may prevent carotenoid oxidation in the gastrointestinal tract. β-Carotene supplements have been reported to decrease, to increase or not to affect plasma tocopherol concentrations (Furr & Clark, 1997).

The results of several large trials of the effects of supplemental β-carotene on the serum concentrations of other carotenoids are now becoming available. Several investigators have reported statistically significant increases in α-carotene concentrations with β-carotene supplementation (Omenn *et al.*, 1993a; Wahlqvist *et al.*, 1994; Albanes *et al.*, 1997; Mayne *et al.*, 1997). [The Working Group noted that small amounts of α-carotene may be present in β-carotene preparations; furthermore, the increases seen could be due to di-*cis* isomers of β-carotene, which are difficult to separate analytically from α-carotene, or they could involve a sparing effect of β-carotene on α-carotene.] The results for the effects of supplemental β-carotene on other carotenoids are less consistent, but there do not appear to be reductions in the concentrations of any of the other major circulating carotenoids.

In a nutritional context, the large differences in the bioavailability of carotenoids make it difficult to define their equivalence as precursors of vitamin A. The molar equivalence between retinol and small amounts of β-carotene in oil is approximately 0.5, whereas that with carotenoids in rapidly stir-fried vegetables is very poor (< 0.05). Carotenoids in fruits seem to be used more efficiently. The results of studies of bioavailability, which are often inconclusive and conflicting, have been reviewed (de Pee & West, 1996).

The absorption of carotenoids and their presence in plasma are influenced by their geometrical isomeric form. The all-*trans* isomer of β-carotene is well absorbed and appears in plasma, whereas the 9-*cis* isomer, although fairly well absorbed, is found in plasma only at low concentrations (Gaziano *et al.*, 1995a). In contrast, the *cis* isomers of lycopene seem to be better absorbed into plasma than the all-*trans* form (Stahl & Sies, 1992). Thus, the 'isomer effect' depends on the carotenoid being studied and the species being used (Olson, 1994; Parker, 1996; Furr & Clark, 1997).

In general, polar carotenoids are absorbed better by humans than non-polar ones. Thus, lutein is absorbed about twice as well as β-carotene (Kostic *et al.*, 1995), and β-apocarotenals and β-apocarotenols seem to be absorbed better than less polar carotenoids (Zeng *et al.*, 1992). The proportions of lutein and zeaxanthin are greater in the chylomicra than in the ingested carotenoid mixture (Furr & Clark, 1997). These conclusions are based on the assumption that the metabolism of carotenoids in the intestinal mucosa represents only a minor part of their transfer into plasma and that their relative rates of clearance from plasma are similar. These assumptions may not hold for all-*trans*-β-carotene or for other provitamin A carotenoids.

When a moderate to large dose of β-carotene is administered orally to humans, most subjects respond by a marked increase in the β-carotene concentration in plasma, which peaks at about 6 h, decreases and then rises to a higher concentration with a second peak at about 24 h (Furr & Clark, 1997). Some subjects, however, show little or no increase in the plasma concentration of β-carotene after a single dose (Furr & Clark, 1997), and they have been called 'poor' or 'non-responders' (Bowen *et al.*, 1993). Of the various explanations that might be given for the lack of response, the most likely is that 'non-responders' are in fact rapid converters of β-carotene into vitamin A. This explanation does not hold for lycopene, however, as the responses of individuals differ (Stahl & Sies, 1996). Different individual responses to lutein were also observed in one small study (O'Neill & Thurnham, 1998), but not in another (Kostic *et al.*, 1995).

3.1.2 *Transport in plasma*
Newly absorbed carotenoids, retinyl ester and small amounts of retinol are transported on chylomicra from the intestinal mucosa via the

lymph into the general circulation. Lipoprotein lipase hydrolyses much of the triglyceride in the chylomicron, resulting in a chylomicron remnant (Furr & Clark, 1997). The latter, which retains apolipoproteins B48 and E on its surface, interacts with receptors on hepatocytes and is taken up by those cells. Small amounts of chylomicron remnants may also be taken up by other tissues. The hepatocytes then incorporate much of the dietary carotenoids into lipoproteins, primarily very-low-density and low-density lipoproteins, whereas xanthophylls are distributed more or less equally between high-density and low-density lipoproteins (Olson, 1994; Furr & Clark, 1997). This distribution accords with the hydrophobicity of the carotenoids and of the lipoproteins. Specific mechanisms of incorporation, such as the α-tocopherol-transport protein of liver, have not been identified for carotenoids. A β-carotene-binding protein has recently been characterized in ferret liver (Rao et al., 1997). If a similar protein exists in human liver, it may play some role in the incorporation of β-carotene into lipoproteins. High-density lipo-proteins may arise both from de-novo synthesis in the liver and from the pinching off of excess surface components from chylomicra in plasma during triglyceride hydrolysis; however, xanthophylls are probably incorporated primarily into high-density lipoproteins in the liver (Olson, 1998).

In plasma, very low-density lipoproteins are rapidly converted by lipoprotein lipase to low-density lipoproteins, which retain the carotenoids and apolipoprotein B100. Receptors for the latter are present on cells of many peripheral tissues and particularly those of the adrenal gland and testes as well as of the liver. High-density lipoproteins pick up cholesterol and possibly xanthophylls from peripheral tissues and apolipoprotein E from other plasma lipoproteins before being taken up by the liver. Except as noted above, carotenoids do not seem to be transferred from one lipid class to another, at least in vitro (Furr & Clark, 1997). Thus, carotenoids are involved in a complex and probably cyclical metabolic pathway involving the intestine, chylomicra, the liver, plasma lipoproteins and peripheral tissues.

3.1.3 Serum carotenoid concentrations

Carotenoids are commonly found in the plasma of fasting subjects. Of the 20 or more carotenoids present (Khachik et al., 1995), the major six, which comprise 60–70% of the total (Barua et al., 1993), are lycopene, lutein, zeaxanthin, β-cryptoxanthin, β-carotene and α-carotene. Because carotenoids are not covalently bound to lipoproteins and apparently are not homeostatically controlled, their concentrations in plasma are highly dependent on the diet. In a more physiological context, their steady-state plasma concentrations depend on the amounts in the diet, their efficiency of intestinal absorption, their uptake by tissues, their release from tissues back into the plasma and their catabolic rates. Plasma carotenoids represent < 10% of the total body pool (40–150 mg; Bendich & Olson, 1989), of which only 10–30% is β-carotene (Thurnham & Flora, 1988; Bendich & Olson, 1989). Because the distribution of carotenoids in a typical population is skewed, median concentrations are generally used in analyses.

The median values for the plasma concentrations of the six main carotenoids in a British and in an American population are summarized in Table 4. The reference ranges are broad since they include individuals who ingest various amounts of carotenoids. Lutein and zeaxanthin, which tend to run closely together on HPLC traces, are grouped; in general, the ratio of lutein to zeaxanthin in the plasma is 4 or 5:1 (Peng et al., 1995). Although the distribution and amounts of carotenoids in individuals differ markedly, each person maintains a fairly constant pattern for up to one year (Cantilena et al., 1992; Peng et al., 1995), probably reflecting a fairly uniform diet during that period, abetted by the presumed buffering effect of tissue carotenoid concentrations. Depending on the variety of dietary sources of carotenoids, there can, however, be marked seasonal changes in serum concentrations (Rautalahti et al., 1993). Carotenoid concentrations measured in the morning were 6–10% higher than those in the evening (Cantilena et al., 1992).

Median carotenoid concentrations also vary with age, but not in the same way for all carotenoids (Briefel et al., 1996). The plasma concentrations of most carotenoids except lycopene tend to increase with age (Thurnham & Flora, 1988; Gregory et al., 1990). In the United States, lycopene is generally found at the highest concentrations in plasma, followed by lutein and zeaxanthin, β-carotene, β-cryptoxanthin and α-carotene, in that order (Briefel et al., 1996). The pattern differs with region, depending on dietary intake. People who ingested canthaxanthin as a tanning agent had canthaxanthin in their plasma (Gunson et al., 1984). Women have higher plasma concentrations of β-carotene, α-carotene and β-cryptoxanthin than men (Stacewicz-Sapuntzakis et al., 1986; Ito et al., 1987; Stryker et al., 1988; Thurnham & Flora, 1988; Thurnham et al., 1988a; Heseker et al., 1991; Olmedilla et al., 1994), while the concentrations of lutein and lycopene tend not to differ between the sexes (Ito et al., 1987; Thurnham & Flora, 1988; Olmedilla et al., 1994). It has been reported that the carotenoid concentrations in women are at their lowest during the menses and that of β-carotene peaks in the late follicular phase,

the other carotenoids following the same trend (Forman et al., 1996); however, other workers have been unable to detect any significant changes associated with menstrual periodicity (Tangney et al., 1991; Rock et al., 1995).

Body mass index and serum glutamyl transferase activity were inversely correlated with both the baseline plasma concentrations of β-carotene and those after supplementation with β-carotene (Albanes et al., 1991), while the serum concentration of cholesterol was positively correlated but only after supplementation. Dietary interventions, including a high intake of vegetables and a low intake of fat, increased the serum concentrations of β-carotene, α-carotene, lycopene and lutein but not that of β-cryptoxanthin (Rock et al., 1997), and the correlations were statistically significant in the case of β- and α-carotene and lutein. In people fed a diet containing few, if any, carotenoids, the plasma concentration decreases in approximately a first-order manner for 14–30 days and then tends to reach slowly declining plateau values (Rock et al., 1992).

Table 4. Median concentrations (μmol/L) of serum carotenoids in adults in Great Britain and the United States

Carotenoid	Men	Women	Reference range (5th–95th percentile)
Great Britain[a]			
Lycopene	0.25	0.25	0.06–0.68
Lutein and zeaxanthin	0.29	0.29	NR
β-Cryptoxanthin	0.13	0.16	0.03–0.51
β-Carotene	0.24	0.32	0.07–0.84
α-Carotene	0.06	0.07	0.02–0.21
United States[b]			
Lycopene	0.47	0.41	0.13–0.82
Lutein and zeaxanthin	0.35	0.35	0.16–0.72
β-Cryptoxanthin	0.13	0.13	0.05–0.38
β-Carotene	0.22	0.28[c]	0.09–0.91
α-Carotene	0.065	0.081[c]	0.02–0.22

NR, not reported
[a] From Gregory et al. (1990)
[b] Based on data from Briefel et al. (1996)
[c] Extrapolated from values for nonsmoking persons

3.1.3.1 Effects of β-carotene supplements

When a single, fairly large supplement (15–30 mg, 28–56 μmol) of all-*trans*-β-carotene is administered orally to adults, the concentrations of β-carotene in plasma increase to a peak (1.5–3-fold higher than baseline) at about 24–30 h and then decline, with a half-life of seven to nine days (Brown et al., 1989). [The Working Group noted that the serum concentrations achieved depend on the composition of the formulation used as a supplement.] The β-carotene concentration returns to a baseline level after about 18 days (Kostic et al., 1995). When large daily supplements of β-carotene (30–300 mg, 56–560 μmol) are given orally, the plasma concentrations increase in a first-order fashion to reach a plateau, usually 7–20-fold higher than baseline, at about 25 days (Meyer et al., 1985; Dimitrov & Ullrey, 1990; Prince et al., 1991; Albanes et al., 1992; Micozzi et al., 1992; Wahlqvist et al., 1994; Manetta et al., 1996; Albanes et al., 1997). The plateau was proportional to the dose given, but interindividual differences in plateau levels have been observed after repeated administration of β-carotene

(Albanes *et al.*, 1992). As already indicated, the bioavailability of β-carotene in oil or in commercial beadlets is far greater than that of β-carotene in vegetables (Micozzi *et al.*, 1992), and ingestion of fat with β-carotene optimizes its absorption. The distribution of carotenoids in the plasma lipoproteins of hypercarotenaemic persons was similar to that in untreated subjects (Mathews-Roth & Gulbrandsen, 1974). Elderly persons may either absorb β-carotene better or clear it more slowly from the plasma than young subjects (Maiani *et al.*, 1989). The concentration of β-carotene in tissues is generally proportional to that in plasma (Dimitrov & Ullrey, 1990; Peng *et al.*, 1995; Manetta *et al.*, 1996).

Supplements of β-carotene might affect the concentrations of other fat-soluble components of the plasma. β-Carotene supplements have little or no effect on plasma retinol concentrations in well-nourished individuals (Albanes *et al.*, 1997), primarily because the plasma retinol concentration is homeostatically controlled. Particular attention has been paid to serum α-tocophenol since the report of Xu *et al.* (1992) that daily doses of β-carotene (15–60 mg per day) for six to nine months lowered α-tocopherol concentrations by 40% in a group of 45 subjects. A similar effect was found in a study of 58 subjects (Mobarhan *et al.*, 1994); however, much larger studies with longer durations of supplementation have shown no effect of β-carotene supplements on serum α-tocophenol concentrations (Albanes *et al.*, 1992; Goodman *et al.*, 1994; Nierenberg *et al.*, 1994; Fontham *et al.*, 1995; Albanes *et al.*, 1997; Mayne *et al.*, 1997).

3.1.3.2 Effects of tobacco smoking

Tobacco smoking has been associated with lowered concentrations of several serum carotenoids, increased turnover of ascorbic acid and a lesser effect on α-tocopherol concentrations. Decreased serum β-carotene concentrations have been reported to be associated with the number of cigarettes smoked per day, the years of smoking and whether the person is a current or an ex-smoker (Stryker *et al.*, 1988; Pamuk *et al.*, 1994; Goodman *et al.*, 1996; Albanes *et al.*, 1997). The concentrations of α-carotene, β-carotene and cryptoxanthin were

lowered by about 30% in heavy smokers (> 10 cigarettes per day), whereas that of lutein/zeaxanthin was less affected, i.e. by 10% (Pamuk *et al.*, 1994; Albanes *et al.*, 1997); the concentrations of lycopene were not affected (Stryker *et al.*, 1988; Thurnham, 1994). Former smokers showed no differences from non-smokers in carotenoid concentrations. Serum retinol concentrations were affected little if at all.

The lowered serum carotenoid concentrations have been attributed to the presence of β-unsaturated aldehydes and of a large number of free radicals, estimated as 10^{15} per puff, in cigarette smoke (Eiserich *et al.*, 1995; Handelman *et al.*, 1996). Protein–carbonyl adduct formation exceeded lipid peroxide formation *in vitro*. The order of disappearance of carotenoids in plasma exposed to gas-phase cigarette smoke *in vitro* was lycopene > β-carotene > lutein/zeaxanthin = cryptoxanthin > retinol (Handelman *et al.*, 1996). α-Tocopherol was affected more *in vitro* than *in vivo*.

3.1.3.3 Effects of alcohol drinking

In the Alpha-Tocopherol, Beta-Carotene Cancer Prevention (ATBC) study (see section 4.1.1.1), consumption of > 12.9 g alcohol per day was associated with a 10–38% decrease in serum carotenoid concentrations, particularly those of α-carotene, β-carotene and β-cryptoxanthin, in both people receiving and not receiving supplements (Albanes *et al.*, 1997). In the Beta-Carotene and Retinol Efficacy Trial (CARET), alcohol consumption was negatively correlated with serum β-carotene concentrations ($r = -0.14$; $p < 0.05$) and positively associated with serum retinol concentrations ($r = 0.10$; $p < 0.05$; Goodman *et al.*, 1996). In a smaller study in Boston, USA, consumption of > 20 g alcohol per day lowered the serum β-carotene concentrations by 24% in men and 11% in women (Stryker *et al.*, 1988). In 98 volunteers in southern France, a negative correlation was reported between the plasma concentration of β-carotene and alcohol intake ($r = -0.35$; $p < 0.001$) (Saintot *et al.*, 1995). No consistent relationship was seen between alcohol intake and plasma β-carotene concentrations in a small group of alcoholics. Supplementation with 30–60 mg/d β-carotene was reported to increase the plasma concentrations, but the people with liver cirrhosis had a lower response than those without (Ahmed *et al.*, 1994). Thus, alcohol ingestion has generally been associated with decreased serum carotenoid concentrations.

3.1.3.4 *Effects of other modulators*
Other factors affect serum carotenoid concentrations, primarily by inhibiting the intestinal absorption of carotenoids. Thus, acidic fibres, like pectins, lower carotenoid absorption in humans (Rock & Swendseid, 1992). The cholesterol-lowering drug, cholestyramine, which binds bile acids, has a similar effect, either by reducing the bile-acid concentration in the lumen or by directly binding carotenoids (Morris *et al.*, 1994). The fat substitute Olestra®, which is not absorbed, reduces serum concentrations of carotenoids, presumably by sequestering the compounds in the lipophilic phase (Peters *et al.*, 1997).

3.1.4 *Tissue carotenoid content*
The tissue concentrations of carotenoids reflect their intake in the diet and/or supplements.

3.1.4.1 *Effects of dietary intake*
Carotenoids are found in all tissues of the body (Blankenhorn, 1957; Stich *et al.*, 1986; Parker, 1988; Dimitrov & Ullrey, 1990; Kaplan *et al.*, 1990; Schmitz *et al.*, 1991; Stahl *et al.*, 1992; Mobarhan *et al.*, 1994; Johnson *et al.*, 1995; Kohlmeier & Kohlmeier, 1995; Peng *et al.*, 1995; Clinton *et al.*, 1996; Nair *et al.*, 1996; Redlich *et al.*, 1996; Virtanen *et al.*, 1996; Sanderson *et al.*, 1997; Table 5). On the basis of the relative weights of tissues in the adult human body (Long, 1961), carotenoids clearly are mainly present in fat, liver, skin and plasma. Some relatively small tissues, such as testes and adrenal glands, and parts of some tissues like the corpus luteum (112 nmol/g) have very high concentrations of carotenoids, whereas some major organs like muscle and brain have very low concentrations. The only major human tissues not cited in Table 5 are those of the skeleton and gastrointestinal tract. The former does not seem to have been studied in this regard, and the latter, which deteriorates rapidly after death, has not been examined in human autopsy specimens.

The total amount of carotenoid in any individual depends of course largely on intake. Thus, the ranges of specific carotenoids in tissues are very broad, and the mean concentrations in fat and liver vary widely in different studies. Some information is available about cells isolated from the gastrointestinal system. Intact buccal mucosal cells have been reported to contain 0.016 nmol of total carotenoids per 10^6 cells (Peng *et al.*, 1995) and exfoliated buccal cells about half as much (Stich *et al.*, 1986). A factor of 40 can be used to convert 10^6 cells to grams wet weight of tissue. Thus, the buccal mucosa contained 0.64 nmol/g, similar to the amount found in other internal organs. Stomach epithelial cells contained 0.5 nmol/g (Sanderson *et al.*, 1997), and colonic and rectal epithelial cells obtained at biopsy contained about 0.060 and 0.040 nmol β-carotene per g (Mobarhan *et al.*, 1994; Maiani *et al.*, 1995). If the ratio of total carotenoids to β-carotene is assumed to be 5, the total carotenoid concentrations in these cells would be 0.30 and 0.20 nmol/g, respectively. Exfoliated colonic cells contained much smaller concentrations of carotenoids, indicating that they are probably incorporated into crypt cells and then are slowly lost during the cell's migration up the villus (Nair *et al.*, 1996). This conclusion is supported by the finding that ingestion of carotenoid-rich vegetables for five to seven days maximizes the carotenoid concentration in exfoliated colonic cells, and this period concords with the migration time in villi. The concentration of total carotenoids in cells obtained by bronchoalveolar lavage (0.52 nmol/g) was similar to that in lung tissue (0.63 nmol/g; Redlich *et al.*, 1996). It has also been shown that β-carotene is secreted into bile at concentrations that reflect those in plasma (Leo *et al.*, 1995).

The total carotenoid concentrations in adipose tissue in various studies were 9.2 (Johnson *et al.*, 1995), 5.7 (Parker, 1988) and 4.2 nmol/g (Virtanen *et al.*, 1996). Because adipose tissue is the main site of storage for carotenoids, biopsies of this tissue are recommended for determining long-term carotenoid status (Kohlmeier & Kohlmeier, 1995). The carotenoid concentration in adipose tissue is higher, however, in women than in men and is inversely associated

Table 5. Estimated carotenoid contents of selected human tissues

Organ	Mean concentration[a] (nmol/g)	Approximate percent of body weight[b]	Mean total amount (µmol)[c]	Percent of total amount[d]
Fat	3.3 (15.6)[e] (0.8)[f]	18.8	42.2	65.39
Liver	5.0 (14.1)[e] (5.1)[f] (21.0)[g]	2.3	7.8	12.09
Muscle	ND[h] (0.07)[i]	42.8	2.04	3.16
Adrenal	33.7 (9.4)[f]	0.02	0.46	0.71
Plasma	ND[h] (1.1)[f] (1.6)[j]	4.9	4.5	6.97
Pancreas	3.7	0.16	0.40	0.62
Spleen	0.96 (5.9)[e]	0.25	0.16	0.25
Kidney	0.98 (1.2)[e] (0.9)f (3.1)[g]	0.41	0.27	0.42
Heart	0.81 (0.84)[e]	0.42	0.23	0.36
Testes	26.3 (7.6)[e]	0.04	0.72	1.12
Lung	ND[h] (1.9)[g]	0.73	0.94	1.46
Thyroid	0.79	0.04	0.021	0.03
Ovary	2.6 (0.9)[f]	0.01	0.018	0.03
Prostate	ND[h] (1.3)[k]	0.024	0.021	0.03
Skin	ND[h] (0.98)[j]	7.0	4.7	7.28
Brain	ND[h] (< 0.04)[f]	2.0	0.054	< 0.08
Total	–	79.9	64.54	100

[a] Mean concentrations, unless otherwise noted, from Kaplan *et al.* (1990). The average molecular mass of mixed carotenoids is assumed to be 543; thus, 1 µg = 1.84 nmol.

[b] From Long (1961); main unlisted tissues are stomach and intestine (7–10%) and skeleton (12–15%)

[c] Based on a reference body weight of 68 kg

[d] Based primarily on Kaplan *et al.* (1990)

[e] From Blankenhorn (1957)

[f] From Stahl *et al.* (1992); plasma concentration in nmol/ml

[g] From Schmitz *et al.* (1991)

[h] Not determined by Kaplan *et al.* (1990)

[i] From Dimitrov & Ullrey (1990)

[j] From Peng *et al.* (1995)

[k] From Clinton *et al.* (1996); lycopene and β-carotene only

with body size and composition, including the body mass index, and with smoking and alcohol consumption. The associations were stronger with some carotenoids than with others, and carotenoid concentrations were little affected by age (mean age, 53 ± 9 years for men and 62 ± 6 years for women); however, a negative correlation with lycopene was seen in men (Virtanen *et al.*, 1996). Negative correlations between plasma lycopene and age were also seen in adults in Great Britain and the USA (Gregory *et al.*, 1990; Brady *et al.*, 1996), but in a study on 46 women with breast cancer and 63 controls, the concentrations of β-carotene, lycopene and lutein/zeaxanthin in breast adipose tissue were not correlated with the respective estimated intakes (Zhang *et al.*, 1997). More than 20 structurally different carotenoids have been detected in the breast milk of lactating women (Khachik *et al.*, 1997), showing that human milk is an important source of carotenoids and vitamin A for infants (Thurnham *et al.*, 1997).

Since ≥ 90% of the carotenoids in the body are found in tissues and < 10% in plasma, the contents of various tissues are of interest.

Lycopene and β-carotene occurred at the highest concentrations in nearly all of the tissues listed in Table 5, lutein/zeaxanthin at intermediate concentrations and cryptoxanthin and α-carotene at lower levels. The pattern of carotenoid concentrations in tissues usually reflects their distribution in plasma. Some exceptions are the preferential accumulation of β-carotene in the pineal gland (Shi *et al.*, 1991) and in the corpus luteum (Moore, 1957) and of lutein/zeaxanthin in the macula of the eye (Handelman *et al.*, 1988).

The relationship between the concentrations of carotenoids in tissues and in plasma is crucial. A significant relationship has been found for both total and specific carotenoids in most studies (e.g. Peng *et al.*, 1995), but a poorer correlation is found between tissue concentrations and dietary intake of carotenoids, possibly because of uncertainties in estimating dietary intakes accurately (Peng *et al.*, 1995). β-Carotene concentrations in the cord blood of fetuses increase from about 0.0019 μmol/L at 20 weeks of gestation to 0.056 μmol/L at 40 weeks. The concentrations in the blood of neonates were lower in mothers who smoked (Moji *et al.*, 1995). The relationship between the concentrations of retinol and β-carotene in maternal serum, cord serum and placentae was assessed at parturition in women whose vitamin A status was adequate (n = 15; serum retinol, > 0.7 μmol/L) and inadequate (n = 16; serum retinol, < 0.7 μmol/L). The concentrations of β-carotene in maternal serum (0.22 mmol/L), cord blood (0.019 μmol/L) and placenta (0.0075 mmol/g) were unaffected by maternal vitamin A status (Dimenstein *et al.*, 1996). A cross-sectional study of 30 women showed that the serum cholesterol concentration was increased during the early follicular phase of the menstrual cycle and that of α-carotene was increased in the mid-luteal phase, but only if uncorrected for total cholesterol. The concentrations of lutein, β-cryptoxanthin, lycopene and β-carotene did not change during the cycle (Rock *et al.*, 1995).

As the concentrations of total and specific carotenoids in plasma and tissues are highly skewed towards lower concentrations (e.g. Stich *et al.*, 1986; Virtanen *et al.*, 1996), either non-parametric methods or log transformation of the data before parametric analysis should be used in statistical analyses.

3.1.4.2 Effect of supplemental intake

Thirteen healthy volunteers were given a daily dose of 30 mg synthetic β-carotene [formulation unspecified] and 7.4 mg of lycopene as vegetable juice for 11 days. The buccal mucosal concentration of β-carotene was increased, but not those of lycopene, lutein, cryptoxanthin or α-carotene (Peng *et al.*, 1994).

The carotenoid concentrations in human lymphocytes were 4.5-fold lower in lung cancer patients (n = 19) than in healthy controls (n = 23), while the serum concentrations were nonsignificantly lower (Bakker Schut *et al.*, 1997). Supplementation with 100 mg/d of crystalline β-carotene in capsules (25 mg, Merck) for 17 days levelled the difference in serum concentrations between one control and two lung cancer patients, but the concentrations of carotenoids in the lymphocytes of cancer patients remained lower. Supplementation with β-carotene (30 mg/d; formulation unspecified) for six weeks markedly increased the concentration in cervicovaginal cells of 24 healthy women (Palan *et al.*, 1992). Patients with cervical intraepithelial neoplasia (n = 30) who received a similar dose for six months also had a significant increase in the β-carotene concentrations of vaginal mucosa over the baseline level (Manetta *et al.*, 1996).

3.1.5 Kinetics

The kinetics of an orally administered dose (73 μmol) of octadeuterated β-carotene *in vivo* has been carefully analysed, although in only one male adult (Novotny *et al.*, 1995, 1996). A model consisting of 11 compartments and a gastrointestinal delay parameter of 4.5 h was devised on the basis of measurements of octadeuterated β-carotene and tetradeuterated retinol in plasma at various times from 0 to 57 days, although measurements were made up to 113 days. A set of fractional transfer coefficients was defined on the basis of several feasible assumptions, with SAAM 31 software (Novotny *et al.*, 1995, 1996). The main features of the model were: slowly and rapidly turning over pools of β-carotene and of retinol in the liver; enterocytic and extrahepatic tissue pools of carotene; pools of β-carotene and retinyl ester in plasma chylomicra; a pool of β-carotene in plasma lipoproteins and a pool of retinol in holo-retinol-binding protein in plasma. The model predicts that 22% of the β-carotene dose will be absorbed, that the hepatic reserves of β-carotene and vitamin A are 7.5 μmol and 324 μmol, respectively, and that 57% of the conversion of β-carotene into vitamin A takes place in the liver and 43% in the intestinal mucosa. With average dietary intakes of 3–7 μmol/d β-carotene, however, the intestine may well play a larger role in the conversion process.

The mean sojourn, or residence, time is defined as the mean time that tracer molecules spend in the system from the moment of entry until the time of irreversible exit. The values were 51 days for β-carotene and 474 days for retinol (vitamin A), which agree well with estimates based on other data. The empirical mean sojourn times in the plasma were only 9–13 days for β-carotene and 26 days for retinol (Novotny *et al.*, 1995, 1996). These differences in mean sojourn time values may well reflect efficient recycling of retinol, and probably of carotenoids as well, in and out of tissue depots. The mean empirical sojourn times for other carotenoids in plasma are similar to that of β-carotene: dimethoxy-β-carotene, six days; ethyl-β-apo-8′-carotenoate, nine days and canthaxanthin, eight days (Zeng *et al.*, 1992; Furr & Clark, 1997). Experimentally, the values for carotenoids are little affected by the dose given (Furr & Clark, 1997).

3.1.6   Metabolism
Carotenoids are oxidized in plants and microorganisms to a variety of compounds with fewer carbon atoms, including β-apocarotenals, abscissic acid, trisporic acid, bixin and crocetin, some of which have important physiological functions in plants (Olson, 1993). Thus, nature can modify carotenoids in a variety of ways at almost every carbon atom in the molecule.

3.1.6.1   β-Carotene
(a) Physiological pathways
β-Carotene was first shown to be converted biologically into vitamin A in mammals in

1930 (Moore, 1957). On the basis of the symmetry of the β-carotene molecules, Karrer and Eugster (1950) suggested that central cleavage was the most logical means for conversion of β-carotene into vitamin A. For many years, however, the pathways for its conversion were unclear, largely because the rate of conversion is relatively slow, cell-free preparations of tissues show little or no activity, β-carotene is rapidly oxidized chemically to various derivatives and the resolving power and sensitivity of the available methods were limited.

In 1960, Glover suggested two pathways for the cleavage of carotenoids into vitamin A, namely, central cleavage to yield two molecules of retinal or asymmetric cleavage to yield a shorter and a longer β-apocarotenal, the latter of which is sequentially shortened by the removal of C_2 and C_3 fragments to yield retinal. The evidence now suggests that central cleavage is the predominant reaction in humans. The possible role of excentric cleavage in human physiology is not known.

(b) Conversion of β-carotene to vitamin A
Because the mechanism for the conversion of carotenoids to vitamin A appears to be similar in humans and animals, data from both sources are referred to in this section. β-Carotene and other provitamin A carotenoids are converted to vitamin A in many tissues of the body. The intestinal mucosa is the main site of conversion after usual dietary intake of carotenoids, but other organs, particularly the liver, convert significant amounts when greater quantities of carotenoids are ingested. Most human tissues contain carotenoids, and retinoic acid, the major retinoid that is biologically active in cellular differentiation, can be formed both from the carotenoids present in a given tissue and from retinol taken up from the plasma.

The only fairly well characterized carotenoid cleavage enzyme in mammals is carotenoid 15,15′-dioxygenase (EC 1.13.11.21). This enzyme, found in many tissues, shows similar properties in various tissues and species (Olson, 1983). It is located in the cytosol, requires molecular oxygen, shows a K_m value for β-carotene of 1–10 μmol/L, has a slightly alkaline optimal pH (7.5–8.5), is inhibited by metal ion chelators and by sulfhydryl-binding reagents and can be activated by glutathione. The activity of the intestinal mucosal enzyme is enhanced by vitamin A deficiency and by treatment with polyunsaturated fatty acids but is depressed by treatment with β-carotene. The activity of the liver enzyme, although seemingly less sensitive to vitamin A status, is increased by treatment with β-carotene or with polyunsaturated fatty acids (van Vliet et al., 1992).

It has been postulated that, in addition to central cleavage, excentric cleavage of β-carotene might occur, yielding apocarotenals of different chain lengths, which might subsequently be shortened by the removal of C_2 and C_3 fragments to yield retinal (Glover, 1960). These fragments are presumed to be oxidized to carbon dioxide. While favouring asymmetric cleavage, Glover found, however, that the amounts of radiolabelled carbon dioxide produced by the metabolism of ^{14}C-β-carotene and ^{14}C-retinol in rats were the same, indicating that asymmetric cleavage is not a major pathway. A few years later, the sole detectable product of ^{14}C-β-carotene was found to be retinal (Goodman & Huang, 1965; Olson & Hayaishi, 1965). Indeed, the stoichiometry of the reaction—the ratio of the moles of retinal formed to those of β-carotene consumed—was found to be 1.1–1.5. Any value greater than 1.0 would, of course, favour central cleavage. The enzyme carotenoid 15,15′-dioxygenase (EC 1.13.11.21) was found to require molecular oxygen.

An interesting challenge to the idea of central cleavage was posed by Hansen and Maret (1988), who, although unable to repeat earlier findings, showed that β-carotene could be converted to β-apocarotenals chemically in the presence of oxygen under normal incubation conditions. In a subsequent re-examination of the cleavage reaction, however, Lakshman et al. (1989) showed that retinal is the primary, if not the sole, product of β-carotene cleavage catalysed by a partially purified enzyme preparation of rabbit and rat intestinal cytosol.

Whether asymmetric cleavage really occurs in mammals then became a key query. Wang and colleagues (Wang, 1994; Wang, X.D. et al.,

1991, 1996) subsequently showed that whole intestinal homogenates convert β-carotene to a group of β-apocarotenals in the presence of oxygen. Of particular interest in this regard was the formation of a pair of β-apocarotenals that are counterparts in a 13′:14′oxidative cleavage reaction. Since retinal was a relatively minor product of the reaction in their studies, they concluded that sequential asymmetric cleavage is a major pathway for the conversion of β-carotene to vitamin A.

The most appropriate way of determining the relative importance of the two pathways is to examine the stoichiometry of the reaction. Central cleavage yields 2 mol of retinal per mole of β-carotene consumed, whereas asymmetric cleavage yields, via β-apocarotenals, a maximum of 1 mol of retinal. Using whole intestinal homogenates similar to those used by Wang, X.-D. et al. (1991), Devery and Milborrow (1994) reported a mean molar ratio of 1.72, and Nagao et al. (1996) reported a molar ratio of 1.88 ± 0.08 (standard deviation [SD]). After correction for the efficiency of solvent extraction, the molar ratio in the latter study was 2.07 ± 0.09 (SD). β-Apocarotenals were detected in only trace amounts, if at all. No stoichiometric studies have been conducted that favour asymmetric cleavage as the major pathway, and the available information indicates that central cleavage is the predominant reaction in mammals. It should be emphasized that the enzyme has not been purified or crystallized.

(c) Retinoic acid formation

The formation of retinoic acid from β-carotene can proceed by central cleavage, followed by conversion of the resulting retinal to retinoic acid by one of several aldehyde dehydrogenases (Blaner & Olson, 1994). As the diterpene aldehyde, citral, inhibits the formation of retinoic acid from retinal (Wang, 1994; Wang, X.-D. et al., 1996), it should inhibit the formation of retinoic acid from β-carotene, if indeed retinal is a free intermediate in the reaction. On the basis of earlier observations that retinoic acid might be produced directly from β-carotene (Napoli & Race, 1988), it was of considerable interest that β-carotene, but not retinal, is converted into retinoic acid in the presence of citral in whole intestinal homogenates and is also found in portal blood derived from ferret intestine perfused with these substrates (Wang, X.-D. *et al.*, 1996). Thus, retinoic acid might be formed by oxidation of retinol or by oxidative cleavage of β-apocarotenoic acids.

The two forms of retinoic acid of physiological interest are all-*trans*- and 9-*cis*-retinoic acid, which are ligands for nuclear retinoid receptors. The 9-*cis* isomer can be formed either by isomerization of all-*trans*-retinoic acid or by oxidative cleavage of dietary 9-*cis*-β-carotene (Nagao & Olson, 1994; Wang, X.-D. *et al.*, 1994) followed by oxidation of 9-*cis*-retinal to 9-*cis*-retinoic acid.

Administration of large amounts of retinol is known to promote the formation of retinoids that are active in gene regulation (Tang & Russell, 1991; Norum, 1993); however, β-carotene does not appear to have an immediate effect on the concentrations of retinoic acid in plasma or adipose tissue. The concentrations in plasma were similar in vegetarians and non-vegetarians and were not changed after administration of 90 mg β-carotene for three weeks, nor were the concentrations in adipose tissue changed over 15 days after administration of 120 mg β-carotene (Johnson *et al.*, 1995).

3.1.6.2 β-Apocarotenoids

β-Apocarotenals can be converted directly to retinal and to an uncharacterized, short-chain aldehyde by the carotenoid 15,15′ dioxygenase (Olson, 1983), although slowly in some cases (Nagao *et al.*, 1996). β-Apo-8′-carotenal, and presumably other analogues, can be reduced to alcohols and then esterified in the human intestine or be oxidized to their corresponding acids (Zeng *et al.*, 1992). Several β-apo-carotenoic acids can also be converted to retinoic acid in ferret liver mitochondria, presumably by β-oxidation (Wang, X.-D. *et al.*, 1996). Ethyl β-apo-8′-carotenoate, however, did not appear to be metabolized in humans (Zeng *et al.*, 1992). This compound bears some resemblance metabolically to etretinate, which is stored in the body for long periods.

3.1.6.3 Other carotenoids

Carotenoid 15,15′-dioxygenase also cleaves the all-*trans* isomers of 3,4,3′,4′-tetradehydro-β-carotene, 5,6-epoxy-β-carotene, 5,8-epoxy-β-carotene, α-carotene, 5,6-epoxy-α-carotene, 5,8-epoxy-α-carotene and 3′,4′-dehydro-β-ψ-caroten-16′-al (Olson, 1983), but usually at rates considerably lower than for all-*trans*-β-carotene. The dioxygenase also cleaves 9-*cis*-β-carotene and possibly 13-*cis*-β-carotene, but again at lower rates than the all-*trans* isomer (Nagao & Olson, 1994; Wang, X.-D. *et al.*, 1994). Carotenoids that are cleaved either at low rates (< 5% that for all-*trans*-β-carotene) or not detectably include 5,6,5′,6′- and 5,8,5′,8′-diepoxy-β-carotene, 3′,4′-didehydro-β-cryptoxanthin, zeaxanthin, lutein, the 5,6 epoxides of several β-apocarotenals and β-apocarotenoic acids (Olson, 1983). Carotenoid 15,15′-dioxygenase has also been reported to cleave β-cryptoxanthin (Sivakumar & Parvin, 1997). The lack of activity of the dioxygenase towards β-apocarotenoic acids accords with the demonstrated β-oxidation of the latter to retinoic acid in mitochondria (Wang, X.-D. *et al.*, 1996).

In humans, 4,4′-dimethoxy-β-carotene is converted to canthaxanthin (4,4′-diketo-β-carotene) and to more polar, unidentified metabolites (Zeng *et al.*, 1992). α-Carotene is cleaved to retinal and α-retinal, presumably by carotenoid 15,15′-dioxygenase (Sivakumar & Parvin, 1997). Lycopene, although absorbed well from oily solutions and taken up by the liver and other organs, is metabolized by poorly understood pathways. Many isomers of lycopene are present in human plasma and tissues, the main ones being all-*trans*- and 5-*cis*-lycopene (Stahl & Sies, 1996). A similar pattern of isomers is found in tomato products; however, the percentage of *cis* isomers of lycopene is 9–21% in tomato products, 58–73% in plasma and 79–88% in prostate tissue (Clinton *et al.*, 1996). Thus, a clear shift from all-*trans* to *cis* isomers takes place *in vivo*, due perhaps to isomerization, preferential uptake of specific isomers or selective extraction of isomers into other liphophilic dietary compounds, such as fat and oil (see section 2.1.3.3).

Canthaxanthin, like lycopene, is not metabolized to detectable products in rats, squirrel monkeys or humans (White *et al.*, 1994).

Lutein may be oxidized *in vivo* in humans to its 3′-keto derivative, isomerized from the 6′R to the 6'S form or converted to 3'-epilutein and zeaxanthin (Khachik *et al.*, 1995). Although the enzymatic reactions have not been clarified, such derivatives appear in human plasma after lutein supplementation. Lutein and zeaxanthin may have a physiological role in the body, since they are specifically found in the retina. Zeaxanthin is concentrated in the macula, while lutein is dispersed throughout the retina (Bone *et al.*, 1988; Handelman *et al.*, 1988). The presence of carotenoids in the eye may improve visual acuity and may also protect against damaging photochemical reactions (Bone *et al.*, 1985, 1993). There is some dispute about the relative amounts of the two carotenoids in the retina: Bone *et al.* (1988) reported that zeaxanthin predominated in more than 90% of human eyes examined, while Handelman *et al.* (1988) reported that the concentration of lutein exceeded that of zeaxanthin in 15/16 whole retinas examined. The total amount of carotenoid recovered in the retina does not appear to be related to age, but the concentration can vary from 3 to 85 ng (Bone *et al.*, 1988) or 35 to 120 ng (Handelman *et al.*, 1988). Zeaxanthin exists as two stereo-isomers in the eye: zeaxanthin itself [(3R,3'R)-β,β-carotene-3,3'-diol] and *meso*-zeaxanthin [(3R,3'S)-β,β-carotene-3,3'diol] (Bone *et al.*, 1993). The presence of lutein and zeaxanthin in the eye does not necessarily imply that lutein undergoes metabolic or structural changes during its absorption and dispersion through the tissues, but lutein usually occurs at considerably greater concentrations than zeaxanthin in the blood of most people in western countries, unless they consume large amounts of yellow corn. These observations led Bone *et al.* (1993) to suggest that *meso*-zeaxanthin arises from lutein by some chemical process in the retina.

Capsanthin, a major carotenoid in paprika, is a dihydroxymonoketo-carotenoid with one five-carbon cyclic ring. When given orally to men, capsanthin is well absorbed, is associated equally with high-density and low-density lipoproteins in plasma and is cleared rapidly from the circulation (Oshima *et al.*, 1997). No metabolites were identified.

9'-*cis*-Bixin, a monomethylester of an acylic C_{24} dicarboxylic acid, and its congeners are found in the seeds of the annatto plant. Extracts of these seeds are used commonly as a food colouring in Spain and Latin America. When ingested by human volunteers, 9-*cis*-bixin is well absorbed but rapidly cleared from plasma. It is both dimethylated to the dicarboxylic acid norbixin and isomerized to all-*trans*-bixin *in vivo* (Levy *et al.*, 1997).

Little is known about the metabolism in mammals of other carotenoids, such as neoxanthin, violaxanthin and astaxanthin. Although found in foods, these carotenoids have not been detected in human plasma (Khachik *et al.*, 1991).

3.1.7 Genetic variation

No clearly defined genetic defects have been observed in the metabolism of carotenoids. Differences in plasma concentrations of carotenoids after an oral dose of β-carotene may represent genetic variability, but the absence of differences in the absorption of other carotenoids complicates the interpretation of relative responsiveness.

3.2 Experimental models

Research on the bioavailability of carotenoids is hampered by the fact that most common laboratory animal species, in contrast to primates, efficiently convert β-carotene to vitamin A, and very little is absorbed intact. The situation in primates has, however, been mimicked in two animal models: the ferret and the preruminant calf. Although both models have some limitations, important information on carotenoid uptake and metabolism have been obtained. Most of the studies on carotenoid uptake, distribution and metabolism in humans and animals have focused on β-carotene, and less information is available for other carotenoids.

3.2.1 Non-human primates

Various carotenoids, including lutein, zeaxanthin, α-cryptoxanthin, β-cryptoxanthin and β-carotene, were detected in plasma, liver and other tissues of monkeys that received the usual, unsupplemented Primate Center diet (Krinsky *et al.*, 1990b; Snodderly *et al.*, 1990), indicating that rhesus monkeys absorb and transport dietary carotenes and xanthophylls in the same way as humans.

When ^{14}C-β-carotene was given at a single dose of 1.26 mg in olive oil to rhesus monkeys, peak accumulation in the serum of labelled retinol derived from the parent was detected after 8–24 h; some unchanged labelled material was also detected. Considerable individual variation was seen in the amount of radiolabel in serum. Most of the absorbed radiolabel was detected in the liver, mainly as retinol, with only 2–8% as unchanged β-carotene. Much less radiolabel was found in other tissues. Rhesus monkeys are thus capable of absorbing β-carotene intact and of using it as a source of retinol. No other β-carotene metabolite was detected in a significant amount (Krinsky et al., 1990b). In contrast, no labelled metabolic products were found when ^{14}C-canthaxanthin or β-lycopene was administered to rhesus monkeys, confirming the finding that neither compound has provitamin A activity. Peak accumulation of radiolabel in plasma was measured at 8–48 h for both compounds, but the clearance of lycopene from plasma appeared to be slower than that of canthaxanthin. The liver was the major depot organ for both carotenoids. Various amounts of the pigments were detected in other tissues, with the highest concentrations in spleen (Mathews-Roth et al., 1990).

When the diet of squirrel monkeys was supplemented with zeaxanthin and β-carotene, rapid plasma responses were measured. After two weeks of increasing zeaxanthin intake, a relatively stable, higher plasma concentration of this compound was reached. In animals given a standard laboratory diet, the plasma concentrations of β-carotene were low and increased only slightly with supplementation. The plasma concentrations of lutein were not affected by zeaxanthin supplementation (Snodderly et al., 1997).

In baboons, the toxicity of ethanol was reported to be enhanced when it was taken together with β-carotene. In animals fed the combination, histological changes in the liver were more pronounced, and increased blood concentrations of the mitochondrial enzyme glutamic dehydrogenase were found as compared with controls that received either ethanol or β-carotene alone. It was suggested that the effect is due to interference by ethanol with the metabolism of β-carotene to retinol and disposition of the carotenoid from the liver. Baboons that received β-carotene and ethanol had higher concentrations of β-carotene in plasma and liver than controls, and the β-carotene-induced increase in liver retinol was lower in animals that received the combination. When β-carotene treatment, was stopped, the plasma concentrations decreased more slowly in the animals fed ethanol. The half-life of β-carotene in plasma was fourfold longer when the slow elimination phase was taken into account. This experiment provides interesting information on the possible interactions between β-carotene and ethanol with respect to bioavailability and metabolism (Leo et al., 1992). [The Working Group noted that the dose of ethanol was very high, supplying 50% of the total energy intake over two to five years.]

The pattern of carotenoids in the macula lutea has also been investigated in monkeys (Handelman et al., 1991; Snodderly et al., 1991). As in humans (Landrum et al., 1997), the main carotenoids are lutein and zeaxanthin, although the ratio between the two xanthophylls differs within different regions of the macula lutea. Macaque monkeys have a consistent pattern of more zeaxanthin than lutein at the foveal centre, and a similar distribution is observed in the macula lutea of adult humans (Bone et al., 1997).

Studies on the conversion of β-carotene to retinoids and apocarotenals have been performed with homogenates from various monkey tissues. β-Carotene was converted to retinoids and apocarotenals by intestine, liver, kidney, lung and adipose tissue (Wang, X.-D. et al., 1991). β-Apo-13-carotenone and β-apo-14'-carotenal were identified after incubation of β-carotene with intestinal preparations from monkeys, rats, ferrets and humans (Tang et al., 1991).

3.2.2 Preruminant calves and cows

The preruminant calf has been introduced as an animal model for the study of carotenoid biokinetics in humans (Hoppe & Schoner, 1987; Poor et al., 1992). Preruminant calves are newborn animals that are maintained in a mono-gastric state by feeding them an all-liquid diet. For most studies of carotenoids, milk substitutes with a low concentration of vitamin A are used (Poor *et al.*, 1992; Hoppe *et al.*, 1996). After a single oral dose of 20 mg β-carotene dissolved in a milk substitute, peak serum concentrations in calves of about 0.4 μmol/L β-carotene were observed after 12–30 h but no significant change in serum vitamin A concentration was found. Relatively high concentrations of β-carotene were found in the adrenal glands, with a maximum 24 h after treatment. High concentrations were found in liver, lung and spleen, also peaking 24 h after administration, whereas the highest concentrations in adipose tissue and kidney were detected 72 and 144 h after dosing, respectively. No significant change in carotenoid concentration was observed in heart or muscle. The serum β-carotene response curves of the calves were similar to those observed in humans after a single dose of β-carotene; however, about 30% of the animals did not show significantly increased serum concentrations after β-carotene administration (Poor *et al.*, 1992). A similar phenomenon has been observed in humans who are designated 'low' or 'poor responders' (Johnson & Russell, 1992; Stahl *et al.*, 1995). There is at least one significant difference between preruminant calves and humans with regard to the biokinetics of carotenoids, which may affect transport and clearance. In human blood, β-carotene is associated mainly with the low-density lipoprotein fraction (Krinsky *et al.*, 1958; Johnson & Russell, 1992), whereas in calves and cows high-density lipoproteins appear to be the major transport form (Schweigert & Eisele, 1990; Bierer *et al.*, 1993, 1995).

The dose–response relationship of β-carotene was also investigated in this model. The compound was administerd orally with a milk substitute to preruminant calves for 28 days at a dose of 0.23, 0.46, 0.92, 1.84 or 3.68 μmol/kg bw per day. Steady-state plasma concentrations were reached on day 28 and were clearly related to the logarithm of dose. At doses between 0.23 and 0.92 μmol/kg bw per day, the relationship with steady-state serum concentrations was linear, but considerable interindividual differences in these concentrations were found, with a calculated coefficient of variation of about 30%. No animals considered to be poor responders were reported. Dose-dependent accumulation of β-carotene was measured in liver, lung, heart, adrenals and adipose tissue. In the liver, the vitamin A concentrations increased with β-carotene intake. All-*trans*-β-carotene was the only isomer present in plasma and the adrenals and the major isomeric form in other tissues (Hoppe *et al.*, 1996).

The absorption and transport of β-carotene, α-carotene, lycopene, canthaxanthin and lutein in preruminant calves were compared after a single oral dose of 20 mg of each carotenoid. The serum responses indicated that all of them were absorbed but in variable amounts; the variations may be due, at least in part, to the use of different vehicles or carotenoid preparations. The peak serum concentrations of canthaxanthin and lutein occurred earlier (8 and 12 h) than those of lycopene, α-carotene and β-carotene (16, 16 and 24 h, respectively). At these times, 70–90% of the serum carotenoids were associated with the high-density lipoprotein fraction. The oxo-carotenoids were cleared more quickly from serum than α-carotene, β-carotene or lycopene, and lycopene and α-carotene had slower disappearance rates than β-carotene (Bierer *et al.*, 1995).

Several studies in humans indicate that heating of a dietary source improves the bioavailability of carotenoids (Micozzi *et al.*, 1992; Stahl & Sies, 1992), but no such effect was seen in the preruminant calf model, in which mild heat treatment had only slight effects on the availability of α- and β-carotene from carrots, as shown by analyses of serum and tissue concentrations (Poor *et al.*, 1993).

β-Carotene is also distributed into the milk of cows. After parenteral administration, elevated concentrations of the parent compound were found in milk and plasma. No increase in the vitamin A concentrations of plasma was observed, whereas the vitamin A concentration of milk increased (Schweigert & Eisele, 1990).

The corpus luteum of both cows and humans has extremely high concentrations of β-carotene. In bovine corpus luteum, the highest concentrations were detected in nuclei, lipids and mitochondria; however, much of the β-carotene was loosely bound in the nuclear and mitochondrial fractions, and in the cytosolic fraction β-carotene was associated with with high-molecular-mass proteins (O'Fallon & Chew, 1984). A study of the intracellular transport of β-carotene in bovine liver and intestine suggested that β-carotene, unlike other lipophilic compounds, is not transported by cytosolic proteins, and other mechanisms such as vesicular transport may be involved (Gugger & Erdman, 1996).

3.2.3 Ferrets

The ferret (*Mustela putorius furo*) has been used to investigate the intestinal absorption, metabolism and storage of carotenoids, and a direct comparison with rats showed that this species is a more appropriate model for humans. In the absence of supplementation, the serum concentration of β-carotene in ferrets was only about 0.01 nmol/ml, and no β-carotene was detected in liver or adipose tissue. After supplementation with 4 or 20 mg/kg bw β-carotene in corn oil for two weeks, the serum concentrations increased to 0.28 and 0.78 nmol/ml, respectively, within the range detected in human serum. Increases in β-carotene concentrations were also measured in liver and adipose tissue, with values in the liver of 1.7 and 7.7 nmol/g tissue after the repeated doses of 4 and 20 mg, respectively (Ribaya-Mercado *et al.*, 1989).

After a single dose of 10 mg/kg bw β-carotene, a peak serum concentration of 0.68 nmol/ml was observed 8 h after ingestion; within 76 h, the compound was essentially cleared from the blood. Peak concentrations of β-carotene in various tissues were detected between 8 and 16 h after administration. The highest concentration was found in the liver (1.2 nmol/g); less was found in the lung (0.04 nmol/g), kidney (0.09 nmol/g) and spleen (0.08 nmol/g). Other polar and nonpolar carotenoids were identified in ferret livers. The results show that this species can absorb carotenoids intact and transport them into various tissues (Gugger *et al.*, 1992).

All-*trans*-β-carotene accumulates preferentially in the serum of ferrets that have ingested an isomeric mixture. Similar effects were observed in humans, suggesting that the ferret is also a suitable model for intestigating the biokinetics of geometric isomers of carotenoids. In the same study, it was shown that less β-carotene is bioavailable from the natural source, carrot juice, than from a commercial beadlet preparations used as a feed additive (White *et al.*, 1993a). Canthaxanthin had specific antagonistic effects on the bioavailability of β-carotene when the two compounds were given concurrently (White *et al.*, 1993b). Furthermore, the biokinetics of carotenoids in ferrets and humans show striking differences. In ferret blood, β-carotene is associated mainly with the high-density lipoprotein fraction, whereas the major transport form in humans is low-density lipoproteins (Ribaya-Mercado *et al.*, 1993).

After long-term supplementation of ferrets with canthaxanthin at 50 mg/kg bw per day, the serum concentrations increased from 0 at baseline to about 0.1 nmol/ml after 12 months. High concentrations of canthaxanthin were also detected in liver, fat, lung and small intestine, but no detectable concentrations were found in the eyes, and the animals showed no clinical signs of toxicity (Tang *et al.*, 1995).

The ferret is also a useful model for studying the bioconversion of β-carotene (Wang *et al.*, 1992; Hebuterne *et al.*, 1995, 1996; Wang, X.-D. *et al.*, 1996). Experiments involving perfusion of the small intestine of ferrets added evidence that geometric isomers of β-carotene are isomer-selective precursors of the respective retinoic acids. After perfusion with all-*trans*-β-carotene, the resulting retinoic acid was mainly in the all-*trans* form; when 9-*cis*-β-carotene was used, about 50% of the retinoic acid formed was the 9-*cis* isomer. Interestingly, the total amount of retinoic acid was similar in the two experiments (Hebuterne *et al.*, 1995).

Interactions of β-carotene with other lipophilic antioxidants have been shown in the ferret model. α-Tocopherol at low doses enhanced the lymphatic transport of β-carotene fourfold, and this effect was even more pronounced at pharmacological doses of vitamin E. It was suggested that α-tocopherol modulates the metabolism of β-carotene and has a positive effect on its intestinal absorption (Wang *et al.*, 1995).

3.2.4 Rats

As rats convert β-carotene and other provitamin A carotenoids to retinol, this species has often been used to study the metabolism of these compounds. For moderate and higher intake, the conversion is inversely related to dose (Brubacher & Weiser, 1985). Fractions of rat tissues have been investigated for their capabilty to cleave carotenoids: after experiments with various fractions of rat liver homogenate, cleavage activity was assigned to the enzyme β-carotene 15,15'-dioxygenase (Olson, 1961; Olson & Hayaishi, 1965). A mechanism for the biosynthesis of vitamin A from β-carotene was postulated on the basis of the results of an investigation of the cleavage products in rat lymph after administration of doubly labelled β-carotene, i.e. that the formation of vitamin A occurs in a dioxygenase-like reaction after cleavage of the central double bond (Goodman *et al.*, 1966b). The primary cleavage product is retinal (Lakshman *et al.*, 1989), as shown in several studies, although the formation of retinal and other retinoids has been challenged in a single report (Hansen & Maret, 1988).

The fate of β-carotene geometric isomers remains an open question. Studies in rats and other species have added evidence that 9-*cis*-β-carotene is an isomer-selective precursor of 9-*cis*-retinal or 9-*cis*-retinoic acid (Nagao & Olson, 1994; Hebuterne *et al.*, 1995). The latter is a high-affinity ligand of retinoic X receptors, which act as ligand-dependent transcription factors (Kliewer *et al.*, 1994). Enzyme preparations partially purified from rat liver and intestine converted all-*trans*, 9-*cis*- and 13-*cis*-β-carotene to an isomeric mixture of all-*trans*, 9-*cis*- and 13-*cis*-retinal (Nagao & Olson, 1994). Relatively more *cis*-retinals were formed when β-carotene *cis* isomers were used as substrates; however, the cleavage rates determined *in vitro* were distinctively lower with 9-*cis*- and 13-*cis*-β-carotene than with the all-*trans* form.

Fewer data are available on the cleavage of carotenoids other than β-carotene in rats. Other provitamin A carotenoids are metabolized to retinal by rat intestinal preparations, but, in comparison with β-carotene, less retinal is formed. Retinal formation from α-carotene and cryptoxanthin was 29 and 55%, respectively, that

of β-carotene. *In vitro*, other carotenoids can influence the efficacy of β-carotene cleavage, as less retinal was formed from β-carotene in the presence of lutein; no effects on β-carotene metabolism were observed in the presence of lycopene (van Vliet *et al.*, 1996a). The highest activity of the enzyme β-carotene 15,15'-dioxygenase within the intestine, investigated in female Wistar rats, was found in the cytosol of mature functional enterocytes harvested from the jejunum. Retinal and retinoic acid were the only metabolites identified in this study; no apocarotenals were detected (Duszka *et al.*, 1996). The absorption and metabolism of β-carotene are affected by the vitamin A and β-carotene concentrations in the diet. The intestinal enzyme activity was higher in rats fed a diet with a low content of vitamin A than in those fed a diet with a low content. The dioxygenase activity was lower when the animals were given a diet supplemented with β-carotene than when they received an unsupplemented diet (van Vliet *et al.*, 1993, 1996b).

No β-carotene was detected in rat serum within 72 h after administration of a single oral dose of ^{14}C-labelled compound; the peak serum concentrations of labelled retinol were measured at 4 h. Small amounts of unchanged β-carotene were found in the liver, but about 90% of the radiolabel in this organ was assigned to the retinol fraction (Krinsky *et al.*, 1990b; Mathews-Roth *et al.*, 1990). Increasing plasma concentrations were reported after a single oral dose of 10 mg/kg bw of all-*trans*- or 9-*cis*-β-carotene, with peak concentrations at 4 h. When the 9-*cis* isomer was administered to rats, higher plasma concentrations of the all-*trans* form (about 0.1 nmol/ml) were measured than after application of the all-*trans* isomer (0.03 nmol/ml), but the 9-*cis* isomer was not detected after administration of the all-*trans* form, and only small amounts of this isomer (0.01 nmol/ml) were found after 9-*cis* supplementation. The results indicate that the 9-*cis* isomer is converted to all-*trans*-β-carotene before or during absorption (Suzuki *et al.*, 1996). Similar observations have been made in humans (Gaziano *et al.*, 1995a; Stahl *et al.*, 1995; You *et al.*, 1996). Rats, like humans, have considerable amounts of 9-*cis*-β-carotene in the liver (Ben-

Amotz *et al.*, 1989). Higher concentrations of *cis* isomers were found in rat liver after administration of 9-*cis*-β-carotene than its 13-*cis* analogue, and an inverse relationship was found between the corresponding liver concentrations of *cis*-β-carotene and the ability to revert symptoms of vitamin A deficiency (Weiser *et al.*, 1993).

Several studies in this animal model indicate that factors which influence the bioavailability of β-carotene in humans also affect their availability in rats. These include bile salts (El-Gorab *et al.*, 1975), fatty acids and pH (Hollander & Ruble, 1978), dietary lipids (Mokady & Ben-Amotz, 1991; Bianchi-Santamaria *et al.*, 1994) and interactions between β-carotene and other carotenoids (High & Day, 1951).

Under normal dietary conditions, very little carotenoid crosses the intestinal mucosa into the systemic circulation. Thus, adipose tissue is usually white, and other organs contain little carotenoid. After long-term supplementation with a large amount (0.2% of diet) of β-carotene, however, β-carotene was found in significant amounts in blood and tissues. Plasma was saturated within three days, whereas saturation was not reached in the liver, adrenal gland or ovary even after 21 weeks of supplementation. The largest amount of β-carotene (9.3 nmol/g) was found in liver (Shapiro *et al.*, 1984). In carcinogenicity experiments as well, long-term dietary supplementation of rodents with large amounts of carotenoids led to appreciable concentrations of the administered carotenoid in the liver and other organs (see section 4.2).

Less is known about the absorption and distribution of carotenoids other than β-carotene in rats. After administration of ^{14}C-labelled lycopene and canthaxanthin, peak accumulation of radiolabel in plasma was detected within 4–8 h. Both pigments accumulated in liver, and small amounts were found in various other tissues (Krinsky *et al.*, 1990b; Mathews-Roth *et al.*, 1990). High concentrations of canthaxanthin and β-carotene were reported in the livers of rats fed a diet containing either 0.2% canthaxanthin or 0.2% β-carotene for two weeks; smaller amounts were measured in the lung (van Vliet *et al.*, 1991).

The results indicate that the rat is not a suitable model for studying the uptake and plasma response of carotenoids, especially β-carotene. Much less of the carotenoid is absorbed unchanged, and the times at which peak concentrations are found in plasma after a single dose differ considerably, being about 4 h in rats and 24–48 h in humans. Since rats efficiently convert β-carotene to retinal, however, this species could be used to investigate the metabolism of provitamin carotenoids; rat tissue preparations are suitable sources for the cleavage enzyme β-carotene 15,15′-dioxygenase. As the fate of geometric isomers of β-carotene appears to be similar in rats and humans, this model may also be used to investigate the metabolism and tissue distribution of geometric isomers in the organism.

Some carotenoids can induce xenobiotic metabolizing enzymes. Canthaxanthin accumulates in rat liver and increases the activities of some drug-metabolizing enzymes, including cytochromes P4501A1 and P4501A2, *para*-nitrophenol-uridine diphosphoglucuronosyl transferase and quinone reductase. Similar but less pronounced effects were detected with astaxanthin. In contrast, β-carotene, lutein and lycopene did not induce the activity of these enzymes (Astorg *et al.*, 1994; Gradelet *et al.*, 1996a).

3.2.5 Other animal species

Several other species have been used to study the bioavailability and metabolism of β-carotene. Low concentrations of β-carotene but increasing amounts of retinol were found in the livers of hamsters fed various concentrations of the compound, indicating that these animals are efficient converters of β-carotene. No carotenoids were detected in the blood of rabbits fed a carotenoid-rich diet, and only small increases were seen in the concentration of vitamin A in liver, indicating that the rabbit is a poor absorber, although preparations of rabbit instestine have been used to investigate the β-carotene cleaving enzyme β-carotene 15,15′-dioxygenase. Preparations of rabbit intestinal mucosa were used to show that lycopene, lutein and astaxanthin competitively inhibit the enzyme and partially protect it from trypsin digestion (Ershov *et al.*, 1994).

The absorption, transport and tissue distribution of β-carotene have been studied in pigs given ^{14}C-labelled compound orally. The amount of radiolabel in plasma increased within 4 h, and, by 24 h, a large amount of radiolabel was found in the liver and lung. In the liver, the label was associated mainly with retinol, while in the lung large amounts of the parent compound (5.4 μg/g tissue) were detected. Thus, pigs absorb the compound intact and accumulate β-carotene in the lung (Schweigert *et al.*, 1995). Studies with preparations of pig intestinal mucosa showed that the major cleavage product of β-carotene is retinal, formed in a molar ratio close to 2, indicating mainly central cleavage. Other retinoids or apocarotenals were not detected (Nagao *et al.*, 1996).

As Mongolian gerbils absorb β-carotene intact, this species could be used to evaluate specific aspects of the biokinetics of carotenoids. After a single oral dose of about 0.15 mg β-carotene, increasing serum concentrations were detected between 0 and 4 h, with a peak concentration of 88 pmol/ml, but the concentration decreased to 0 within 72 h. In tissues, the highest β-carotene concentrations were found in liver and spleen; low concentrations were also detected in kidney, lung and adipose tissue (Pollack *et al.*, 1994).

Studies on the bioavailability of β-carotene and its geometric isomers have been performed in chickens given an isomeric mixture extracted from the alga *Dunaliella bardawil*. Chicks were fed either synthetic β-carotene (all-*trans* isomer) or β-carotene from the alga (containing about equal amounts of the all-*trans* and 9-*cis* isomers) at equivalent levels of total β-carotene. The absolute amount of β-carotene in chick liver was higher when the natural source was used, but no difference was found in the content of retinol. The ratio of 9-*cis*-β-carotene to its all-*trans* analogue exceeded that of the natural source, indicating preferential accumulation of 9-*cis*-β-carotene in chick livers. Similar data were obtained when purified isomers were used (Mokady *et al.*, 1990). In chick liver, the highest concentration of β-carotene was detected in the mitochondrial fraction, followed by lysosomes, microsomes and nuclei (Mayne & Parker, 1986).

3.2.6 Conclusion

No animal species provides a model suitable for studying all aspects of the biokinetics of carotenoids in humans. The preruminant calf and the ferret appear to be the most suitable species. The results of studies with non-human primates are promising, but more studies are needed to evaluate these models. Other species may be considered for the investigation of specific aspects of the biokinetics of carotenoids, such as their metabolism.

4. Preventive Effects

4.1 Humans
4.1.1 Studies of cancer occurrence
4.1.1.1 Observational studies based on blood and other tissue measures of carotenoids
(a) Methodological comments

The concentrations of carotenoids in blood and tissue discussed in this section are markers of exposure to carotenoids in the diet. Several problems are involved in estimating exposure to carotenoids on the basis of circulating levels: The measure of the carotenoid, e.g. plasma concentration, may not be representative of the concentration in the appropriate tissue; and plasma or serum concentrations measured at one time may not be sufficiently characteristic of exposure to carotenoids over decades but rather indicators of more recent dietary intake (Olson, 1984; LeGardeur *et al.*, 1990). The reproducibility of measures in blood over periods of up to two years may, however, be better than that of dietary measures of intake (Kaaks *et al.*, 1997). The value of serum concentrations as a marker of true internal exposure is still uncertain. There are clearly individual differences in the metabolism and kinetics of β-carotene, and the relationship between serum concentrations and those in specific tissues is still not known. One source of error is the possible degradation of carotenoids in serum samples during storage, especially at temperatures above –70 °C (Craft *et al.*, 1988; Comstock *et al.*, 1993; Ocké *et al.*, 1995); carotenoids in serum samples that are repeatedly thawed and refrozen are particularly sensitive to degradation.

In case–control studies, carotene intake or the concentrations of carotenoids in the tissues of the cancer patients may have been altered by the cancer, due either to treatment of the disease or to changes in dietary habits or metabolism caused by the disease. For this reason, cohort and nested case–control studies are more reliable, since information on carotenoid status is collected before diagnosis of cancer. In such studies, the disease process can still affect carotenoid status, but its effect can be minimized by excluding cancer cases that occur during the first years of follow-up. This source of bias is of particular concern with regard to cancers of the lung, stomach and liver.

The strength of the association between exposure to carotenoids and cancer risk may depend on the balance between the amount of carotenoids available and the extent of exposure to other risk factors, such as cigarette smoking. Thus, the association may differ according to the concentrations of other factors, making it difficult to assess associations between carotenoid status and cancer risk. The concentrations of carotenoids in blood and adipose tissue have been associated with several factors potentially related to the risk for cancer (Roe, 1987; Stryker *et al.*, 1988; Albanes *et al.*, 1992; Hebert *et al.*, 1994; Margetts & Jackson, 1996; Berg *et al.*, 1997). Various foods, nutrients and dietary patterns may also confound the relationships between carotenoid measures and disease. Intake of carotenoids, for example, is strongly associated with intake of several potentially protective nutrients, such as fibre, vitamin E, vitamin C and flavonoids, both because they are included in the same foods and because of clustering of dietary behaviour. Therefore, carotenes may simply be markers of fruit and vegetable intake.

The measure of carotenoids most widely used in studies on cancer is the β-carotene concentration in serum or plasma (Tables 6–8). Other predominant circulating carotenoids in humans, i.e. α-carotene, lycopene, lutein, cryptoxanthin and total carotenoids have also been determined. The carotenoid concentration in adipose tissue was used in one study (van't Veer *et al.*, 1996).

In cohort studies with nested case–control analyses (that is, studies based on a cohort in which biological specimens for all cases and for a sample of non-cases were analysed), the concentrations of total carotenoids, β-carotene and, in two populations, α-carotene, cryptoxanthin, lutein and lycopene were determined in serum or plasma samples collected at the time of a baseline survey, stored frozen (at –20 to –75 °C) and thawed for analysis at the end of the follow-up period (Table 7). The carotenoids were determined by HPLC, the laboratory personnel being unaware of the case or control status of the samples. The coefficients of variation for the determinations of β-carotene, reported in some of the studies, usually varied from 2 to 6%, and those for other carotenoids were 7–17%. The mean serum or plasma β-carotene concentrations, available for eight populations, ranged from 5 to 38 µg/dl (0.09–0.71 µmol/L) in the control samples. The range for the samples stored at –70 °C or lower was 17–38 µg/dl (0.32–0.54 µmol/L), and that for samples stored at above –70 °C was 5–22 µg/dl (0.09–0.41 µmol/L). The corresponding range in cohort studies in which blood samples from all participants were analysed shortly after collection was 17–36 µg/dl (0.32–0.67 µmol/L).

Most of the case–control studies reviewed were based on concentrations of circulating β-carotene; other carotenoids were also determined in some studies (Table 8). The commonest method for determining circulating carotenoids was HPLC with UV–visible detection. Measurements of total carotenoids in tissue extracts by spectrophotometry were used in a small number of studies. The concentrations of β-carotene in controls varied from 17 to 141 µg/dl (0.32–2.63 µmol/L); the coefficients of variation, with few exceptions, were not reported. The comparability of cases and controls is an additional concern.

(b)   Results
The main results from analytical observational epidemiological studies on the association between tissue concentrations of carotenoids and the occurrence of cancer that were published not earlier than 1980 are presented

Table 6. Description of cohort studies of the association between serum or plasma concentrations of carotenoids and cancer

Study, country	Study cohort	Cohort size	Age (years)	Starting year	Length of follow-up (years)	Cancer end-point	Site of cancer	No. of cancer cases
ATBC Study (Alpha-Tocopherol, Beta Carotene Cancer Prevention Study Group, 1994a), Finland	Smokers in southwestern Finland	7287 M	50–69	1985–88	5–8	Incidence	Lung	208
Basel Study (Eichholzer et al., 1996), Switzerland	Employees of three pharmaceutical companies	2974 M	20–79	1971–73	17	Mortality	All	290
							Lung	87
							Stomach	28
							Prostate	30
							Colon	22
							Pancreas	15
Skin Cancer Prevention Study (Greenberg et al., 1996), USA	Basal-cell or squamous-cell carcinoma patients from 4 clinical centres	1188 M, 532 F	< 85	1983–86	7–10	Mortality	All	82
CARET (Omenn et al., 1996a), USA	Smokers or asbestos-exposed workers	12 025 M, 6289 F	45–74	1985–94	1–9	Incidence	Lung	275
Nutrition Status Survey (Sahyoun et al., 1996), USA	Non-institutionalized residents of Massachusetts	254 M, 471 F	≥ 60	1981–84	9–12	Mortality	All	45
Hokkaido (Ito et al., 1997), Japan	Rural Japanese residents	929 M, 1424 F	≥ 40	1986–89	2–8	Mortality	All	44
							Stomach	10

ATBC, Alpha-Tocopherol Beta-Carotene; CARET, Beta-Carotene and Retinol Efficacy Trial; M, male; F, female

Table 7. Description of nested case–control studies of the association between serum or plasma concentrations of carotenoids and cancer

Study, country	Reference	Cohort size	Sex	Age (years)	Starting year	Length of follow-up (years)	Site of cancer	Numbers of cancer cases/ controls	Matching variables
Guernsey, UK	Wald et al. (1984)	5004	Female	28–75	1968–75	7–14	Breast	39/78	Age, menopausal status, parity, family history of breast cancer, history of benign breast disease
Hypertension Detection and Follow-up Program, USA	Willett et al. (1984)	4480	Both	30–69	1973–74	5	All, lung, breast, prostate, leukaemia and lymphoma, gastrointestinal	111/210	Age, sex, race, smoking, time of blood collection, blood pressure, use of anti-hypertensive medication, random assignment, parity and menopausal status
Honolulu Heart Program, USA	Nomura et al. (1985)	6860	Male	52–75	1971–75	10	Lung, stomach, colon, rectum, urinary bladder	284/302	Randomly selected controls in age strata
	Nomura et al. (1997)					20	Oral and pharyngeal, laryngeal, oesophageal	69/138	Age, time of blood collection, smoking, alcohol intake
Washington County, USA	Menkes et al. (1986)	25 802	Both	≥ 18	1974	9	Lung	99/196	Age, sex, race, smoking, time of blood collection, length of fasting, time since last menstrual period, menopausal status[a]
	Schober et al. (1987)		Both			9	Colon	72/143	
	Burney et al. (1989)		Both			12	Pancreas	22/44	
	Helzlsouer et al. (1989)		Both			12	Urinary bladder	35/70	
	Hsing et al. (1990)		Male			12	Prostate	103/103	
	Comstock et al. (1991)		Both			9	Rectum	34/68	
			Female			9	Breast	30/59	
	Batieha et al. (1993)	(15 161)	Female			16	Cervix	50/100	
	Zheng et al. (1993)		Both			16	Oral and pharyngeal	28/112	
	Breslow et al. (1995)		Both			–	Basal skin, squamous skin, melanoma	99/198	
	Helzlsouer et al. (1996)	(20 305)	Female			15	Ovary	35/67	

IARC Handbooks of Cancer Prevention

Table 7 (contd)

Study, country	Reference	Cohort size	Sex	Age (years)	Starting year	Length of follow-up (years)	Site of cancer	Numbers of cancer cases/ controls	Matching variables
British United Provident Association, UK	Wald et al. (1988)	22 000	Male	35–64	1975–82	2–9	All, lung, colorectal, stomach, urinary bladder, skin, central nervous system	271/533	Age, smoking, duration of storage
Multiple Risk Factor Intervention Trial, USA	Connett et al. (1989)	12 866	Male	35–57	1973–75	8–10	All, lung, colon, oesophagus, urinary bladder, kidney	156/311	Age, smoking, clinical centre, treatment group, date of randomization
Mobile Clinic Health Survey, Finland	Knekt et al. (1990)	36 265	Both	15–99	1968–72	6–10	All, stomach, colon, rectum, pancreas, lung, prostate, basal skin, lymphoma and leukaemia, breast, cervix, endometrium, ovary	766/1419	Age, sex, place of residence
	Knekt et al. (1991)						Oral cavity and pharynx, larynx, oesophagus, liver, kidney, urinary bladder, melanoma, brain		
Kaiser Permanente Medical Care Program, USA	Orentreich et al. (1991)	–	Both	26–78	1969–73	5–9	Lung	123/246	Age, sex, skin colour, smoking, date of health check-up, storage duration
Skin Cancer Prevention Study, USA	Karagas et al. (1997)	1805	Both	35–84	1983–86	3–5	Squamous skin	129/250	Age, sex, study centre

[a] The matching variables varied from one study to another.

68

Table 8. Description of case–control studies of the association between tissue concentrations of carotenoids and cancer

Reference, country	Population base	Time period	Sex	Age (years)	Site of cancer	No. of cases/ controls	Controls Type	Matching variables
Pastorino et al. (1987), Italy	Instituto Nazionale di Tumori and Consorio Provinciale Antitubercolare, Milan	NR	Female	62 (10) [a]	Lung	47/159	Hospital	NR
Gerber et al. (1988), Italy, France	Instituto Nazionale Tumori, Milan and Paul Lamarque Cancer Center, Montpellier	1982–85	Female	25–65	Breast	306/314	Hospital	NR
Hayes et al. (1988), Netherlands	Hospitals in the Rotterdam region	1982–85	Male	50–79	Prostate	134/130	Hospital	NR
Palan et al. (1988), USA	Bronx Municipal Hospital Center, New York	NR	Female	NR	Cervix	32/37	Volunteer	NR
Palan et al. (1991), USA	Bronx Municipal Hospital Center, New York	1988	Female	28 (8) [a]	Cervix	10/36	Volunteer	NR
Palan et al. (1992), USA	Bronx Municipal Hospital Center, New York	NR	Female	16–69	Cervix	10/26	Volunteer	NR
Kune et al. (1989), Australia	Repatriation General Hospital, Melbourne	1984–85	Male	NR	Lung	64/63	Hospital	NR
Kune et al. (1992), Australia	Repatriation General Hospital, Melbourne	1984–85	Male	70 (8) [a]	Skin, basal-cell, squamous-cell	88/88	Hospital	Sex
Kune et al. (1993), Australia	Repatriation General Hospital, Melbourne	1982	Male	64 (8) [a]	Oral and pharynx	41/88	Hospital	Sex
Potischman et al. (1990), USA	Roswell Park Memorial Institute and two surgeons in Buffalo, New York	1985–86	Female	30–80	Breast	83/113	Hospital	NR
Stryker et al. (1990), USA	Massachusetts General Hospital	1982–85	Both	≥ 18	Melanoma	204/248	Hospital	NR

Table 8 (contd)

Reference, country	Population base	Time period	Sex	Age (years)	Site of cancer	No. of cases/ controls	Selection of controls Type	Selection of controls Matching variables
Ramaswamy et al. (1990), India	Bangalore	NR	Both	NR	Oral cavity, head and neck, gastrointestinal tract, lung, breast, cervix	285/50	Hospital, volunteer	Age, sex, socioeconomic status
Ramaswamy & Krishnamoorthy (1996), India	Bangalore	NR	Female	30–65	Cervix, breast	200/100	Volunteer	Age
Harris et al. (1991), UK	Churchill and John Radcliffe Hospitals, Oxford	1979–81	Male	62 (8) [a]	Lung	171/97	Hospital	NR
Potischman et al. (1991a), USA	Four Latin American countries	NR	Female	NR	Cervix	387/670	Hospital, population	NR
Potischman et al. (1994), USA	Four Latin American countries	1986–87	Female	< 70	Cervix	696/1217	Hospital, population	Age
Smith & Waller (1991), New Zealand	Wellington Hospital	1981–84	Both	20–80	All, oesophagus, stomach, small intestine, colon, rectum, larynx, lung, basal skin, squamous skin, melanoma, breast, uterus, ovary, cervix, urinary bladder, kidney, prostate, haematopoietic, thyroid, brain	389/391	Hospital	Age, sex, date of admission

Table 8 (contd)

Reference, country	Population base	Time period	Sex	Age (years)	Site of cancer	No. of cases/ controls	Selection of controls — Type	Selection of controls — Matching variables
London et al. (1992) USA	Five teaching hospitals in the Boston, Massachusetts, area	1986–88	Female	58–69	Breast	377/403	Hospital	None
Malvy et al. (1993), France	Paris, Lyon, Lille, Bordeaux, Tours, Nancy	1986–89	Both	0–16	Leukaemia, lymphoma, central nervous system, sympathetic nervous system, renal, bone, soft tissue	418/632	Population	Age, sex, residence
Pan et al. (1993), China	Chang-Gung Memorial Hospital	1988–89	Male	NR	Hepatocellular carcinoma	59/101	Hospital	Age
Jinno et al. (1994), Japan	NR	NR	Both	NR	Hepatocellular carcinoma	60/40	Hospital	Age
Torun et al. (1995), Turkey	NR	NR	Both	NR	All, breast, head and neck, genitourinary, lung, gastrointestinal	208/156	NR	NR
van't Veer et al. (1996), Germany, France, The Netherlands, Spain, Switzerland	Berlin, Coleraine, Zeist, Malaga, Zürich	NR	Female	50–74	Breast	347/374	Population	Age

NR, not reported
[a] Mean (SD)

in Tables 9–11, by study design. The small numbers of cases may be one reason for failure to detect associations in some studies, and the results of studies based on ≥ 40 cases were given particular emphasis. The relative risk (RR) between high and low concentrations of carotenoids and the mean differences between the concentrations of carotenoids in cases and controls are also tabulated.

(c)   Cohort studies
The Alpha-Tocopherol Beta-Carotene Cancer Prevention (ATBC) study involved 29 133 men aged 50–69 (median, 57), out of 54 171 potentially eligible participants, in southwestern Finland who currently smoked five or more cigarettes per day (median, 20). The median duration of smoking was 36 years. Subjects were excluded if they were taking more than a predefined dose of supplements of vitamins E or A or β-carotene, had a history of cancer other than non-melanoma skin cancer or serious debilitating disease or were being treated with anticoagulants. The lung cancer incidence among untreated men was 47 per 10 000 person–years. Eighty-nine percent of the subjects drank alcohol, mostly beer and spirits, with a median ethanol intake was about 11 g/d. The baseline plasma concentrations of retinol, α-tocopherol, β-carotene, vitamin C and high-density lipoprotein were determined in most participants and were consistent with those reported in other western populations (e.g. median serum β-carotene, 0.32 μmol/L). The cancer cases that occurred during a median follow-up of 6.1 years were identified by the Finnish Cancer Registry. Advice on stopping smoking was provided to all participants at entry, and 22%, equally distributed in the study groups, quit during the follow-up. The incidence of lung cancer was lower among subjects in the highest quartile of serum β-carotene concentrations than among those in the lowest; the relative risk between the extreme quartiles, adjusted for age and amount of smoking, was calculated by the Working Group to be 0.81 (Table 9). Similar associations were observed in the entire trial population and when they were grouped into those receiving β-carotene as part of the intervention and those not receiving the

supplement (Alpha-Tocopherol Beta-Carotene Cancer Prevention Study Group 1994a,b; Albanes *et al.*, 1996).

In the study in Basel, Switzerland, 2974 healthy male employees at three pharmaceutical companies were followed up from 1971, initially for 12 years (Stähelin *et al.*, 1991) and later for 17 years (Eichholzer *et al.*, 1996; Table 6). According to the death certificates from the Swiss Federal Office of Statistics, 290 of the men died of cancer during the 17-year follow-up period. All of those who developed cancer and those with lung or stomach cancer had had significantly lower plasma carotene concentrations before diagnosis (20% α-carotene, 80% β-carotene) than the non-cases, with mean case–control differences of 18, 30 and 30%, respectively (Table 9), as calculated by the Working Group. A strong gradient was observed for stomach cancer, with an estimated relative risk of 0.30 (95% confidence interval [CI], 0.13–0.70) between the highest and lowest quartiles of the distribution of β-carotene concentrations, after exclusion of the first two years of follow-up [calculated by the Working Group]. Individuals with low plasma concentrations of both carotene and retinol had strongly increased rates of death from all cancers and from lung cancer. This association persisted after exclusion of men who developed cancer during the first two years of follow-up and after adjustment for age, smoking and serum lipids. The relative risks for individuals in the higher quartiles of carotene and retinol concentrations in comparison with those in the lowest quartiles were 0.28 (95% CI, 0.11–0.70) for lung cancer and 0.47 (95% CI, 0.32–0.68) for all cancers combined [calculated by the Working Group]. Further adjustment for plasma concentrations of vitamins C and E did not materially alter the results.

The Skin Cancer Prevention Study was a multicentre, double-blind clinical trial in the United States, comprising 1720 men and women under 85 years of age who had had at least one basal-cell or squamous-cell skin carcinoma diagnosed from a biopsy speciment (Greenberg *et al.*, 1996; Table 6). The participants had no known genetic predisposition to skin cancer. During the 7–10-year follow-up, 82 persons were ascertained

Table 9. Results of cohort studies on the association between serum or plasma concentrations of carotenoids and cancer

Reference, country	No. of cancer cases	Site of cancer	Exposure Type	Exposure Category	Highest versus lowest category RR	95% CI	p value for trend	Controlled variables	Mean (µg/dl)	Difference between cases and non-cases (%) [a]
Alpha-Tocopherol Beta Carotene Cancer Prevention Study Group (1994b), Finland	208	Lung	SBC	Quartile	0.81		NR	Age, smoking	17[b]	NR
Eichholzer et al. (1996), Switzerland	290	All	PTC				NR	Age, smoking, lipids	24	-18**
	87	Lung	PTC				NR			-30**
	28	Stomach	PTC	Quartile[c]	0.47	0.20-2.94	NR			-30**
	30	Prostate	PTC	Quartile[c]	1.23	0.52-2.94	NR			-20
	22	Colon	PTC	Quartile[c]	1.92	0.61-5.88	NR			+5
	15	Pancreas	PTC	NR	NR		NR			-18
Greenberg et al. (1996), USA	82	All	PBC	Quartile	0.78	0.42-1.46	0.26	Age, sex, smoking, body mass index, study centre	18	NR
Omenn et al. (1996a), USA	275	Lung	SBC	Median	0.69	0.54-0.88	0.003	NR	15	NR
Sahyoun et al. (1996), USA	45	All	PTC	Quintile	0.72	0.25-2.02	0.34	Age, sex, lipids, disease status, disabilities	135	NR
Ito et al. (1997), Japan	44	All	SBC	Tertile	0.33	0.14-0.75	NR	Age, smoking, alcohol consumption	36	-35***
			SAC	Tertile	0.75	0.35-1.62	NR		7	-30**
			SLY	Tertile	0.67	0.32-1.44	NR		20	-24**
	10	Stomach	SBC	Tertile	0.45	0.73-2.78	NR	Age, sex, smoking, alcohol consumption, vegetable intake	NR	NR

NR not reported; SBC, serum β-carotene; SAC, serum α-carotene; SLY, serum lycopene; PTC, plasma total carotenoids; PBC, plasma β-carotene
[a] Unadjusted; test for difference from zero: ** $p < 0.01$, *** $p < 0.001$; estimated as [(case mean − control mean)/control mean] x 100
[b] Median
[c] Higher versus lowest quartile, first two years of follow-up excluded

from death certificates to have died of cancer. Plasma β-carotene concentration at the beginning of the study was inversely related to cancer mortality, the relative risk between the highest and lowest quartiles being 0.53 (95% CI, 0.30–0.94). The relative risk for cancer was not statistically significant after adjustment for age, sex, smoking, body mass index and study centre: 0.78 (95% CI, 0.42–1.5; p for trend = 0.26; Table 9).

The Beta-Carotene and Retinol Efficacy Trial (CARET) involved 14 254 current or former smokers (7965 men and 6289 women) and 4060 asbestos-exposed workers, aged 50–69, resident in six areas of the United States, who were recruited from answers to more than 1 400 000 letters sent to establish eligibility and to obtain informed consent. Of these workers, 1153 had already participated in pilot studies in which treatment with lower doses of β-carotene was initiated (Goodman et al., 1993; Omenn et al., 1993b). The mean age of the asbestos-exposed workers was 57 years, and that of smokers was 58 years. No women had been exposed to asbestos, while they represented about one-half of the smokers. The incidence of lung cancer in the untreated group was 46 per 10 000 person–years. Subjects with a history of cancer other than non-melanoma skin cancer during the previous five years, aspartate aminotransferase and alkaline phosphatase activities above the 99% upper limits, a history of cirrhosis or hepatitis during the previous 12 months, unwillingness to limit supplementation with vitamin A or β-carotene, a Karnowski index of < 70 and women who had undergone menopause less than one year previously were excluded. Only 3% of the asbestos-exposed workers were nonsmokers, while 58% were former smokers. Among the smokers, about two-thirds were current smokers of a mean number of 24 cigarettes per day. The ex-smokers had stopped smoking an average of three years before recruitment; before quitting, they had smoked a mean of 28 cigarettes per day. Among the asbestos-exposed workers in the pilot study, the ex-smokers had quit an average of 19 years before recruitment; their mean duration of exposure to asbestos had been 35 years, and they had spent an average of 25 years in high-risk trades in insulating, shipyards, use of plasterboard, plumbing, shipscaling, shipfitting and sheetmetal work (Omenn et al., 1993b). Sixty-six percent of the asbestos-exposed workers, 67% of the male smokers and 62% of the female smokers drank alcoholic beverages, the median alcohol intake being 12, 12 and 9 g/d, respectively. The baseline plasma concentrations of retinol, α-tocopherol, β-carotene and retinyl palmitate were determined in a subset of 1182 participants and were consistent with those reported for other western populations (e.g. mean serum β-carotene, 0.27 µmol/L). Advice on stopping smoking was provided to the whole study group, resulting in a 5% rate of quitting per year, equally distributed among the subgroups (Grizzle et al., 1991; Omenn et al., 1991; Goodman et al., 1992; Omenn et al., 1994, 1996a). During a mean follow-up of four years, 275 confirmed cases of lung cancer occurred, and a statistically significant inverse association between baseline serum β-carotene concentration and lung cancer incidence was observed (Table 9). The relative risk for lung cancer among people with a serum β-carotene concentration above the median was 0.69 (95% CI, 0.54–0.88; p for trend = 0.003) among all participants and 0.62 (95% CI, 0.46–0.82; p for trend = 0.0008) among heavy smokers, when compared with people with a concentration below the median. The association was similar in the subgroup of individuals who received β-carotene and retinol supplements and in the placebo group, as well as in current and former smokers. No association was seen in the population that had been exposed to asbestos.

The Nutrition Status Survey conducted in Boston, Massachusetts, USA, during 1981–84 comprised 725 non-institutionalized people aged 60–101 who were free of terminal wasting disease or severe metabolic disorders; they were healthier and better educated than the general population. During the 9–12-year follow-up, 45 of them died of cancer. The relative risk for death from cancer between the highest and lowest quintiles of plasma carotenoid status, adjusted for age, sex, serum cholesterol, disease status and disabilities, was 0.72 (not significant) (Sahyoun et al., 1996).

The population involved in the study carried out in Hokkaido, Japan, comprised 2353 healthy men and women over 39 years of age living in rural areas. During the two- to eight-year follow-up, 44 deaths from malignant neoplasms were confirmed from death certificates. After adjustment for age, smoking and alcohol consumption, an inverse association was observed with serum β-carotene concentration (Table 9), but no differences were observed in the concentrations of α-carotene and lycopene. The relative risk between the highest and lowest tertiles of serum β-carotene concentration was 0.33 (95% CI, 0.14–0.75). The corresponding relative risk for stomach cancer after further adjustment for intake of green and yellow vegetables was 0.45 (95% CI, 0.73–2.8) (Ito *et al.*, 1997).

(d)   Cohort studies with nested case–control analyses

The association between blood carotenoid status and cancer risk has been studied in nested case–control studies in nine populations (Table 7). The cohorts ranged in size from 1805 to 36 265 persons, and the number of cancer cases occurring during the 2–20-year follow-up periods ranged from 39 to 766.

On Guernsey, United Kingdom, during 1968–75, 5004 women aged 28–75 volunteered a plasma sample, which was stored at –20 °C (Wald *et al.*, 1984) and analysed for β-carotene. During a 7–14-year follow-up, 39 new cases of breast cancer were found by general practitioners. On the basis of the plasma concentrations of β-carotene in the cancer cases and in two matched controls per case, the relative risk between the highest and lowest quintiles of plasma β-carotene was 0.36 but was not significant (Table 10); the association was stronger for premenopausal women. The women in this group had a 28% lower ($p < 0.05$) age-adjusted mean concentration of β-carotene than the corresponding controls. Exclusion of those cancer cases occurring during the first two years of follow-up did not notably alter the results. The β-carotene concentrations were very low (mean, 5 μg/dl, 0.09 μmol/L), probably due to degradation during storage, as the serum samples were thawed several times (Wald *et al.*, 1988). [The Working Group noted that the method for

determining serum β-carotene and the reliability of the method were not reported.]

In the Hypertension Detection and Follow-up Program, a trial of treatment for hypertension at 14 centres in the United States, serum samples were collected during 1973–74 from 4480 men and women aged 30–69 with a diastolic blood pressure of at least 90 mm Hg (Table 7). The serum samples were stored at –70°C. During a five-year follow-up, 111 cases of cancer (excluding non-melanoma skin cancer) occurred among participants with no history of cancer. The cases were confirmed by a review of hospital records, pathology reports and death certificates, and each case was matched with two controls. The coefficient of variation for the determinations of carotenoid was 8.7%. No significant association was found between serum carotenoid concentration and the occurrence of cancers at all sites combined (Table 10). When the mean carotenoid concentrations adjusted for lipids were compared for cases of cancer at various sites and for the corresponding controls, a significant, 36% higher mean concentration was found in cases of leukaemia and lymphoma combined than among controls ($p = 0.05$). No association was seen for cancers of the lung, breast or prostate or for all cancers of the gastrointestinal tract (Willett *et al.*, 1984).

A total of 6860 men of Japanese ancestry, 52–75 years of age, participated in the Honolulu Heart Program in Hawaii, United States, during 1971–75 (Table 7), in which serum samples were taken and were stored at –75 °C. During the 10-year follow-up, 81 cases of cancer of the colon, 74 of the lung, 70 of the stomach, 32 of the rectum and 27 of the urinary bladder were recorded in the Hawaii Tumor Registry. Each cancer case was confirmed by histological examination of tissue obtained at surgery or biopsy. An age-stratified random sample of controls was selected from among those men who did not develop cancer during the follow-up. A significant inverse gradient was found between serum β-carotene concentration and the occurrence of lung cancer, and the relative risk between the highest and lowest quintiles was 0.45 (95% CI, 0.17–1.2 [calculated by the Working Group]; Table 10) after adjustment for age and smoking, with a *p* value of 0.04 for trend. Further adjustment for alcohol intake and serum cholesterol, retinol and vitamin E concentrations did not alter the results. The association was found for men with various intensities of smoking but was strongest in heavy smokers. It persisted throughout the 10-year follow-up period. The median concentration of β-carotene was significantly lower in men with squamous- and small-cell carcinomas (but not those with adenocarcinomas) than in controls. The coefficient of variation of the β-carotene determinations was very high (33%), perhaps due to the low mean concentration in the controls. An inverse association with stomach cancer was also reported between the highest and lowest tertiles of serum β-carotene concentration, with an age-adjusted relative risk of 0.3 (95% CI, 0.2–0.7). This association was seen mainly in patients whose cancer was diagnosed within the first five years of follow-up (*p* = 0.001). No association was observed for cancers of the colon (Nomura *et al.*, 1985).

At a later stage of the study, 28 cases of cancer of the oesophagus, 23 of the larynx and 18 of oral–pharyngeal cancer occurred during a follow-up of 20 years. These 69 cases were matched to 138 controls. The mean concentrations of α- and β-carotene were lower in the cases than in the controls after adjustment for age, smoking and alcohol consumption. When data for the three sites of cancer were combined, a strong association was found. The relative risk between the highest and lowest tertiles was 0.19 (95% CI, 0.05–0.75) for α-carotene, 0.10 (95% CI, 0.02–0.46) for β-carotene, 0.25 (95% CI, 0.06–1.0) for β-cryptoxanthin and 0.22 (95% CI, 0.05–0.88) for total carotenoids. A significant gradient was observed for all four variables, and the associations were still present after the 10-year follow-up (Nomura *et al.*, 1997).

Serum samples were collected in 1974 from 25 802 men and women, representing about 30% of the population of Washington County, Maryland, United States, who were 18 years of age or over. The serum samples were stored at −73 °C (Menkes *et al.*, 1986; Table 7). During the follow-up, ending in 1983–90, the incidences of cancers of the lung (Menkes *et al.*,

1986), colon (Schober *et al.*, 1987), pancreas (Burney *et al.*, 1989), urinary bladder (Helzlsouer *et al.*, 1989), prostate (Hsing *et al.*, 1990), rectum and breast (Comstock *et al.*, 1991), cervix (Batieha *et al.*, 1993), oral cavity (Zheng *et al.*, 1993), skin (Breslow *et al.*, 1995) and ovary (Helzlsouer *et al.*, 1996) among originally cancer-free persons were obtained from the Washington County Cancer Register. One, two or four controls were drawn from among people who were alive and had no history of cancer, except skin cancer, and were matched to persons in the subgroups with cancers at specific sites for age, sex and race. Matching was also perfomed in some studies for time of blood collection (Menkes *et al.*, 1986; Schober *et al.*, 1987; Comstock *et al.*, 1991; Batieha *et al.*, 1993; Zheng *et al.*, 1993; Helzlsouer *et al.*, 1996), time since the previous meal (Burney *et al.*, 1989; Helzlsouer *et al.*, 1989; Comstock *et al.*, 1991; Batieha *et al.*, 1993; Zheng *et al.*, 1993; Helzlsouer *et al.*, 1996), smoking (Menkes *et al.*, 1986) and menopausal status (Batieha *et al.*, 1993; Helzlsouer *et al.*, 1996).

An inverse association was found between serum β-carotene concentration and lung cancer occurrence (Menkes *et al.*, 1986; Table 10), the relative risk for lung cancer (99 cases) between the highest and lowest quartiles of concentrations of the micronutrient being 0.45 (*p* = 0.04) [calculated by the Working Group]. Adjustment for potential confounding factors—education, marital status, occupation, time since last meal, treatment of hypertension, intake of vitamin supplements, smoking history, hormone use (in women) and socioeconomic indicators—did not alter the relationship. A strong inverse association was observed for squamous-cell carcimoma, with a relative risk of 0.23 [calculated by the Working Group] (95% CI, 0.07–0.72) between persons with serum β-carotene concentrations over and below the median. No significant association was observed for small-cell carcinoma, adenocarcinoma or large-cell carcinoma or for unspecified carcinomas of the lung combined.

In a complementary study based on a larger study population, 157 male and 101 female cases of lung cancer were found during a maximum follow-up of 19 years. In comparison with 515 controls matched for race, sex, age, date of blood collection and subpopulation, a significant inverse association was seen between lung cancer occurrence and the concentration of carotenoids, with the exception of lycopene. The relative risks between the highest and lowest quintiles were 0.48 (p for trend = 0.01) for serum α-carotene, 0.44 (p = 0.002) for β-carotene, 0.29 (p < 0.001) for cryptoxanthin, 0.41 (p < 0.001) for lutein/zeaxanthin and 1.0 (p = 0.99) for lycopene. The results were similar for men and women. The associations, with the exception of that with cryptoxanthin concentration, disappeared after adjustment for smoking (Comstock *et al.*, 1997). The serum β-carotene concentration was not significantly associated with the risk for colon cancer (n = 72) (Schober *et al.*, 1987; Table 10). The serum lycopene concentration was inversely associated with the risk for pancreatic cancer (n = 22), the relative risk between the highest and lowest tertiles of concentrations of the micronutrient being 0.19 [calculated by the Working Group] (p for trend < 0.05; Burney *et al.*, 1989; Table 10). Adjustment for total carotenoids, β-carotene, selenium and vitamin E in serum and for education and smoking history did not noticeably alter the results. The association was independent of length of follow-up, suggesting that latent cancers had not contributed to the finding, and was strongest for nonsmokers. The total serum concentration of carotenoids or of β-carotene was not significantly associated with the risk for pancreatic cancer. A nonsignificant inverse association was found between serum lycopene concentration and the risk for cancer of the urinary bladder (n = 35; Helzlsouer *et al.*, 1989; Table 10), the relative risk between the highest and lowest tertiles, adjusted for history of cigarette smoking and intake of vitamin supplements, being 0.50 (95% CI, 0.15–1.6) [calculated by the Working Group] (p for trend = 0.06).

No evidence was found for associations between the serum concentrations of β-carotene, lycopene or total carotenoids and the risk for prostatic cancer (n = 103; Hsing *et al.*, 1990; Table 10). The mean difference between cases and controls varied between –6 and +4%.

Adjustment for time since the last meal, smoking and education did not alter the results. No interaction was observed between β-carotene concentration and age, and the concentrations were similar for latent (n = 18) and clinically apparent (n = 85) cancer cases. No association was present between the serum β-carotene concentration and the occurrence of rectal (n = 34) or postmenopausal breast (n = 30) cancer (Comstock *et al.*, 1991; Table 10), the relative risks between persons in the highest and lowest tertiles of concentrations of the micronutrient being 1.2 and 1.1, respectively [calculated by the Working Group]. A nonsignificant inverse association was, however, seen between the serum lycopene concentration and risk for rectal cancer, the relative risk being 0.36 [calculated by the Working Group] (p for trend = 0.10).

The concentrations of several carotenoids were inversely associated with the risk for cervical cancer (n = 50; Batieha *et al.*, 1993; Table 10). The relative risks between the highest and lowest tertiles [calculated by the Working Group] were 0.37 (p for trend = 0.02) for total carotenoids, 0.32 (p = 0.01) for α-carotene, 0.33 (p = 0.02) for β-carotene, 0.43 (p = 0.07) for cryptoxanthin and 0.40 (p = 0.08) for lycopene. The associations were not altered by exclusion of cancer cases that occurred during the first years of follow-up. Education, marital status, oral contraceptive use, smoking and serum concentrations of retinol, lutein, α-tocopherol, γ-tocopherol or selenium did not confound the results. Similar patterns of risk were observed for the 32 cases of carcinoma *in situ* and for the 18 cases of invasive cancer, although the associations were generally weaker for invasive cancer. Serum lutein concentration was not associated with cervical cancer risk. [The Working Group noted that no information was available on known strong risk factors such as human papillomavirus infection and sexual behaviour.]

Low serum concentrations of various carotenoids were nonsignificantly associated with the occurrence of oral or pharyngeal cancer (n = 28) (Zheng *et al.*, 1993; Table 10). The association was significant for total carotenoids, the unadjusted relative risk between the highest and lowest tertiles of concentrations being 0.33 (*p* for trend = 0.05). The relative risks for β-carotene, α-carotene, cryptoxanthin, lutein and lycopene ranged from 0.33 to 0.65. No association was found between serum β-carotene or lycopene concentration and the incidence of melanoma (*n* = 30) or basal-cell (*n* =32) or squamous-cell (*n* = 37) carcinoma of the skin (Breslow *et al.*, 1995; Table 10). The relative risks between the highest and lowest tertiles of the distribution of concentrations varied from 0.8 to 1.4. No significant inverse association was found between total serum carotenoids, α-carotene, β-carotene, cryptoxanthin, lutein or lycopene and the occurrence of ovarian cancer (*n* = 35; Helzlsouer *et al.*, 1996; Table 10). The unadjusted relative risks between the tertiles of distribution varied from 0.66 to 2.0.

The British United Provident Association Medical Centre in London undertook medical examinations of 22 000 men aged 35–64 years during 1975–82 (Wald *et al.*, 1988; Table 7). The serum samples were stored at –40 °C. The diagnoses of cancer or death were received from the Office of Population Censuses and Surveys. During the two- to nine-year follow-up, 271 cancer cases occurred. The relative risk for cancers at all sites combined between the highest and lowest quintiles of serum β-carotene concentration was 0.60 [calculated by the Working Group] (*p* for trend = 0.01). The incidence of lung cancer (*n* = 50) showed a significant inverse trend (*p* = 0.008) and a relative risk of 0.41 [calculated by the Working Group]. The association was not dependent on the length of follow-up and was still present after follow-up for five years or more. No significant association was observed for cancers of the colorectum (*n* = 30), stomach (*n* = 13), urinary bladder (*n* = 15), skin (*n* = 56) or central nervous system (*n* = 17).

The Multiple Risk Factor Intervention Trial comprised 12 866 men, 35–57 years of age, who were at high risk for coronary heart disease and who were selected from several clinical centres in the USA covering a population of 361 662 (Multiple Risk Factor Intervention Trial Research Group, 1982; Table 7). About 63% of the participants were cigarette smokers (Connett *et al.*, 1989). A nested case–control

study was conducted on the basis of serum samples collected during 1973–75 from randomized participants and stored at –50 to –70 °C. During the 10-year follow-up, 156 individuals died of cancer; all of the deaths were reviewed by a committee. The relative risk for lung cancer (*n* = 66) between the highest and lowest quintiles of total serum carotenoid concentrations was 0.54 [calculated by the Working Group] (*p* for trend = 0.03; Table 10). A nonsignificant association with serum β-carotene concentration was observed (*p* for trend = 0.08), with a relative risk of 0.43 [calculated by the Working Group]. The associations were not due to age, smoking status, alcohol consumption, obesity or plasma lipids and were strongest during the first five years of follow-up. No significant association was observed for cancers at all sites combined.

The Finnish Mobile Clinic conducted health examinations on 36 265 men and women, 15 years of age or over, in 25 cohorts in various parts of Finland during 1968–72 (Knekt *et al.*, 1990; Table 7). Serum samples were taken and were stored at –20 °C. During the 6–10-year follow-up, 766 cancer cases occurred among persons who had originally been cancer-free. Cancers at 19 sites were studied: stomach, colon, rectum, pancreas, lung, prostate, breast, cervix, endometrium and ovaries combined, basal-cell carcinoma of the skin, lymphomas and leukaemias combined (Knekt *et al.*, 1990), larynx, oesophagus, kidney, urinary bladder, brain, oral and pharyngeal cancers combined, liver and gall-bladder combined and melanoma (Knekt *et al.*, 1991). The relative risks for cancers at all sites, adjusted for smoking, between the highest and lowest quintiles of serum β-carotene concentrations were 0.77 (95% CI, 0.48–1.1) [calculated by the Working Group] (*p* for trend = 0.01) for men and 1.0 (95% CI, 0.59–2.0) [calculated by the Working Group] (*p* for trend = 0.26) for women (Table 10). The relationship for men persisted after exclusion of cancer cases that occurred during the first two years of follow-up and after adjustment for potential confounding factors. No interaction with smoking or serum concentrations of cholesterol, α-tocopherol or selenium was observed. Significantly lower mean concentrations of β-

Table 10. Results of nested case–control studies including more than 10 cases of cancer on the association between serum or plasma concentrations of carotenoids and cancer

Reference, country	Site of cancer	No. of cases	No. of controls	Exposure Type	Exposure Category	RR (95% CI) for highest versus lowest category	p value for trend	Control mean (µg/dl)	Difference between cases and controls (%)[a]
Willett et al. (1984), USA	Lung	17 M/F	28 M	STC	NR	NR	NR	112	+8
Nomura et al. (1985), USA	Lung	74 M	302 M	SBC	Quintile	0.45 (0.17–1.25)	0.04	29	–31 **
Menkes et al. (1986), USA	Lung	99 M/F	196 M/F	SBC	Quintile	0.45	0.04	29	–14 ***
Wald et al. (1988), UK	Lung	50 M	99 M	SBC	Quintile	0.41	0.008	20	–22
Connett et al. (1989), USA	Lung	66 M	131 M	STC / SBC	Quintile / Quintile	0.54 / 0.43	0.03 / 0.08	99 / 12	–12 * / –23
Knekt et al. (1990), Finland	Lung	144 M	270 M	SBC	Quintile[b]	1.00 (0.52–2.00)	NR	8	–21 **
Orentreich et al. (1991), USA	Lung	123 M/F	246 M/F	SBC	Quintile	0.33	0.01	6	–15
Knekt et al. (1991), Finland	Larynx	11 M/F	17 M/F	SBC	Standard units[c]	0.88	0.82	8	–7
Nomura et al. (1997), USA	Larynx	23 M	138 M	STC / SBC / SAC / SCR / SLU / SLY / SZE	–	–	–	92 / 15 / 5 / 11 / 16 / 22 / 3	–12 / –15* / –23 / +12 / –12 / –16 / –12
Knekt et al. (1991), Finland	Oral and pharynx	20 M/F	37 M/F	SBC	Standard units[c]	0.42	0.16	10	–18

Table 10 (contd)

Reference, country	Site of cancer	No. of cases	No. of controls	Exposure Type	Exposure Category	RR (95% CI) for highest versus lowest category	p value for trend	Control mean (μg/dl)	Difference between cases and controls (%)[a]
Zheng et al. (1993), USA	Oral and pharynx	28 M/F	112 M/F	STC	Tertile	0.33	0.05	94	−17*
				SBC	Tertile	0.50	0.17	15	−24*
				SAC	Tertile	0.37	0.06	3	−17
				SCR	Tertile	0.33	0.07	10	−16
				SLU	Tertile	0.61	0.37	23	−19
				SLY	Tertile	0.65	0.46	6	−7
Nomura et al. (1997) USA	Oral and pharynx	18 M	138 M	STC	–	–	–	92	−3
				SBC	–	–	–	16	−5
				SAC	–	–	–	4	−16*
				SCR	–	–	–	14	−24
				SLU	–	–	–	17	−1
				SLY	–	–	–	21	+4
				SZE	–	–	–	3	+6
Nomura et al. (1997) USA	Oesophagus	28 M	138 M	STC	–	–	NR	104	−23*
				SBC	–	–	–	19	−44*
				SAC	–	–	–	5	−42*
				SCR	–	–	–	17	−36*
				SLU	–	–	–	16	−6
				SLY	–	–	–	21	−7
				SZE	–	–	–	3	−21
Nomura et al. (1995), USA	Stomach	70 M	302 M	SBC	Tertile	0.3 (0.2–0.7)	0.08	29	−21
Wald et al. (1988), UK	Stomach	13 M	26 M	SBC	–	–	NR	25	−27
Knekt et al. (1990), Finland	Stomach	48 M 28 F	90 M 48 F	SBC SBC	Quintile [b] Quintile [b]	1.25 (0.36–5.00) 1.11 (0.26–5.00)	NR	8 10	−10 +27

Table 10 (contd)

Reference, country	Site of cancer	No. of cases	No. of controls	Exposure Type	Exposure Category	RR (95% CI) for highest versus lowest category	p value for trend	Control mean (µg/dl)	Difference between cases and controls (%)[a]
Willett et al. (1984), USA	Gastro-intestinal	11 M/F	22 MF	STC	–	–	NR	112	+9
Nomura et al. (1985), USA	Colon	81 M	302 M	SBC	–	–	NR	29	–19
	Rectum	32 M	302 M	SBC	–	–	–	29	–4
Schober et al. (1987), USA	Colon	72 M/F	143 M/F	SBC	Quintile	0.83 (0.31–2.00)	NR	34	–4
Wald et al. (1988), USA	Colorectum	30 M	59 M	SBC	–	–	NR	23	–11
Knekt et al. (1990), Finland	Colon	13 F	24 F	SBC	Quintile[b]	3.33 (0.62–10.0)	NR	8	+13
	Rectum	15 M	29 M	SBC	Quintile[b]	2.00 (0.29–10.0)	–	7	+24
		22 F	42 F	SBC			–	16	–23
Connett et al. (1989), USA	Colon	14 M	28 M	STC	–	–	NR	110	–2
				SBC	–	–	–	12	–8
Comstock et al. (1991), USA	Rectum	34 M/F	68 M/F	SBC	Tertile	1.25	0.26	20	+16
				SLY	Tertile	0.36	0.10	37	–18
Burney et al. (1989), USA	Pancreas	22 M/F	44 MF	STC	Tertile	0.72	NS	121	+3
				SBC	Tertile	0.82	NS	38	+4
				SLY	Tertile	0.19	< 0.05	50	–32*
Knekt et al. (1990), Finland	Pancreas	17 M	28 M	SBC	Quintile[b]	1.67 (0.24–10.0)	NR	7	+6
		11 F	19 F	SBC	–	–	–	15	–9
Knekt et al. (1991), Finland	Liver and gall-bladder	12 M/F	22 M/F	SBC	Standard unit[c]	0.68	0.45	9	–17

Table 10 (contd)

Reference, country	Site of cancer	No. of cases	No. of controls	Exposure Type	Category	RR (95% CI) for highest versus lowest category	p value for trend	Control mean (µg/dl)	Difference between cases and controls (%)[a]
Wald et al. (1988), UK	Skin	56 M	107 M	SBC		–	NR	23	–3
Knekt et al. (1990), Finland	Basal cell	49 M / 38 F	93 M / 69 F	SBC / SBC	Quintile[b] / Quintile[b]	0.32 (0.09–1.11) / 2.50 (0.59–10.0)	NR / –	10 / 11	–13 / +13
Knekt et al. (1991), Finland	Melanoma	10 M/F	18 M/F	SBC	Standard units[c]	0.03	< 0.01	12	–52**
Breslow et al. (1995), USA	Basal-cell	32 M/F	64 M/F	SBC / SLY	Tertile / Tertile	1.3 (0.4–4.0) / 1.4 (0.4–4.0)	0.72 / –	21 / 29	0 / +7
	Squamous-cell	37 M/F	74 M/F	SBC / SLY	Tertile / Tertile	1.4 (0.5–4.0) / 1.0 (0.3–3.1)	– / –	25 / 27	+7 / +4
	Melanoma	30 M/F	60 M/F	SBC / SLY	Tertile / Tertile	0.8 (0.2–2.3) / 1.1 (0.4–3.2)	– / –	21 / 39	–11 / +6
Karagas et al. (1997), USA	Squamous-cell	129 M/F	250 M/F	PBC	Quartile	0.73 (0.38–1.41)	0.37	17	–9
Wald et al. (1984), UK	Breast	39 F	78 F	PBC	Quintile	0.36	NS	5	–28
Willett et al. (1984), USA	Breast	14 F	31 F	STC	–	–	NR	112	+8
Knekt et al. (1990), Finland	Breast	67 F	123 F	SBC	Quintile[b]	3.33 (1.00–10.0)	NR	14	–13
Comstock et al. (1991), USA	Breast	30 F	59 F	SBC / SLY	Tertile / Tertile	1.11 / 0.71	0.43 / 0.29	22 / 30	–10 / –16
Knekt et al. (1990), Finland	Ovary	16 F	29 F	SBC	Quintile[b]	0.77 (0.14–5.00)	NR	11	–12

Table 10 (contd)

Reference, country	Site of cancer	No. of cases	No. of controls	Exposure Type	Exposure Category	RR (95% CI) for highest versus lowest category	p value for trend	Control mean (µg/dl)	Difference between cases and controls (%)[a]
Helzlsouer et al. (1996), USA	Ovary	35 F	67 F	STC	Tertile	0.88 (0.3–2.3)	NR	108	–8
				SAC	Tertile	1.95 (0.6–6.0)	0.24	2	+21
				SBC	Tertile	0.93 (0.4–2.4)	–	18	–9
				SCRLSS	Tertile	0.66 (0.3–1.8)	0.40	9	–7
				LU	Tertile	1.97 (0.7–5.9)	–	19	+15
				SLY	Tertile	1.36 (0.4–4.3)	0.59	31	–17
Knekt et al. (1990), Finland	Endometrium	12 F	21 F	SBC	–	–	NR	9	+15
Knekt et al. (1990), Finland	Cervix	23 F	44 F	SBC	–	–	NR	18	–10
Batieha et al. (1993), USA	Cervix	50 F	99 F	STC	Tertile	0.37 (0.16–0.89)	0.02	93	–15 *
				SAC	Tertile	0.32 (0.13–0.79)	0.01	3	–42 *
				SBC	Tertile	0.33 (0.12–0.86)	0.02	14	–23
				SCR	Tertile	0.43 (0.17–1.08)	0.07	9	–27 *
				SLU	Tertile	0.85 (0.38–1.92)	0.71	19	–6
				SLY	Tertile	0.40 (0.15–1.04)	0.08	35	–12
Willett et al. (1984), USA	Prostate	11 M	21 M	STC	–	–	NR	112	+4
Hsing et al. (1990), USA	Prostate	103 M	103 M	STC	Median	1.06 (0.54–2.10)	NR	104	+4
				SAC	Median	0.80 (0.21–2.98)	–	4	–3
				SBC	Quartile	1.08 (0.45–2.62)	0.94	24	0
				SLY	Quartile	0.50 (0.20–1.29)	0.26	32	–6
Knekt et al. (1990), Finland	Prostate	37 M	68 M	SBC	Quintile[b]	5.00 (1.11–10.0)	–	7	–1
Nomura et al. (1985), USA	Bladder	27 M	302 M	SBC	–	–	–	29	0
Helzlsouer et al. (1989), USA	Bladder	35 M/F	70 M/F	SBC	Tertile	0.63 (0.19–2.00)	0.35	33	+11
				SLY	Tertile	0.50 (0.15–1.59)	0.06	45	–7

Table 10 (contd)

Reference, country	Site of cancer	No. of cases	No. of controls	Exposure Type	Exposure Category	RR (95% CI) for highest versus lowest categories	p value for trend	Control mean (μg/dl)	Difference between cases and controls (%)[a]
Wald et al. (1988), UK	Bladder	15 M	29 M	SBC	–	–	–	23	–9
Knekt et al. (1991), Finland	Bladder	15 M/F	29 M/F	SBC	Standard unit[c]	1.72	0.22	8	+31
Knekt et al. (1991), Finland	Kidney	20 M/F	38 M/F	SBC	Standard unit[c]	0.32	0.06	12	–38
Willett et al. (1984)	Leukaemia and lymphoma	11 M/F	23 M/F	STC	–	–	NR	112	+36*
Knekt et al. (1990), Finland	Leukaemia and lymphoma	19 M 13 F	36 M 25 F	SBC SBC	– Quintile[b]	– 5.00 (0.36 -)	NR –	8 12	–2 –12
Wald et al. (1988), UK	Central nervous system	17 M	34 M	SBC	–	–	NR	21	–10
Knekt et al. (1991), Finland	Brain	18 M/F	34 M/F	SBC	Standard unit[c]	1.44	0.34	10	+15
Willett et al. (1984), USA	All	111 M/F	210 M/F	STC	Quintile[b]	1.5	0.49	112	+7
Wald et al. (1988), UK	All	271 M	533 M	SBC	Quintile[b]	0.60	0.01	22	–10**
Connett et al. (1989), USA	All	156 M	311 M	STC SBC	– –	– –	NR ·	96 10	–4 –6
Knekt et al. (1990), Finland	All	453 M 313 F	841 M 578 F	SBC SBC	Quintile[b] Quintile[b]	0.77 (0.48–1.11) 1.00 (0.59–2.00)	0.01 0.26	8 13	–14*** –6

M, male; F, female; NR, not reported; STC, serum total carotenoids; SBC, serum β-carotene; SAC, serum α-carotene; SCR, serum cryptoxanthin; SLY, serum lycopene; SLU, serum lutein; PBC, plasma β-carotene; SZE, serum zeaxanthine; NS, not significant

[a] Estimated as [(case mean–control)/control mean] x 100: test for difference from zero: * p < 0.05, ** p < 0.01, *** p < 0.001

[b] Higher versus lowest quintile, first two years of follow-up excluded

[c] Difference from mean divided by standard deviation

carotene were found only for men with lung cancer (n = 144; 21%) [calculated by the Working Group] (p = 0.005) and men and women with melanoma (n = 10; 58%) [calculated by the Working Group] (p < 0.01). A non-significant interaction was found between smoking and β-carotene concentration with respect to lung cancer: the relative risks between the highest and lowest tertiles of β-carotene concentration [calculated by the Working Group] were 0.37 (95% CI, 0.09–1.4) for non-smoking men and 1.1 (95% CI, 0.45–2.5) for men who smoked. The association disappeared after adjustment for smoking. The smoking-adjusted relative risk [calculated by the Working Group] for prostatic cancer (n = 32) between the highest and lowest quintiles of β-carotene concentrations was 5.0 (95% CI, 1.1–10), and the corresponding risk for breast cancer (n = 52) was 3.3 (95% CI, 1.0–10). [The Working Group noted that the serum samples were stored for a long time at –20 °C, and that the β-carotene concentrations may therefore have decreased.]

During 1969–73, serum samples were obtained from 453 men and women in a cohort of 143 574 persons, 26–78 years of age, who were participating in multiphasic health check-ups at the Kaiser Permanente Medical Care Program in San Francisco, USA (Friedman *et al.*, 1986); the serum samples were stored at –40 °C. The relative risk between the highest and lowest quintiles of serum β-carotene concentrations in the 123 patients with lung cancer in whom such concentrations were determined was 0.33 [calculated by the Working Group] (p = 0.01; Table 10; Orentreich *et al.*, 1991). [The Working Group noted the low concentrations of β-carotene and the fact that it was found in only 17% of the sera assayed, suggesting loss during storage.]

A nested case–control study was included in the Skin Cancer Prevention Study, a multi-centre, randomized trial in the USA (Karagas *et al.*, 1997; Table 7). The study population consisted of 1805 men and women, 35–84 years of age, each of whom had at least one basal-cell or squamous-cell skin carcinoma before entry into the study. Serum samples were collected at the beginning of the study and stored at –75 °C. During the three- to five-year follow-up, 129 new cases of squamous-cell skin cancer occurred. The smoking-adjusted relative risk for squamous-cell carcinoma of the skin between the highest and lowest quintiles of serum β-carotene concentrations was 0.73 (95% CI = 0.38–1.4), with a p value for trend of 0.37.

(e)   Case–control studies
Case–control studies of blood carotenoid status published since 1980 are summarized in Table 8. About 30 such studies have been published, covering populations in 15 countries and about 20 cancer sites. The most frequently studied sites are the lung, cervix, breast and skin. The numbers of cases in the studies varied from 10 to 696. In most of the studies, the controls were hospital patients; in about 50% of them, the controls were selected by matching for age and sometimes for some other factors. The results are shown in Table 11.

(i) Several sites of cancer
A total of 285 clinically and histopathologically confirmed carcinomas of the oral cavity (n = 50), [other] head and neck (n = 50), gastrointestinal tract (n = 50), lung (n = 35), breast (n = 50) and uterine cervix (n = 50) were studied at the Kidwai Memorial Institute of Oncology in Bangalore, India (Table 8). Fifty persons free from disease were selected from among the hospital staff and attenders of patients by matching for sex, age and socioeconomic status. The cancer patients had significantly lower total carotenoid concentrations than the controls (p < 0.01), whatever site of cancer was involved (Table 11; Ramaswamy *et al.*, 1990). [The Working Group noted that only total carotenoids could be measured with the spectrophotometric methods used and that the comparability of the case and control groups was unclear.]

In a later study, the total serum carotenoid concentrations of 100 patients with cancer of the breast and 100 with cancer of the uterine cervix were compared with those of 50 healthy controls and 25 patients with benign diseases of the breast and cervix (Table 8). The cancer patients had lower concentrations than the patients with benign disease, while the healthy controls had the highest values. In the cancer patients, a significant trend was observed towards lower serum carotenoid concentrations

Table 11. Results of case–control studies (including > 10 cases) of the association between tissue concentrations of carotenoids and cancer

Reference, country	Site of cancer	No. of cases	No. of controls	Exposure Type	Exposure Category	RR (95% CI) for highest versus lowest category	p value for trend	Control Mean (µg/dl)	Difference between cases and controls (%)[a]
Pastorino et al. (1987), Italy	Lung	47 F	159 F	PBC	Tertile	0.20 (0.04–0.87)	< 0.05	39	–29 **
Kune et al. (1989), Australia		64 M	63 M	SBC	–	–	NR	84	–33 ***
Ramaswamy et al. (1990), India		25 M, 10 F	25 M,25 F	SBC	–	–	NR	142	–43 ***
Smith & Waller (1991), New Zealand		39 M/F	391 M/F	SBC	Quartile	0.15 (0.04–0.53)	NR	75	–30 **
Torun et al. (1995) Turkey		12 M/F	50 M, 106F	SBC	–	–	–	75	–42**
Ramaswamy et al. (1990), India	Oral cavity	50 M/F	50 M/F	STC	–		NR	142	–42 ***
Kune et al. (1993), Australia	Oral cavity and pharynx	41 M	88 M	SBC	–	–	NR	89	–29 ***
Smith& Waller (1991), New Zealand	Stomach Colon Rectum	10 M/F 32 M/F 20 M/F	391 M/F 391 M/F 391 M/F	SBC SBC SBC	– – –	– – –	NR NR -	75 75 75	–47 ** +5 –14*
Pan et al. (1993), China	Hepatocellular carcinoma	59 M	101 M	SBC	Quartile	0.20 (0.08–0.52)	0.02	25	36 ***
Jinno et al. (1994), Japan		41 M, 19 F	20 M, 20 F	SBC	–	–	NR	36	–55 **
Smith & Waller (1991), New Zealand	Basal-cell carcinoma	72 M/F	391 M/F	SBC	–	–	NR	75	+10
Smith & Waller (1991), New Zealand	Squamous-cell carcinoma	32 M/F	391 M/F	SBC	–	–	NR	75	+17
Kune et al. (1992), Australia	Basal-cell and squamous-cell carcinoma	88 M	88 M	SBC	–	–	NR	89	–24 ***
Stryker et al. (1990), USA	Melanoma	96 M, 108 F	96 M, 152 F	PAC PBC PLY	Quintile Quintile Quintile	1.1 (0.6–1.9) 0.9 (0.5–1.5) 1.0 (0.5–1.7)	0.7 0.6 0.9	5 19 34	+11 9 –1

Table 11 (contd)

Reference, country	Site of cancer	No. of cases	No. of controls	Exposure Type	Category	RR (95% CI) for highest versus lowest category	p value for trend	Control Mean (µg/dl)	Difference between cases and controls (%)[a]
Smith & Waller (1991), New Zealand		15 M/F	391 M/F	SBC	–	–	–	75	+18
Gerber et al. (1988), Italy, France	Breast	306 F	314 F	SBC	–	–	–	44	+5
Potischman et al. (1990), USA		83 F	113 F	PBC	Quartile	0.32 (0.09–1.11)	0.02	14	-19 **
				PAC	Quartile	1.59 (0.34–7.69)	0.19	3	-11
				PLY	Quartile	0.63 (0.19–2.00)	0.43	26	-15 *
Ramaswamy et al. (1990), India		50 F	25 F	SBC	–	–	–	141	-25 ***
Smith & Waller (1991), New Zealand		48 F	391 M/F	PBC	–	–	–	75	-5
London et al. (1992), USA		377 F	403 F	SBC	Quintile	1.2 (0.7–1.9)	0.97	24	-1
				SAC	Quintile	1.2 (0.7–1.9)	0.71	4	0
				SLY	Quintile	1.0 (0.7–1.7)	0.82	32	-5
Torun et al. (1995), Turkey		59 F	59 F	SBC	–	–	–	77	-20 *
van't Veer et al. (1996), The Netherlands	Cervix	347 F	374 F	ABC	Tertile	0.74 (0.45–1.23)	0.31	0.94 (mg/g)	-3
Orr et al. (1985), USA		78 F	240 F	PBC	–	–	NR	79	-38 ***b
Harris et al. (1986), UK		32 F	226 F	SBC	Quintile	0.90 (0.20–5.00)	NR	29	+1
Palan et al. (1988), USA		32 F	37 F	PBC	–	–	NR	23	-68 **
Palan et al. (1991), USA		10 F	36 F	PBC	–	–	NR	29	-59 ***
Palan et al. (1992), USA		10 F	26 F	PBC	–	–		31	-58 ***
Ramaswamy et al. (1990), India		50 F	25 F	STC	–	–	NR	141	-25 ***
Potischman et al. (1991a), USA		387 F	670 F	SBC	Quartile	0.72 (0.5–1.2)	0.05	26	-13
				SAC	Quartile	0.92 (0.6–1.5)	0.29	9	-11
				SCR	Quartile	0.77 (0.4–1.3)	0.14	19	+2
				SLY	Quartile	1.14 (0.8–2.1)	0.69	15	
				SLU	Quartile	0.89 (0.5–1.5)	0.93	20	

Table 11 (contd)

Reference, Country	Site of cancer	No. of cases	No. of controls	Exposure Type	Category	RR (95% CI) for highest versus lowest category	p value for trend	Control mean (μg/dl/l)	Difference between cases and controls (%)[a]
Smith & Waller (1991), New Zealand		15 F	391 F	SBC	–	–	NR	75	–25 *
Smith & Waller (1991), New Zealand	Prostate	20 M	391 M/F	SBC	–	–	NR	75	–4
Hayes et al. (1988), The Netherlands	Prostate: clinical focal	94 M 40 M	130 M	PBC	Quintile Quintile	0.77 0.77	0.47 0.36	17	–16 * –6
Smith & Waller (1991), New Zealand	Bladder	14 M/F	391 M/F	SBC	–	–	NR	75	+13
Malvy et al. (1993), France	Renal	13 M/F	632 M/F	SBC	Quintile	0.06 (0.02–0.91)	NR	58	–69
Malvy et al. (1993), France	Leukaemia	158 M/F	632 M/F	SBC	Quintile	0.36 (0.20–0.64)	NR	58	–28 ***
	Lymphoma	66 M/F	632 M/F			0.23 (0.10–0.56)		58	–32 ***
	Central nervous system	57 M/F	632 M/F			0.12 (0.03–0.40)	NR	58	–30 ***
	Sympathetic nervous system	23 M/F	632 M/F			–	NR	58	+4
	Bone	42 M/F	632 M/F		Quintile	0.06 (0.01–0.29)	NR	58	–45 ***
	Soft-tissue sarcoma	30 M/F	632 M/F		–	–	NR	58	–27
	All	418 M/F	632 M/F		Quintile	0.26 (0.17–0.39)	NR	58	–33 ***
Smith & Waller (1991), New Zealand	All	389 M/F	39 M/F	SBC	–	–	NR	75	–2
Torun et al. (1995), Turkey		50 M 106 F	156 M/F	SBC	–	–	NR	75	–34 *

M, male; F, female; STC, serum total carotenoids; SBC, serum β-carotene; SAC, serum α-carotene; SCR, serum cryptoxanthin; SLU, serum lutein; SLY, serum lycopene; PTC, plasma total carotenoids; PBC, plasma β-carotene; PAC, plasma α-carotene; PLY, plasma lycopene; ABC, adipose tissue β-carotene; NR, not reported

[a] Estimated as [(case mean–control mean)/control mean] x 100; test for difference from zero: * $p < 0.005$, ** $p < 0.01$, *** $p < 0.001$.

[b] Percentage of cancer patients with β-carotene level below normal

with increasing stage of the disease (Ramaswamy & Krishnamoorthy, 1996). [The Working Group noted that the results were not adjusted for use of tobacco.]

The concentrations of β-carotene in 389 patients in Wellington Hospital, New Zealand, with recently diagnosed cancer were compared with those in 618 family members of the patients and 675 control patients. Cancers at 20 sites—oesophagus, stomach, small intestine, colon, rectum, larynx, lung, skin (basal-cell, squamous-cell, melanoma), breast, uterus, cervix, ovary, urinary bladder, kidney, prostate, haematopietic, thyroid, brain—were studied. Low concentrations of β-carotene were observed for individuals with cancers of the lung ($n = 39$), stomach ($n = 10$), oesophagus ($n = 6$), rectum ($n = 20$) and cervix ($n = 15$) (Table 11), the mean differences between cases and controls, adjusted for age, sex and length of sample storage, being 25–47%. Similar results were obtained for relatives of the patients with lung, stomach or cervical cancer, with differences of 10–20%. The relative risk between the highest and lowest quartiles of β-carotene concentrations for lung cancer, excluding the adenocarcinomas, was 0.15 (95% CI, 0.04–0.53) [calculated by the Working Group]. Patients with cancers of the colon, skin, breast, urinary bladder or prostate and relatives of these patients did not have lower β-carotene concentrations than the controls (Smith & Waller, 1991).

The serum β-carotene concentrations of 418 children with newly diagnosed, histologically confirmed malignancies were compared with those of 632 cancer-free controls in six cities in France (Table 8). The controls were healthy children, recruited by the school health-care service or undergoing routine health examinations in general paediatrics wards, and were matched for sex, age and residence. The age- and sex-adjusted serum concentrations showed a significant inverse association with the incidence of all cancers combined (Table 11); the relative risk between the highest and lowest quintiles of concentrations was 0.26 (95% CI, 0.17–0.39) [calculated by the Working Group]. Corresponding, significant, inverse associations [odds ratios calculated by the Working Group] were observed for leukaemia

($n = 158$; odds ratio, 0.36), lymphoma ($n = 66$; odds ratio, 0.23), central nervous system cancer ($n = 57$; odds ratio, 0.12), renal tumours ($n = 13$; odds ratio, 0.06) and bone tumours ($n = 42$; odds ratio, 0.06). No significant differences were observed for cancer of the sympathetic nervous system or soft-tissue sarcoma (Malvy et al., 1993).

In a comparison of 208 cancer patients in Turkey with 156 healthy subjects, a 34% [calculated by the Working Group] lower serum β-carotene concentration was seen in the cancer cases than in the controls ($p < 0.05$; Tables 8 and 11). When the mean concentrations were studied by site, significantly lower concentrations were found for cancers of the breast ($n = 59$), lung ($n = 12$), head and neck ($n = 38$), genitourinary organs ($n = 46$) and gastrointestinal tract ($n = 20$; $p < 0.05$) (Torun et al., 1995). [The Working Group noted that the control group was not described, and no adjustments for confounding were performed.]

(ii) Lung cancer

Forty-seven female patients in Italy with pathologically proven lung cancer were compared with 159 female hospital patients over 40 years of age who had been admitted for causes unrelated to cancer or any chronic disease (80% suffered from musculoskeletal disease) (Table 8). The lung cancer patients had significantly lower mean plasma β-carotene concentrations than the controls (Table 11). The relative risk for lung cancer between the highest and lowest tertiles of plasma β-carotene concentrations was 0.20 (95% CI, 0.04–0.87) [calculated by the Working Group], after adjustment for age, smoking, plasma cholesterol and plasma triglycerides. The relative risk, calculated by the Working Group, was 0.11 for nonsmokers and 0.42 for smokers (Pastorino et al., 1987).

The mean serum β-carotene concentration was 33% lower [calculated by the Working Group] in 64 men in Australia with histologically confirmed lung cancer than in 63 randomly selected controls admitted to the same hospital for small surgical operations (Table 8). The difference was statistically significant after adjustment for age and smoking ($p < 0.001$; Table 11; Kune et al., 1989).

[The Working Group was aware of, but did not further consider, a number of studies in which smoking was not adjusted for.]

(iii) Hepatocellular carcinoma

The serum β-carotene concentrations of 59 male patients in China with cytologically or pathologically confirmed hepatocellular carcinoma were compared with those of 101 age-matched controls (Table 8). The controls were selected from among patients who, according to ultrasonography, did not have liver cirrhosis or any other observable lesion; both cases and controls were hepatitis B virus carriers. An inverse association was noted between serum β-carotene concentration and the occurrence of hepatocellular carcinoma (Table 11), the relative risk between the highest and lowest quartiles of β-carotene concentrations being 0.20 [calculated by the Working Group] (p for trend = 0.02). The association persisted after adjustment for age, education, ethnicity, occupation, alcohol intake, smoking status and dietary intake of β-carotene (Pan *et al.*, 1993).

The serum β-carotene concentrations of 60 Japanese patients with hepatocellular carcinoma and 85 patients with liver cirrhosis tended to be lower than those of 40 age-matched patients with chronic hepatitis (Tables 8 and 11; Jinno *et al.*, 1994) . [The Working Group noted that only age was controlled for.]

(iv) Skin cancer

Comparison of the highest and lowest quintiles of concentrations of β-carotene, α-carotene and lycopene resulted in relative risks of 0.9, 1.1 and 1.0, respectively, in a comparison of 204 cases of histologically confirmed malignant melanoma and 248 melanoma-free controls, after adjustment for age, sex, plasma lipids, hair colour and ability to tan (Stryker *et al.*, 1990).

In a study of the association between serum β-carotene concentration and basal-cell and squamous-cell carcinoma of the skin among men in Australia, 88 surgical patients without previous skin cancer were selected as unmatched controls. The mean concentrations of serum β-carotene were 24% lower [calculated by the Working Group] in the carcinoma patients than in controls ($p < 0.001$). An inverse trend was also seen between serum β-carotene concentration and skin cancer risk ($p < 0.0001$) (Kune *et al.*, 1992).

(v) Breast cancer

A hospital-based case–control study was conducted in Milan, Italy, and Montpellier, France, involving 314 cases of breast cancer and 306 controls of similar ages (Table 8). No significant difference in the lipid-adjusted plasma β-carotene concentrations was found between breast cancer patients and controls (Table 11; Gerber *et al.*, 1988).

Women in Buffalo, New York, USA, were evaluated for the presence of a breast mass but had no previous history of cancer. Consequently, 83 were classified histologically as breast cancer patients and 113 as controls free from breast cancer (Table 8). An inverse association was seen between β-carotene concentration and breast cancer occurrence (Table 11). The relative risk between quartiles of concentrations was 0.32 (95% CI, 0.09–1.1) [calculated by the Working Group] (p for trend = 0.02) after adjustment for age, age at first birth, family history, age at menarche, body mass index, parity, age at menopause, income, marital status and plasma lipids. This association was restricted to postmenopausal women (p for trend < 0.001). The associations for α-carotene and lycopene were not significant (Potischman *et al.*, 1990, 1991b).

The relationship between serum concentrations of β-carotene, α-carotene and lycopene and the risks for breast cancer and proliferative benign breast disease were addressed in a case–control study of postmenopausal women in Boston, Massachusetts, USA (Table 8). A total of 377 women with newly diagnosed stage I or II breast cancer, 173 women with proliferative benign breast disease and 403 controls were available. No inverse association was observed between the serum concentrations of any of the carotenoids and the occurrence of breast cancer (Table 11). The relative risks for breast cancer between the highest and lowest quintiles were, after adjustment for age, alcohol intake, age at first birth, parity, family history of breast cancer, age at menarche, body weight and prior history of benign breast disease, 1.2 (95% CI,

0.7–1.9) for α-carotene, 1.2 (95% CI, 0.7–1.9) for β-carotene and 1.0 (95% CI, 0.7–1.7) for lycopene (London *et al.*, 1992).

In a study of the β-carotene concentrations in adipose tissue and breast cancers in post-menopausal women in five European countries, 347 patients were recruited from the surgical units of the participating hospitals, and 374 population controls with no history of breast cancer were selected by matching for age (Table 8). The mean β-carotene concentration was similar in the two groups; the relative risk for the highest versus the lowest tertile of β-carotene concentration, adjusted for age, study centre, reproductive factors, alcohol, body mass index and smoking, was 0.74 (95% CI, 0.45–1.2; Table 11; van't Veer *et al.*, 1996).

(vi) Cervical carcinoma

The plasma β-carotene concentrations of 78 patients with untreated uterine cervical cancer were compared with the values for 240 healthy controls (Table 8). Of the cervical cancer patients, 38% had concentrations lower than normal *(p < 0.0005;* Table 11; Orr *et al.*, 1985). [The Working Group noted that confounding factors were not adjusted for in the analysis.]

The serum β-carotene concentrations of 43 patients with dysplasia, 38 with carcinoma *in situ* and 32 with invasive cervical carcinoma were compared with those of 226 hospital controls in the United Kingdom (Table 8). The concentrations in women with invasive disease were similar to that of controls after adjustment for age, smoking, use of oral contraceptives, number of sexual partners and social class, but a reduced concentration was observed in women with preinvasive disease, and the reduction was significant for those with carcinoma *in situ* (Table 11; Harris *et al.*, 1986).

In a series of studies, the plasma β-carotene concentrations in patients with cervical cancer or cervical dysplasia were found to be significantly lower than in healthy controls in the USA (Palan *et al.*, 1988, 1991, 1992; Table 8). [The Working Group noted that confounding factors were not adjusted for.]

Two studies of patients in four Latin American countries addressed the association between the serum concentrations of various carotenoids and invasive cervical cancer (Table 8). In the first study, which concentrated on early stages of the disease in 387 cases and 670 controls, the age-adjusted associations with β-carotene, α-carotene and cryptoxanthin concentrations were significant, the relative risks between the highest and lowest quartile of serum concentrations (*p* value for trend) being 0.61 (0.0005), 0.79 (0.04) and 0.82 (0.05), respectively. No association was seen for lycopene (RR, 1.1) or lutein (RR, 1.1). After further adjustment for age at first sexual intercourse, number of sexual partners, number of pregnancies, presence of human papillomavirus 16/18, interval since last cervical Papanicolaou smear, number of household facilities and serum lipids, a significant inverse trend for β-carotene (RR, 0.72) remained, but all of the other associations became nonsignificant (Potischman *et al.*, 1991a; Table 11). The second study added cases of more advanced disease (*n* = 309) and showed results similar to those of the study of early-stage cancers, except that patients with more advanced disease had slightly lower lycopene and lutein concentrations. The concentrations of β-carotene, α-carotene and cryptoxanthin showed no trend with advancing disease. Adjustment for smoking, alcohol intake or oral contraceptive use did not alter the observed relationships (Potischman *et al.*, 1994).

(viii) Prostatic cancer

The concentrations of β-carotene were determined in 94 patients with clinically diagnosed prostatic cancer, 40 with focal prostatic cancer, 130 with benign prostatic hyperplasia and 130 hospitalized for minor surgical interventions and with no history of cancer (controls) in The Netherlands (Hayes *et al.*, 1988; Table 8). The age-adjusted mean β-carotene concentrations were significantly [(16%) calculated by the Working Group] lower in clinically diagnosed prostatic cancer patients than in controls (Table 11). No significant trends were found, however, either for clinically diagnosed prostatic cancer or for all prostatic cancers combined. The relative risks for the highest versus the lowest quintile of plasma β-carotene concentration were 0.77 for both cancer groups [calculated by the Working Group]. The lowest serum β-carotene concentrations were observed in patients whose blood had been drawn before treatment or who had advanced stages of the disease. After exclusion of those patients whose blood had been obtained after treatment, the values for subjects with advanced clinical disease were significantly lower than those for controls.

(f)   Summary of findings
The findings presented in Tables 6–11 are summarized by cancer site and study design in Table 12. The consistency, strength and any dose–response relationship of the associations are described.

The results for lung cancer were remarkably consistent, almost all studies showing an inverse association between blood β-carotene or total carotene status and lung cancer risk. All seven studies in which the possible presence of a gradient between carotene concentration and lung cancer occurrence was examined gave significant results. Although some studies showed that the strongest association was for squamous-cell carcinoma, this was not a consistent finding. In general, no associations were found for adenocarcinomas.

The positive results in cohort studies in which cases diagnosed early were excluded indicate that the explanation cannot be metabolic effects of undiagnosed cancer. Although the methods used to measure carotenoids were of variable precision, imprecision would tend to obscure rather than to account for the observed association between carotenoid concentrations and lung cancer occurrence. All of the studies considered included control for tobacco and other factors; incomplete adjustment due to mis-measurement or omission of factors remains a concern, however. There has been some suggestion of effect modification due to smoking, but relatively little information is available. The combination of carotene with other micronutrients may have a greater effect than a specific carotene alone.

The results of the few studies on cervical and oral and pharyngeal cancer are also consistent. For other sites, the aggregate results are less compelling, and the evidence for an inverse association is less strong.

4.1.1.2   *Observational studies based on dietary questionnaires*
(a)   Methodological comments
The quality of the dietary information used in epidemiological analyses is determined by the dietary assessment instrument, the method of administration, the choice of study subjects and the database used to convert information on food intake into nutrient estimates. In most epidemiological studies, food frequency questionnaires are used to glean information about the usual intake of a number of food items over a defined period of time. The more comprehensive the list of vegetables, fruits and mixed or prepared dishes containing vegetables and fruits (e.g. juices, stews, pizza and salads), the better the estimate of carotenoid intake becomes. In particular, identification of the major sources of carotenoids from national nutrition surveys appropriate for a country or ethnic population and their inclusion in a dietary interview improves its quality. Since many vegetables and fruits are consumed seasonally, inclusion of seasonal intake in an interview is important. Information on portion size, obtained for each food from specific examples or photographs, may also contribute to the quality of an interview, especially for mixed or prepared dishes. Several epidemiologial studies have been based on dietary histories rather than food frequency questionnaires. Since dietary histories include foods in the order and combinations in which they are generally eaten, they can improve the quality of the dietary information.

Structured dietary assessment instruments can be administered by trained interviewers in person or by phone. Because of the length of dietary interviews and the large number of participants in many cohort and case–control studies, however, interviews are frequently mailed, to be completed by the participant at home. In these situations, the clarity of the interview and the literacy and commitment of the study participant become critical in determining the quality of the information obtained.

In nearly all epidemiological studies of carotenoid intake and cancer published before

Table 12. Summary of results from studies (of more than 10 cases) of the association between serum or plasma concentrations of β-carotene and cancer

Site of cancer	Design	No. of studies	No. with inverse association[a]	No. with strong inverse association[b]	No. with dose–response association[c]
All	Cohort	4	2	2	–
	Nested case–control	4	2	0	2/2
	Case–control	3	2	2	1/1
Lung	Cohort	3	3	2	1/1
	Nested case–control	7	6	5	5/5
	Case–control	5	5	5	1/1
Larynx	Cohort	0	–	–	–
	Nested case–control	2	1	–	–
	Case–control	0	0	–	–
Oral and pharynx	Cohort	0	–	–	–
	Nested case–control	3	2	1	1/2
	Case–control	2	2	2	–
Oesophagus	Cohort	0	–	–	–
	Nested case–control	1	1	–	–
	Case–control	0	–	–	–
Stomach	Cohort	2	1	1	–
	Nested case–control	3	1	1	1/1
	Case–control	1	1	1	–
Colorectum	Cohort	1	0	–	–
	Nested case–control	8	0	–	–
	Case–control	2	1	0	–

Table 12 (contd)

Site of cancer	Design	No. of studies	No. with inverse association [a]	No. with strong inverse association [b]	No. with dose–response association [c]
Pancreas	Cohort	1	0	–	–
	Nested case–control	2	0	1	1/1
	Case–control	0	–	–	–
Liver	Cohort	0	–	–	–
	Nested case–control	1	0	–	–
	Case–control	2	2	2	1/1
Skin	Cohort	0	–	–	–
	Nested case–control	7	1	1	1/1
	Case–control	5	1	0	–
Breast	Cohort	0	–	–	–
	Nested case–control	4	0	–	–
	Case–control	7	3	1	1/1
Endometrium	Cohort	0	–	–	–
	Nested case–control	1	0	–	–
	Case–control	0	0	–	–
Ovary	Cohort	0	–	–	–
	Nested case–control	2	0	–	–
	Case–control	0	0	–	–
Cervix	Cohort	0	–	–	–
	Nested case–control	2	1	1	1/1
	Case–control	6	5	3	1/1

Table 12 (contd)

Site of cancer	Design	No. of studies	No. with inverse association[a]	No. with strong inverse association[b]	No. with dose–response association[c]
Prostate	Cohort	1	0	–	–
	Nested case–control	3	0	–	–
	Case–control	2	1	0	–
Bladder	Cohort	0	–	–	–
	Nested case–control	4	0	–	–
	Case–control	1	0	–	–
Kidney	Cohort	0	–	–	–
	Nested case–control	1	1	1	1/1
	Case–control	0	–	–	–
Leukaemia and lymphoma	Cohort	0	–	–	–
	Nested case–control	2	0	0	–
	Case–control	2	2	1	–
Brain, central nervous system and sympathetic nervous system	Cohort	0	–	–	–
	Nested case–control	2	0	–	–
	Case–control	2	1	1	–

[a] > 30% reduction in cancer risk or significantly reduced mean carotene level

[b] At least a 50% reduction in cancer risk or a 30% reduction in mean carotene among the studies reporting an inverse association

[c] Significant gradient; x/x, number of studies reporting a gradient per number of studies investigating a gradient among the studies reporting an inverse association

1990, the databases used to estimate the carotenoid content of specific foods were based on the food composition tables of the US Department of Agriculture (1976–94) or those of McCance and Widdowson (Paul & Southgate, 1976). Both of these sources focus on the provitamin A carotenoid content of foods, since vitamin A activity was the subject of their estimations. The laboratory techniques used, however, were for measurement of β-carotene, α-carotene, lycopene and other minor hydrocarbon carotenoids (Simpson, 1990). The estimates of most vegetables and fruits in food composition tables are reasonable estimates of β-carotene, since it is the hydrocarbon carotenoid that occurs at the highest concentration. In epidemiological studies in which these databases were used, the carotenoids estimated are referred to variously as 'carotenoids', 'provitamin A carotenoids', 'carotene' and 'β-carotene'.

Databases on the major individual carotenoids in common foods have now been published in Finland (Heinonen, 1990) and the United States (Chug-Ahuja et al., 1993; Mangels et al., 1993), specifically for lutein/zeaxanthin, β-cryptoxanthin, lycopene, α-carotene and β-carotene. In other countries, such as Spain (Olmedilla et al., 1990), this information is being incorporated and expanded for national food composition tables. The carotenoid databases rely on laboratory analyses and a selection of values from the published literature; however, the estimates of individual carotenoid concentrations are still limited by lack of information on certain vegetables and fruits and by variations in carotenoid content due to genetic manipulation of crops, agricultural practices and food processing and preparation techniques.

The validity of measurements of carotenoid intake made with food frequency questionnaires is difficult to evaluate. Correlation with blood β-carotene concentrations ranges from 0.2 to 0.3 (Roidt et al., 1988), but blood β-carotene concentrations are affected by absorption and metabolism and may be imperfect measures of biological activity at the sites of carcinogenesis. Clearly, measures of dietary intake at one time may not reflect the usual patterns of intake during

the decades that may elapse between initiation of carcinogenesis and clinical detection. Most important, intake of β-carotene and other carotenoids correlates with total vegetable and fruit intake, making it difficult to know whether any reduction in cancer risk associated with increased carotenoid intake is attributable to specific carotenoids, other phytochemicals found in vegetables and fruit or dietary patterns associated with increased vegetable and fruit intake.

Carotene intake and risks for cancers at various sites have been evaluated in a large number of studies in which intake was inferred from questionnaires on fruit and vegetable intake, without quantification of carotene intake. Those studies are not included. Others give estimates of the total carotenoid composition of the diet on the basis of a nutrient database, but fail to distinguish the intake of individual carotenoids. These studies are summarized in the Tables 13–23.

Studies based on a dietary assessment or a dietary database that provide a quantitative estimate of intake of one or more carotenoid are also summarized in the text for illustrative purposes, if they included sufficient subjects to ensure reasonable power, i.e. cohort studies with at least 50 cases per site and case–control studies with at least 100 cases.

These criteria do not necessarily enable distinction of a specific effect of a dietary carotenoid from the effect of other components of fruits and vegetables; however, the findings of investigators who attempted to resolve this issue are summarized.

(b)   Cohort studies

Table 13 summarizes the major cohort studies in which intake of carotenoids was measured.

In a study of 35 215 women aged 55–69 years in Iowa, USA, 212 new cases of cancer of the colon were documented between 1986 and 1990. The risk for colon cancer was evaluated in relation to the intake of certain nutrients, as assessed from a questionnaire on food frequency that was completed on entry and from a nutrient database [type unspecified]. No effect of total β-carotene derived from supplements and the diet was found (Bostick et al., 1993).

A self-administered semi-quantitative food frequency questionnaire was completed by 57 837 women in the Canada, and the cohort was subsequently followed from 1982 to 1987. During that period, 519 new cases of breast cancer were diagnosed. These patients were compared in a nested case–control design with 1182 women who did not have breast cancer at the time the case was diagnosed. The intake of nutrients was estimated from a database developed for other studies (Risch et al., 1988; Jain et al., 1990). Estimated β-carotene consumption was not found to have a protective effect (Rohan et al., 1993).

Responses to a semi-quantitative food frequency questionnaire were used to examine the relationship between intake of various carotenoids, vegetables and fruits and the risk for prostatic cancer in a cohort of 47 894 US male health professionals, aged 40–75 years. In this cohort, 773 cases of prostatic cancer other than stage A1 were identified, 87% of which were confirmed by medical records. The carotenoid contents of specific foods were estimated from the database of the US Department of Agriculture (Mangels et al., 1993). The intakes of β-carotene, α-carotene, lutein and β-cryptoxanthin were not associated with an increased risk. Only lycopene intake was related to a lower risk, with an age- and energy-adjusted relative risk of 0.79 (95% CI, 0.64–0.99) for high versus low quintile of intake (p for trend, 0.04). Similar patterns of risk with these five carotenoids were seen for advanced stages C and D of the disease (Giovannucci et al., 1995).

In the Finnish Mobile Clinic Health Survey, 9235 men and women were interviewed about their diet at the time of enrolment during the preceding year; 117 cases of lung cancer were found among men and 88 cases of breast cancer among women during a maximal 25-year follow-up. The composition of nutrients at baseline was estimated by reference to Finnish food composition tables. The results suggest that carotenoid intake is associated with the incidence of lung cancer in nonsmokers but not in smokers, with relative risks between the lowest and highest tertiles of 2.5 (p for trend = 0.04) and 1.1 (p for trend

= 0.91), respectively. The β-carotene, α-carotene, lycopene and lutein intakes were not significantly lower in men with lung cancer than in those without (Knekt et al., 1991). No significant associations were observed between β-carotene, lycopene or lutein intake and the incidence of breast cancer (Järvinen et al., 1997).

In a cohort study in The Netherlands of 62 573 women who had completed a self-administered dietary questionnaire on entry, 650 breast cancer cases were identified after 4.3 years of follow-up. Nutrient intake was estimated by reference to Dutch food composition tables. No association was found with the estimated intake of β-carotene (Verhoeven et al., 1997).

(c)   Case–control studies
  (i) Lung cancer
The main case–control studies of lung cancer and carotene intake are summarized in Table 14. In nearly all of them, the risk for lung cancer was lower among people with a high dietary intake of carotenoids. A clear majority of the studies, however, found stronger inverse trends with vegetable and fruit intake than with estimated carotenoid intake. Even among the Finnish men participating in the ATBC trial, who used tobacco and alcohol heavily, the dietary intake of β-carotene at baseline was inversely related to the incidence of lung cancer in both those receiving β-carotene and those receiving placebo (Albanes et al., 1996).

In the two population-based case–control studies of lung cancer in which newly documented data from the US Department of Agriculture on the content of the five major carotenoids in foods was used, statistically significant or marginally significant inverse trends in risk were seen in association with intake of lutein, α-carotene and β-carotene (Le Marchand et al., 1993; Ziegler et al., 1996). Although intake of these carotenoids was highly correlated in both populations, the analyses suggested that individual carotenoids may have independent effects.

Inverse associations with intake of carotene were observed in both ex-smokers and current smokers in all of the studies that included people

Table 13. Cohort studies (including case-control studies nested within cohorts) of the association between dietary carotenoids and cancer

Reference, country	Site of cancer	Size of cohort	No. of cases	Exposure Carotenoid	Exposure Database*	Category	RR[a]	95% CI	p for trend
Shekelle et al. (1981), USA	Lung	2 107	33	Carotene index	USDA	Quartiles	[0.59]		0.003
Kromhout (1987), Netherlands	Lung	872 men	63 (deaths)	β-Carotene	Dutch	Quartile	0.68	0.35–1.34	
Knekt et al. (1991), Finland	Lung Smokers Nonsmokers	4 538 men	93 24	Carotenoids	Finnish	Tertiles	[0.93] [0.40]		0.91 0.04
Shibata et al. (1992a), USA	Lung Male Female	11 580	94 70	β-Carotene	USDA	Tertiles	1.07 0.59	0.66–1.74 0.32–1.07	
Shibata et al. (1992b), USA	Lung	5 080 men	125	β-Carotene	USDA	Tertiles	0.98	0.59–1.63	
Steinmetz et al. (1993), USA	Lung	41 837 women	179	β-Carotene	USDA	Quartiles	0.81	0.48–1.38	0.39
Bandera et al. (1997), USA	Lung Males Females	27 544 20 456	395 130	Carotenoids	USDA	Tertiles	0.73 0.82	0.58–0.94 0.52–1.29	0.03 0.35
Ocké et al. (1997), Netherlands	Lung	561 men	54	β-Carotene	Dutch	Dichotomy	[0.96]	0.55–1.67]	
Yong et al. (1997), USA	Lung	10 068	248	Carotenoids	USDA	Quartile	0.74	0.52–1.06	0.14
Zheng et al. (1995), USA	Upper digestive tract Stomach	34 691 women	33 26	Carotene	USDA	Tertiles	0.7 0.3	0.3–1.8 0.1–1.0	0.44 <0.05
Heilbrun et al. (1989), Hawaii	Colon Rectum	8 006	102 60	β-Carotene Other carotenes β-Carotene Other carotenes	USDAM	Quintiles	[0.72] [0.74] [0.83] [0.93]		0.11 0.15 0.42 0.40
Shibata et al. (1992a), USA	Colon Male Female	11 580	97 105	β-Carotene	USDA	Tertiles	1.40 1.10	0.86–2.27 0.68–1.77	

Table 13 (contd)

Reference, country	Site of cancer	Size of cohort	No. of cases	Exposure Carotenoid	Exposure Database*	Categories	RR**	(95% CI)	P for trend
Bostick et al. (1993), USA	Colon	35 215	212	β-Carotene	NR	Quintiles	0.80	0.52–1.22	0.27
Shibata et al. (1994), USA	Pancreas	13 979	65	β-Carotene	USDA	Tertiles	0.78	0.44–1.37	
Graham et al. (1992), USA	Breast	18 586	344	Carotene	USDA	Quintiles	0.89	0.63–1.26	
Shibata et al. (1992a), USA	Breast	[~7300]	219	β-Carotene	USDA	Tertiles	0.79	0.57–1.10	
Hunter et al. (1993), USA	Breast	89 494	1439	Carotene	USDA	Quintiles	0.89	0.76–1.05	0.08
Rohan et al. (1993), Canada	Breast	56 837	519	β-Carotene	USDAM	Quintiles	0.77	0.53–1.10	0.12
Kushi et al. (1996), USA	Breast	34 387	879	Carotenoids	NR	Quintiles	0.88	0.70–1.12	0.98
Järvinen et al. (1997), Finland	Breast	4 697	88	β-Carotene Lycopene Lutein	Finnish	Tertiles	[1.01] [0.99] [1.19]		
Verhoeven et al. (1997) Netherlands	Breast	62 573	650	β-Carotene	Dutch	Quintiles	1.01	0.72–1.42	0.96
Hsing et al. (1990), USA	Prostate age < 75 age > 75	17 633	(deaths) 78 71	β-Carotene	USDA	Quartiles	1.9 0.2	1.0–3.7 0.1–0.6	< 0.05 < 0.01
Shibata et al. (1992a), USA	Prostate	[~4300]	208	β-Carotene	USDA	Tertiles	1.09	0.78–1.51	
Giovannucci et al. (1995), USA	Prostate	47894	773	α-Carotene β-Carotene β-Cryptoxanthin Lycopene Lutein	New	Quintiles	1.09 1.05 0.94 0.79 1.10	0.87–1.36 0.83–1.32 0.75–1.17 0.64–0.99 0.88–1.37	0.77 0.70 0.76 0.04 0.34
Shibata et al. (1992a) USA	Bladder Male	[~4 300]	71	β-Carotene	USDA	Tertiles	1.32	0.73–2.40	

McW, McCance and Widdowson (Paul & Southgate, 1976); McWM, McCance and Widdowson, modified by reference to country data; USDA, derived from US Department of Agriculture (1976–94); USDAM, derived from US Department of Agriculture, modified by reference to country data; Dutch, derived from Dutch food composition tables; Finnish, derived from analyses of Finnish foods (Heinonen, 1990); New = recently released data on carotenoids (Mangels et al., 1993); NR, not reported

[a] Relative risk for highest relative to lowest consumption

who had never smoked, with effects similar in magnitude to that generally observed among smokers. Diet has not been sufficiently investigated in occupationally exposed populations with increased risks for lung cancer. Inverse associations between carotenoid intake and risk have been seen consistently in men and women and in many countries but less consistently across racial subgroups, with less evidence for an effect in blacks and Hispanics than in whites and Asians. Most studies of histological specificity found inverse associations of comparable magnitude with squamous-cell, small-cell and adenocarcinoma.

Several case–control studies have been conducted on the dietary intake of individual carotenoids and lung cancer.

In a study of 106 cases of epidermoid lung cancer and 212 hospital controls, a food frequency questionnaire was administered by nutritionists, and estimates of β-carotene consumption were derived by reference to standard French food tables. The odds ratio for low versus high consumption of β-carotene was 4.1 (95% CI, 2.1–7.4). Introduction of tobacco consumption into a logistic regression analysis did not modify these associations (Dartigues *et al.*, 1990). [The Working Group noted that the measure of β-carotene used may have included other carotenoids.]

In a study of 839 cases and 772 controls, an attempt was made to recruit equal numbers of women and men by matching each female case identified with a male selected at random from among men in the Toronto, Canada, metropolitan area. A detailed, quantitative dietary history was elicited, and nutrient intake was derived by reference to a database comprising information from the US Department of Agriculture supplemented by data from Canadian sources. The estimated β-carotene consumption had no protective effect, either in models adjusted for cigarette smoking or in strata of nonsmokers or smokers (Jain *et al.*, 1990). [The Working Group noted that the measure of β-carotene used may have included other carotenoids.]

A newly available database on individual carotenoids was used to reanalyse the dietary data from a case–control study reported earlier (Le Marchand *et al.*, 1989), which involved 230 men and 102 women with lung cancer and 597

male and 268 female controls. After adjustment for smoking, inverse associations of comparable magnitude and statistically significant trends (all $p < 0.04$) were seen for dietary β-carotene, α-carotene and lutein for both men and women, while no consistent associations were found for dietary lycopene or β-cryptoxanthin. The smoking-adjusted relative risks for men and women in the lowest quartile of intake relative to those in the highest were 2.1 and 3.8, respectively, for β-carotene, 2.3 and 2.2 for α-carotene and 1.8 and 3.6 for lutein. Intake of the individual carotenoids was highly correlated, so that identification of independent effects was difficult; however, high intake (above the median) of two of these carotenoids was generally more protective to men and women combined than high intake of one, whereas high intake of all three did not confer additional protection (Le Marchand *et al.*, 1991, 1993).

Three of the case–control studies of lung cancer focused on nonsmokers, including ex-smokers and people who had never smoked. Cohort studies of lung cancer generally have too few people in the latter category to evaluate the effects of diet.

A total of 124 cases of lung cancer in nonsmoking women and 263 community-based controls were identified by random-digit dialling, and dietary histories were collected by telephone with a reduced version of the US National Cancer Institute food frequency questionnaire; nutrient intake was estimated from the National Cancer Institute data bank derived from US Department of Agriculture sources. In univariate analyses, estimated intake of β-carotene, α-carotene, cryptoxanthin and lycopene had protective effects. In an analysis with adjustment for age, education, total calories and fruit consumption, the odds ratio for vegetable consumption was 0.3 (95% CI, 0.1–0.5); the association with β-carotene intake was weaker (after adjustment for vitamin C consumption instead of fruit consumption), with an odds ratio of 0.5 (95% CI, 0.3–0.9) (Candelora *et al.*, 1992).

A population-based case–control study of lung cancer among nonsmoking white women in Missouri, USA, involved both women who had never smoked and former smokers who

Table 14. Case–control studies of the association between lung cancer and dietary carotenoids

Reference, country	Site (subgroup if any)	No. of cases	No. of controls	Exposure Carotenoid	Exposure Database	Category	OR[a]	95% CI	p for trend
Hinds et al. (1984), USA		364	627	Carotene	USDAM	Quartiles	[0.6	0.4–0.9	
Wu et al. (1985), USA	Adenocarcinoma	149 F	149 F	β-Carotene	USDA	Quartiles	[0.4	0.2–0.9]	
	Squamous cell	71 F	71 F			Dichotomy	[0.7	0.3–1.7]	
Bond et al. (1987), USA		308 M	308[b]	Carotenoid index	NR	Tertiles	[0.85	0.52–1.37]	0.001
		308 M	308[c]				[0.42	0.23–0.74]	0.32
Byers et al. (1987), USA		296 M	587	Carotene	USDAM	Quartiles	[0.56]		
		154 F	315				[0.77]		
Pastorino et al. (1987), Italy		47F	159	Carotene	McWM	Tertiles	[0.34]		
Humble et al. (1987), USA	Non-Hispanic	335	548	Carotene	USDA	Tertiles	[0.6	0.4–1.0]	
	Hispanic	132	234				[1.1]	0.6–2.0]	
Pierce et al. (1989), Australia		71 M	71	β-Carotene	McWM	Dichotomy	[0.85]	0.38–1.89]	
Fontham et al. (1988), USA		1253	1274	Carotene	USDA	Tertiles	0.88	0.70–1.11	0.29
Ho et al. (1988), Singapore		50 M	50 M	β-Carotene	NR	Quartiles	[0.3]	0.1–1.0]	0.06
Koo (1988), Hong Kong	Nonsmokers	88	137	β-Carotene	NR	Tertiles	[0.73]		0.27
Mettlin (1989), USA		569	569	β-Carotene	USDA	Quintiles	0.5		
Dartigues et al. (1990), France		106	212	β-Carotene	McWM	Dichotomy	[0.24]	0.14–0.48]	
Jain et al. (1990), Canada		839	772	β-Carotene	USDAM	Quartiles	0.89		0.95
Kalandidi et al. (1990), Greece	Nonsmokers	91	120	β-Carotene	USDAM	Quartiles	1.01	0.64–1.5	
Candelora et al. (1992), USA	Never smokers	124	263	Carotene	USDAM	Quartiles	0.3	0.1–0.6	0.0004
				β-Carotene			0.4	0.2–0.8	0.06

Table 14 (contd)

Reference, country	Site (subgroup if any)	No. of cases	No. of controls	Exposure Carotenoid	Database	Categories	OR[a]	(95% CI)	p for trend
Candelora et al. (1992) (contd)				α-Carotene			0.2	0.1–0.4	0.0005
				Lutein			0.9	0.5–1.7	0.52
				Cryptoxanthin			0.4	0.2–0.4	0.02
				Lycopene			0.6	0.3–1.2	0.13
Alavanja et al. (1993), USA	Nonsmokers	429	1021	Total	Prelim	Quintiles	0.80		0.85
				β-Carotene		Quintiles	1.00		0.83
Dorgan et al. (1993), USA		1951	1238	Carotenoids	USDA	Tertiles	[0.79]	0.64–0.97]	<0.05
Le Marchand et al. (1993), Hawaii, USA		230 M	597	β-Carotene	New	Quartiles	[0.48]		0.001
				α-Carotene			[0.43]		0.001
				Lutein			[0.56]		0.04
				Lycopene			[0.67]		0.07
				β-Cryptoxanthin			[0.91]		0.81
		102 F	268	β-Carotene			[0.26]		0.003
				α-Carotene			[0.45]		0.02
				Lutein			[0.28]		0.002
				Lycopene			[0.77]		0.83
				β-Cryptoxanthin			[0.91]		0.99
Mayne et al. (1994), USA	Nonsmokers	413	413	β-Carotene	USDA	Quartile	0.70	0.50–0.99	
Ziegler et al. (1996), USA		763	564	α-Carotene	New	Quartiles	[0.45]	0.27–0.75]	0.004
				β-Carotene			[0.63]	0.38–1.02]	0.04
				β-cryptoxanthin			[1.22]	0.76–1.92]	0.13
				Lutein/zeaxanthin			[0.62]	0.39–0.97]	0.07
				Lycopene			[0.93]	0.58–1.49]	0.87
Hu et al. (1997), China		227	227	β-Carotene	Chinese	Quartiles	0.8	0.4–1.3	0.40

Chinese, derived from Chinese food composition tables; McW, McCance and Widdowson (Paul & Southgate, 1976) tables; McWM; McCance and Widdowson tables modified by reference to country data; USDA, derived from US Department of Agriculture (1976–94); USDAM, derived from US Department of Agriculture data modified by reference to country data; Prelim, preliminary new USDA data on carotenoids (Smucker et al., 1989); New, recently released USDA data on carotenoids (Mangels et al., 1993).
[a] Odds ratio for highest relative to lowest consumption
[b] Dead controls
[c] Living controls

had quit 15 years earlier. A total of 429 cases, including 211 (49%) of adenocarcinoma, and 1021 controls were identified. A 60-item, self-administered food frequency questionnaire with semi-quantitative questions on portion size was used to characterize usual diet four years earlier, and a preliminary US Department of Agriculture database was used to estimate carotenoid intake. Interviews were conducted by proxy for the 58% of patients who had died or were too ill to be interviewed. No trends in risk by quintile of intake of β-carotene or of total carotenoids were observed, either before or after adjustment for calories (Alavanja *et al.*, 1993). [The Working Group noted that the large proportion of proxy interviews might have jeopardized the reliability of the dietary measures.]

In a population-based study of nonsmokers, 413 individually matched pairs of lung cancer cases and controls were selected from a motor vehicle license file. A food frequency questionnaire was administered by interview with about two-thirds of the lung cancer patients and by proxy for the remaining one-third; consumption of nutrients were estimated from the US National Cancer Institute database. The odds ratio for estimated consumption of β-carotene was 0.70 (95% CI, 0.50–0.99); however, the estimated consumption of raw fruits and vegetables showed a stronger effect (Mayne *et al.*, 1994).

A recently published database on individual carotenoids in US foods was used in a reanalysis of the results of a population-based case–control study of lung cancer in men in New Jersey, USA, which involved 763 patients and 564 controls, 43% of whom had to be interviewed by proxy. The usual frequency of consumption of 44 food items, including the major sources of carotenoids, about four years previously had been assessed from an interviewer-administered questionnaire. An increased risk for lung cancer was associated with low vegetable and fruit intake but was restricted to current and recent cigarette smokers and pipe and/or cigar users. The smoking-adjusted risk of current and recent smokers in the lowest quartile of α-carotene intake was more than twice that of smokers in the highest quartile of intake, whereas the corresponding risks associated with intakes of β-carotene and of lutein/zeax-

anthin were increased by 60% (Ziegler *et al.*, 1996). [The Working Group noted that the large proportion of proxy interviews might have jeopardized the reliability of the dietary measures.]

(ii) Upper aerodigestive tract cancer

The major case–control studies of upper aerodigestive tract cancer and carotene intake are summarized in Table 15. Inverse associations with carotene intake were generally not seen for oral cancer but were often significant for laryngeal and oesophageal cancer.

A study was carried out in six regions of Europe which included 1147 men with laryngeal cancer and 3057 population controls. A dietary questionnaire was administered, and the consumption of nutrients was estimated by reference to European food composition tables. Although there was a suggestion of an inverse association between cancer of the epilarynx or endolarynx and β-carotene intake in multivariate analyses, the effect disappeared after adjustment for vitamin C, although there was an inverse association with consumption of fruits, vegetables and vegetable oil (Estève *et al.*, 1996). [The Working Group noted that the measure of β-carotene used might have included other carotenoids.]

A population-based study was conducted in a high-incidence population in the north of France which comprised 743 cases (704 male and 39 female) and 1975 controls (922 male and 1053 female). Diet was defined from a questionnaire, and β-carotene intake was estimated from British food composition tables (Paul & Southgate, 1976). A significant reduction in risk was seen in association with high carotene intake (odds ratio, 0.53; *p* = 0.03) (Tuyns *et al.*, 1987a). [The Working Group noted that the measure of β-carotene used might have included other carotenoids.]

(iii) Gastric cancer

The major case–control studies of gastric cancer and carotene intake are summarized in Table 16. In general, a consistent reduction in risk with increasing consumption of foods containing carotenes was seen; however, the effect of carotene tended to be attenuated when vitamin C intake was included in the statistical model.

Table 15. Case–control studies of the association between upper aerodigestive tract cancer and dietary carotenoid

Reference, country	Site of cancer	No. of cases	No. of controls	Exposure Carotenoid	Exposure Database**	Categories	OR[a]	95% CI	p for trend
McLaughlin et al. (1988), USA	Oral and pharyngeal	571 M 300 F	642 M 337 F	Carotene	USDA	Quartiles	0.8 0.8		0.11 0.44
Rossing et al. (1989), USA	Pharyngeal	166	547	Carotenoids	USDA	Quartiles	[0.8	0.4–1.4]	0.3
Gridley et al. (1990), USA	Oral and pharyngeal (blacks)	142 M 48 F	139 M 62 F	Carotene	USDA	Quartiles	0.2 1.5		0.001 0.64
Zheng et al. (1992a), China	Oral and pharyngeal	115 M 89 F	269 M 145 F	Carotene	Chinese	Tertiles	1.31 1.37		0.34 0.29
Kune et al. (1993), Australia	Oral and pharyngeal	41 M	398 M	β-Carotene	McWM	Tertiles	0.36	0.1–0.9	0.03
Mackerras et al. (1988), USA	Larynx	151	178	Carotene	USD	Tertiles	[0.5	0.2–0.9]	
Freudenheim et al. (1992), USA	Larynx	250	250	Carotenoids	USDAM	Quartiles	0.40	0.20–0.83	0.06
Zheng et al. (1992b), China	Larynx	201	414	Carotene	Chinese	Tertiles	0.8	0.5–1.3	0.28
Estève et al. (1996), SW Europe	Larynx Endolarynx Hypolarynx/ epilarynx	1147 727 399	3057	Carotene	McWM	Quintiles	[0.60] [0.76]	0.41–0.88] 0.48–1.23]	
Ziegler et al. (1981), USA	Oesophagus	120 (deaths)	250 (deaths)	Carotene	USDA	Tertiles	[0.8]		

Table 15 (contd)

Reference, country	Site of cancer	No. of cases	No. of controls	Exposure Carotenoid	Exposure Database**	Categories	OR[a]	95% CI	p for trend
Decarli et al. (1987), Italy	Oesophagus	105	348	Carotene	USDAM	Tertiles	0.23	0.12–0.46	< 0.001
Tuyns et al. (1987a), France	Oesophagus	743	1975	Carotene	McWM	Quartiles	0.53		0.026
Brown et al. (1988), USA	Oesophagus	207	422	Carotene	USDAM	Tertiles	0.8	0.5–1.6	
Graham et al. (1990a). USA	Oesophagus	178	174	Carotene	USDA	Quartiles	0.66	0.36–1.23	0.10
Valsecchi (1992), Italy	Oesophagus	211	712	β-Carotene	USDA	Tertiles	[0.4	0.3–0.6]	
Gao et al. (1994), China	Oesophagus	624 M	851 M	Carotene	Chinese	Quartiles	0.5		< 0.001
		278 F	701 F				0.6		0.09
Hu et al. (1994), China	Oesophagus	196	392	β-Carotene	Chinese	Quartiles	0.7	0.4–1.4	0.10
Tavani et al. (1994), Italy	Oesophagus (non-smokers)	46	230	β-Carotene	Italian	Tertiles	0.4	0.2–0.9	< 0.05
Zhang et al. (1997), USA	Oesophagus and gastric cardia	95	132	β-Carotene	USDA	Quartiles	0.8	0.6–1.2	0.26

Chinese, derived from Chinese food composition tables; Italian, derived from Italian food composition tables; McW, McCance and Widdowson (Paul & Southgate, 1976) tables; McWM, McCance and Widdowson tables modified by reference to country data; USDA, derived from US Department of Agriculture (1976–94); USDAM, derived from USDA data modified by reference to country data

[a] Odds ratio for highest relative to lowest consumption

A case–control study of diet and gastric cancer carried out in four regions of Spain comprised 354 cases and 354 matched controls. Information on diet was derived from dietary history questionnaires and nutrient values from British and Spanish food composition tables. High carotene intake was associated with a modest, nonsignificant reduction in risk (odds ratio, 0.66; $p = 0.31$) (Gonzalez et al., 1994). [The Working Group noted that the method used to measure β-carotene might have included other carotenoids.]

A quantitative dietary history was administered to 246 patients with gastric cancer and 246 population controls in Canada, and intake of nutrients was estimated from a database comprising US Department of Agriculture data modified from Canadian sources. The odds ratio was 0.33 (95% CI, 0.15–0.71) for high consumption of β-carotene and 0.39 (95% CI, 0.03–4.52) for consumption of other carotenes. The effect of β-carotene disappeared when vitamin C and/or dietary fibre intake was included in the statistical model (Risch et al., 1985). [The Working Group noted that the method used to measure β-carotene might have included other carotenoids.]

In a case–control study of 1016 patients with gastric cancer and 1159 population controls, the concentrations of nutrients were determined from a food frequency questionnaire based on Italian food tables, supplemented by English data. Although there was a suggestion of an inverse association with β-carotene intake in a univariate analysis, this disappeared in a multivariate analysis that also included intake of protein, nitrites, ascorbic acid and α-tocopherol, with an odds ratio of 0.9 (95% CI, 0.7–1.1) for the highest consumption quintile in comparison with the lowest (Buiatti et al., 1990). [The Working Group noted that the method used to measure β-carotene might have included other carotenoids.]

In a population-based case–control study of gastric cancer, 338 patients and 679 controls were interviewed with a food frequency questionnaire; nutrient intake was estimated from Swedish food composition tables. Although there was an inverse association between estimated β-carotene intake 20 years previously and during adolescence, this large-ly disappeared in a multivariate analysis that incorporated estimated intake of ascorbic acid, α-tocopherol and nitrates, with an odds ratio for the highest consumption quartile of β-carotene in comparison with the lowest of 0.73 (95% CI, 0.45–1.18; p for trend, 0.1) (Hansson et al., 1994).

(iv)   Colorectal cancer

The major case–control studies of colorectal cancer and carotene intake are summarized in Table 17. The findings were not consistent: only about one-half of the studies that reported intake of carotenes showed an inverse association; many of the other studies that failed to find an effect of carotenes, however, found inverse associations with fruit and vegetable intake.

A self-administered dietary questionnaire was used in a study in which 419 patients with colorectal cancer and 732 controls were selected from an electoral register and nutrient composition was estimated from a database largely derived from British sources. The effect of β-carotene was evaluated in strata of cases of colon and rectal cancer, subdivided by sex. The only association found was an increased risk for colon cancer among women (Potter & McMichael, 1986). [The Working Group noted that the measure of β-carotene used might have included other carotenoids.]

In a case–control study of 715 patients with colorectal cancer and 727 community controls, a quantitative dietary history was elicited and nutrient consumption was estimated by reference to Australian food tables. The frequency of β-carotene consumption, presented by quintiles, did not affect the risk in a multivariate model (Kune et al., 1987). [The Working Group noted that the measure of β-carotene used might have included other carotenoids.]

In a hospital-based study in Singapore, 203 patients with colorectal cancer and 425 controls were asked about their diet one year previously on the basis of a quantitative food frequency questionnaire. Intake of nutrients was estimated from food composition tables compiled from tables for East Asian foods designed by the United Nations Food and Agricultural Organi-

Table 16. Case–control studies of the association between gastric cancer and dietary carotenoids

Reference, country	Subgroup	No. of cases	No. of controls	Exposure Carotenoid	Exposure Database	Category	OR[a]	95% CI	p for trend
Correa et al. (1985), USA	Whites	71	90	Total carotenoids	USDA	Dichotomy	0.68	0.43–1.08	
	Blacks	101	110				1.08	0.67–1.73	
Risch et al. (1985), Canada		246	246	β-Carotene	USDAM	Unit (10 000 IU/day)	0.33	0.15–0.71	0.004
				Other carotenes			0.39	0.03–4.52	
You et al. (1988), China		564	1131	Carotene	Chinese	Quartiles	0.5	0.3–0.6	
Buiatti et al. (1990), Italy		1016	1159	β-Carotene	McWN	Quintiles	0.9	0.7–1.1	
Graham et al. (1990b), USA		186 M	181 M	Carotene	USDA	1 standard deviation	0.59	0.45–0.77	
		107 F	104 F				0.71	0.51–0.99	
Boeing et al. (1991), Germany		143	579	Carotene	German	Quintiles	1.42	0.88–2.93	
La Vecchia et al. (1937a,1994), Italy		723	2024	β-Carotene	McWM	Quintiles	0.27	0.19–0.38	< 0.001
Gonzalez et al. (1994), Spain		354	354	Carotene	McWM	Quartiles	0.66		0.31
Hansson et al. (1994), Sweden		338	679	β-Carotene	McWM	Quartiles	0.73	0.45–1.18	0.10
Munoz et al. (1997), Italy	Positive family history	88	103	β-Carotene	McWM	Tertiles	0.27	0.11–0.65	< 0.05

Chinese, derived from Chinese food composition tables; German, derived from German food composition tables; McWM, McCance and Widdowson (1976) tables modified by reference to country data; USDA, derived from US Department of Agriculture data (1976–94); USDAM, derived from US Department of Agriculture data modifed by reference to country data

[a] Odds ratio for highest relative to lowest consumption

zation and the US Department of Health, Education, and Welfare. No consistent protective effect of β-carotene was found. Although the odds ratio for the medium tertile compared to the lowest estimated consumption of β-carotene for rectal cancer was significantly reduced, the odds ratio for the highest tertile was not and the *p* for trend was not significant (Lee *et al.*, 1989). [The Working Group noted that the measure of β-carotene used might have included other carotenoids.]

The semi-quantitative food frequency questionnaire developed for cohort studies by Willett *et al.* (1985) was administered by interview in a study of 746 cases of colon cancer and an equal number of neighbourhood controls. No association was found with estimated intake of β-carotene (Peters *et al.*, 1992). [The Working Group noted that the measure of β-carotene used might have included other carotenoids.]

In a study of 231 cases of colon cancer and 391 controls identified by random digit dialling, a dietary history questionnaire was administered at home. Consumption of nutrients was estimated from a database derived from US Department of Agriculture sources. An inverse association was found with the estimated consumption of β-carotene, the adjusted odds ratios being 0.4 (95% CI, 0.2–0.8) for the highest quartile compared with the lowest in men and 0.5 (0.2–1.0) in women (West *et al.*, 1989). [The Working Group noted that the measure of β-carotene used might have included other carotenoids.]

In a population-based case–control study of colon cancer among French Canadians living in Montreal, patients aged 35–79 and diagnosed during 1989–93 were identified at five major teaching hospitals in Montreal covering > 90% of the French-speaking colon cancer patients in the city. Controls were selected by a modified random digit dialling method. Finally, 200 male and 202 female cases ([55%] of those eligible) and 239 male and 429 female controls matched by age, telephone exchange and language (50% of those eligible) were interviewed at home, assisted by relatives if necessary, about their annual diet two years previously. Frequency and amount were

derived from models for more than 200 food items (Jain *et al.*, 1980a), and the intake of nutrients was estimated from a database developed for other studies (Jain *et al.*, 1990). When men and women in the highest quartile of intake were compared with those in the lowest, the relative risks associated with both β-carotene (0.72; 95% CI, 0.49–1.06) and other carotenoid intake (0.76; 95% CI, 0.52–1.11) were suggestively but not significantly reduced. Neither test for trend reached statistical significance (Ghadirian *et al.*, 1997). [The Working Group noted that the measure of β-carotene used might have included other carotenoids.]

(v) Pancreatic cancer

The major case–control studies of pancreatic cancer and carotene intake are summarized in Table 18. In the most of these studies, interviews to estimate usual dietary intake before diagnosis had to be conducted by proxy. Several reported an inverse association between estimated β-carotene intake and the risk for pancreatic cancer.

As part of the IARC SEARCH programme, five case–control studies of diet and pancreatic cancer were conducted in Australia, Canada, the Netherlands and Poland. The data from the five studies were combined in an overview analysis, resulting in a total of 802 patients and 1669 controls, 60 and 25% of whom, respectively, were interviewed by proxy. A significant inverse association was found for estimated consumption of β-carotene, adjusted for energy intake, the odds ratio for the highest quintile in comparison with the lowest being 0.37 (*p* for trend, < 0.0001) (Howe *et al.*, 1992). [The Working Group noted that the measure of β-carotene used might have included other carotenoids. In addition, it noted the difficulty in obtaining reliable data on diet from proxy interviews.]

Family members of 212 white men who had died of cancer of the pancreas and 220 controls identified by random digit dialling were interviewed about the subjects' dietary intake two years before death or the interview. Nutrient intake was estimated by reference to the database of the University of Minnesota (USA). An inverse association was found with β-carotene

Table 17. Case–control studies of the association between colorectal cancer and dietary carotenoids

Reference, country	Site	No. of cases	No. of controls	Exposure Carotenoid	Exposure Database	Category	OR[a]	95% CI	p for trend
Potter & McMichael (1986), Australia	Colon	121 M 99 F	241 M 197 F	β-Carotene	McWM	Quintiles	0.8 2.2	0.4–1.6 1.0–4.7	
	Rectum	124 M 75 F	248 M 148 F				0.9 1.5	0.4–1.7 0.6–3.6	
Kune et al. (1987), Australia	Colorectal	388 M 327 F	398 M 329 F	β-Carotene	McWM	Quintiles	[0.50] [0.38]		0.001 0.001
Tuyns et al. (1987b), Belgium	Colon Rectum	453 365	2851 2851	β-Carotene	Dutch	Quartiles	0.98 0.82		0.68 0.40
La Vecchia et al. (1988a), Italy	Colon Rectum	339 236	778 778	Carotenoids	USDAM	Tertiles	0.61 0.59		< 0.01 < 0.01
Lee et al. (1989), Singapore	Colorectal	203	425	β-Carotene	FAOM	Tertiles	0.85	0.55–1.29	
West et al. (1989), USA	Colon	112 M 119 F	185 M 206 F	β-Carotene	USDAM	Quartiles	0.4 0.5	0.2–0.8 0.2–1.0	
Whittemore et al. (1990), N. American Chinese	Colon	293	~880	β-Carotene	USDAM	'Unit'	0.89	0.82–0.95	
Freudenheim et al. (1991), USA	Colon	205 M 223 F	205 M 223 F	Carotenoids	USDA	Quartiles Quartiles	0.83 0.65	0.46–1.48 0.37–1.16	
	Rectum	293 M 151 F	277 M 146 F			Quartiles Tertiles	0.34 0.48	0.20–0.59 0.24–0.93	< 0.001
Howe et al. (1992),	Colorectal	4564	9408	β-Carotene	USDAM	Quintiles	0.89	0.75–1.05	0.07

Table 17 (contd)

Reference, country	Site	No. of cases	No. of controls	Exposure Carotenoid	Exposure Data base	Category	OR[a]	95% CI	p for trend
Peters et al. (1992), USA	Colon	746	746	β-Carotene	USDA	Quintiles	0.99 (per unit)	0.93–1.05	
Meyer & White (1993), USA	Colon	238 M	224 M	β-Carotene / Other carotenes	FAO	Quartiles	1.20 / 1.23		
		186 F	190 F	β-Carotene / Other carotenes			0.65 / 0.66		
Zaridze et al. (1993), Russia	Colorectum	217	217	β-Carotene	Russian	Quartiles	0.21	0.09–0.48	0.002
Fernandez et al. (1997), Italy	Colorectum (with family history)	112	108	β-Carotene	Italian	Tertiles	0.5	0.2–1.0	< 0.05
Ghadirian et al. (1997), Canada	Colon	402	668	β-Carotene / Other carotenes	USDAM	Quartiles	0.72 / 0.76	0.49–1.06 / 0.52–1.11	0.20 / 0.07
Slattery et al. (1997), USA	Colon	1099 M / 894 F	1290 M / 1120 F	β-Carotene	USDA	Quintiles	1.1 / 1.3	0.8–1.5 / 0.9–1.8	0.40 / 0.16

Dutch, derived from Dutch nutrient data bank; German, derived from German food composition tables; Italian, derived from Italian food composition tables; Russia, derived from Russian food composition tables; FAO, WuLeung et al. (1972); FAOM, WuLeung et al. (1972), modified by reference to Britishe, 1978) and local sources; McW, McCance and Widdowson (Paul & Southgate, 1976) tables; McWM, McCance and Widdowson tables modified by reference to country data; USDA, derived from US Department of Agriculture (1976–94); USDAM, derived from US Department of Agriculture data modified by reference to country data

[a] Odds ratio for highest relative to lowest consumption

Table 18. Case–control studies of the association between pancreatic cancer and dietary carotenoid

Reference, country	No. of cases	No. of controls	Exposure		Category	OR[a]	95% CI	p for trend
			Carotenoid	Database				
Falk et al. (1988), USA	203 M 160 F	890 M 344 F	Carotene	USDA	Tertiles	0.8 1.65		
Howe et al. (1990), Canada	249	505	β-Carotene	USDAM	Quartiles	0.93	0.57–1.51	0.77
Baghurst et al. (199*), Australia	104	253	β-Carotene	McWM	Quartiles	0.45	0.22–0.92	0.025
Bueno de Mesquita et al. (1991), Netherlands	164	480	β-Carotene	McWM	Quintiles	0.61	0.38–0.97	
Ghadirian et al. (1991), Canada	179	239	β-Carotene	USDAM	Quartiles	0.69	0.32–1.48	
Olsen et al. (1991), USA	212	220	β-Carotene	USDA	Quartiles	0.6	0.3–1.0	< 0.03
Howe et al. (1992), various	802	1669	β-Carotene	Various	Quintiles	0.37		< 0.0001

McWM, McCance and Widdowson (Paul & Southgate, 1976) tables modified by reference to country data; USDA, derived from US Department of Agriculture (1976–94); USDAM, derived from US Department of Agriculture data modified by reference to country data
[a] Odds ratio for highest relative to lowest consumption

intake in a model with adjustment for energy intake, but the association was not significant when the analysis was restricted to information derived from spouses only (Olsen *et al.*, 1991). [The Working Group noted that the measure of β-carotene used might have included other carotenoids and the difficulty in obtaining reliable data on diet from proxy interviews.]

(vi) Breast cancer

The main case–control studies of breast cancer and carotene intake are summarized in Table 19. Most reported no association with carotene intake.

In a study in which the serum concentrations of micronutrients were assessed, 214 women with breast cancer and 215 hospital controls were administered a dietary frequency questionnaire, and consumption of nutrients was estimated by reference to Italian and British sources. No protective effect of β-carotene was found (Marubini *et al.*, 1988). [The Working Group noted that the measure of β-carotene used might have included other carotenoids.]

In a population-based study, 451 case–control pairs completed a self-administered dietary questionnaire. The intake of nutrients was estimated from a database derived from British and Australian sources. Risk decreased with increasing estimated consumption of β-carotene, the relative risk at the highest concentration relative to the lowest being 0.76 (95% CI, 0.50–1.18; *p* for trend, 0.03) (Rohan *et al.*, 1988). [The Working Group noted that the measure of β-carotene used might have included other carotenoids.]

A dietary history questionnaire was administered to 250 women with breast cancer and 499 controls sampled from the general population. Nutrient intake was derived from a database based on French and British sources, supplemented by local data. No protective effect from estimated consumption of β-carotene was found (Toniolo *et al.*, 1989). [The Working Group noted that the measure of β-carotene used might have included other carotenoids.]

In a study of 150 women with breast cancer and equal numbers of hospital and neighbourhood controls, a food frequency questionnaire was administered and nutrient intake was estimated by reference to Argentine food composition tables. A weak inverse association was found with estimated β-carotene intake, adjusted for daily caloric intake, which was a major risk factor in this study. The odds ratio in comparison with neighbourhood controls was 0.90 (95% CI, 0.80–1.0), and that in comparison with hospital controls was 0.92 (0.84–1.0) (Iscovich *et al.*, 1989). [The Working Group noted that the measures of β-carotene used might have included other carotenoids.]

In a combined analysis of the original data from 12 case–control studies of diet and breast cancer comprising 4427 cases and 4341 population and 1754 hospital controls, intake of nutrients was estimated from the databases used in the original studies. An inverse association was found for the estimated consumption of β-carotene (odds ratio, 0.87; *p* < 0.007), but this was weaker than that seen with vitamin C (odds ratio, 0.69; *p* < 0.0001) (Howe *et al.*, 1990). [The Working Group noted that the measures of β-carotene used might have included other carotenoids.]

Dieticians interviewed 133 women with newly diagnosed breast cancer and 238 population controls using a structured diet history. Nutrient intake was estimated from the Dutch nutrient data bank. No significant trend with estimated consumption of β-carotene was seen (van't Veer *et al.*, 1990). [The Working Group noted that the measure of β-carotene used might have included other carotenoids.]

A quantitative food frequency questionnaire was used to assess diet one year previously for 200 women with breast cancer and 420 hospital controls. Intake of nutrients was estimated from food composition tables compiled from tables for East Asian foods, as in the study of diet and colorectal cancer (Lee *et al.*, 1989). Premenopausal women appeared to be protected by their estimated consumption of β-carotene, with an odds ratio of 0.39 (95% CI, 0.16–0.69) for the higher tertile of consumption compared with the lower (*p* for trend, 0.02), in a model that included consumption of red meat, polyunsaturated fatty acids, soya or total protein and β-carotene. In postmenopausal women, there was no significant effect of any dietary variable (Lee *et al.*, 1991). [The Working Group noted that the measure of β-carotene used might have included other carotenoids.]

In a case–control study based on a mammography screening programme, 265 women with breast cancer and 432 controls completed a self-administered food frequency questionnaire; intake of nutrients was derived by reference to Swedish food composition tables. Estimated β-carotene intake had a protective effect in a logistic regression model after adjustment for age, county of residence, month of mammography and total energy intake, the odds ratio for the highest quartile of consumption relative to the lowest being 0.6 (95% CI, 0.4–0.9; *p* for trend, 0.03) (Holmberg *et al.*, 1994). [The Working Group noted that the measure of β-carotene used might have included other carotenoids.]

In a population-based case–control study of premenopausal, white women aged ≥ 40 in western New York State, USA, cases of breast cancer diagnosed during 1986–91 were identified from pathology records at hospitals in two counties; controls matched on age and county of residence were selected from motor vehicle registers. Personal interviews were conducted with 297 patients (66% of those eligible) and 311 controls (62%). Diet was assessed by asking about the usual intake of 172 food items two years previously, and the intake of individual carotenoids was estimated from the US Department of Agriculture database for vegetables, fruits and multi-ingredient foods (Chug-Ahuja *et al.*, 1993; Mangels *et al.*, 1993). The relative risks, adjusted for known risk factors for breast cancer, for the highest quartile of intake relative to the lowest were 0.67 (95% CI, 0.42–1.08) for α-carotene, 0.46 (95% CI, 0.28–0.74) for β-carotene and 0.47 (95% CI, 0.28–0.77) for lutein/zeaxanthin; statistically significant inverse trends (all *p* values for trend, < 0.002) were seen for all three carotenoids. Little evidence of an association was seen with β-cryptoxanthin or lycopene. Comparable reductions in risk and statistically significant trends were noted for total vegetable intake (similarly adjusted RR, 0.46; 95% CI, 0.28–0.74) (Freudenheim *et al.*, 1996). [The Working Group noted the relatively low rates in both cases and controls.]

In another report from the same study, the role of family history was evaluated in relation to that of antioxidant intake. β-Carotene appeared to have no effect in women with a family history of breast cancer but had an inverse association in women with no such history (odds ratio for highest quartile compared with lowest, 0.5; 95% CI, 0.3–0.7; *p* for trend, < 0.01) (Ambrosone *et al.*, 1995). [The Working Group noted that the measure of β-carotene used might have included other carotenoids.]

(vii) Prostatic cancer

The main case–control studies of prostatic cancer and carotene intake are summarized in Table 20. Inverse associations with estimated carotene intake were reported in a few studies, but these were generally not consistent. The role of lycopene was addressed in a few studies, with mixed results.

In a study of 100 men with prostatic cancer, 100 cases of benign prostatic hypertrophy and 100 hospital controls, a quantitative food frequency questionnaire was administered, and nutrient consumption was estimated by reference to Japanese food tables. An association with estimated β-carotene consumption was found in comparisons with both patients with benign prostatic hypertrophy and hospital controls, the odds ratios for the lowest quartile of consumption relative to the highest (corrected for kcal consumption) being 2.9 (95% CI, 1.3–6.4) and 3.5 (1.52–8.06), respectively. The associations were stronger in men aged 70–79 than in those aged 50–69 (Ohno *et al.*, 1988). Similar findings from this study were presented by Oishi *et al.* (1988). [The Working Group noted that the measure of β-carotene used might have included other carotenoids.]

In a study of 358 cases of prostatic cancer and 679 controls selected by random digit dialling, the subjects were interviewed at home with a dietary history; nutrients were estimated by reference to a database derived from US Department of Agriculture sources. No associations were found with β-carotene intake when the data were stratified by age and aggressiveness of tumours (West *et al.*, 1991). [The Working Group noted that the measure of β-carotene used might have included other carotenoids.]

Table 19. Case–control studies of the association between breast cancer and dietary carotenoids

Reference, country	Subgroup	No. of cases	No. of controls	Exposure Carotenoid	Exposure Database	Category	OR[a]	95% CI	p for trend
Katsouyanni et al. (1988), Greece		120	120	Carotene	USDAM	Centiles	0.56	0.32–0.98	< 0.1
Marubini et al. (1988), Italy		214	215	β-Carotene	McWM	Quintiles	1.2	0.6–2.5	0.72
Rohan et al. (1988), Australia		451	451	β-Carotene	McWM	Quintiles	0.76	0.50–1.18	0.03
Iscovich et al. (1989), Argentina		150	150[b] 150[c]	Carotene	USDAM	Dichotomy	0.90 0.92	0.80–1.00	0.84–1.02
Toniolo et al. (1989), Italy		250	499	β-Carotene	McWM	Quartiles	1.0		
Ewertz & Gill (1990), Denmark		1486	1336	β-Carotene	Danish	Quartiles	1.17	0.93–1.47	0.16
Howe et al. (1990), several countries		4427	4341	β-Carotene	USDAM & McWM	Quintile	0.85		0.007
van't Veer et al. (1990), Netherlands		133	238	β-Carotene	Dutch	Quartiles	0.63		0.23
Graham et al. (1991), USA		439	494	Carotene	USDA	Quartiles	0.56	0.38–0.82	0.08
Ingram et al. (1991), Australia		99	209	Carotene	McWM	Dichotomy	0.8	0.5–1.4	
Lee et al. (1991), Singapore		200	420	β-Carotene	FAOM	Tertiles	0.33	0.16–0.69	0.003
Richardson et al. (1991), France		409	515	β-carotene	McWM	Tertiles	1.0	0.7–1.5	
London et al. (1992), USA		313	349	Carotene	USDA	Quintile	0.6	0.3–1.1	0.17
Levi et al. (1993a), Switzerland		107	318	β-Carotene	USDA	Tertiles	0.4		< 0.01
Zaridze et al. (1991), Russia	After menopause	81	85	β-Carotene	USSR	Quartiles	0.09	0.02–0.49	< 0.001
Holmberg et al. (1994), Sweden		265	432	β-Carotene	McWM	Quartile	0.6	0.4–0.9	0.03

Table 19 (contd)

Reference, country	Subgroup (if any)	No. of cases	No. of controls	Exposure Carotenoid	Exposure Database	Categories	OR[a]	95% CI	p for trend
Ambrosone et al. (1995), USA	Family history	38	22	β-Carotene	USDAM	Quartiles	1.0	0.4–3.0	0.3
	Family history	263	294				0.5	0.3–0.7	< 0.01
Yuan et al. (1995), China		834	834	Carotene	Chinese	Unit (90%)	0.6	0.4–0.9	
Freudenheim et al. (1996), USA		297	311	α-Carotene	New	Quartiles	0.67	0.42–1.08	0.002
				β-Carotene			0.46	0.28–0.74	< 0.001
				β-Cryptoxanthin			1.05	0.65–1.67	0.89
				Lycopene			0.87	0.55–1.39	0.24
				Lutein + zeaxanthin			0.47	0.28–0.77	< 0.001
Negri et al. (1996), Italy		2569	2588	β-Carotene	Italian	Quintiles	0.84	0.7–1.0	< 0.05
Braga et al. (1997), Italy	Age: < 45	470	472	β-Carotene	Italian	Quartiles	0.72	0.6–0.9	< 0.01
	45–54	772	694				0.77	0.7–0.9	< 0.01
	55–64	799	802				0.82	0.7–1.0	
	> 65	528	620				0.85	0.7–1.0	

Chinese, derived from Chinese food composition tables; Danish, derived from Danish food composition tables; Dutch, derived from Dutch nutrient data bank; Italian, derived from Italian food composition tables; USSR, derived from USSR food composition tables; FAOM, WuLeung et al. (1972), modified by reference to British and local sources; McWM, McCance and Widdowson (Paul & Southgate, 1976) tables modified by reference to country data; USDA, derived from US Department of Agriculture (1976–94); USDAM, derived from US Department of Agriculture data modified by reference to country data; New, recently released US Department of Agriculture on carotenoids (Mangels et al., 1993)

[a] Odds ratio for highest relative to lowest consumption
[b] Neighbourhood controls
[c] Hospital controls

Table 20. Case–control studies of the association between prostatic cancer and dietary carotenoids

Reference, country	Subgroup (if any)	No. of cases	No. of controls	Exposure Carotenoid	Exposure Database	Category	OR[a]	95% CI	p for trend
Ross et al. (1987), USA	Blacks	142	142	β-Carotene	SDA	Tertiles	0.6		
	Whites	142	142				1.0		
Kolonel et al. (1987, 1988), Hawaii	Age < 70	189	391	β-Carotene	FAO	Quartiles	1.0	0.6–1.6	0.55
				Other Carotenes			0.9	0.5–1.5	0.32
	Age > 70	263	508	β-Carotene			1.5	0.9–2.3	0.09
				Other Carotenes			1.6	1.0–2.5)	0.08
Ohno et al. (1988), Japan		100	100[b] 100[c]	β-Carotene	FAO	Quartiles	[0.34	0.15–0.76]	0.002
Mettlin et al. (1989), USA	Age < 68	169	180	β-Carotene	USDA	Quintiles	0.30	0.13–0.66	
	Age > 68	202	191				0.96	0.50–1.85	
Le Marchand et al. (1991), Hawaii	Age < 70	189	391	Lycopene	FAO	Quartiles	0.9		0.35
				Lutein			0.7		0.21
	Age > 70	263	508	Lycopene			1.1		0.57
				Lutein			1.3		0.39
West et al. (1991), USA	Age 45–67	179	385	β-Carotene	USDAM	Quartiles	0.8	0.5–1.2	
	Age 68–74	179	29				1.4	0.9–2.4	
Rohan et al. (1995), Canada		207	207	β-Carotene	USDAM	Quartiles	0.94	0.53–1.65	0.5
				Other Carotenes			0.68	0.38–1.20	0.2
Key et al. (1997), United Kingdom		328	328	Carotene	McWN	Tertiles	0.83	0.57–1.21	0.35
				Lycopene			0.99	0.68–1.45	0.88

FAO, WuLeung et al. (1972); McWN,1991 edition of McCance and Widdowson tables (Holland et al.,1991a); USDA, derived from US Department of Agriculture (1976–94); USDAM, derived from US Department of Agriculture data modified by reference to country data

[a] Odds ratio for highest relative to lowest consumption
[b] Benign prostatic hypertrophy controls
[c] Hospital controls

The results of dietary analyses in a population-based case–control study of prostatic cancer in Hawaii, USA, have been published in three articles (Kolonel *et al.,* 1987, 1988; Le Marchand *et al.,* 1991). The cases were identified through the Hawaii Tumor Registry during the period 1977–83. Among men < 70 years of age, no clear relationship between risk for prostatic cancer and intake of β-carotene or of other carotenoids was observed, but among the men aged > 70 years, the risk tended to increase with increasing intake of both β-carotene and other carotenoids. Further analysis by Le Marchand *et al.* (1991) indicated that consumption of papaya, which contributed 16% of the β-carotene intake in this population, accounted entirely for this finding. [The Working Group noted that the measure of β-carotene might have included other carotenoids.]

In a population-based case–control study in England, men aged < 75 with prostatic cancer and age-matched controls were interviewed, for a total of 328 cases (77% of those eligible) and 328 controls (81% were the first potential control identified). The usual intake of 83 food items during the previous five years was assessed from an adapted food frequency questionnaire (Bingham *et al.,* 1994). Intake of provitamin A carotenoids (referred to as 'carotene') and of lycopene was also estimated (Holland *et al.,* 1991a,b). In matched analyses, the risk for prostatic cancer was lower in men with higher provitamin A carotenoid intake, the odds ratios, adjusted for social class, being 0.69 (95% CI, 0.47–1.1) and 0.83 (95% CI, 0.57–1.2) for the middle and upper thirds of intake, respectively (*p* for trend, 0.35). Lycopene intake did not appear to be associated with an increased risk (Key *et al.,* 1997). [The Working Group noted that the measure of β-carotene used may have included other provitamin A carotenoids and that the estimate of lycopene was crude.]

(viii) Cancers of the urinary tract

The main case–control studies of cancers of the urinary bladder and kidney and carotene intake are summarized in Table 21.

In a large population-based case–control study in Canada, the role of β-carotene and other provitamin A carotenoids was evaluated for all men and women, 35–79 years of age, living in Alberta, south–central Ontario or Toronto in whom urinary bladder cancer had been diagnosed during 1979–82. Controls were matched to cases on age, sex and area ofresidence. Interviews conducted at home were used to assess diet (Howe *et al.,* 1986). The intake of neither β-carotene nor other carotenoids was associated with risk (Risch *et al.,* 1988). [The Working Group noted that the measure of β-carotene might have included other carotenoids.]

In a study of 432 men with urinary bladder cancer and 792 population and hospital controls, the questionnaire used in the study of Estève *et al.* (1996) was administered, and nutrient intake was estimated from a database derived for this study, modified by data from Spanish sources. There was no association with estimated intake of carotene (Riboli *et al.,* 1991). [The Working Group noted that the measure of β-carotene might have included other carotenoids.]

(ix) Cancers of the female genital tract

The major case–control studies of invasive cervical cancer, endometrial cancer and ovarian and vulvar cancers and carotene intake are summarized in Table 22. Several showed inverse associations. In only a few, however, was it possible to analyse the effect of other dietary factors or, in the studies of cervical cancer, the major potential confounder, human papillomavirus infection.

In a large case–control study of invasive cervical cancer among mestizos (65%), whites (30%) and other races in four Latin American countries, 748 female patients (99% of those eligible) and 1411 hospital and community controls (96%) were interviewed about their frequency of consumption as adults of 58 food items, excluding any recent dietary changes. The hospital controls were randomly selected from lists of admissions to general hospitals serving the populations from which cases were derived; the community controls were randomly selected from current census listings for the county of residence of the corresponding case.

The intakes of β-carotene and other carotenoids were estimated on the basis of typical portion sizes and Latin American food composition tables (Flores *et al.*, 1969). Risk was increased among women in the highest quartile of intake of β-carotene and other carotenoids relative to women in the lowest. The relative risks, adjusted for age, study site, presence of human papillomavirus 16/18, sexual and reproductive behaviour, screening practices and socioeconomic status, were 0.68 (95% CI, 0.5–1.0) for β-carotene and 0.61 (95% CI, 0.4–0.9) for other carotenoids, with significant *p* values for trend of 0.02 and 0.003 (Herrero *et al.*, 1991). [The Working Group noted that the measure of β-carotene used might have included other carotenoids.]

In a study in which the serum concentrations of various carotenoids were also measured, 102 women with cervical intraepithelial neoplasia and controls with normal Papanicolaou smears completed a food frequency questionnaire. Their intake of various carotenes was estimated from a programme of the US National Cancer Institute (Block *et al.*, 1994). The risk increased with decreasing consumption of nearly all of the carotenoids examined, but the adjusted odds ratio showed a significant trend (*p* = 0.02) only for lycopene consumption, with an odds ratio for the lowest to the highest quartile of consumption of 5.4 (95% CI, 1.3–23.3) (van Eewyk *et al.*, 1991). [The Working Group noted that the measure of β-carotene used might have included other carotenoids.]

The diets of 201 women with vulvar cancer diagnosed between 1985 and 1987 and 342 community controls frequency-matched on age, race and residence were assessed by interview about the usual frequency of intake of 61 food items, selected to include the major food sources of carotenoids in the diets of whites, blacks and Hispanics in the USA, on the basis of preliminary determinations of the major carotenoids in common fruits and vegetables from the US Department of Agriculture and published reports (Smucker *et al.*, 1989). The risk for vulvar cancer, adjusted for number of sexual partners, cigarette smoking and age, was inversely related to α-carotene intake, the relative risk for women in the lowest quartile of

intake relative to the highest being 1.7 (95% CI, 1.0–3.0; *p* for trend, 0.09). The intakes of β-carotene, lutein, lycopene, cryptoxanthin and all carotenoids were not related to risk. Further adjustment for duration and intensity of cigarette smoking, a history of genital infections, a previous abnormal Papanicolaou smear, socioeconomic status, race and study area did not change these results substantially (Sturgeon *et al.*, 1991).

(x) Cancers at other sites

The main case–control studies of carotene intake and cancers at other sites, including the liver and lymphoma and malignant melanoma, are summarized in Table 23.

The relationship between dietary intake of β-carotene and other carotenoids and the risk for malignant melanoma was examined in a population-based case–control study in three counties in western Washington State, USA. The study comprised 234 cases diagnosed during 1984–87 among white men and women aged 25–65 years and 248 controls, frequency-matched on age, sex and county. The subjects completed a mailed food frequency questionnaire covering the intake of 71 foods or food groups seven years earlier (Roidt *et al.*, 1988). Portion sizes of vegetables were estimated from pictures, and the intakes of β-carotene and other carotenoids were estimated on the basis of the assumptions of a WHO Expert Committee about (WHO, 1966) the distribution of vitamin A activity in various foods. The risk for malignant melanoma among men and women in the three highest quartiles of β-carotene intake, relative to those in the lowest quartile, was increased by 40–50%; however, neither the risk for the fourth quartile nor the test for trend was statistically significant. The positive relationship was strongest for men. Intake of other provitamin carotenoids was not associated with risk (Kirkpatrick *et al.*, 1994).

4.1.1.3 Intervention trials

Only β-carotene has been tested for cancer-preventive activity in intervention trials. The results of five studies involving β-carotene supplementation alone or in association with other agents have been published: the two

Table 21. Case–control studies of the association between urinary tract cancer and dietary carotenoids

Reference, country	Site of cancer	No. of cases	No. of controls	Exposure Carotenoid	Database	Category	OR[a]	95% CI	p for trend
Risch et al. (1988), Canada	Bladder	826	792	β-Carotene Other carotenes	USDAM	Quartiles	0.97 0.97	0.85–1.11 0.85–1.12	
La Vecchia et al. (1989), Italy	Bladder	163	181	Carotenoids	USDAM	Tertiles	0.31		< 0.10
Steineck et al. (1990), Sweden	Urothelial tract	323	392	Carotene	Swedish	Tertiles	0.9	0.6–1.5	
Nomura et al. (1991), Hawaii	Lower urinary tract Men Women	195 66	390 132	Carotenoids	FAO	Quartiles	0.7 0.5	0.4–1.2 0.2–1.3	0.45 0.31
Riboli et al. (1991), Spain	Bladder	432	792	Carotene	McWM	Quartiles	1.31	0.89–1.94	0.18
Vena et al. (1992), USA	Bladder (males) Age < 65 Age > 65	171 180	449 406	Carotene	USDA	Quartiles	0.45 0.72	0.26–0.78 0.41–1.27	< 0.01 0.14
Bruemmer et al. (1996), USA	Bladder	262	405	β-Carotene	FAO	Quartiles	1.08	0.64–1.82	0.86
McLaughlin et al. (1984), USA	Kidney Males Females	313 182	428 269	Carotene	NR	Quartiles	0.8 1.3		
Maclure & Willett (1990), USA	Kidney Incident Prevalent	605 203 207		β-Carotene	USDA	Quintiles	0.81 1.08	0.48–1.4 0.65–1.8	0.39 0.94

Swedish, derived from Swedish food composition tables; FAO, WuLeung et al. (1972); McWM, McCance and Widdowson (Paul & Southgate, 1976) tables modified by reference to country data; USDA, derived from US Department of Agriculture (1976–94); USDAM, derived from US Department of Agriculture data modified by reference to country data; NR, not reported

[a] Odds ratio for highest relative to lowest consumption

Table 22. Case–control studies of the association between cancers of the female genital tract and dietary carotenoids

Reference, country	Site of cancer	No. of cases	No. of controls	Exposure Carotenoid	Exposure Database	Category	OR[a]	95% CI	p for trend
Marshall et al. (1983), USA	Cervix	513	490	β-Carotene	USDA	1 standard deviation	0.86		
La Vecchia et al. (1988b),Italy	Cervix	392	392	β-Carotene	Italian	Tertiles	[0.18]	0.12–0.27]	< 0.001
Verreault et al. (1989), USA	Cervix	189	227	Carotene	McWM	Quartiles	0.6	0.3–1.2	0.11
Slattery et al. (1990), USA	Cervix	266	408	β-Carotene	USDA	Quartiles	0.99	0.56–1.76	
Ziegler et al. (1990), USA	Cervix	218	498	Carotenoids	USDA	Quartiles	[0.98]		0.72
Herrero et al. (1991), Latin America	Cervix	748	1411	β-Carotene Other carotenoids	McWM	Quartiles	0.68	0.5–1.0	0.02
La Vecchia et al. (1986), Italy	Endometrium	206	206	Carotene	USDAM	Tertiles	0.61 0.27	0.4–0.9 0.12–0.60	0.003 0.001
Barbone et al. (1993), USA	Endometrium	103	236	Carotene	USDA	Tertiles	0.4	0.2–0.8	0.007
Levi et al. (1993b), Switzerland & Italy	Endometrium	274	572	β-Carotene	McWM	Tertiles	0.49		< 0.01
Shu et al. (1993), China	Endometrium	268	268	Carotene	Chinese	Quartiles	1.3		0.72
Byers et al. (1983), USA	Ovary	274	1034	Carotene	USDA	Tertiles	[0.77]		
La Vecchia et al. (1987b), Italy	Ovary	455	1385	Carotene	USDA	Tertiles	0.94	0.55–1.61	0.17
Shu et al. (1989),China	Ovary	172	172	Carotene	Chinese	Quartiles	1.1		0.97
Slattery et al. (1989), USA	Ovary	85	492	Carotene	USDA	Tertiles	0.5	0.3–1.0	
Engle et al. (1991), USA	Ovary	71	141	β-Carotene	USDA	Quartiles	0.3	0.1–0.8	< 0.07
Risch et al. (1994), Canada	Ovary	450	564	β-Carotene Other carotenes	USDAM	4000 IU 1000 IU	0.87 0.90	0.77–0.99 0.85–0.96	0.017 0.001
Sturgeon et al. (1991), USA	Vulva	201	342	α-Carotene β-Carotene Lutein Lycopene Cryptoxanthin	Prelim	Quartiles	[0.57 [0.79 [1.02 [1.27	0.3–1.0] 0.5–1.4] 0.6–1.7] 0.8–2.0]	0.09 0.23 0.81 0.76
							[1.03	0.6–1.7]	0.36

Chinese, derived from Chinese food composition tables; Italian, derived from Italian food composition tables; McWM, McCance and Widdowson (Paul & Southgate, 1976) tables modified by reference to country data; USDA, derived from US Department of Agriculture (1976–94); USDAM, derived from US Department of Agriculture data modified by reference to country data; Prelim, preliminary new USDA data on carotenoids (Smucker et al., 1989)
[a] Odds ratio for highest relative to lowest consumption

Table 23. Case–control studies of the association between cancers at other sites and dietary carotenoids

Reference, country	Site of cancer	No. of cases	No. of controls	Exposure Carotenoid	Exposure Database	Category	OR[a]	95% CI	p for trend
La Vecchia et al. (1988c), Italy	Liver	151	1051	Carotenoids	USDAM	Tertiles	0.5		
Pan et al. (1993), Taiwan	Liver	59	101	β-Carotene	Taiwan	Quartiles	0.6	[0.2–1.4]	
Stryker et al. (1990), USA	Melanoma	204	248	Carotene	USDA	Quintiles	0.7	0.4–1.2	0.2
Kirkpatrick et al. (1994), USA	Melanoma	234	248	β-Carotene	USDA	Quartile	1.43	0.80–2.54	0.32
				Other carotenes			1.25	0.72–2.16	0.54
Tavani et al. (1997), Italy			1157	β-Carotene	Italian	Tertiles			
	Hodgkin's disease	158					0.7		
	Non-Hodgkins lymphoma	429					0.6		< 0.01
	Multiple myeloma	141					0.6		< 0.05
	Soft-tissue sarcoma	101					0.5		< 0.05

Italian, derived from Italian food composition tables; Taiwan, derived from Taiwanese food composition tables; USDA, derived from US Department of Agriculture (1976–94); USDAM , derived from US Department of Agriculture data modified by reference to country data

[a] Odds ratio for highest relative to lowest consumption

Linxian trials (Linxian1, Linxian2), the ATBC cancer prevention study, the CARET, the Physicians' Health Study (PHS) and the Skin Cancer Prevention Study (SCPS). The designs and results of the five trials are summarized here. The treatment strategies, dimensions and end-points of the first four studies are somewhat similar and are compared in the tables; the last study is considered separately.

(a) Populations (Table 24)
Linxian trials: The first study (Linxian1) involved 29 584 male and female residents of the Chinese county of Linxian aged 40–69, out of 50 000 potentially eligible participants. Subjects with debilitating diseases and prior oesophageal or gastric cancer were excluded (Blot *et al.*, 1993). The second (Linxian2) involved 3318 subjects from the same population who were found by mass balloon cytology to have oesophageal dysplasia before the start of the trial (Blot *et al.*, 1995). About one-half of the participants in each trial were men, most aged less than 60. Very high mortality rates from oesophageal (oesophagus and cardia) and gastric cancer had previously been reported in the area (Blot *et al.*, 1993); however, the rate for lung cancer in the untreated subjects was extremely low (Blot *et al.*, 1994; 2.7 per 10 000 person–years [calculated by the Working Group]). Most of the subjects were nonsmokers (70%) and nondrinkers (77%). The baseline plasma concentrations of retinol, riboflavin, ascorbic acid and β-carotene, assessed in a limited number of subjects at recruitment, were lower than those reported in western populations, as in previous surveys (Blot *et al.*, 1993).

ATBC trial: The ATBC cancer prevention study involved 29 133 residents of southwestern Finland, all men aged 50–69, all currently smoking five or more cigarettes per day, out of 54 171 potentially eligible participants. Subjects taking more than a predefined dose of supplements of vitamins E or A or β-carotene, those with a history of cancer (other than non-melanoma skin cancer) or serious debilitating disease and those treated with anticoagulants were excluded. The median age was 57 years, the median number of cigarettes smoked was 20 per day, and the median duration of smoking

was 36 years. In untreated subjects, the incidence of lung cancer was 47 per 10 000 person–years. Eighty-nine percent of the subjects drank alcoholic drinks, mostly beer and spirits, with a median ethanol intake of about 11 g/d. The baseline plasma concentrations of retinol, α-tocopherol, β-carotene, vitamin C and high-density lipoprotein cholesterol were determined for most participants and were consistent with those reported for other western populations (e.g. median serum β-carotene, 0.32 µmol/L). Advice on how to stop smoking was provided to all participants at entry, and 22% of men in each group stopped smoking during the follow-up (Alpha-Tocopherol Beta-Carotene Cancer Prevention Study Group, 1994a,b).

CARET: The Beta-Carotene and Retinol Efficacy Trial involved 14 254 current or former smokers and 4060 asbestos-exposed workers resident in six United States areas, aged 50–69, recruited by sending more than 1 400 000 letters to determine eligibility and asking for informed consent. Of these persons, 1153 had already participated in previous pilot studies, during which treatment was initiated (Goodman *et al.*, 1993; Omenn *et al.*, 1993b). The mean age was 57 years for asbestos-exposed workers and 58 years for the smokers. None of the asbestos-exposed workers were women, while they represented about one-half of the smokers. The incidence rate of lung cancer in the untreated group was 46 per 10 000 person–years. Subjects who had had cancer during the previous five years (other than non-melanoma skin cancer), aspartate aminotransferase and alkaline phosphatase activity greater than the 99% upper limits, a history of cirrhosis or hepatitis within the past 12 months, were unwilling to limit supplementation of vitamin A or β-carotene or had a Karnowski index of less than 70 and women who had undergone menopause less than one year previously were excluded. Only 3% of asbestos-exposed workers were nonsmokers, while 58% were former smokers. Of the smokers, about two-thirds were current smokers, of a mean of 24 cigarettes per day. The ex-smokers had stopped smoking on average three years before recruitment and, before quitting, had smoked a mean of 28 cigarettes per day. Of the asbestos-exposed workers

Table 24. Populations involved in four intervention trials: demographic characteristics, smoking and alcohol consumption baseline incidence or mortality for lung cancer, baseline levels of micronutrients

Variable	Linxian1	ATBC	CARET Asbestos-exposed	CARET Smokers	PHS
Number	29 584	29 133	4060	14 254	22 071
Men	13 313 (45%)	29 133	4060	7982 (56%)	22 071
Women	16 271 (55%)	–	–	6272 (44%)	–
Age	40–69	50–69	50–69	50–69	40–84
Smoking					
No	70%	–	3%	–	50%
Ex			58%	34%	39%
Current	30%	100%	39%	66%	11%
Cig./day	≥ 6/month	20 (median)	~25 (mean)	~25 (mean)	
Lung cancer incidence (per 10 000 person-years)	[2.1] (mortality)	48	43	47	6
Alcohol					
No	77%	11%	34%	33–38%	
Yes	23%	89%	66%	62–67%	
g/day (median)		11	12	9–12	
Serum micronutrients					
β-Carotene (µmol/L)	[0.11, 0.13][a]	[0.39[b] 0.32][c]	[0.21] [b]	[0.28] [b]	0.56[b]
α-Tocopherol (µ/mol/L)		[26.2[b] 26.7]	[31.1] [b]	[31.8] [b]	
Retinol (mg/dL)	35.7, 35.5[a]	58.7[b]	[62.7] [b]	[62.5] [b]	
Stopped smoking during the trial		22%	5% / year	5% year	

ATBC, Alpha-Tocopherol Beta-Carotene Cancer Prevention Study; CARET, β-Carotene and Retinol Efficiency Trial; PHS, Physicians' Health Study
[a] Mean, baseline in treatment and placebo group
[b] Mean, overall at baseline
[c] Median

in the pilot study, the ex-smokers had stopped smoking an average of 19 years before recruitment; they had been exposed to asbestos for a mean of 35 years and had spent an average of 25 years in high-risk trades such as insulating, shipyard work, plasterboard use, plumbing, shipscaling, shipfitting and sheetmetal work (Omenn et al., 1993a). Sixty-six percent of the asbestos-exposed workers, 67% of the male smokers and 62% of the female smokers drank alcoholic beverages, the median alcohol intakes being, respectively, 12, 12 and 9 g/d. The baseline plasma concentrations of retinol, α-tocopherol, β-carotene and retinyl palmitate were determined in a subset of 1182 participants and were consistent with those reported for other western populations (e.g. mean serum β-carotene, 0.27 µmol/L). Advice on stopping smoking was provided to the whole study group, resulting in a 5% quitting smoking per year, equally distributed among the study groups (Grizzle et al., 1991; Omenn et al., 1991; Goodman et al., 1992; Omenn et al,. 1994, 1996a).

PHS: The Physicians' Health Study involved 22 071 US male physicians aged 40–84, out of 261 248 potentially eligible participants and 33 211 participating in a six-month running-in phase. People with a history of cancer (excluding non-melanoma skin cancer), myocardial infarct, stroke or transient cerebral ischaemia, current hepatic or renal disease, peptic ulcer, gout, other contraindications to aspirin consumption, current use of aspirin or platelet-active drugs or nonsteroidal anti-inflammatory agents and current use of vitamin A supplement were excluded. At baseline, 11% were current smokers and 39% former smokers. The incidence of lung cancer in untreated subjects was very low: 6 per 10 000 person–years. The baseline plasma concentrations of β-carotene were quite high—0.56 µmol/L on average— almost twice as high as those in the ATBC and CARET studies (Hennekens & Eberlein, 1985; Hennekens *et al.*, 1996).

(b)   Study designs (Table 25)
Linxian: In the Linxian1 trial, a fractional factorial design was used, with treatments of: (a) retinol palmitate plus zinc oxide, (b) riboflavin plus niacin, (c) ascorbic acid plus molybdenum–yeast complex or (d) β-carotene (15 mg/d) plus selenium–yeast plus α-tocopherol. Seven treatment groups, ab, ac, ad, bc, bd, cd and abcd, and one placebo group resulted from the design. Each factor was thus administered to one-half of the population (Li, B. *et al.*, 1993). In the Linxian2 study, one group was assigned to receive a multiple vitamin supplement and the other the placebo. The daily supplementation included one multivitamin, multimineral tablet and one β-carotene capsule (15 mg/d) (Li, J.-Y. *et al.*, 1993). Treatment was for about five years in both trials. The predefined end-points were the incidence of and mortality from oesophageal and gastric cancer.
ATBC: The study had a 2 x 2 factorial design, with three treatment groups and one placebo: DL-α-tocopheryl acetate, 50 mg/d; β-carotene, 20 mg/d; β-carotene plus α-tocopherol and placebo. Treatment lasted five to eight years (median, six years). The predefined primary end-point was the incidence of and mortality from lung cancer, and the secondary end-points were the incidences of other major cancers (Alpha-Tocopherol Beta-Carotene Cancer Prevention Study Group 1994a,b; Albanes *et al.*, 1996).

CARET: This randomized, double-blinded, placebo-controlled investigation followed two pilot studies, one on asbestos-exposed workers, the other on smokers, based on treatment with 15 mg/d β-carotene plus 25 000 IU retinol or placebo and a factorial design: 30 mg β-carotene, 25 000 IU retinol, both or placebo. Treatment in the pilot studies lasted 1.5–3.3 years. The eligible subjects in these two studies were then recruited into the full-scale study, in which the intervention was daily administration of a combination of 30 mg β-carotene and 25 000 IU vitamin A as retinyl palmitate, planned for a period of six years but interrupted 21 months earlier (mean, four years). The predefined primary end-point was the incidence of lung cancer; the secondary end-points were the incidences of other cancers, including mesothelioma and prostatic cancer (Omenn *et al.*, 1991, 1994, 1996b).
PHS: This study was a 2 x 2 factorial trial of β-carotene, aspirin and placebo. The 22 071 subjects were randomly assigned to aspirin, 325 mg on alternate days; β-carotene, 50 mg on alternate days; β-carotene plus aspirin or placebo. The first component was terminated after six years because of early signs of prevention of myocardial infarct (Steering Committee of the Physicians' Health Study Research Group, 1988). The β-carotene component was continued, reaching an average of 12 years of intervention. The predefined end-points were cardiovascular disease for aspirin and cancer incidence for β-carotene (Hennekens & Eberlein, 1985; Hennekens *et al.*, 1996). All contacts with the participants were based on postal questionnaires.

(c)   Compliance, dropouts and plasma concentrations of micronutrients (Table 26)
Linxian: Compliance was assessed by monthly counts of pills and by biochemical measurements, the latter on a random subsample, at baseline and every three months (Blot *et al.*, 1993, 1995). In Linxian1, the overall rate of pill disappearance was 93% (range, 92–93% among study groups). Only 5% of the subjects were poor compliers (< 50% pill disappearance), equally distributed among the subgroups. At baseline, the plasma concentrations of micronu-

Table 25. Study design, treatment (type, dose and duration) and predefined end-points in four intervention trials

	Linxian1	Linxian2	ATBC	CARET	PHS
Study design	Fractional factorial: combination of 4 types of supplements for 7 treatment and 1 placebo groups	Randomized, double-blind, placebo-controlled: 1 treatment and 1 placebo group	2 × 2 factorial: 3 treatment and 1 placebo groups	Randomized, double-blind, placebo-controlled: 1 treatment and 1 placebo groups	2 × 2 factorial: 3 treatment and 1 placebo groups
Treatment and dose	Daily: – retinol palmitate 5000 IU + zinc oxide 22.5 mg – riboflavin 3.2 mg + niacin 40 mg – ascorbic acid 120 mg + moly-bdenum 30 μg – β-carotene 15 mg + selenium 50 μg + α-tocopherol 30 mg	Daily: β-carotene 15 mg, vitamin A acetate 10 000 IU, α-tocopherol 60 IU, ascorbic acid 180 mg, folic acid 800 μg, vitamin B complex, micro-elements, including selenium 50 μg and zinc 45 mg	Daily: α-tocopherol 50 mg or β-carotene 20 mg or α-tocopherol + β-carotene	Daily: retinol 25 000 IU + β-carotene 30 mg	On alternate days: aspirin 325 mg or β-carotene 50 mg or aspirin + β-carotene
Duration	5 years	5 years	6 years (median)	4 years (mean)	11–12 years (for β-carotene)
Predefined end-points	Oesophageal and stomach cancer, incidence and mortality	Oesophageal and stomach cancer, incidence and mortality	Lung cancer and other major cancers, incidence	Lung and other cancers, incidence	Cardiovascular disease and lung cancer, incidence

ATBC, Alpha-Tocopherol Beta-Carotene cancer prevention study; CARET, β-Carotene and Retinol Efficiency Trial; PHS, Physicians' Health Study trients were similar in all subgroups, but during treatment the concentrations of retinol, ascorbic acid and β-carotene increased in both the placebo and treatment groups, significantly more in subjects treated with the particular supplement. The plasma β-carotene concentration in the treated group (1.7 μmol/L) was 14.5-fold higher than at entry (Blot *et al.*, 1993).

ATBC: Compliance was assessed by counting capsules at a follow-up visit every four months and by plasma measurements at baseline, in random samples during the study and systematically after three years of treatment. The average overall rate of pill disappearance during the study was 93% (range, 93.1–93.4% among study groups). Dropouts, including deaths, accounted for 31.1% of the whole study group. The median plasma concentrations of micronutrients were similar at baseline in the treatment and placebo groups, but after three years of supplementation, the ratio to baseline concentration was 17.6 (up to 5.6 μmol/L) for β-carotene (Alpha-Tocopherol Beta-Carotene Cancer Prevention Study Group, 1994b). Supplementation with β-carotene did not affect the serum retinol concentrations.

CARET: Compliance was assessed in 85% of subjects by weighing the returned bottles to estimate the number of remaining capsules; in 15% of cases, assessment was based on the subjects' own estimates. Blood was collected annually from participants in the pilot study and every two years from the others (Omenn *et al.*, 1996b,c). The percent of dropouts at 36 months after randomization was 14–20% across study groups. During supplementation, the median serum concentration of β-carotene increased by 12.4-fold to 3.8 μmol/L. The retinol concentration in the treated group exceeded that in the placebo group by 10% ($p > 0.01$) (Omenn *et al.*, 1996c).

PHS: Compliance was assessed on the basis of the subjects' own reports on capsule disappearance. At the end of the 12-year follow-up, 80% of participants reported that they were still taking the pills. The blood concentrations of β-carotene were measured in a subsample of participants resident in three areas, who were visited without announcement at their offices. The average plasma concentration of people receiving β-

carotene was four times higher (2.2 μmol/L) than that of people not given the supplement (Hennekens *et al.*, 1996).

(d)   Results (Table 26)
Linxian: In the Linxian1 study, a protective effect of supplemental β-carotene, vitamin E and selenium of borderline significance was reported with regard to the incidence and mortality rates of gastric cancer (based on 539 cases and 331 deaths) when compared with untreated subjects; the relative risk for death from gastric cancer was 0.79 (95% CI, 0.64–0.99) and that for incidence was 0.84 (95% CI, 0.71–1.0). The mortality ($n = 360$) and incidence ($n = 640$) of oesophageal cancer were not affected by supplementation (mortality: RR, 0.96; 95% CI, 0.78–1.2; incidence: RR, 1.0; 95% CI, 0.87–1.2). The difference in cumulative cancer deaths began after one year of treatment for oesophageal cancer and after two years for gastric cancer. The protective effect was slightly greater in women (RR, 0.79; $p < 0.05$ versus 0.93 in men) (Blot *et al.*, 1993, 1995). The mortality rate from lung cancer was lower in the β-carotene-supplemented group but not significantly so (RR, 0.55; 95% CI, 0.26–1.1, based on 31 deaths) (Blot *et al.*, 1994).

In the Linxian2 trial, the relative risk for cancer mortality was 0.97 in men and 0.92 in women (not significant). The risk differed slightly by age in both trials, being lower in people under 55 (not significant) (Li, J.-Y. *et al.*, 1993; Blot *et al.*, 1995).

ATBC: At the end of follow-up, 894 newly diagnosed, confirmed cases of lung cancer and 553 deaths from lung cancer were reported to the Finnish Cancer Registry or on death certificates. The numbers of lung cancer cases by intervention group were: α-tocopherol, 204; β-carotene, 242; α-tocopherol plus β-carotene, 240; placebo, 208. The relative risk for lung cancer was 0.99 (95% CI, 0.87–1.1) among people receiving α-tocopherol and 1.2 (95% CI, 1.0–1.3) for those receiving β-carotene, as compared with those who did not receive the particular supplement. The cumulative incidence of cancer was similar in groups receiving and not receiving α-tocopherol, while a difference was seen in the β-carotene-treated subjects after

Table 26. Compliance (mean pill consumption), dropout rates, changes in serum β-carotene levels and effect of β-carotene supplementation on lung cancer incidence or mortality (relative risk and 95% CI) in cancer prevention trials

	Linxian 1	ATBC	CARET	PHS
Compliance	93%	93%	93%	78%
Dropout rate		31.1% (including deaths)	15% (asbestos-exp.) 20% (smokers)	20%
Change in serum β-carotene level (μmol/L)	1.5 (14.5x)	5.3 (17.6x)	3.6 (12.4x)	1.7 (4x)
Lung cancer				
Mortality	0.55 (0.26–1.14)			
Incidence				
Overall		1.16 (1.02–1.33)	1.36 (1.07–1.73)	
By smoking				
Nonsmokers		NA	NA	0.78 (0.34–1.79)
Former smokers		NA	asbestos-exposed: 2.34 (1.17–4.68) non-asbestos-exposed: 0.80 (0.44–1.45)	
Current overall		1.16 (1.02–1.33)	1.40 (1.10–1.80)	0.90 (0.58–1.40)
< 20 cig/d		0.97 (0.76–1.23)		
20–29 cig/d		1.25 (1.04–1.51)		
> 29 cig/d		1.28 (0.97–1.70)		
By alcohol consumption				
Non-drinkers		1.05 (0.82–1.35)	1.07 (0.76–1.51)	
Drinkers[a]		1.41 (1.07–1.87)	1.90 (1.11–3.24)	

ATBC, Alpha-Tocopherol, Beta-Carotene cancer prevention study; CARET, β-Carotene and Retinol Efficiency Trial; PHS, Physicians' Health Study; NA, not applicable

[a] 25.6 g/d in ATBC and > 30 g/d in CARET, as ethanol

three years of follow-up. After 7.5 years, the group receiving β-carotene had a 16% higher cumulative incidence of lung cancer than those not given β-carotene (95% CI, 2–33%). The duration of intervention was not, however, relevant when categories < 1, 1–3 and > 3 years of follow-up were considered. A similar pattern was seen for mortality from lung cancer, although the difference between the treated and untreated groups was not significant (Alpha-Tocopherol Beta-Carotene Prevention Study Group, 1994b; Albanes *et al.*, 1996).

The results of a further analysis (Albanes *et al.*, 1996) suggested that the excess risk associated with β-carotene supplementation was concentrated mainly among people who currently smoked more than 20 cigarettes per day (RR = 0.97 for 5–19 cigarettes per day (95% CI, 0.76–1.2); 1.2 for 20–29 cigarrettes per day (95% CI, 1.0–1.5) and 1.3 for > 30 cigarettes per day (95% CI, 0.97–1.7; *p* for trend = 0.15)) and who drank more than 11 g/d of ethanol (RR = 1.05 for an ethanol intake < 2.6 g/d ('non-drinkers'; 95% CI, 0.82–1.4) 1.0 for 2.60–10.9 g/d (95% CI, 0.79–1.4), 1.3 for 11.0–25.6 g/d (95% CI, 0.95–1.7) and 1.4 for > 25.6 g/d (95% CI, 1.1–1.9; *p* for trend = 0.08)). The serum concentration of β-carotene at baseline did not influence the effect of supplementation, while a high dietary intake of vitamin E (but not its baseline serum concentrations) tended to be inversely associated with the risk associated with β-carotene (p for trend = 0.03). The incidence of lung cancer in treated and untreated groups was, however, lower in people with higher baseline β-carotene plasma concentrations, as in the observational studies (Alpha-Tocopherol Beta-Carotene Prevention Study Group, 1994b; Albanes et al., 1996). The incidences (per 10 000 person–years) of cancers of the prostate (16.3 versus 13.2) and stomach (8.3 versus 6.6) were higher among people receiving β-carotene supplementation than among those who did not. Supplementation had no effect on the incidences of cancers of the urinary bladder (9.3 versus 9.0) or colorectum (9.0 versus 8.6).

CARET: By the end of the follow-up, 388 participants had developed lung cancer, of whom 254 had died. The relative risk for lung cancer incidence was 1.3 (95% CI, 1.0–1.6; p = 0.02) in the treated group, 1.4 (95% CI, 0.95–2.1) in the asbestos-exposed group, 1.4 (95% CI, 1.1–1.9) among current smokers with no exposure to asbestos and 0.80 (95% CI, 0.48–1.3) among ex-smokers with no exposure to asbestos. The heterogeneity of the relative risks was not statistically significant. The cumulative incidences in the treated and placebo groups were virtually identical for the first 18 months and then tended to diverge. Mortality rates from lung cancer followed similar patterns, the relative risk for the whole cohort being 1.5 (95% CI, 1.1–2.0) (Omenn et al., 1996b,c).

A subsequent analysis (Omenn et al., 1996c), based on a stratified, weighted log-rank statistic, with the weight function raising linearly from 0 at time of randomization to 1 at two years and thereafter, and on unweighted and weighted Cox regression models for relative risk estimates, gave the following main results: weighted analysis, relative risks for lung cancer incidence and 95% CI—all participants, 1.4 (1.1–1.7); asbestos-exposed, 1.8 (1.2–2.8); current smokers at baseline, 1.4 (1.0–1.9); former smokers at baseline (not exposed to

asbestos), 0.80 (0.44–1.4); former smokers exposed to asbestos, 2.3 (1.2–4.7); non-drinkers at baseline, 1.2 (0.80–1.8) and drinkers of > 30 g/d of ethanol, 2.0 (1.1–3.8). The excess in lung cancer risk was thus confirmed and was shown to be concentrated in people exposed to asbestos, in current smokers and in drinkers. Ex-smokers not exposed to asbestos showed no excess risk (RR, 0.80; CI, 0.44–1.4). The increase in risk tended to be constant with years of follow-up. In all groups, a baseline β-carotene plasma concentration above the median was associated with a protective effect against lung cancer (Goodman et al., 1996).

The risk tended to be concentrated among cases of large-cell carcinoma (weighted analysis not adjusted for multiple comparisons, RR = 2.2; 95% CI, 1.1–4.3, based on 63 cases). No significant difference among groups was reported for cancers at other sites. A total of 23 mesotheliomas were found, with 14 in the treated group and nine in those given the placebo (Omenn et al., 1996c). [The Working Group noted that treatment was stopped early on the basis of an interim analysis, and the risk may therefore be overestimated.]

PHS: After an average of 12 years of follow-up, there were 2562 malignant neoplasias, of which 1272 (49.6%) were in the group receiving β-carotene. A total of 169 lung cancers developed in this low-risk population, of which 82 (49%) were in the treated group. The relative risks and 95% confidence intervals associated with β-carotene supplementation were: non-smokers, 0.78 (0.34–1.8); former smokers, 1.0 (0.62–1.6) and current smokers, 0.90 (0.58–1.4). The relative risk for all cancers was 0.98 (0.91–1.1). No significant modification in risk was found by year of follow-up (categories 1–4, 1–2, 3–4, 5–9) (Fontham et al., 1995; Hennekens et al., 1996).

(e)   The Skin Cancer Prevention Study

The Skin Cancer Prevention Study involved 1188 men and 532 women with a mean age of 63.2 years from among 5232 potentially eligible subjects in four US medical centres. One aim of the study was to test the effect of oral treatment with β-carotene at 50 mg/d in the secondary prevention of non-melanoma skin cancer in people from whom a skin cancer had recently been removed. A second aim was to test the effectiveness of β-carotene in reducing the average number of new skin cancers per person–year of observation. The trial was double-blinded, placebo-controlled and randomized. About 45% of subjects had had one previous skin cancer, 20% had had two and about 34% had had three or more. About 20% were current smokers, 36% were nonsmokers and about 45% were ex-smokers. At baseline, the median β-carotene plasma concentration was 0.33 μmol/L in the group receiving treatment and 0.34 μmol/L in that given a placebo. The median duration of treatment was 4.3 years. At least 80% of the subjects had taken more than 50% of the capsules by the fourth year of treatment. Supplementation with β-carotene increased the plasma concentration by about 10-fold (to 3.3 mmol/L), while the retinol concentrations did not change. β-Carotene supplementation had no effect overall or in any subgroup of sex, age, smoking, medical centre, number of previous skin cancers, skin type, baseline plasma β-carotene or baseline plasma retinol, among the 702 participants who developed at least one new skin cancer (340 on placebo and 362 on β-carotene), and no effect was found of year of follow-up. In a subsequent report based on further follow-up, the relative risk for all deaths from cancer in the treated group was 0.83 (95% CI, 0.54–1.3). Among the smokers, the relative risk for skin cancer was 1.4 (95% CI, 0.99–2.1) (Greenberg *et al.*, 1990, 1996).

(f)   Conclusions from the five trials

With the exception of the protective effect of β-carotene at 15 mg/d in combination with selenium and α-tocopherol against gastric cancer in the main Linxian trial, which was of borderline significance, none of the studies provided evidence of a protective effect of β-carotene, alone or in combination with α–tocopherol or retinol, against any of the predefined endpoints. The reduction in gastric cancer risk reported in the Linxian trial was not confirmed in the ATBC study. The reduction began after one year of observation and may thus be attributable to an effect on very late stages of carcinogenesis or, more probably, on already

existing preclinical gastric cancers. The Linxian study also showed a nonsignificant reduction in the risk for lung cancer, which was not consistent with the results of the ATBC study or the CARET, which, on the contrary, showed excess risks for lung cancer among people given β-carotene after 18–36 months of follow-up. These findings are discussed in section 6.1. In the PHS, the incidence of lung cancer was virtually identical in the treated and untreated groups. The ATBC study and the CARET, which comprised a total of nearly 1600 cases of prostatic cancer and nearly 600 cases of colorectal cancer, showed no protective effect.

The Working Group noted several differences in the populations and study designs of the trials. The underlying incidence of lung cancer in the groups that did not receive β-carotene differed widely across studies, consistent with the different prevalences of exposure to tobacco and asbestos. The two studies that did not show an increased risk for lung cancer (Linxian and PHS) had limited power to detect a modest increase (Omenn, 1996).

The baseline plasma concentrations of β-carotene in the Linxian study were less than one-half those in the ATBC study, the CARET and the SCPS and less than one-quarter those in the PHS (see Table 24). When the inverse associations between overall mortality, cancer mortality (SCPS) and lung cancer incidence (ATBC, CARET) and baseline concentrations of β-carotene were considered independently from the treatment, they were consistent with the results of the observational studies; however, the variation in baseline β-carotene concentration was not related to the effect of β-carotene supplementation in the subgroup analyses in the ATBC study and the CARET (Albanes *et al.*, 1996; Omenn *et al.*, 1996c). The trials involved different doses and preparations of β-carotene, which may have resulted in differences in bioavailability and therefore in different plasma concentrations (see section 6.1.4). It should also be noted that β-carotene was combined with selenium and α-tocopherol in the Linxian study and with retinol in the CARET study and that the duration of treatment and of follow-up varied across the studies from four to 12 years.

The Working Group considered the possibility that differences in knowledge about their supplementation status among subjects in the ATBC study and the CARET could have resulted in the observed adverse effects on lung cancer incidence and mortality. Subjects who developed skin yellowing would be aware that they were receiving supplement. It is highly improbable, however, that any subsequent change in smoking habits or diet would have been sufficiently rapid and of such magnitude to result in the changes in lung cancer incidence and mortality observed. Further, the reports by the investigators suggest that relevant changes in lifestyle did not occur selectively.

4.1.2 Studies of intermediate end-points
Almost all of the studies with end-points other than cancer in humans have involved β-carotene rather than other carotenoids, and most have entailed experimental as opposed to epidemiological approaches. The end-points considered include: neoplasms such as colorectal adenomas that clearly are part of the carcinogenic process; other changes, including leukoplakia and cervical dysplasia, that are precursors of invasive cancer; changes in cell proliferation and induction of chromosomal damage, which play important roles in carcinogenesis and physiological or biochemical measures, such as immunological function, which may reflect susceptibility or resistance to carcinogenesis.

4.1.2.1 Observational studies of dietary and serum carotenoids
The most extensive database on this topic relates to cervical intraepithelial neoplasia (CIN). A recent review of all published analytical epidemiological studies of carotenoid measurements and the risks for CIN1, CIN2 and CIN3 (Potischman & Brinton, 1996) covered five studies in which plasma concentrations of individual carotenoids were measured; in six, dietary intake was estimated through questionnaires. Inverse associations were found in several studies for estimated concentrations of carotenoids other than lutein. Confounding and effect modification by the presence of human papillomavirus was not adequately evaluated. In a subsequent case–control study, five types of carotenoids were evaluated in the sera of women persistently infected with this virus and women who were either not persistently or not infected. After statistical adjustment, lower serum concentrations of β-caro-tene, β-crypoxanthin and lutein were found to be significantly associated with persistent infection (Giuliano et al., 1997).

The roles of various micronutrients in the etiology of colorectal adenoma were evaluated in an analysis of cohorts of health professionals. Adenomatous polyps of the left colon or rectum had been diagnosed in 564 of 15 964 women and 331 of 9490 men who had undergone endoscopy during 10- and four-year follow-up periods, respectively. The odds ratio for adenoma of the distal colon in association with the highest consumption of β-carotene as opposed to the lowest was 0.79 (95% CI, 0.58–1.1) after control for folate intake (Giovannucci et al., 1993).

The association between dietary intakes of α- and β-carotene, β-cryptoxanthin, lutein plus zeaxanthin and lycopene and the prevalence of colorectal adenomas observed by sigmoidoscopy was investigated among 488 matched pairs of men and women aged 50–74. After adjustment for other known risk factors for colorectal adenoma, no association was found (Enger et al., 1996).

In a case–control study of 472 California (USA) residents with at least one adenomatous polyp found at screening sigmoidoscopy and 502 matched controls with no polyps at screening, the plasma concentrations of six-carotenoids and of all carotenoids were evaluated. The odds ratios, adjusted for several factors including fruit and vegetable intake, revealed no association with the prevalence of polyps (Shikany et al., 1997).

The relationship between serum concentrations of micronutrients including β-carotene and precancerous gastric lesions was investigated in 3433 persons in China (Zhang et al., 1994). Among a random sample of 600 asymptomatic men and women without cancer, aged 35–64 years, the serum β-carotene concentration was strongly and independently associated with the risk for intestinal metaplasia, the risk in the highest tertile of serum β-carotene concentrations being 40% lower than that in the lowest tertile (odds ratio, 0.6; 95% CI, 0.4–0.9; *p* for trend = 0.01). More detailed analyses suggested that the major effect of serum β-carotene is on the transition from chronic atrophic gastritis, almost universal in the study population, to intestinal metaplasia but not on progression to dysplasia. The combination of high serum ascorbic acid and β-carotene concentrations was most strongly related to the risk for intestinal metaplasia (odds ratio, 0.16; 95% CI, 0.1–0.4).

In two earlier studies from Colombia (Haenszel *et al.*, 1985) and the United Kingdom (UK Subgroup of the ECP-EURONUT-IM Study Group, 1992), among 857 people who had undergone gastroscopy, serum β-carotene concentrations were also inversely associated with dysplasia. In the latter report, the inverse association between serum β-carotene and intestinal metaplasia was not statistically significant.

Among 624 men from various areas of Japan, the plasma concentrations of β-carotene were associated with a lower risk for atrophic gastritis (adjusted *p* value for trend = 0.01). Although the risk also tended to be lower with higher concentrations of plasma lycopene, the relationship was not statistically significant (adjusted *p* value for trend = 0.25) (Tsugane *et al.*, 1993).

4.1.2.2 *Experimental studies of colorectal adenoma*

Two published clinical trials specifically addressed the prevention of colorectal adenoma in patients in whom an adenoma had previously been diagnosed and removed. Both studies had a factorial design in which other nutritional interventions were assessed simultaneously with β-carotene supplementation. Neither trial provided evidence of a protective effect of β-carotene after four years of intervention. The Polyp Prevention Study (Greenberg *et al.*, 1994) was conducted at six United States academic medical centres and involved 864 patients, who were randomized by a 2 x 2 factorial design in which the factors were 25 mg/d β-carotene and a combination of vitamins C and E. The study was double-blinded, and follow-up consisted of colonoscopy performed one year and four years after enrolment. The

principal end-point of interest was the occurrence of new colorectal adenomas between the first and the final follow-up colonoscopy; about 35% of the patients had a new adenoma. β-Carotene appeared to have no effect in the 751 patients who completed the full four years of the study (RR, 1.0; 95% CI, 0.85–1.2). There was also no evidence of efficacy in subgroups defined by lower initial serum concentration of β-carotene or in subgroups stratified by age, sex, proximal or distal site of adenoma in the colorectum or number of prior adenomas.

The Australian Polyp Prevention Trial (MacLennan *et al.*, 1995) also included patients with a recently removed colorectal adenoma who were randomized by a 2 x 2 x 2 factorial design to 20 mg/d β-carotene, fat reduction or supplemental wheat bran fibre. Follow-up colonoscopy was conducted two years and four years after randomization. Of the 424 randomized patients, 390 completed the two-year examination and 306 the four-year examination; an adenoma was diagnosed in about 30% at the four-year examination. There was no evidence of a reduction in incidence in the group receiving β-carotene (odds ratio, 1.3; 95% CI, 0.8–2.2). The adenomas in the group receiving β-carotene tended to be larger than 1 cm, but there were relatively few such lesions, and the results were not statistically significant.

A report of a third, somewhat smaller trial has been published only in abstract form (Kikendall *et al.*, 1990, 1991).

4.1.2.3 *Experimental studies of cellular dysplasia and atypia*

The effects of β-carotene supplementation on the progression or regression of cellular dysplasia or atypia in the cervix, oesophagus or lung have been examined in seven trials. None showed clear evidence of efficacy. In a trial in the Netherlands (de Vet *et al.*, 1991), 278 patients were randomized to receive 10 mg/d β-carotene or a placebo for three months. All of the patients had cervical dysplasia at entry into the study, and they were randomized in strata according to the severity of the dysplasia. The recorded outcome was progression or regression of cellular changes. When a relatively liberal definition of regression was used and adjustment was made for various prognostic variables, there was no evidence that β-carotene-treated patients were more likely to have regressed lesions (odds ratio, 0.68; 95% CI, 0.28–1.6). When strict criteria for regression were used, patients receiving β-carotene seemed slightly less likely to have regression (odds ratio, 1.2; 95% CI, 0.43–3.4), but neither of the results was statistically significant. An analysis in which compliance with the medication was taken into account still gave no evidence of a greater probability of regression in the group receiving β-carotene.

In an uncontrolled trial in the United States, reported in preliminary form (Meyskens & Manetta, 1995), 30 patients with cervical dysplasia were given 30 mg/d β-carotene for three months; those whose severity of dysplasia did not change or regress were treated for an additional three months. There were no control patients. The authors reported a 70% probability of remission at six months; at 12 months (six months after stopping β-carotene), only 33% of the patients had a lesser degree of dysplasia than at entry into the study.

In the large community intervention in Linxian, China, β-carotene (15 mg/d) was given in combination with vitamin E and selenium to more than 29 000 randomized patients. In 391 patients who underwent oesophageal and gastric endoscopy in a search for occult cancer and dysplasia, no significant difference was observed among people receiving and not receiving the supplement; 16 of 214 untreated patients had dysplasia as opposed to 13 of 177 patients treated with the combination (Wang, G. *et al.*, 1994). A total of 3318 men and women participating in the trial of dysplasia had grade 1 or 2 oesophageal dysplasia at baseline and were subsequently given supplementation with 25 vitamins and minerals, including 15 mg β-carotene, for six years. The supplemented group was significantly more likely to have reversion of dysplasia at the end of follow-up as compared with the placebo group (odds ratio, 1.2; 95% CI, 1.1–1.4) (Mark *et al.*, 1994).

In a study of 755 men and women in Texas, USA, exposed to asbestos, 50 mg/d β-carotene was administered with 25 000 IU retinol on alternate days. Patients were randomized, with stratification by the presence of atypia in spu-

tum. The median length of follow-up was about five years. The authors reported no difference in the frequency of cytological abnormalities: 46 of 349 β-carotene-treated patients versus 37 of 338 placebo-treated patients had moderate atypia or worse at the end of the intervention, as assessed by cytology (McLarty, 1995).

4.1.2.4 *Experimental studies of oral leukoplakia*

Perhaps the largest number of intervention studies that suggest a beneficial effect of β-carotene involved treatment of patients with oral leukoplakia, a lesion with a definite, though modest, probability of progressing to invasive cancer (Garewal, 1995). In these studies, the measured end-point has usually been regression of the size of the visible leukoplakia, which is largely subjective, although assessment based on histological evidence is also difficult because of the usually patchy distribution of the lesion. The published intervention studies have entailed relatively short periods of supplementation with β-carotene (three to nine months), and only a few involved a placebo-treated comparison group; randomization was not often performed, and in most the investigators were aware of the treatment the patients were receiving.

In a randomized, placebo-controlled, double-blinded trial in Uzbekistan, six months of treatment with a combination of β-carotene, retinol and vitamin E led to a significant reduction in the prevalence odds ratio for oral leukoplakia (odds ratio, 0.62; 95% CI, 0.39–0.98). The risk for progression or no change versus regression was reduced by 40% by this intervention, although not statistically significantly (odds ratio, 0.60; 95% CI, 0.23–1.6) (Zaridze *et al.*, 1993).

In a study of chewers of tobacco and betel quid in Kerala (India), 130 people with oral leukoplakia were assigned to treatment with 180 mg β-carotene per week, β-carotene plus vitamin A or placebo, for six months. Regression of leukoplakia was assessed by marking the location and dimensions of the lesions on a chart of the oral cavity and by examining photographs. The assessed end-points were either complete remission of leukoplakia or the appearance of new lesions. Three and six months after the beginning of therapy, there was no statistically significant difference between the group receiving β-carotene alone and the group receiving placebo with regard to remission or development of new leukoplakia. At six months, however, there was a modestly lower, but not statistically significant, risk for new leukoplakia, which was seen in four of 27 patients receiving β-carotene and seven of 33 patients receiving placebo. At six months, four of 27 patients given β-carotene and one of 33 on placebo showed evidence of remission. A statistically significantly larger proportion of patients receiving β-carotene plus vitamin A showed regression of leukoplakia than in the group receiving placebo (Stich et al., 1988).

In another study in the same area of India, 160 men and women with oral leukoplakia were randomized to receive either vitamin A (300 000 IU per week, $n = 50$), β-carotene (360 mg/week, $n = 55$) or placebo ($n = 55$) for 12 months. Complete regression was achieved in 10% of those on placebo, 52% of those given vitamin A and 33% given β-carotene. Homogeneous leukoplakias and smaller lesions responded better than non-homogeneous and larger lesions. One-half of the group on β-carotene and two-thirds of those given vitamin A showed relapse after withdrawal of the supplementation (Sankaranarayanan et al., 1997).

Other intervention studies of β-carotene and oral leukoplakia did not involve placebo controls. Among 24 patients treated in Arizona (USA) with 30 mg/d β-carotene for three months (Garewal et al., 1990), two had complete remission and 15 partial remission at the end of treatment. In an uncontrolled study in Canada, 18 patients were treated with 120 mg/d β-carotene for three months. Four patients had a complete or partial remission, and one appeared to have worsening of the oral lesions. Seventeen of these patients were continued for an additional three months on β-carotene. By the end of the study, eight patients were found to have an improvement in their oral leukoplakia, and nine were assessed as stable. The authors suggested that smokers had a better response to β-carotene (Malaker et al., 1991). In a study in Italy, 18 evaluable patients received 90 mg/d β-carotene for nine

months, when six showed complete remission and two, partial remission. The patients were followed-up after the end of treatment for between two and seven months. After β-carotene supplementation was stopped, an additional four patients were found to have complete remission of their leukoplakia, and one had a partial response (Toma et al., 1992).

In the United States, 79 patients with leukoplakia received a combination of 30 mg/d β-carotene with 1 g vitamin C and 800 IU vitamin E, for nine months. At the end of treatment, 56% of the patients had clinical improvement, which was greatest in those who had diminished their use of alcohol and tobacco (Kaugars et al., 1994).

4.1.2.5 Experimental studies of cell proliferation

Measures of the proportion of proliferating cells in the rectal crypt, such as the labelling index, have been suggested for use as indicators of risk for colorectal cancer. The effect of β-carotene, alone or in combination with other vitamins, on these measures of proliferation has been assessed in three intervention studies.

Within a randomized, multifactorial trial of polyp prevention in Australia, 24 patients were given 30 mg/d β-carotene and 17 were given placebo; all underwent rectal mucosal biopsy two to four years after randomization. Cell proliferation was determined by staining for proliferating cell nuclear antigen in five rectal mucosal crypts. No significant difference in total labelling index was found between the group receiving β-carotene and that receiving placebo, but patients taking β-carotene had a significantly lower proportion of labelled cells in the top 40% of the crypt (Macrae et al., 1991). It has been suggested that a higher proportion of proliferating cells in the upper crypt represents initial evidence of neoplastic transformation (Lipkin et al., 1994).

A subsequent report from Ireland indicated that β-carotene supplementation significantly ($p < 0.005$, signed rank sum test) reduced the total labelling index in the rectal crypt. Among 10 patients randomly assigned to receive 9 mg/d β-carotene, the labelling index in 10 rectal crypts dropped from 7.1% before the trial to 3.9% after the one-month intervention. The control group showed only a modest change in labelling index, from 6.9 to 6.6% after the intervention. The decrease in proliferation was seen only in the lower 60% of the crypt, and there was no significant reduction in proliferating cells in the higher 40% (Cahill *et al.*, 1993). [The Working Group noted that the authors reported only measures before and after intervention and no formal assessment of the difference between the treated and placebo groups.]

The largest trial of the effects of β-carotene in mucosal crypt labelling was reported from Illinois, USA, and involved 41 individuals who had had colorectal cancer and 40 who had had an adenoma. The participants were assigned at random to receive 30 mg/d β-carotene or placebo for 90 days. The labelling index, determined for proliferating cell nuclear antigen in at least three crypts per biopsy, was assessed before randomization and after three months, at the end of the intervention. β-Carotene had no significant effect on the total labelling index, and no significant difference was found in labelling in the lower, middle or upper third of the crypt compartment (Frommel *et al.*, 1995). [The Working Group noted the large fluctuations in the before-and-after measures of labelling among groups and that the proportion of labelled cells was substantially higher (> 20%) than in the other reports discussed here.]

Biochemical measures that may reflect cell proliferation include ornithine decarboxylase activity and excretion of N-acetylspermidine. Both measures were assessed in the study in Illinois summarized above (Frommel *et al.*, 1995), with no consistent evidence of an effect of β-carotene. An earlier report from the USA, however, found a significant decrease in ornithine decarboxylase activity from pretreatment values among 20 men who had previously had colon cancer and were assigned to receive 30 mg/d β-carotene for six months (Phillips *et al.*, 1993). [The Working Group noted that no control subjects were included.]

In a study in the Russian Federation, 44 patients with chronic atrophic gastritis were treated with 20 mg/d β-carotene for three weeks. Ornithine decarboxylase activity in the gastric mucosa was significantly lower than before treatment and than in 19 control patients who did not receive β-carotene (Bukin *et al.*, 1993). [The Working Group noted that treatment was not assigned at random and that few data were presented on the comparability of these groups.]

4.1.2.6 Experimental studies of chromosomal damage

Chromosomal damage includes micronuclei and sister chromatid exchange, which are generally evaluated in cell scrapings or sputum specimens. Almost all of the studies were based on oral and bronchial mucosal specimens.

Most of the studies of micronucleus formation have come from one group of investigators at the British Columbia Cancer Research Centre in Canada. They initially conducted a pilot study (described above in the discussion of leukoplakia) among betel chewers in Kerala, India. People given 180 mg β-carotene weekly for four months showed a significant decrease in the number of micronuclei per cell (Stich *et al.*, 1988, 1990a). In a similar study, in which the independent effects of β-carotene, canthaxanthin and retinol were compared, a significant decrease was noted in micronucleus counts after administration of β-carotene and retinol, but no change was observed with canthaxanthin (Stich *et al.*, 1984). A pilot study was also conducted among Inuits who used tobacco snuff regularly. Their oral mucosa contained ample amounts of retinol but relatively small amounts of β-carotene. A statistically significant ($p < 0.001$) decrease in micronucleus count, from 1.9 to 0.7%, was seen in 23 people given 180 mg β-carotene per week for 10 weeks, whereas no significant change was found in 10 people given a placebo (Stich *et al.*, 1985).

In a randomized double-blinded trial of the effects of β-carotene on sister chromatid exchange, 70 healthy male smokers in The Netherlands were assigned to receive 20 mg/d β-carotene for 14 weeks and 73 to placebo. Sister chromatid exchange was evaluated as the mean number per lymphocyte. The counts were similar at the end of treatment: 4.4 versus 4.2, respectively. [The Working Group noted that the reliability of the measurement of sister chromatid exchange in this trial was questionable; the absolute count decreased in both treated and control groups and the standard deviation of the counts after treatment was reduced by more than one-half.] In the same study, 14 weeks of supplemental β-carotene at 20 mg/d significantly reduced the micronucleus counts in sputum from 114 heavy smokers: the counts decreased by 16% in the 61 men receiving placebo and by 27% in those receiving β-carotene ($p < 0.05$), after adjustment for the initial concentrations (van Poppel *et al.*, 1992).

A study among cigarette smokers in South Africa involved random assignment of 60 subjects to three treatment groups: 40 mg/d β-carotene, 900 IU/d vitamin E or placebo. After six weeks of treatment, no change was observed in the frequency of sister chromatid exchange in peripheral blood lymphocytes (Richards *et al.*, 1990).

4.1.2.7 Experimental studies of immunological end-points

The effect of carotenoid supplementation on immunological function in humans has been examined in studies with various end-points. The results have been mixed: some studies indicate increased immunological function after supplementation and others no change. Relatively few of the studies had a randomized, placebo-controlled design, and most were simple comparisons of measures taken before and after treatment. The studies have focused exclusively on β-carotene.

Nine men with Barrett's oesophagus in Tucson (USA) had a statistically significant increase in the proportion of lymphocytes with natural killer (NK) and HLA-DR markers after two months' treatment with 30 mg/d β-carotene. They also had a nonsignificant increase in the proportion of cells with T-helper, interleukin (IL)-2R and transferrin receptor markers (Prabhala *et al.*, 1991). A further report from the same group, on 20 healthy men and women, indicated that the increase in T-helper (CD4+) cells was significant at doses of, e.g. 30, 45 and 60 mg/d but not at 15 mg/d, and that there had been a possibly similar dose-dependent increase in cells with NK, transferrin receptor and IL-2 receptors (Watson *et al.*, 1991). [The Working Group noted that only four patients were randomized to each dose and the comparisons were of status before and after rather than of changes between patients receiving β-carotene and those receiving placebo.]

A randomized controlled trial of 50 adults in Michigan (USA), however, showed no evidence of a change in immunological markers with β-carotene treatment. Groups of 10 received β-carotene at a dose of 15, 45, 180 or 300 mg/d or placebo for four weeks. No significant change was found in the total number or percentage of peripheral B cells, T cells, T-cell subsets, NK cells or HLA-DR- or IL-2R-expressing cells, and there was no significant change in the proliferative response after OKT3-antibody stimulation or in the production of IL-2 by stimulated peripheral blood mononuclear cells (Ringer *et al.*, 1991). [The Working Group noted that some of the differences between these results and those noted above may have been due to the shorter duration of the latter study; in Tucson, immunological changes were found only after two months of treatment.]

Mixed findings were also reported from Japan in a study of 20 university-age volunteers who were randomized to 20 mg/d β-caroteneor placebo for nine months. A significant increase was found in the CD4:CD8 ratio but no change in NK cells, virgin T cells, cytotoxic T cells or memory T cells (Murata *et al.*, 1994).

Exposure to UV light has been reported to suppress delayed-type hypersensitivity in the skin. In a study in New York (USA), 24 healthy men were assigned randomly to 30 mg/d β-carotene or placebo. After 28 days, all received dermal exposure to UV light, and their responses to antigens were assessed over the next 21 days. Men on placebo showed a statistically significant decrease in delayed-type hypersensitivity, whereas those on β-carotene showed only a slight, nonsignificant decrease (Fuller *et al.*, 1992). [The Working Group noted that the diminution in delayed-type hypersensitivity was not compared directly in the treated and control groups; however, the data indicate that the difference was probably not statistically significant.]

A group of 45 male cigarette smokers in The Netherlands were randomized to receive 20 mg/d β-carotene or placebo for 14 weeks. No effect of the treatment was noted on lymphocyte subpopulations in peripheral blood, as measured by 10 markers; however, the proliferative response to phytohaemagglutinin was 12% higher in the group receiving β-carotene, and this difference was statistically significant. The response pertained only to cells stimulated in plasma; it appeared even to be decreased in cells in fetal calf serum, and there was no change in the response to concanavalin A (van Poppel *et al.*, 1993). [The Working Group noted that many immunological end-points were measured, and the multiplicity of comparisons was not taken into acount in calculating the *p* values.]

A report from the Physicians' Health Study involved a subset of 59 male physicians chosen from among participants in the Boston (USA) area, 29 of whom had been randomized to receive 50 mg β-carotene every other day for about 10 years and 30 of whom had received placebo. Participants ≥ 65 years had lower NK cell activity than younger men; however, older men receiving β-carotene had significantly greater NK activity than those on placebo. No treatment-associated differences were seen in men under 65. The older men showed no differences in the proportion of NK cells or in IL-2 receptor expression (Santos *et al.*, 1996). In a subsequent report from this group of investigators, the effects of β-carotene were evaluated in 11 healthy elderly women assigned to receive 90 mg/d β-carotene for three weeks. No difference in delayed-type hypersensitivity skin responses was seen in comparison with 12 control women receiving placebo. Similarly, there were no differences in a variety of other immunological measures, including proportions of lymphocyte subpopulations, lymphocyte proliferation *in vitro* and production of IL-2 (Santos *et al.*, 1997).

The effects of β-carotene in conjunction with other supplements or as a component of diet have been addressed in three studies. The delayed hypersensitivity response was reported to be stronger after 12 months of supplementation with multivitamins which included β-carotene (Bogden *et al.*, 1994); and among participants in the Linxian trial, the group receiving β-carotene, vitamin E and selenium had significantly higher T-lymphocyte mitogenic responsiveness *in vitro* (Zhang *et al.*, 1995). In a group of nine healthy women who were placed on a β-carotene-depleted diet for 68 days and then given 15 mg/d β-carotene, no effects were seen on the numbers of immunological cells or on the peripheral blood mononuclear cell proliferative response to phytohaemagglutinin or concanavalin A (Daudu *et al.*, 1994) .

A randomized trial in England involved 25 participants who received either 15 mg/d β-carotene or placebo for 28 days and were then crossed over to the other treatment. Blood was collected for the analysis of a number of immunological measures at baseline and at the end of each of the two intervention periods. There was a statistically significant increase in the activity of tumour necrosis factor-α after supplementation, and an increase was seen in the proportion of monocytes expressing HLA-DR, intracellular adhesion molecule-1 and leukocyte function-associated antigen-3 (Hughes *et al.*, 1997).

In a randomized trial in Illinois (USA), 40 patients with a history of colorectal polyps and 40 with a prior colorectal cancer received 30 mg/d β-carotene or placebo for three months. At the end of the intervention, the counts of CD4+ T cells and IL-2R-expressing lymphocytes were significantly increased among the cancer patients given β-carotene but not among the patients with polyps. There were no clear changes in other measures, including CD8+ counts, CD4:CD8 ratios or NK cell counts (Kazi *et al.*, 1997). [The Working Group noted the loss of some blood specimens and the lack of direct statistical comparisons of treated and control groups.]

4.1.2.8 *Summary*

The effects of β-carotene (and, to a lesser extent, canthaxanthin) on possible antecedents of malignancy have been addressed in a substantial number of investigations. They provide strong evidence of a lack of efficacy of short-term supplementation with β-carotene in preventing colorectal adenomas, a neoplasm that can be a precursor for invasive cancer, but the interventions were of relatively brief duration. The reports of clinical studies generally show regression of oral leukoplakia; however, in most of the trials, the design was not randomized or double-blinded and the assessment of leukoplakia was often subjective. The results of studies of other measures of possible relevance to carcinogenesis, such as cytogenetic abnormalities, have also been inconsistent. On balance, intervention studies of carotenoids and premalignant lesions show no consistent pattern of protection.

4.2   Experimental models
4.2.1   Experimental animals
4.2.1.1   β-Carotene
(a)   Skin (Table 27)

Mouse: Two groups of two-month old albino hairless mice (University of California strain [sex unspecified]) received intraperitoneal injections of β-carotene (beadlets containing 10% β-carotene dissolved in distilled water at a concentration of 250 mg/ml) or placebo (filler of the beadlets) dissolved in distilled water three times a week for six months. During the first month, 61 mice given β-carotene and 56 mice given the placebo received 0.4-ml injections, providing 10 mg β-carotene for the supplemented animals; for the remaining five months they received 0.2-ml injections, providing 5 mg β-carotene One month after the start of the injections, UV irradiation at 6.5×10^3 J/m^2 (mainly UV-B) was initiated and continued three times a week for the duration of the study, 15 months. Skin tumours > 4 and > 50 mm^3 were registered. Eight of the mice with large tumours, five receiving β-carotene and three receiving the placebo, were killed, and the tumours were examined histologically. The tumours were all relatively well-differentiated squamous-cell carcinomas which had invaded the dermis and subcutaneous tissue. Mortality was relatively high, amounting to 18/61 and 35/61 animals receiving β-carotene and 12/56 and 32/56 controls after two and seven months, respectively. The first tumours > 4 and > 50 mm^3 were found in mice on β-carotene after 7.75 and 8 months, respectively, and both sizes of tumour were found in controls after 7.25

months. After 12 months, 53 and 40% of the tumours in mice given β-carotene and 80 and 75% of the those in controls were > 4 and > 50 mm^3, respectively. The numbers of mice per survivors with tumours > 4 mm^3 were 2/24 after 40 weeks, 6/21 after 47 weeks ($p = 0.03$; χ^2 test for 2 x 2 contingency tables) and 8/15 after 52 weeks ($p = 0.0761$) among animals given β-carotene, and 2/22, 13/21 and 17/21, respectively, in controls. The numbers of mice per survivors with tumours > 50 mm^3 were 1/24 and 1/22 after 40 weeks, 5/21 and 10/21 after 47 weeks ($p = 0.1074$) and 6/15 and 16/21 after 52 weeks ($p = 0.0281$) in animals given β-carotene and placebo, respectively (Epstein, 1977).

Four groups of 75 female Swiss albino 955 mice, nine to ten weeks old, were painted on a clipped, mid-dorsal area of the skin with 0.02 ml of a 0.5% solution of benzo[*a*]pyrene in acetone (0.1 mg benzo[*a*]pyrene per painting), twice a week for 60 weeks. Two of the four groups were kept in the dark except during treatment and observation; the other two groups were also kept in the dark but were exposed to long UV irradiation (300–400 nm; 5890 erg/cm^2 per s) for 2 h immediately after each skin painting. One of the groups kept in the dark and one of the groups subjected to UV irradiation were fed a normal rodent diet, while the other two groups were fed a diet containing 500 mg/kg β-carotene from 10% β-carotene-containing beadlets [use of placebo beadlets unspecified]. After one month, the animals fed the β-carotene-supplemented diet received an additional dose of 100 mg/kg bw crystalline β-carotene as a 1% solution in arachis oil by stomach tube twice a week [duration unspecified]. Two additional groups of 75 mice were fed a normal rodent diet and kept either continuously in the dark or subjected to UV irradiation for 2 h twice a week. These mice did not develop any skin tumours, and β-carotene had no consistent or significant effect on the incidence of benzo[*a*]pyrene-induced skin tumours in mice kept continuously in the dark during the final half of the experiment; however, during the last 20 weeks of the study, β-carotene significantly reduced the incidence of skin tumours in mice kept in the dark, from about 56 to 30% at 40 weeks and from about 67 to

Table 27. Effects of β-carotene on skin tumorigenesis in experimental mice

Strain, sex	No. of animals/group	Carcinogen (dose)	β-Carotene (dose, route)	Treatment relative to carcinogen	Preventive efficacy	Reference
Hairless [sex unspecified]	56–61	UV irradiation; 6.5 x 10³ J/m²	5/10 mg/mouse, intraperitoneally, 3 times/week	Before and during	Skin tumour size: 35–47% [SU] Skin tumour incidence after 47 weeks: 50% (p = 0.1074) –54% (p =0.03)	Epstein (1977)
Swiss Albino, female	75	B[a]P, 0.1 mg/skin painting; UV (300–400 nm) 5890 erg/cm² per s	500 mg/kg diet + 100 mg/kg bw by gavage twice/week	Before and during	Tumours, incidence B[a]P, 19–30% (p < 0.005) B[a]P/UV: 47% (SU)	Santamaria et al. (1981, 1983a,b, 1988); Santamaria & Bianchi (1989)
SKH/hr, female	24	UV-B (7.2 kJ/m²)	6.68 g/kg bw per day, diet	Before and during	Onset of skin tumours: 22% (p < 0.01)	Mathews-Roth (1982)
SKH/hr female	24	DMBA [dose unspecified]; croton oil	6.68 g/kg bw per day, diet	Before and during	Onset of skin tumours: 17% (p < 0.025) Tumour yield: 78% after 10 weeks (p < 0.01); 71% after 20 weeks (p < 0.01)	Mathews-Roth (1982)
SKH/hr, female	24	DMBA [dose unspecified]; UV-B (2.7 kJ/m²)	6.68 g/kg bw per day, diet	Before and during	Onset of skin tumours: 33% (p < .05)	Mathews-Roth (1982)
SKH/hr, [sex unspecified]	[about 25]	UV-B, 3.6 kJ/m², 3 times/week	33 g/kg diet	After	Papillomas/carcinomas Incidence After 10 weeks: 52% (NS) After 16 weeks: 39% (NS) After 20 weeks: none (NS)	Mathews-Roth (1983)
SKH/hr [sex unspecified	7 or 9	UV-B, 8 x 10⁴ J/m², single fluence	33 g/kg diet	Before and after	Papillomas/carcinomas Incidence: 34% (NS) Number: 60% (NS)	Mathews-Roth (1983)
SKH/hr-1, female	24	UV-B, total dose of 8 x 10⁴ J/m²	0.01, 0.07, 2/3.3% in diet; beadlets	Before and during	Papillomas/carcinomas Incidence Low dose: none (NS) Mid dose: 48% (p < 0.0125) High dose: 25% (p < 0.025) Multiplicity: none (NS)	Mathews-Roth & Krinsky (1985)

Table 27 (contd)

Species, strain, sex	No. of animals/group	Carcinogen (dose)	β-carotene, dose, route	Treatment relative to carcinogen	Preventive efficacy	Reference
SKH/hr-1, female	24	UV-B, one dose of 8 × 10⁴ J/m²	0.1% in diet; beadlets	Before, during and after	Papillomas Incidence Only before: 36% ($p < 0.1$) Only after: 79% ($p < 0.025$) Before and after: 50% ($p < 0.05$)	Mathews-Roth & Krinsky (1987)
HRA/SKH, female	40	DMBA (2.56 µg/mouse); TPA (1 µg twice/week)	290 and 1430 IU/kg bw/day, oral gavage	Before and during	Papillomas Incidence: 19–22% (NS)[b] Multiplicity: 44–46% ($p < 0.05$) Carcinomas: none (NS)	Steinel & Baker (1990)
HRA/SKH, female	16–19 (survivors)	DMBA (2.56 µg/mouse); TPA (1 µg twice/week)	1430 IU/kg bw per day, gavage	After	Tumours: none (NS)	Steinel & Baker (1990)
SKH:hr-1, female	30	DMBA (150 µg; TPA (5 µg twice/week)	2.8% as beadlets in diet	Before, during and after	Cumulative number of tumours: 29% ($p = 0.057$)	Lambert et al. (1990)
SKH:hr-1, female	30	DMBA (150 µg; TPA (5 µg twice/week)	2.6%, crystalline in diet	Before, during and after	Cumulative number of tumours: 39% ($p = 0.05$)	Lambert et al. (1990)
CR:ORL Sencar, female	30	DMBA (4 µg; TPA, (1.4 µg once/week)	2.8% as beadlets in diet	Before, during and after	Cumulative number of tumours: 25% (NS)	Lambert et al. (1990)
CR:ORL Sencar, female	30	DMBA (4 µg; TPA, (1.4 µg once/ week)	2.6%, crystalline in diet	Before, during and after	Cumulative number of tumours: 22% (NS)	Lambert et al. (1990)
Swiss, male and female	30	DMBA (100 nmol/painting, twice weekly, 8 weeks)	1 mg, painted on skin, 5 times/week, 24 weeks	Before, during and after	Tumours Survival: 233% [SU] Incidence: 37% (NS) Latency: 75% (NS) Number/mouse: 86% ($p < 0.001$)	Azuine et al. (1991)
Hairless Swiss nude, male	20	DMBA (100 nmol/painting, twice weekly, 8 weeks)	1 mg, painted on skin, 5 times/week, 24 weeks	Before, during and after	Tumours Survival: 67% [SU] Incidence: 50% (NS) Latency: 143% (NS) Number/mouse: 94% ($p < 0.001$)	Azuine et al. (1991)

Table 27 (contd)

Species, strain, sex	No. of animals/group	Carcinogen (dose)	β-carotene, dose, route	Treatment relative to carcinogen	Preventive efficacy	Reference
ICR, [sex unspecified]	16	DMBA, 100 μg; single application (1 μg twice/week)	200 and 400 nmol, skin application, twice/week	After	Papillomas Incidence: high dose, 64% (NS); low dose, 55% (NS) Multiplicity: high dose, 65% [SU]; low dose, 21% [SU] Latency: none [SU]	Murakoshi et al. (1992); Nishino (1995)
Sencar, male, female	13–25	20 μg DMBA, single application; 2 μg TPA, 20 weekly applications	0.6, 6, 60 and 600 mg/kg diet	During and after	Papillomas Incidence and yield: none [rather an increase] Conversion of papilloma to carcinoma: males, 87% (significant [p value unspecified]); females, 64% (NS) to 86% (significant [p value unspecified])	Chen et al. (1993)
CD-1, female	10	DMBA [dose unspecified]	200 mg/kg bw per day, gavage	After	Cumulative papilloma size, after 7 days: 11% ($p < 0.05$); after 14 days: 18% ($p < 0.05$)	Katsumura et al. (1996)

UV, ultraviolet; B[a]P, benzo[a]pyrene; DMBA, 7,12-dimethylbenz[a]anthracene; TPA, 12-O-tetradecanoylphorbol 13-acetate; NS, nonsignificant; SU, statistics unspecified

54% at 60 weeks ($p < 0.05$ [statistics unspecified]). In comparison with benzo[a]pyrene alone, the combination with UV irradiation increased the skin tumour incidence by two- to sevenfold at different times. β-Carotene reduced the incidence of benzo[a]pyrene- and UV-induced skin tumours considerably, e.g. from about 12 to 2% at 20 weeks, from about 47 to 21% at 28 weeks, from about 61 to 34% at 38 weeks, from about 68 to 35% at 40 weeks and from about 95 to 65% at 60 weeks. At the end of the study, 10–20% of the skin tumours were papillomas and 80–90% were squamous epitheliomas in the various groups [no information was provided on statistics] (Santamaria *et al.*, 1981, 1983a,b, 1988; Santamaria & Bianchi, 1989).

β-Carotene (33 g/kg diet; 6.68 g/kg bw per day; from carotenoid-containing beadlets) was administered in the diet to three groups of 24 female hairless Philadelphia Skin and Cancer Hospital SKH/hr mice, five to eight weeks of age, for 30–32 weeks. Three groups of mice received placebo beadlets. After 10 weeks on the respective diets, skin tumours were induced by one of three methods, each being applied to one of the β-carotene-treated groups and to one of the placebo control groups. In the first method, the mice were irradiated with UV-B (7.2 kJ/m^2 of total energy, 54% of which was between 285 and 320 nm) three times a week for 22 weeks. In the second method, a 0.5% solution of DMBA in acetone was painted twice at an interval of two weeks onto the entire back of each mouse, followed—three weeks after the second DMBA treatment—by painting two drops of a 0.5% solution of croton oil in acetone on the entire back twice weekly for 16 weeks. In the third method, the DMBA treatment was followed two weeks later by UV-B irradiation (2.7 kJ/m^2 of total energy, 54% of which was between 285 and 320 nm) three times per week [period of treatment unspecified]. Representative skin tumours from about 30% of the mice were studied histologically. Each method of tumour induction resulted in both squamous-cell carcinomas and papillomas. β-Carotene significantly delayed the time to appearance, but not the yield, of skin tumours induced by UV-B irradiation alone, the first tumour > 1 mm^3 appearing in weeks 11

and 9 in the mice given β-carotene and in controls, respectively ($p < 0.01$; life-table analyses with χ^2 test). β-Carotene delayed the onset of skin tumours induced by DMBA and croton oil, the first 15 tumours appearing significantly later in the mice on β-carotene than in those on placebo ($p < 0.025$; life-table analyses with χ^2 test). β-Carotene also significantly ($p < 0.01$; life-table analyses with χ^2 test) reduced the yield of skin tumours induced by DMBA and croton oil, the average number of tumours per mouse being 1.74 in animals given β-carotene and 8.0 in those on placebo after 10 weeks of treatment and 3.40 and 11.6 after 20 weeks. The onset of the first skin tumour > 1 mm^3 induced by DMBA and UV-B was also delayed by β-carotene, the first tumour appearing six weeks after the start of treatment in those on placebo and after eight weeks in the β-carotene-fed group ($p < 0.05$; life-table analyses with χ^2 test). β-Carotene had no effect on the average number of skin tumours per animal induced by DMBA and UV-B (Mathews-Roth, 1982).

An unspecified number of Philadelphia Skin and Cancer Hospital SKH/hr mice, five to eight weeks of age, were fed normal mouse chow and were irradiated with UV-B (3.6 kJ/m^2) for 20 min, three times per week for an unspecified period [at least 24 weeks]. As soon as a mouse developed a skin tumour ≥ 1 mm^3, it was allocated at random to a β-carotene-supplemented diet (33 g/kg diet from β-carotene-containing beadlets) or to placebo beadlet-supplemented control diet. There was a nonsignificant trend for a delayed appearance of new skin papillomas and carcinomas in mice fed the β-carotene-supplemented diet; e.g. the seventh skin tumour developed after 10 weeks in 20% of β-carotene-fed mice and 42% of those on placebo, after 16 weeks in 43% on β-carotene and 70% on placebo and after 20 weeks in 79% of each group [incidences estimated from a figure]. There was also a statistically insignificant trend for inhibition by β-carotene of the development of skin tumours > 4 mm^3 ($p < 0.3$; Student's t test) and > 50 mm^3 ($p < 0.1$; Student's t test) [not further specified]. In a second experiment, groups of mice received the β-carotene-supplemented diet (seven mice) or the placebo diet (nine mice) for 34 weeks. After 10 weeks on their respective diets, all mice were subjected to a large single fluence of UV-B irradiation (8×10^4 J/m^2) and were observed for 43 weeks [apparently, all mice were fed a normal diet during the last nine weeks of this period]. There was no intercurrent mortality. The first skin tumours were seen five weeks after exposure to UV-B, and no new skin tumours developed 21 weeks after exposure. β-Carotene did not significantly reduce the incidence or total number of skin tumours > 1 mm^3, the incidences being 2/7 and 4/9 and the total numbers 2 and 5 in the β-carotene and control groups, respectively (Mathews-Roth, 1983).

Six groups of 24 female hairless Philadelphia Skin and Cancer Hospital SKH/hr-1 mice, five to seven weeks old, were fed diets supplemented with β-carotene or placebo beadlets. Groups 1 and 2 were fed rodent chow supplemented with 3.3% β-carotene (3.3 g/kg diet) in beadlets or placebo beadlets for 16 weeks and then 2% β-carotene (2 g/kg diet) for another 22 weeks; groups 3 and 4 were fed a diet containing 0.07% β-carotene (700 mg/kg diet) or placebo beadlets for 30 weeks; groups 5 and 6 were fed diets containing 0.01% β-carotene (100 mg/kg diet) or placebo for 26 weeks and four days. All mice were subjected to UV-B irradiation (total dose, 10.8 J/m^2) for 16 weeks [schedule of irradiation unspecified], starting after 12 weeks on their diets for groups 1 and 2, after one month for groups 3 and 4 and after four days for groups 5 and 6. The animals were killed 10 weeks after irradiation. At the end of the study, the β-carotene content of the epidermis was found to be increased in a dose-related manner. β-Carotene at dietary concentrations of 3.3/2% and 0.07% prevented or delayed the appearance of UV-B-induced skin tumours; e.g. the percentages of mice with skin tumours 21 weeks after the start of the irradiation were 63% at the high dose and 84% with placebo ($p < 0.025$; Student's t test), 44% at the intermediate dose and 85% with placebo ($p < 0.0125$; Student's t test) and 65% at the low dose and 56% with placebo. The average numbers of tumours per mouse were also lower (but not statistically significantly) in those on β-carotene than in the respective placebo groups; e.g. 21 weeks after the start of the irradiation,

1.83 at the high dose and 2.65 with the placebo, 1.27 at the intermediate dose and 1.70 with the placebo and 1.29 at the low dose and 1.30 with the placebo (Mathews-Roth & Krinsky, 1985)

Groups of 24 female hairless Philadelphia Skin and Cancer Hospital SKH/hr-1 mice, five to seven weeks old, were fed a diet containing 0.1% β-carotene in beadlets, and two other groups received the same diet supplemented with placebo beadlets for six weeks. All mice then received a single exposure to 8×10^4 J/m^2 UV-B radiation for 220 min. Immediately after exposure, one of the groups on the β-carotene-supplemented diet was switched to the placebo diet and one of the placebo groups was switched to the β-carotene-supplemented diet, while the two other groups were continued on their respective diets. The animals were observed for 24 weeks after treatment. At the end of the study, β-carotene was detected in the skin even of animals that received the pigment before irradiation. There was no intercurrent mortality. The first tumours appeared five weeks after irradiation, some growing to 50 mm^3 but most measuring 1–4 mm^3. When β-carotene was fed before or after or only after exposure to UV-B, the incidences of skin tumours (mainly papillomas) were significantly reduced, being 14/24 for the group continuously fed the placebo diet, 7/24 for the group fed the β-carotene diet ($p < 0.05$; Fisher's exact test) and 3/24 for the group fed the placebo diet before and the β-carotene-supplemented diet after exposure to UV-B ($p < 0.0025$; Fisher exact test). The skin tumour incidence in the group fed the β-carotene-supplemented diet only before UV-B exposure was 9/24, which was not statistically significantly lower than that (14/24) in the group continuously fed the placebo diet (Mathews-Roth & Krinsky, 1987).

From three weeks of age, 120 inbred female HRA/Skh mice were fed a vitamin A- and β-carotene-free diet (8% sucrose, 27% dextrose, 30% corn flour, 21% soya protein, 5% cellulose, 6% peanut oil and 3% vitamin–mineral premix without vitamin A). At 42–49 days of age, 2.56 mg (10 nmol) DMBA in 50 μl acetone were applied over the lower half of the dorsal skin surface of each mouse. One week later, 1 mg (1.6 nmol) 12-O-tetradecanoylphorbol 13-

acetate (TPA) in 50 ml acetone was applied over the same skin surface, twice weekly for a further 19 weeks. At the same time, the mice were divided into three groups of 40 mice and were given 100 ml peanut oil or 10 or 50 IU β-carotene (290 or 1430 IU/kg bw per day) in 100 ml peanut oil on five days per week for 39 weeks. The mice were held for a further 12 weeks for observation. A group of 20 mice was similarly treated with DMBA and TPA but received normal feed throughout the study. β-Carotene had no effect on body weight, but all of the mice on the vitamin A- and β-carotene-free diet had statistically significantly reduced body weights ($p < 0.0001$ [method of statistical analysis unspecified]). The incidence of skin papillomas was reduced from 97% in the control group to 77% in both β-carotene-treated groups at week 20 and from 68% in the control group to 50 and 52% in the groups at the low and high doses of β-carotene, respectively, at week 40. The incidences of papillomas in the group fed normal feed were 100% at week 20 and 78% at week 40, and the maximum number of papillomas per mouse found during weeks 6–14 was significantly reduced ($p < 0.05$; two-tailed unpaired t test) from 3.5 ± 1.6 in the control group to 2.5 ± 2.1 and 2.5 ± 2.4 in mice at the low and high doses of β-carotene, respectively, and 4.9 ± 1.8 in the group given normal feed. The incidences of squamous-cell carcinomas and carcinomas *in situ* of the skin in mice still alive at the end of the study (week 52) ranged from 7/38 to 7/25 in the various groups and did not differ significantly (two-tailed unpaired t test). In order to investigate the effect of β-carotene on established skin tumours, mice on normal feed were treated with DMBA and TPA as described above and were distributed randomly into two groups at week 20. Both groups received the vitamin A- and β-carotene-free diet in weeks 20–40, and one group received the high dose of β-carotene and the other group only peanut oil. There was no significant difference between the two groups with regard to papilloma yield or the occurrence of skin carcinomas, the incidences of carcinomas being 3/19 and 6/16 in controls and β-carotene-treated groups, respectively [no further details given] (Steinel & Baker, 1990).

Four groups of 30 female CR:ORL Sencar mice and 30 female Skh:HR-1 mice, 10–13 weeks of age, were maintained on standard rodent pellet diet, finely ground rodent standard diet containing 2.8% β-carotene (from 10% β-carotene-containing beadlets), 2.6% crystalline β-carotene (type 1, *trans*, synthetic) or placebo beadlets at a concentration equal to that of the diet containing 2.8% β-carotene. In week 11, a single dose of 4 mg DMBA in 0.2 ml acetone was applied to the skin of the back of each Sencar mouse and 150 mg DMBA in 0.2 ml acetone to Skh mice. One week later, all mice received a first application of TPA: Sencar mice received 1.4 mg TPA in 0.2 ml acetone once a week for 11 weeks, while Skh mice received 5 mg TPA in 0.2 ml acetone twice a week for 18 weeks. No significant difference in body weight was found between the groups. The Sencar mice given the β-carotene beadlets had a statistically nonsignificant (Kruskal-Wallis test), 25% decrease in the cumulative number of skin tumours (total number of tumours in survivors), with 414 tumours in those given the placebo and 312 in those given β-carotene, whereas Skh mice had a statistically significant ($p = 0.057$; Kruskal-Wallis test), 29% decrease in the cumulative number of skin tumours, with 315 tumours in those on placebo and 223 with the beadlets. Sencar mice fed the crystalline β-carotene supplement had a 22% decrease in the cumulative number of skin tumours (284 versus 366 with placebo), while Skh mice had a 39% decrease (174 versus 287; $p = 0.05$; Kruskal-Wallis test). At one time (week 11), significantly fewer tumour-bearing animals were found among the Sencar mice fed the beadlets than the placebo ($p < 0.05$; Fisher's exact test), while no such significant difference was seen between the group fed the crystalline β-carotene supplement. Significantly fewer tumour-bearing Skh mice among those fed the beadlets than among those receiving the placebo ($p < 0.05$; Fisher's exact test) were found at two times, and fewer tumour-bearing mice mice fed the crystalline β-carotene diet were found at four times [statistics unspecified]. There was a statistically significant delay in the time to appearance of tumours in Skh mice fed either the beadlet or the crystalline supplement ($p < 0.05$; Kruskal-Wallis test), but no statistically significant difference was seen in Sencar mice (Lambert *et al.*, 1990).

Two groups of 30 Swiss mice of each sex [number per sex unspecified], six to eight weeks old, were painted on the shaven back skin with 100 nmol DMBA in 0.1 ml acetone twice weekly from week 3 to week 11. One of the groups received 1 mg β-carotene in 0.1 ml acetone topically on the back skin on five days per week from week 1 to week 24 (end of the study), while the other group received no further treatment. A third group of animals was treated with acetone alone or with 1 mg β-carotene in acetone. β-Carotene increased the survival rate from [8/30] to [27/30] and the mean latency of skin tumours from 8 to14 weeks and reduced the incidence of skin tumours from [30/30] to [19/30] (not significant; Student's *t* test) and the number of skin tumours per mouse from 13.1 ± 1.7 to 1.8 ± 0.3 ($p < 0.001$; Student's *t* test). None of the animals treated with acetone alone or with 1 mg β-carotene in acetone died, and no skin tumours were found (Azuine *et al.*, 1991).

Groups of 20 male inbred hairless Swiss nude mice were treated in a study of similar design but with 50 nmol DMBA. β-Carotene increased the survival rate from [12/20] to [22/20] [statistics unspecified] and the mean latency of skin tumours from 7 to 17 weeks, and it reduced the incidence from [20/20] to [10/20] (not significant; Student's *t* test) and the number of skin tumours per mouse from 46.4 ± 5.1 to 2.6 ± 0.4 ($p < 0.001$; Student's *t* test). None of the animals treated with acetone alone or with 1 mg β-carotene in acetone died, and no skin tumours were found (Azuine *et al.*, 1991).

The backs of 48 ICR mice [sex unspecified], seven weeks old, were shaved and two days later given a single application of 0.1 mg DMBA [vehicle unspecified]. One week later, 1 mg (1.62 nmol) TPA was painted on the shaven skin twice weekly for 20 weeks. Groups of 16 mice received 200 or 400 nmol β-carotene in 0.2 ml acetone at the same time as each application of TPA, or the vehicle in acetone. There was no significant difference in body weight among the groups. The first skin tumours (papillomas) appeared within nine weeks after the start of application of TPA in both control and treated groups [time to tumour appearance not further specified]. At 20 weeks, the percentages of mice bearing papillomas [estimated from a figure] were 69, 31 and 25 [statistics unspecified], and the average numbers of skin tumours were 3.73, 2.94 and 1.31 [standard deviations unspecified] (not significant; Student's *t* test) in controls and in those given the low and high doses of β-carotene, respectively. The tumours were smaller in the β-carotene-treated animals than in controls; e.g. the average numbers of tumours 1–2 mm in diameter per mouse were 2.20, 1.81 and 1.06 [standard deviations unspecified] in the three groups, respectively. Furthermore, no tumours > 4 mm in diameter were seen in β-carotene-treated mice, whereas 0.26 such tumours per mouse [standard deviation unspecified] were seen in the control group [statistics unspecified]. The study was repeated with similar results [no further details presented] (Murakoshi *et al.*, 1992; Nishino, 1995).

After pregnant Sencar mice had delivered their pups, they were placed on a vitamin A-deficient diet (TD85239) supplemented with 0.6, 6, 60 or 600 mg/kg β-carotene (crystalline; > 95% pure). At the age of three weeks, the pups were weaned onto the same diets as their mothers: 18, 20, 13 and 25 females on diets supplemented with 0.6, 6, 60 and 600 mg/kg β-carotene, respectively, and 22 and 25 males on diets supplemented with 60 and 600 mg/kg β-carotene, respectively. At the age of three weeks, all mice received a single skin application of 20 mg DMBA in 0.2 ml acetone, followed one week later by 20 weekly topical applications of 2 mg TPA in 0.2 ml acetone. There was no significant difference in body weight or survival between the groups. β-Carotene did not significantly affect the number of skin papillomas in female mice. Significantly more male mice aged 11–15 weeks developed skin papillomas when given the high dose (about 86% at 14 weeks) than the low dose (about 33% at 14 weeks; Fisher-Irwin exact test [*p* values unspecified]). The maximal number of papillomas in mice at the high dose (553 in females and 315 in males) was statistically significantly higher than in those at the lower dose: 149–339 in females and 169 in males (Wilcoxon rank sum test [*p* values unspecified]). The conversion of papillomas to carcinomas—(total number of carcinomas per maximal number of papillomas) x 1000—was much lower in mice at the high dose (0.4 for females and 0.6 for males) than at the lower doses (1.1–3.5 for females and 4.7 for males), the differences being statistically significant in males and for two of the three groups of females (Fisher-Irwin exact test and log-rank test [*p* values unspecified]). There was no significant difference in the time to appearance of carcinomas between the groups (log-rank test) (Chen *et al.*, 1993). [The Working Group noted the use of vitamin A-deficient animals.]

Two groups of 45 female hairless Crl:Skh1 (hr/hr) BR mice, 80 days old, were fed standard mouse chow or chow fortified with 0.5% (w/w) β-carotene (type 1, all-*trans*, synthetic, crystalline) for 32 weeks. In week 11, all mice received a single application of 150 mg DMBA in acetone on the dorsal skin; one week later, 5 mg TPA in acetone were applied twice weekly for 11 weeks and once weekly for another nine weeks. There was no significant difference in body weight between the groups. The levels of β-carotene in mice that received the supplement were significantly increased in liver and skin but remained near the limit of detection in serum throughout the study. Nearly all mice had developed skin tumours towards the end of the study. In weeks 17 and 18, the incidence of skin tumours in those given β-carotene was statistically significantly lower than that in the control group ($p < 0.05$; Fisher's exact test [no further details given]). The time to appearance of the first skin tumour was statistically significantly longer in mice given β-carotene than in the controls ($p < 0.05$; Kruskal-Wallis test [no further details given]). The cumulative number of skin tumours and their time to appearance were significantly lower in the β-carotene group ($p = 0.03$; analysis of variance) (Lambert *et al.*, 1994).

Skin papillomas were induced in 20 female CD-1 mice, eight weeks old, by dermal application of DMBA for 60 days, until 10–20 papillomas had developed in each mouse. Two groups of 10 mice were then given 200 mg/kg bw per day β-carotene in 0.1 ml peanut oil or peanut oil alone. By day 14, the β-carotene level was 0.006 μmol/L in serum, 0.6 nmol/g tissue in liver and 0.12 nmol/g tissue in skin papillomas, whereas no β-carotene was detected in controls. Mean food intake and mean body weights were not affected by β-carotene. The cumulative size of the skin papillomas (number of papillomas x diameter of each papilloma), measured in each animal on days 7 and 14 after the start of β-carotene administration, was 96.8 ± 7.6% of the size at the start of the β-carotene treatment at day 7 and 96.4 ± 5.6% at day 14, the sizes in the control group being 109.0 ± 5.4% at day 7 and 117.2 ± 10.9% at day 14 ($p < 0.05$; Dunnett's *t* test) (Katsumura *et al.*, 1996).

(b)   Colon (Table 28)

Mouse: Groups of female inbred Swiss Webster (ICR) mice [initial number of mice unspecified], 10 weeks old, were fed diets containing 2 or 22 mg/kg of diet (ppm) β-carotene (type III, dissolved in corn oil). After five weeks, half of the animals at each dose received seven weekly subcutaneous injections of 20.5–31 mg/kg bw 1,2-dimethylhydrazine (DMH) as the dihydrochloride in 1 mmol/L neutralized EDTA, for a total dose of DMH of 196 mg/kg bw. At week 17, 10 or 12 mice in each group given DMH and all mice not treated with DMH were killed and examined for hyperplastic colonic lesions; and at week 36, 31 animals at the low dose and 32 at the high dose were killed and examined for colon tumours. The remaining 30 mice at the low dose and 27 at the high dose were observed for an additional 13 weeks and killed when moribund. Mice fed the high dose gained significantly more weight (37.0 ± 4.0 g) than those fed the low dose of β-carotene (34.4 ± 3.4 g; $p < 0.05$; Student's *t* test). Food intake was similar in all groups. DMH induced mild hyperplasia of the colonic epithelium, and β-carotene did not appear to moderate this effect. Mice fed the high dose of β-carotene had fewer colon tumours than those fed the low dose. Adenomas were reduced in both incidence (low dose: 19/31, high dose: 12/32; not significant; χ^2 test) and multiplicity (low dose: 1.96 ± 1.72, high dose: 1.17 ± 0.39; $p < 0.05$; Student's *t* test). Adenocarcinomas were reduced in both

Table 28. Effects of β-carotene on colon tumorigenesis in experimental animals

Species, strain, sex	No. of animals/group	Carcinogen (dose)	β-Carotene (dose, route)	Treatment relative to carcinogen	Preventive efficacy	Reference
Mouse, Swiss Webster (ICR)	10–32	1,2-Dimethylhydrazine; total dose 196 mg/kg bw; subcutaneous	22 mg/kg diet	Before, during and after	Hyperplasia: none Adenoma: incidence, 38% (NS); multiplicity, 40% ($p < 0.05$) Adenocarcinoma: incidence, 96% ($p < 0.001$); Multiplicity, 86% ($p < 0.05$)	Temple & Basu (1987); Basu et al. (1988)
Rat, Holtzman, male	28	1,2-Dimethylhydrazine; 30 mg/kg bw, subcutaneous, total dose, 480 mg/kg bw	1% in diet	Before, during and after	Tumours/cancers in colon: None (NS)[a]	Colacchio et al. (1989); Colacchio & Memoli (1986)
Rat, Wistar Crl, male	36	MNNG, 2 mg/rat, intrarectally twice weekly for 3 weeks	0.2/0.4% in diet	Before, during and after	Adenocarcinoma Incidence: none (NS) Adenoma: none (NS)	Jones et al. (1989)
Rat, Fischer 344 [sex unspecified]	25–30	Azoxymethane; 2 x 15 mg/kg bw, subcutaneous	90 mg/kg in diet	After	Large aberrant crypt foci: number, 51% ($p < 0.05$) Tumours: incidence, 26% ($p < 0.05$)	Shivapurkar et al. (1995)
Rat, Sprague-Dawley, male	20–30	1,2-Dimethylhydrazine 12 weekly doses of 20 mg/kg bw; subcutaneous	0.005% in diet	Before and during	Carcinomas Incidence: 44% [SU]	Yamamoto et al. (1994)
Rat, Fischer-344, male	20	Azoxymethane; 2 doses of 15 mg/kg bw, subcutaneous	1, 10 and 20 mg/kg diet (high-fat, low-fibre diet)	Before, during and after	Aberrant crypt foci Low dose: 20% (NS); mid-dose: 53% ($p < 0.05$); high dose: 71% ($p < 0.05$) Tumours Low dose: 36% (NS); mid-dose: 73% ($p < 0.05$); High dose: 73% ($p < 0.05$)	Alabaster et al. (1995, 1996)
Rat, Fischer 344, male	15	Azoxymethane; 3 x 15 mg/kg bw, subcutaneous	50 and 200 mg/kg bw/day, orally	Before, during, after	Aberrant crypt foci: low dose: 26% ($p < 0.01$); high dose: 37% ($p < 0.01$)	Komaki et al. (1996)
Rat, Sprague-Dawley, female	6	MNU, 30 x 4 mg intrarectally	0.24, 1.2 and 6 mg; gavage, daily for 2 weeks	After	Aberrant crypt foci; number/colon Low dose: none (NS) Mid dose: none (NS) High dose: none (NS)	Narisawa et al. (1996)

NS, not significant; MNNG, N-methyl-N-nitro-N-nitrosoguanidine; SU, statistics unspecified; MNU, N-methyl-N-nitrosourea incidence, by 96% (low dose: 10/31, high dose: 1/32; $p < 0.01$; χ^2 test), and multiplicity, by 86% (low dose: 0.57 ± 0.73, high dose: 0.08 ± 0.29; $p < 0.05$; Student's t test). The mortality rate of mice on the high-β-carotene diet was about half (19%) that of mice on the low-β-carotene diet (40%), but the difference was not statistically significant (Temple & Basu, 1987; Basu *et al.*, 1988).

Rat: Two groups of 28 weanling male Holtzman rats were fed regular chow supplemented with either 1% β-carotene (w/w; from beadlets containing 10% β-carotene) or 10% placebo beadlets for 24 weeks. After four weeks, all rats received 16 weekly subcutaneous injections of 30 mg/kg bw symmetrical DMH dissolved in neutral sodium hydroxide-corrected phosphate-buffered saline (total dose, 480 mg/kg bw). At 24 weeks, the animals were killed and examined for intestinal tumours. All rats had colon cancers, and β-carotene had no effect on the tumour response: 3.79 colon cancers per rat in the β-carotene group and 3.71 in the group given placebo (not significant; Colacchio & Memoli, 1986; Colacchio *et al.*, 1989).

Two groups of 36 weanling male Wistar Crl rats, three weeks old and weighing about 50 g, were fed a powdered basic diet (NIH-07 containing 10 000 IU vitamin A and 1.4 mg carotene per kg) supplemented with either 0.4% β-carotene (from beadlets containing 10% β-carotene) or placebo beadlets (4%) for two weeks. The β-carotene and placebo contents of the diets were then reduced by a factor of two, and these diets were fed until termination of the study at 25 weeks. At five weeks of age, 2 mg N-methyl-N'-nitro-N-nitrosoguanidine (MNNG; 0.15 ml of a solution of 13.4 mg/ml distilled water, pH 5) were administered intrarectally twice weekly for three weeks. Two additional groups of 18 rats did not receive MNNG and served as β-carotene and placebo control groups, respectively; a further group of eight rats served as untreated controls. There were no significant differences among the groups in body weight. β-Carotene did not affect the incidence of MNNG-induced colorectal cancer: 34/36 rats receiving β-carotene had adenocarcinomas and 17/36 had adenomas, whereas

34/35 MNNG-treated controls had adenocarcinomas and 24/35 had adenomas ($p = 0.12$; χ^2 test). The locations of the tumours were similar in the two groups (Jones *et al.*, 1989).

Fifty-five Fischer 344 rats [sex and age unspecified] were fed a 'high-risk' diet, high in fat and low in fibre, with the following composition: casein, 194.9 g/kg; DL-methionine, 2 g/kg; dextrose, 256.5 g/kg; sucrose, 256.5 g/kg; wheat bran, 25.6 g/kg; fat mixture (44.2% lard, 46.2% corn oil, 9.6% hydrogenated coconut oil, 200 g/kg); calcium-free AIN76 salt mix, 35 g/kg; modified AIN76A vitamin mix, 10 g/kg; choline bitartrate, 2 g/kg and calcium carbonate, 17.5 g/kg. After two weeks, the rats were given two subcutaneous injections of 15 mg/kg bw azoxymethane [interval between injections unspecified]. After another six weeks, 25 rats were given the diet supplemented with 90 ppm β-carotene [formulation unspecified]. Five rats fed the unsupplemented diet were killed at 10 weeks, five rats from each group at 14 and 18 weeks, and the remaining rats 30 weeks after the start of the study. There were no significant differences between the groups in body weight. β-Carotene significantly reduced the number of aberrant crypt foci ($p < 0.05$; Student's t test) and the incidence and multiplicity of colonic adenomas and adenocarcinomas. Thus, the ratio of the number of aberrant crypt foci with eight or more aberrant crypts per focus in the unsupplemented group and in the β-carotene-supplemented group at week 18 was 2.06, and colonic tumours had occurred by the end of the study in 74% of the unsupplemented and 55% of the β-carotene-supplemented groups ($p < 0.05$; Fisher exact test) [incidences estimated from a figure] at multiplicities of 1.35 and 0.70 ($p < 0.05$; Student's t test), respectively (Shivapurkar *et al.*, 1995).

Male Sprague-Dawley rats, five weeks old, were fed CE-2 basic diet either as such for 26 weeks (30 animals) or supplemented with 0.005% β-carotene (type III, from carrot [formulation in the diet unspecified]) for 14 weeks, followed by CE-2 basic diet for the final 12 weeks (20 animals). From day 3, all rats were given weekly subcutaneous injections of 20 mg/kg bw DMH for 12 weeks. At the end of week 26, all rats were killed and examined for the presence of colon carcinomas. A group of 20 rats fed CE-2 basic diet for 26 weeks served as untreated controls. No significant differences in body weight were seen among the groups. β-Carotene reduced the incidence of colon adenocarcinomas, mucinous adenocarcinomas and signet-ring cell carcinomas from 24/30 to 9/20 [statistics unspecified] (Yamamoto et al., 1994).

Four groups of 20 male Fischer 344 rats, four weeks old, were fed a high-fat (20% fat), low-fibre (1% wheat bran) diet containing 0, 1, 10 or 20 mg/kg β-carotene for 30 weeks [formulation in the diet unspecified]. All rats were given two subcutaneous injections of 15 mg/kg bw azoxymethane, one in week 3 and one in week 4. After 10 weeks, five rats per group were killed and examined for the presence of aberrant crypt foci in the colon. The remaining rats were continued on their respective diets for an additional 20 weeks and examined for the presence of colon tumours. Four comparable groups of rats were kept on the same diets and received a subcutaneous injection of saline only in weeks 3 and 4. There was no significant difference in body weight among the groups. β-Carotene reduced the number of aberrant crypt foci per rat from 44.0 ± 4.18 in the control group to 35.0 ± 3.29 in rats at 1 mg/kg β-carotene, 20.6 ± 0.68 in those at 10 mg/kg and 12.8 ± 1.96 in those at 20 mg/kg; the differences from the controls were statistically significant ($p < 0.05$; Student's t test) for the two highest doses. In addition, β-carotene reduced the incidence of colon adenoma and adenocarcinoma from 11/15 in controls to 7/15 in those at 1 mg/kg β-carotene, [3/15] in those at 10 mg/kg and [3/15] in those at 20 mg/kg, the differences from controls again being statistically significant only at the two highest doses. No aberrant crypt foci or colon tumours were found in controls not treated with azoxymethane (Alabaster et al., 1995, 1996) [The Working Group noted discrepancies between the two publications in the total number of aberrant crypt foci and the incidence of colon adenomas.]

Three groups of 20 male Fischer 344 rats, five weeks old, were kept on a semi-purified diet (20% casein, 59% sucrose, 4% cellulose, 0.15% choline, 4% mineral mixture, 1% vitamin mixture and 12% olive oil) and received β-carotene at 0, 50 or 200 mg/kg bw per day in distilled water for five weeks. At six, seven and eight weeks of age, 10 rats in each group were injected subcutaneously with 15 mg/kg bw azoxymethane; the other 10 animals in each group served as controls. All rats were killed at 10 weeks of age, and the colons of five azoxymethane-treated rats and five that did not receive azoxymethane were examined for the presence and number of colonic aberrant crypts and foci. Mean food intake and mean body weight were not significantly affected by β-carotene administration. No neoplasms were found. No aberrant crypt foci were observed in the colons of controls that did not receive azoxymethane, but all rats given the carcinogen had foci. In rats given β-carotene, both the number of foci per colon and the number of crypts per colon were statistically significantly decreased ($p < 0.01$; Dunnett's t test) as compared with the control group; the numbers of aberrant crypt foci per colon were 217 ± 23.5, 159.8 ± 16.4 and 135.4 ± 16.3 in controls and those at 50 and 200 mg β-carotene, and the numbers of aberrant crypts per colon were 381.2 ± 38.1, 267.0 ± 33.8 and 223.6 ± 27.5, respectively. The numbers of aberrant crypts per focus were also lower in rats receiving β-carotene than in controls, but the differences were not statistically significant (Komaki et al., 1996). [The Working Group noted that a positive effect was noted even though β-carotene was administered in distilled water.]

Twenty four female Sprague-Dawley rats, seven weeks old, received three intrarectal instillations of 4 mg N-methyl-N-nitrosourea (MNU) in 0.5 ml distilled water in week 1 and were then divided into four groups of six animals which received 0.2 ml corn oil containing 0, 0.24, 1.2 or 6 mg β-carotene by intragastric gavage daily during week 2 and week 5. In week 6, all rats were killed and their colons were examined for aberrant crypt foci. The numbers of aberrant crypt foci per colon were not significantly reduced by administration of β-carotene (56.1 ± 10.0 at the high dose) but were in fact slightly higher in rats at the low (74.5 ± 3.9) and intermediate (67.7 ± 3.9) doses than in the control group (62.7 ± 7.2) (Narisawa et al., 1996).

(c)   Respiratory tract (Table 29)
Mouse: Two groups of 16 male, specific pathogen-free, ddY mice, six weeks old,

Table 29. Effects of β-carotene on tumorigenesis in organs other than skin, salivary glands, buccal pouch, colon and liver

Organ	Species, strain, sex	No. of animals/group	Carcinogen (dose, route)	β-Carotene (dose, route)	Treatment relative to carcinogen	Preventive efficacy	Reference
Lung	Mouse, ddY, male	16	4-NQO, 10 mg/kg bw, single s.c. injection Glycerol (10%) in drinking-water	0.05% in drinking-water (3.27 mg/mouse per day)	During and after	Type II adenoma Incidence: none (NS) Multiplicity: none (NS)	Murakoshi et al. (1992)
Lung	Mouse, N:GP(S), male and female	38–41	0.5 mg B[a]P, single dose, s.c.	500 mg/kg diet	After	Adenoma Incidence: males, none (NS); females, 34% (NS) Multiplicity: males, 17% (NS); females, 40% (NS)	Yun et al. (1995)
Respiratory tract	Hamster, male and female	40–60	64 mg B[a]P/animal; intratracheally + 8 mg Fe₂O₃	56 mg/kg diet	Before, during and after	(Pre)neoplasia None (some weak indication of enhancement)	Beems (1987)
Respiratory tract	Hamster, male	?	NDEA, 17.8 mg/kg bw, s.c. twice weekly, 20 weeks	1.5 mg s.c. twice weekly for 21 weeks	Before and during	Tumour incidence, 48% (NS)	Moon et al. (1994)
Respiratory tract	Hamster, male	50	10 doses of 8 mg B[a]P + 8 mg Fe₂O₃ over 12 weeks	56 mg/kg diet	Before, during and after	(Pre)neoplasia None (some weak indication of enhancement)	Wolterbeek et al. (1995a)
Urinary bladder	Mouse, B6D2F₁ [sex unspecified]	24	NBHBA, 10 weekly doses of 1.5 or 3.0 mg; gavage	5 mmol/kg diet	After	Hyperplasia and carcinomas: none (SU)	Hicks et al. (1984)
Urinary bladder	Mouse, B6D2F₁	24	5 mg NBHBA, gavage, twice/week	0.1% in diet	Before, during and after	Carcinoma: incidence, 47% (p < 0.05)	Mathews-Roth et al. (1991)
Urinary bladder	Rat, Fischer 344 [sex unspecified]	About 70	NBHBA; total dose, 635 mg/rat [route unspecified]	3 mmol/kg diet	Before, during and after	Hyperplasia and carcinomas: none (SU)	Pedrick et al. (1990)
Forestomach	Mouse, Swiss, female	20	B[a]P; 1 mg, twice weekly, 4 weeks; gavage	4.7 mmol/animal per day, gavage	Before, during and after	Gross tumour incidence, 85% (p < 0.001)	Azuine et al. (1992)

Table 29 (contd)

Organ	Species, strain, sex	No. of animals/group	Carcinogen (dose, route)	β-Carotene (dose, route)	Treatment relative to carcinogen	Preventive efficacy	Reference
Stomach, small intestine	Rat, Wistar Crl, male	36	MNNG; 3.82–4.10 mg/kg bw per day in drinking- water	0.2/0.4% in diet	Before, during and after	Stomach, adenocarcinoma, incidence: 43% (NS) Small intestine, incidence, multiplicity: none (rather, a small increase)	Jones et al. (1989)
Small intestine	Rat, Holtzman, male	28	DMH; 30 mg/kg bw s.c.; total dose, 480 mg/kg bw	1% in diet	Before, during and after	Tumours: none (NS)	Colacchio & Memoli (1986); Colacchio et al. (1989)
Small intestine	Rat, Sprague-Dawley, male	20–30	DMH; 12 weekly doses of 20 mg/kg bw s.c.	0.005% in diet	Before and during	Carcinomas Incidence: none [SU]	Colacchio & Memoli (1986); Colacchio et al. (1989)
Pancreas	Rat, Bor(WISW, Cob) Wistar, female	40	Azaserine, 30 mg/kg bw, two i.p. injections	60 mg/kg diet	After	Preneoplasia: Number: 27% (NS – 43% ($p < 0.05$)	Appel et al. (1991)
Pancreas	Rat, Wistar, male	15?	Azaserine, 3 x 30 mg/kg bw; i.p.	100 and 1000 mg/kg diet	After	Preneoplasia High dose: 29% ($p < 0.05$) Tumours: None (NS)	Appel & Woutersen (1996)
Pancreas	Rat, Wistar, male	15?	Azaserine, 3 x 30 mg/kg bw; i.p.	100 and 1000 mg/diet diet	Before and during	Preneoplasia High dose: 42% ($p < 0.05$) Tumours: None (NS)	Appel & Woutersen (1996)
Pancreas	Hamster, male	40	NBOPA, 3 weekly doses of 20 mg; s.c.	60 mg/kg diet	After	Preneoplasia and carcinomas: none (NS)	Appel et al. (1996)
Multiple organs	Rat, F344/DUCrj Fischer, male	10–20	DMH, 40 mg/kg bw; two s.c. injections; MNU, 20 mg/kg bw, 4 i.p. injections,	0.2% in diet	After	Preneoplasia/cancers Liver cell foci: 25% (NS) Colonic carcinoma: 56% (NS) Nephrobastoma: 56% (NS)	Imaida et al. (1990)

4-NQO, 4-nitroquinoline 1-oxide; NS, not significant; B[a]P, benzo[a]pyrene; NBHBA, N-nitrosobutyl(4-hydroxybutyl)amine; NBOPA, N-nitrosobis(oxopropyl)amine; MMNG, N-methyl-N-nitro-N'-nitrosoguanidine; DMH, 1,2-dimethylhydrazine; s.c., subcutaneously; i.p. intraperitoneally; MNU, N-methyl-N-nitrosourea; SU, statistics unspecified received drinking-water containing 0.05% β-carotene (as an emulsion containing 0.5% sucrose ester P-1750, 1% Sansoft 8000, 0.2% L-ascorbyl stearate and 4% peanut oil; mean β-carotene intake, 3.27 mg/d per mouse) or the emulsion without β-carotene for four weeks. On the first day, all mice received a single subcutaneous injection of 10 mg/kg bw 4-nitroquinoline 1-oxide (4-NQO) dissolved in a 20:1 mixture of olive oil and cholesterol (about 0.3 mg 4-NQO per mouse). During weeks 5–25, the drinking-water of all mice contained 10% glycerol. The mice were killed at week 30. There was no significant difference in water intake or body weight between the two groups. The percentages of mice with lung tumours (type II adenoma) were 94 and 93, and the mean numbers of lung tumours per mouse were 4.06 ± 0.18 in controls and 4.93 ± 0.28 in those given β-carotene. The size of the lung tumours [not further specified] was similar in the two groups. The study was repeated with almost similar results [no further details presented] (Murakoshi et al., 1992; Nishino, 1995).

Two groups of newborn male and female N:GP(S) mice, less than 24 h old, received a single subcutaneous injection into the scapular region of 0.02 ml of a suspension of 0.5 mg benzo[a]pyrene in 1% aqueous gelatin or 0.02 ml of the 1% aqueous gelatin alone. After weaning, the mice received NIH 7-open formula diet either alone (41 males and 39 females given benzo[a]pyrene; 39 male and 40 female controls) or containing 500 mg/kg β-carotene (40 males and 40 females given benzo[a]pyrene; 40 male and 38 female controls) for six weeks. Nine weeks after the benzo[a]pyrene injection, all mice were killed and examined for lung tumours. β-Carotene did not significantly affect the incidence of lung tumours (adenoma), which occurred in [15/41] males and [22/39] females given benzo[a]pyrene and [15/40] males and [15/40] females given benzo[a]-pyrene plus β-carotene (χ^2 test); nor did it affect the multiplicity, which was 1.02 ± 2.17 in males and 1.38 ± 2.08 in females given benzo[a]pyrene and 0.85 ± 1.42 in males and 0.83 ± 1.81 in females given benzo[a]pyrene plus β-carotene (Student's t test). No lung tumours were found in mice fed only β-carotene, while 1/39 males

and 1/40 females in the group on unsupplemented diet developed a pulmonary adenoma (Yun et al., 1995).

Hamster: β-Carotene was added at a dose of 56 mg/kg to a semisynthetic diet as water-dispersible beadlets containing 10% pure β-carotene and administered to a group of weanling Syrian golden hamsters [age not further specified], initially consisting of 40 males and 40 females, for 374 days to females and 429 days to males. A group of 60 male and 60 female hamsters fed the same diet without β-carotene served as controls [use of placebo beadlets unspecified]. After an adaptation period of 30 days on the diets, all hamsters received an intratracheal instillation of 8 mg benzo[a]-pyrene and 8 mg ferric oxide suspended in 0.2 ml sterile saline once every two weeks for 16 weeks. At the end of the study, the serum concentrations of β-carotene and serum retinol (free and bound to retinol-binding protein) were higher in the animals given β-carotene than in controls; however, the concentrations of both β-carotene and vitamin A in the liver were statistically significantly increased ($p < 0.01$; analysis of variance). Body weight and food intake were not affected by β-carotene. At the end of the experiment, the survival rate in one of the groups had dropped below 25% [mortality not further specified]. β-Carotene did not clearly affect the tumour response (predominantly epidermoid carcinomas, epidermoid papillomas, adenosquamous carcinomas and adenomas) in the respiratory tract, the incidences of tumours in males being 34/57 in controls and 26/38 in those given β-carotene and those in females being 37/57 and 25/36, respectively. When the tumour incidences were analysed by a method that took into account differences in mortality between the groups, however, the tumour response in the respiratory tract tended to increase in animals of each sex given β-carotene rather than to decrease ($p = 0.07$ for positive trend), and the incidences of epidermoid papillomas in the trachea, bronchi and larynx in these animals were statistically significantly increased ($p = 0.04$), as were those of all types of laryngeal tumours combined ($p = 0.03$ [incidences of tumours at these sites unspecified]). The incidence and severity of preneoplastic changes in the respiratory tract—dysplasia in the larynx, metaplasia in the trachea and bronchi, alveolar bronchiolization in the lungs—were not affected by β-carotene (Beems, 1987).

Groups of 10–20 male Syrian golden hamsters, five to six weeks of age, were given subcutaneous injections of 1.5 mg β-carotene (micellar form dispersed in an aqueous solution, 40 mg/ml) twice a week. After one week, the animals received NDEA at 17.8 mg/kg bw by subcutaneous injection 24 h after every β-carotene injection for 20 weeks. At termination of the study after 25 weeks on the test diets, the entire respiratory tree was removed, and incidence of tumours was examined. β-Carotene reduced the tumour incidence by 48% (not significant) (Moon et al., 1994).

Two groups of 50 male Syrian golden hamsters [age unspecified] were fed a pelleted diet containing 4000 IU/kg retinyl palmitate with or without 1% (w/w) β-carotene. After one month, all of the hamsters received 10 intratracheal instillations of 8 mg benzo[a]pyrene and 8 mg ferric oxide particles suspended in 0.2 ml saline for 12 weeks, while two groups of 20 hamsters received 10 intratracheal instillations of ferric oxide only. One week after the last instillation, six to eight hamsters in each group given benzo[a]pyrene were killed; the remaining survivors were killed five weeks later. The incidences of preneoplastic and neoplastic changes in the larynx, trachea and lungs were not reduced by β-carotene but on the contrary were almost twice as high in hamsters fed the β-carotene-supplemented diet: Squamous-cell carcinomas of the larynx, carcinomas in situ, squamous-cell carcinomas of the trachea and papillomas, squamous-cell carcinomas, adenosquamous carcinomas, adenocarcinomas and carcinosarcomas of the lungs or bronchi occurred in 15/41 animals, in comparison with 8/39 in hamsters on the control diet; however, the difference was not statistically significant ($p = 0.15$; two-sided Fisher exact probability test). The average time to appearance of the tumours was 19 weeks in animals receiving β-carotene and 18 weeks in controls. No respiratory-tract tumours were found in hamsters that were not treated with benzo[a]pyrene (Wolterbeek et al., 1995a).

(d)   Urinary bladder (Table 29)

Mouse: Groups of 23–25 B6D2F$_1$ mice [sex and age unspecified] were given N-nitrosobutyl(4-hydroxybutyl)amine (NBHBA) in ethanol or ethanol alone by stomach tube: two groups received 10 weekly doses of 1.5 mg NBHBA (total dose, 15 mg), two groups received 10 weekly doses of 3.0 mg NBHBA (total dose, 30 mg), and two groups received alcohol alone [volume unspecified]. For the next six months, one group on each treatment was maintained on standard diet, while the other three groups received standard diet supplemented with 5 mmol/kg β-carotene [method and dose not further specified]. No significant effect of β-carotene was observed on the incidence of either hyperplasia or carcinoma of the urothelium, the incidences being 0/24, 7/23, 16/25, 18/24 13/25 and 12/25 for hyperplasia and 0/24, 0/23, 6/25, 4/24, 12/25 and 11/25 for carcinoma in the vehicle controls, the β-carotene controls, the mice fed the low dose of NBHBA, those fed the low dose of NBHBA plus β-carotene, those fed the high dose of NBHBA and those given the high dose of NBHBA plus β-carotene, respectively [statistics unspecified] (Hicks et al., 1984)

Two groups of 24 male B6D2F$_1$ mice, five to seven weeks old, were fed powdered rodent chow supplemented with either 10% β-carotene-containing beadlets (0.1% β-carotene in the diet) or the same amount of placebo beadlets, for about seven months. After five weeks, all mice received 5 mg NBHBA in saline (total dose, 90 mg) by gastric tube twice weekly for nine weeks. The mice were killed six months after the first instillation of NBHBA. β-Carotene did not affect body weight, but it reduced the incidence of urinary bladder tumours (carcinoma in situ and transitional-cell carcinoma) from 15/24 to 8/24 ($p < 0.05$; χ^2 test) (Mathews-Roth et al., 1991).

Rat: A total of 285 weanling Fischer 344 rats [age and sex unspecified] were randomized into four groups [number of rats per group not specified], two of which received a basic vitamin A-deficient diet while the other two received the same diet with added vitamin A palmitate [amount unspecified] for 46 days. At day 46, the diets of one of the groups on the basic diet and one of the groups with added vitamin A were supplemented with 3 mmol/kg β-carotene [not further specified]; the other group on basic diet received a low level of vitamin A palmitate in the drinking-water to maintain a healthy but vitamin A-deficient condition. After day 102, the rats were dosed [route unspecified] with 635 mg per rat NBHBA in five weekly portions, except for one-half of the rats on vitamin A-deficient basic diet with added vitamin A palmitate and β-carotene and half the rats on vitamin A-deficient basic diet receiving vitamin A palmitate in their drinking-water, which were treated with the NBHBA vehicle [unspecified] only. All rats were killed 42 weeks later, and the urinary bladders were examined histologically. The urothelium of vehicle-treated rats was normal. β-Carotene did not reduce the incidence of hyperplasia or carcinoma of the bladder epithelium in NBHBA-treated rats, hyperplasia being seen in 16/26, 16/26, 20/28 and 16/33 and carcinomas in 10/26, 10/26, 8/28 and 17/33 rats on the vitamin A-deficient basic diet with added vitamin A palmitate and β-carotene, the vitamin A-deficient basic diet with added vitamin A palmitate, the vitamin A-deficient basic diet with β-carotene and the vitamin A-deficient basic diet with vitamin A palmitate in the drinking-water, respectively (Pedrick et al., 1990) [The Working Group noted the absence of information on mortality and intercurrent deaths.]

(e) Liver (see also Table 30)

Mouse: Groups of 17 eight-week-old male C3H/He mice, which have a high spontaneous incidence of liver tumours, received 0.005 or 0.05% β-carotene mixed with the drinking-water as an emulsion containing 0.5% sucrose ester P-1750, 1% Sansoft 8000, 0.2% L-ascorbyl stearate and 4% peanut oil, to give mean β-carotene intakes of 0.24 and 2.47 mg/d per mouse, respectively, or the emulsion without β-carotene for 40 weeks, at the end of which the mice were killed. There was no significant difference in body weight or water intake between the groups. All of the mice developed well-

differentiated hepatocellular carcinomas. β-Carotene did not significantly reduce the mean number of liver tumours per mouse, although relatively few occurred in animals at the high dose: 6.31 ± 0.62 in controls, 7.38 ± 0.83 at the low dose and 4.71 ± 0.39 at the high dose. The size [not further specified] and histological appearance of the tumours did not differ among the groups (Murakoshi et al., 1992).

Rat: Groups of 15 male albino Wistar rats, 50 days old and weighing about 150 g, were fed an adequate basal diet gelatinized with a 3% agar solution (water content of the diet, 50%) and another was fed the basal diet supplemented with 1 mg/kg β-carotene. After seven days, all animals receiving β-carotene and those in one of the two groups given unsupplemented basal diet received a single dose of 500 mg aflatoxin B_1 dissolved in 0.2 ml dimethylsulfoxide by stomach tube, while the other group on basal diet received 0.2 ml dimethylsulfoxide only. Three weeks after aflatoxin B_1 administration, the animals fed the β-carotene-supplemented diet were switched to basal diet. The experiment was terminated at 24 months, when all survivors were killed and examined for liver lesions. The incidence of hepatocellular carcinomas in the group treated with aflatoxin B_1 and given unsupplemented diet was 12/15; no liver tumours were found in the vehicle controls or in the group treated with aflatoxin B_1 and fed the β-carotene-supplemented diet. In these groups, 14/15 rats survived for 24 months, whereas in the group treated with aflatoxin B_1 and fed the basal diet only 7/15 animals survived (Nyandieka et al., 1990). [The Working Group noted the absence of statistical analysis.]

Two groups of Wistar rats [age unspecified], weighing 90–100 g, were kept on a commercial natural diet containing 5 μg/g diet vitamin A and 0.08 μg/g diet β-carotene; a group of 10 received corn oil and a group of 12 received corn oil containing β-carotene (trans, type I; 70 mg/kg bw) intragastrically every other day for eight weeks. After two weeks, all rats received a single intraperitoneal injection of 200 mg/kg bw N-nitrosodiethylamine (NDEA) in 0.9% saline. Two weeks later, all rats received a single dose of 20 mg/kg bw 2-acetylaminofluorene

Table 30. Effects of β-carotene on liver tumorigenesis in experimental animals

Species, strain, sex	No. of animals/group	Carcinogen (dose/route)	Carotenoid (dose/route)	Treatment period	Preventive efficacy	Reference
Mouse, C3H/He, male	17	–	0.005 and 0.05% in drinking-water (0.24 and 2.47 mg/mouse per day)	–	Liver carcinomas Incidence: none (NS) Multiplicity: low dose, none (NS); high dose, 25% (NS)	Murakoshi et al. (1992)
Rat, Wistar, male	15	500 mg AFB1, single dose by gavage	1 µg/kg diet	Before and during	Hepatocellular carcinomas: 100% [SU]	Nyandieka et al. (1990)
Rat, Wistar, male	10–12	NDEA, 200 mg/kg bw, single dose, i.p. 2-AAF, 10–20 mg/kg bw, 5 daily doses, gavage; partial hepatectomy	70 mg/kg bw, gavage; 8 weeks	Before, during and after	Preneoplasia Incidence: 75% ($p < 0.005$); Number: 95% ($p < 0.05$); Area: 85% ($p < 0.01$)	Moreno et al. (1991)
Rat, Wistar, male	7–11	NDEA, 200 mg/kg bw, single dose, i.p. 2-AAF, 10–20 mg/kg bw, 5 daily doses, gavage; partial hepatectomy	70 mg/kg bw, gavage; 8 weeks	Before	Preneoplasia Incidence: 55% ($p < 0.05$) Number: 87% ($p < 0.05$) Area: 77% ($p < 0.01$)	Moreno et al. (1991)
Rat, Wistar, male	11	NDEA, 200 mg/kg bw, single dose, i.p.; 2-AAF, 10–20 mg/kg bw, 5 daily doses, gavage	70 mg/kg bw, gavage; 8 weeks	During and after	Preneoplasia Incidence: none Number: 25% (NS) Area: 55% (NS)	Moreno et al. (1991)
Rat, Fischer, male	13–15	IQ (100 mg/kg bw), single dose, gavage	0.02% in diet	Before and during	GST-P+ foci: Number 45% ($p < 0.001$) Area 30% ($p < 0.05$)	Tsuda et al. (1994)

Table 30 (contd)

Species, strain, sex	No. of animals/group	Carcinogen (dose/route)	Carotenoid (dose/route)	Treatment period	Preventive efficacy	Reference
Rat, Sprague-Dawley, male	10–14	2-AAF, 0.05% in diet	100 mg/kg diet	Before and during; before; after	Hyperplastic liver-cell nodules Before and during: Incidence, 77% [SU] Number, 99% [SU] Before: Incidence, 60% [SU] Number, 97% [SU] After: Incidence, 37% [SU] Number, 84% [SU]	Sarkar et al. (1994)
Rat, Fischer, male	15–16	NDEA (200 mg/kg bw), single dose, i.p.	0.1% in the diet	After	None (NS)	Hirose et al. (1995)
Rat, Fischer, male	15–16	NDEA (200 mg/kg bw), single dose, i.p. + Glu-P-1 (0.03% in diet)	0.1% in the diet	After	GST-P+ foci, Number: 26% ($p < 0.01$) Area: 48% ($p < 0.05$)	Hirose et al. (1995)
Rat, Fischer, male	15–16	NDEA (200 mg/kg bw) + NDMA (0.002% in drinking-water)	0.1% in the diet	After	None (rather an increase)	Hirose et al. (1995)
Rat, Sprague-Dawley, male	8–12	3'-Met-DAB, 0.06% in diet	120 mg/kg diet	Before, during and after	Hyperplastic liver-cell nodules Before and during: Incidence, 75% [SU] Number, 97% [SU] Multiplicity, 92% ($p < 0.001$) Before: Incidence, 58% [SU] Number, 92% [SU] Multiplicity, 87% ($p < 0.001$) After: Incidence, 37% [SU] Number, 71% [SU] Multiplicity, 67% ($p < 0.001$)	Sankar et al. (1995a)

Table 30 (contd)

Species, strain, sex	No. of animals/group	Carcinogen (dose/route)	Carotenoid (dose/route)	Treatment period	Preventive efficacy	Reference
Rat, Sprague-Dawley, male	12–14	NDEA, 200 mg/kg bw, single dose, i.p. Phenobarbital, 0.05% in drinking-water for 12 weeks	120 mg/kg diet	Before, during and after	Preneoplasia Incidence: significant [% unspecified] Number: 75% ($p < 0.001$) Volume: 66% ($p < 0.001$)	Sarkar et al. (1995b)
Rat, Sprague-Dawely, male	12–14	NDEA, 200 mg/kg bw, single dose, i.p. Phenobarbital, 0.05% in drinking-water for 12 weeks	120 mg/kg diet	Before	Preneoplasia Incidence: significant [% unspecified] Number: 58% ($p < 0.001$) Volume: 62% ($p < 0.001$)	Sarkar et al. (1995b)
Rat, Sprague-Dawely, male	12–14	NDEA, 200 mg/kg bw, single dose, i.p. Phenobarbital, 0.05% in drinking-water for 12 weeks	120 mg/kg diet	After	Preneoplasia Incidence: significant [% unspecified] Number: 41% ($p < 0.001$) Volume: 34% ($p < 0.05$)	Sarkar et al. (1995b)
Rat, Wistar, male	6	NDEA, 200 mg/kg bw, single dose, i.p. 2-AAF, 20 mg/kg bw, 6 daily doses, gavage; partial hepatectomy	70 mg/kg bw, gavage; 8 weeks	Before, during and after	Preneoplasia Incidence: 50% [SU] Number: 46% ($p < 0.05$) Area: 72% ($p < 0.05$)	Moreno et al. (1995)
Rat, SPF Wistar, male	10	NDEA, 200 mg/kg bw, single dose, i.p. 2-AAF, 50 mg/kg diet Phenobarbital, 500 ppm in diet	300 mg/kg diet, 3 weeks	Before and during	Preneoplastic foci: None (NS)	Astorg et al. (1996)

Table 30 (contd)

Species, strain, sex	No. of animals/group	Carcinogen (dose/route)	Carotenoid (dose/route)	Treatment period	Preventive efficacy	Reference
Rat, SPF Wistar, male	9–10	NDEA, 200 mg/kg bw, single dose, i.p. 2-AAF, 50 mg/kg diet Phenobarbital, 500 ppm in diet	9 doses of 10 mg/kg bw; i.p.	Before and during	Preneoplastic foci: None (NS)	Astorg et al. (1996)
Rat, Fischer 344, male	12	AFB_1 (0.25 mg/kg bw, intragastrically, for 2 weeks)	Carotenoid-rich food extract, 250 mg/kg bw intragastrically	Initiating or post-initiating phase	Decrease in foci diameter ($p < 0.05$), decrease in number of foci/cm³ ($p < 0.05$)	He et al. (1997)
Rat, SPF Wistar, male	7–9	2-Nitropropane 6 x 100 mg/kg bw, i.p.	300 mg/kg diet	Before and during	Fraction of liver volume occupied by GST-P+ foci: none (NS)	Astorg et al. (1997)
Rat, SPF Wistar, male	9–10	NDEA, 100 mg/kg bw, single dose, i.p.	300 mg/kg diet	Before and during	Fraction of liver volume occupied by GST-P+ foci: 58% (NS)	Astorg et al. (1997)
Rat, SPF Wistar, male	9–10	AFB_1, 2 x 1 mg/kg bw, i.p.	300 mg/kg diet	Before and during	Fraction of liver volume occupied by GST-P+ foci: 83% ($p < 0.05$)	Gradelet et al. (1998)

From Appel & Woutersen (1996)
NS, not significant; AFB1, aflatoxin B₁; SU, statistics unspecified; NDEA, N-nitrosodiethylamine; i.p., intraperitoneally; 2-AAF, 2-acetylaminofluorene; IQ, 2-amino-3-methylimidazo [4,5-f]quinoline;
GST-P⁺, glutathione S-transferase placental form-positive; Glu-P-1, 2-amino-6-methyldipyrido[1,2-α: 3′2′-d]imidazole; NDMA, N-nitrosodimethylamine; 3′-Met-DAB, 3′-methyl-4-dimethylaminoazobenzene

(2-AAF) dissolved in corn oil by gavage for four consecutive days and were subjected one day later to a two-thirds hepatectomy. Four days later, a last dose of 10 mg/kg bw 2-AAF was given by gavage. All rats were killed eight weeks after the start of the experiment. The body weights were statistically significantly higher in the β-carotene group (309 ± 31g) than in the control group (264 ± 30 g; $p < 0.005$; Student's t test). The hepatic concentration of β-carotene was enhanced in animals that received it for eight weeks (1.79 ± 0.42) in comparison with controls (0.84 ± 0.14) and in those that received it for six weeks after initiation (2.23 ± 1.71; 1.57 ± 1.89 in controls) but not in those that received β-carotene only for two weeks in the initiation study (0.72 ± 0.07; 1.34 ± 1.44 in controls). β-Carotene reduced the incidence of hyperplastic nodules from 10/10 to 3/12 ($p < 0.005$; Student's t test), the total number of nodules from 581 to 8, the number of nodules per cm^2 from 33.7 ± 29.3 to 1.7 ± 1.4 ($p < 0.05$; Student's t test) and the total area of the nodules from 0.62 ± 0.24 to 0.10 ± 0.09 mm^2 ($p < 0.005$; Student's t test) (Moreno et al., 1991).

Two groups of male rats were similarly treated, except that β-carotene in corn oil was administered to 11 rats and corn oil to seven rats only during the first two weeks of the experiment (initiation study). There was no significant difference in body weight between the two groups. β-Carotene reduced the incidence of hyperplastic nodules from 7/7 to 5/11 ($p < 0.05$; Student's t test), the total number of nodules from 302 to18, the number of nodules per cm^2 from 14.3 ± 18.5 to 1.9 ± 2.0 ($p < 0.05$; Student's t test) and the total area of the nodules from 0.35 ± 0.20 to 0.08 ± 0.07 mm^2 ($p < 0.005$; Student's t test).

Another two groups of 11 male rats were treated similarly, except that administration of corn oil with or without β-carotene was begun after two weeks and NDEA was administered on the first day of the experiment (selection–promotion study). There was no significant difference in body weight between the two groups. β-Carotene had no significant effect on the selection–promotion phase of liver carcinogenesis: the incidences of hyperplastic nodules were 7/11 in both groups, the total number of

nodules was 1143 in controls and 138 in the β-carotene group, the number of nodules per cm^2 was 18.9 ± 18.8 in controls and 14.2 ± 19.5 in the β-carotene group (not significant; Student's t test), and the total area of the nodules was 0.38 ± 0.33 in controls and 0.17 ± 0.14 mm^2 in the β-carotene group (not significant; Student's t test) (Moreno et al., 1991).

Two groups of 13 or 15 male, six-week old Fischer rats were given basal diet containing 0 or 0.02% β-carotene for eight days [formulation in diet unspecified]. On day 7, each rat was given a single dose of 100 mg/kg bw 2-amino-3-methylimidazo[4,5-f]quinoline (IQ) by gavage 12 h after a two-thirds hepatectomy. After two weeks on basal diet without added β-carotene, all rats were fed basal diet containing 0.05% phenobarbital for eight weeks. One week after the start of the phenobarbital feeding, each rat received a single intraperitoneal injection of 100 mg/kg bw D-galactosamine. Two additional groups of five rats each, fed basal diet with or without 0.02% β-carotene, did not receive the intragastric dose of IQ but were otherwise treated in the same way as the two other groups. At 11 weeks, all survivors were killed, and the livers were examined for the presence of placental glutathione S-transferase-positive (GST-P+) foci (areas > 70 mm in diameter). The body weights of the rats treated with β-carotene and IQ were slightly, statistically significantly lower than those of the rats treated only with IQ ($p < 0.05$; Student's t test). β-Carotene significantly reduced both the number per cm^2 and the area (mm^2/cm^2) of GST-P+ foci, the numbers being 14.54 ± 4.04 and 7.99 ± 3.14 ($p < 0.001$; Student's t test) and the areas being 107 674 ± 42 178 and 74 949 ± 33 221 ($p < 0.05$; Student's t test) for the rats given IQ and those given β-carotene plus IQ, respectively. No significant induction of GST-P+ foci was found in the rats not given IQ (Tsuda et al., 1994).

trans-β-Carotene administered at a dose of 100 mg/kg diet before and during the initiation and selection–promotion phase (20 weeks), only during the initiation phase (four weeks) or only during the selection–promotion phase (10 weeks) to groups of 10–14 male Sprague-Dawley rats weighing 130–150 g [age unspecified] reduced the incidence and total number of hyperplastic nodules induced in liver cells by 2-AAF at 0.05% in the diet for 16 weeks. The incidences of nodules were 13/13, 3/13, 4/10 and 7/11 and the total numbers were > 600, 8, 18 and 94 in the 2-AAF-treated animals and the groups receiving the β-carotene-supplemented diet before and during the initiation and selection–promotion phase, only during the initiation phase or only during the selection–promotion phase, respectively [no statistical analysis reported]. In each group receiving β-carotene, the β-carotene content of the liver was two to four times higher than that in controls (0.35 μg/g liver) (Sarkar et al., 1994).

trans-β-Carotene administered at a dose of 120 mg/kg diet before and during the initiation and selection–promotion phase (20 weeks), only during the initiation phase (four weeks) or only during the selection–promotion phase (10 weeks) to groups of 8–12 male Sprague-Dawley rats weighing 130–150 g [age unspecified] reduced the incidence, total number and multiplicity of hyperplastic nodules induced in the liver by 3′-methyl-4-dimethylaminoazobenzene (3′-Met-DAB) at 0.06% in the diet for 16 weeks. The incidence, total number and multiplicity (average number of nodules per nodule-bearing liver) of hyperplastic nodules in the three groups were: incidence: 8/8, 3/12, 5/12 and 7/11; numbers: 350, 10, 28 and 102; and multiplicity: 43.75 ± 11.31, 3.3 ± 1.15, 5.6 ± 2.07 and 14.57 ± 2.99 (for the last measure, $p < 0.001$ for all three groups; Student's t test [no statistical analysis reported for incidence or total number of nodules]). In the groups receiving β-carotene, the level of this carotenoid in the liver was two to four times higher than that in controls (0.39 μg/g liver) (Sarkar et al., 1995a).

Seven groups of 15 or 16 male Fischer 344 rats, six weeks old, with an average body weight of 150.2 g, were given a single intraperitoneal injection of 200 mg/kg bw NDEA and were fed basal diet for two weeks. Two of the groups received unsupplemented basal diet for another six weeks, and the other five groups received the basal diet supplemented with 0.1% β-carotene (in gelatin as coating material), 0.03% 2-amino-6-methyldipyridol[1,2-α:3′,2′-d]imidazole (Glu-P-1), 0.3% Glu-P-1 plus 0.1% β-carotene, 0.002% N-nitrosodimethylamine

(NDMA) or 0.002% NDMA plus 0.1% β-carotene for six weeks. At the end of week 3, all rats were subjected to a two-thirds hepatectomy. There were no significant differences in body weight or relative liver weight between the groups, except for a statistically significantly reduced liver weight in rats fed the diet with Glu-P-1 plus β-carotene (3.34 g/100 g bw) as compared with that in rats fed the diet with Glu-P-1 alone (3.60 g/100 g bw) ($p < 0.05$), which in turn was significantly greater than that of rats fed the unsupplemented basal diet (3.20 g/100 g bw) ($p < 0.001$ [statistical test unspecified]). β-Carotene significantly reduced the development of NDEA plus Glu-P-1-induced GST-P$^+$ foci in the liver, the numbers and areas of the foci in rats fed β-carotene plus Glu-P-1 being 34.4 ± 10.5/cm^2 and 6.2 ± 2.8 mm^2/cm^2 versus 46.8 ± 11.0/cm^2 and 12.0 ± 5.6 mm^2/cm^2 in those fed Glu-P-1, respectively ($p < 0.01$ for the number and < 0.05 for the area [statistical test unspecified]). β-Carotene significantly increased the development of NDEA plus NDMA-induced GST-P$^+$ foci, the numbers and areas of foci in the animals fed β-carotene plus NDMA being 20.9 ± 5.1/cm^2 and 2.9 ± 1.2 mm^2/cm^2 versus 16.5 ± 3.9/cm^2 and 2.1 ± 1.0 mm^2/cm^2 in those treated with NDMA, respectively ($p < 0.05$ for the number; the difference is not significant for the area [statistical test unspecified]). β-Carotene did not affect the development of GST-P$^+$ foci induced by NDEA alone, the numbers and areas of foci in rats fed β-carotene plus NDEA being 3.5 ± 1.5/cm^2 and 0.3 ± 0.3 mm^2/cm^2 versus 3.8 ± 1.6/cm^2 and 0.4 ± 0.2 mm^2/cm^2 in those treated with NDEA, respectively [statistical test unspecified] (Hirose et al., 1995).

Two groups of 12–14 male Sprague-Dawley rats weighing 130–150 g [age unspecified] were fed a purified basal diet alone or supplemented with 120 mg/kg β-carotene for 20 weeks, followed by the unsupplemented diet during the final two weeks of the study. After four weeks, all rats received a single intraperitoneal injection of 200 mg/kg bw NDEA in 0.9% saline. Four weeks later, all rats were given drinking-water containing 0.05% phenobarbital for 12 weeks; during the final two weeks of the study, all rats received unsupplemented drinking-water. At 22 weeks, the rats were killed and examined for hyperplastic nodules in the liver. β-Carotene significantly decreased (Student's t test) the incidence of nodules and the total area of the liver parenchyma occupied by the nodules [no further data presented]. Moreover, β-carotene reduced the number of hyperplastic nodules per cm^3 liver from 1664.75 ± 184.49 to 421 ± 46.24, and the volume per 0.1 mm^3 from 1.90 ± 0.19 to 0.64 ± 0.17 ($p < 0.001$ for both number and volume; Student's t test). Similar results were found in additional groups of rats treated comparably but fed the β-carotene-supplemented diet only during the first four weeks of the study, before the NDEA injection (initiation study) or only during weeks 10–20 (selection–promotion study). The number of hyperplastic nodules per cm^3 liver was reduced from 1664.75 ± 184.49 to 702.75 ± 24.12 and the volume per 0.1 mm^3 from 1.90 ± 0.19 to 0.73 ± 0.10 ($p < 0.01$ for both number and volume; Student's t test) in the initiation study. In the selection–promotion study, the number was reduced from 1664.75 ± 184.49 to 989.25 ± 83.77 ($p < 0.001$; Student's t test) and the volume per 0.1 mm^3 from 1.90 ± 0.19 to 1.26 ± 0.43 ($p < 0.05$; Student's t test) (Sarkar et al., 1995b).

Two groups of six male Wistar rats weighing 60–70 g [age unspecified] were kept on regular chow pellets containing 0.24 μg/g diet β-carotene and 20 μg/g diet vitamin A and received either corn oil or corn oil containing 70 mg/kg bw trans-β-carotene (type I) by gavage for eight weeks. After two weeks, each rat received a single intraperitoneal injection of 200 mg/kg bw NDEA in 0.9% saline. Two weeks later, all rats were given 20 mg/kg bw 2-AAF dissolved in corn oil by gavage on four consecutive days, followed on the fifth day by a two-thirds hepatectomy; two and four days later, all rats again received 20 mg/kg bw 2-AAF in corn oil by gavage. Eight weeks after the start of the study, all rats were killed. The average body weight of rats fed β-carotene (266.8 ± 10.1 g) was significantly higher than that of the controls (244.3 ± 17.8 g) ($p < 0.05$; Student's t test). The concentration of β-carotene in the liver was increased from 0.06 ± 0.06 μg/g liver in controls to 0.34 ± 0.40 μg/g liver in rats fed β-carotene. β-Carotene reduced the incidence

of hyperplastic nodules from 6/6 to 3/6, the total number of nodules from 1691 to 23, the number of hepatocyte nodules per cm^2 from 37.1 ± 9.7 to 20.1 ± 12.5 ($p < 0.05$; Student's t test) and the total area of the nodules from 0.54 ± 0.39 to 0.15 ± 0.06 mm^2 ($p < 0.05$; Student's t test) (Moreno et al., 1995).

Two groups of 10 male SPF Wistar rats, 24–27 days old, were fed a semiliquid purified diet containing 10% corn oil and 6000 IU/kg vitamin A and supplemented with 300 mg/kg β-carotene from a 10% dispersible powder or the same diet supplemented with placebo powder for 21 days, followed by the same diet with no supplement for 21 days. On day 15, all rats were injected intraperitoneally with 200 mg/kg bw NDEA in 0.9% saline. 2-AAF was added to the diet at 50 mg/kg on days 42–56. On day 49, all rats were subjected to a two-thirds hepatectomy. From day 56 to the end of the experiment (day 70), the diets were supplemented with 500 ppm phenobarbital. The liver β-carotene content in the group fed this compound was 30.4 ± 3.0 μg/g after 15 days of feeding and remained significant on day 49 (4.7 ± 0.9 μg/g liver) and at the end of the experiment (1.1 ± 0.3 μg/g liver), indicating good absorption of the compound. There was no significant difference in body weight between the two groups. β-Carotene did not significantly inhibit (one-sided Dunnett's test and one-sided t test) the number of γ-glutamyltranspeptidase-positive (GGT$^+$) liver foci (28.7 ± 3.1 versus 28.4 ± 2.3 in controls), the number of GST-P$^+$ foci (51.2 ± 5.3 versus 51.4 ± 7.6 in controls), the mean area of GGT$^+$ foci (0.156 ± 0.02 mm^2 versus 0.145 ± 0.017 mm^2 in controls), the mean area of GST-P$^+$ foci (0.167 ± 0.027 mm^2 versus 0.146 ± 0.023 mm^2 in controls), the area occupied by GGT$^+$ foci (4.88 ± 0.90% versus 4.39 ± 0.82% in controls) or the area occupied by GST-P$^+$ foci (7.64 ± 1.02% versus 7.49 ± 1.45% in controls) (Astorg et al., 1996).

Male SPF Wistar rats, 24–27 days old, were fed a semiliquid purified diet containing 10% corn oil, 6000 IU/kg vitamin A and 3 g/kg carotenoid placebo powder for 21 days, followed by the same diet with no supplement for 21 days. Ten animals were then injected intraperitoneally with 10 mg/kg bw emulsified β-carotene three times per week during the first three weeks of the experiment (total β-carotene dose, 90 mg/kg bw), while nine controls were injected with the placebo emulsion. On day 15, all rats were injected intraperitoneally with 200 mg/kg bw NDEA bw in 0.9% saline. 2-AAF was added to the diet at 50 mg/kg on days 42–56. On day 49, all rats were subjected to a two-thirds hepatectomy. From day 56 to the end of the experiment (day 70), the diets were supplemented with 500 ppm phenobarbital. There was no significant difference in body weight between the two groups. The β-carotene content of the liver in the group fed this compound was 43.0 ± 3.4 μg/g on day 15 of the experiment and remained significant on day 49 (2.1 ± 0.9 μg/g liver) and at the end of the experiment ($0.4 \pm$ μg/g liver), indicating good incorporation into the liver. β-Carotene did not significantly inhibit (one-sided Dunnett's test and one-sided t test) the number of GGT^+ foci (31.4 ± 3.5 versus 37.1 ± 2.5 in controls), the number of $GST-P^+$ foci (52.1 ± 7.7 versus 47.1 ± 4.6 in controls), the mean area of GGT^+ foci (0.149 ± 0.041 mm^2 versus 0.150 ± 0.015 mm^2 in controls), the mean area of $GST-P^+$ foci (0.151 ± 0.037 mm^2 versus 0.153 ± 0.013 mm^2 in controls), the area occupied by GGT^+ foci ($4.59 \pm 1.09\%$ versus $5.58 \pm 0.59\%$ in controls) or the area occupied by $GST-P^+$ foci ($6.93 \pm 1.15\%$ versus $7.22 \pm 0.87\%$ in controls) (Astorg et al., 1996).

Male Fischer 344 rats, weighing 40–50 g, were acclimatized for two weeks and then randomized into experimental groups of 12 animals each. As the initiation stage, aflatoxin B_1 was administered intragastrically at daily doses of 0.25 mg/kg bw, dissolved in tricaprylin at a concentration of 250 mg/ml, for two periods of five days each with two days between dosing periods. Carotenoid-rich food extracts were prepared by repeated chloroform extraction of tomato paste (rich in lycopene), orange-juice concentrate (rich in β-cryptoxanthin) or tinned sliced carrots (rich in α- and β-carotene). The carotenoid content of each extract was estimated by high-performance liquid chromatography; solvents were removed under nitrogen, and the extracts were diluted to 500 mg/ml with tricaprylin. The carotenoid extracts were given by gavage at a dose of 250 mg/kg bw

during the initiation phase immediately after the aflatoxin B_1; after a one-week recovery period, they were given by gavage every second day for 12 weeks (i.e. the post-initiation phase, experimental weeks 3–15). At experimental week 15, GGT^+ foci in liver were measured as an indicator of hepatocarcinogenesis. The foci were significantly smaller in the groups treated with extracts of carrot (129 mm) and tomato (132 mm) during the post-initiation phase than in the control group (309 mm; $p < 0.05$). The number of foci per cm^3 was significantly lower in the groups treated with extracts of carrot (0.002), tomato (0.06) and orange (0.0001) during the initiation phase than in the control group (1.86; $p < 0.05$). The final body weights varied slightly among the groups, but administration of carotenoids during the initiation phase resulted in higher weights (He et al., 1997).

Wistar rats, 24–27 days old, were fed either a semiliquid purified diet containing 10% corn oil and 6000 IU/kg vitamin A supplemented with 300 mg/kg β-carotene from a 10% dispersible powder or the same diet supplemented with placebo powder for 28 days, followed by the same diet with no supplement for 21 days. On days 14, 16, 18, 21, 23 and 25, all rats were injected intraperitoneally with 100 mg/kw bw 2-nitropropane in 2% Tween 20. 2-AAF was added to the diet at 50 mg/kg on days 49–63. On day 56, all rats were subjected to a two-thirds hepatectomy. From day 63 to the end of the experiment (day 70), the rats received unsupplemented diet. The β-carotene content of the livers of rats fed this carotenoid was still 1.9 ± 0.5 μg/g liver at the time of partial hepatectomy, i.e four weeks after cessation of β-carotene feeding. β-Carotene did not significantly inhibit the onset of preneoplastic foci in the liver, as seen from the number of GGT^+ foci per cm^3 liver (407 ± 67 versus 371 ± 53 in controls), the number of $GST-P^+$ foci (1000 ± 230 versus 703 ± 120 in controls), the mean volume (10^{-3} mm^3) of GGT^+ foci (31.7 ± 7.5 versus 62.4 ± 20.6 in controls), the mean volume of $GST-P^+$ foci (34.1 ± 3.9 versus 59.9 ± 13.5 in controls), the fraction of the liver volume (mm^3/cm^3) occupied by GGT^+ foci (10.0 ± 4.2 versus 15.7 ± 5.5 in controls) or the fraction of the liver volume occupied by GST$^+$ foci (30.3 ± 11.0 versus 33.4 ± 8.6 in controls (Astorg *et al.*, 1997).

In a similar study, the animals were fed the same diets for 21 days, followed by the diet with no supplement for 21 days. On day 14, all rats were injected intraperitoneally with 100 mg/kw bw NDEA in 0.9% saline; 2-AAF was added to the diet at 50 mg/kg on days 42–56; all rats were subjected to a two-thirds hepatectomy on day 49; and the rats received unsupplemented diet from day 56 to the end of the experiment on day 63. β-Carotene did not significantly inhibit the number of GGT$^+$ foci/cm^3 liver (251 ± 66 versus 205 ± 40 in controls) or the number of GST-P$^+$ foci (1991 ± 285 versus 1853 ± 327 in controls); it decreased (not significantly) the mean volume (10^{-3} mm^3) of GGT$^+$ foci (23.4 ± 6.3 versus 61.0 ± 14.1 in controls), the mean volume of GST$^+$ foci (13.4 ± 3.4 versus 27.1 ± 8.4 in controls), the fraction of the liver volume (mm^3/cm^3) occupied by GGT$^+$ foci (5.4 ± 2.4 versus 10.8 ± 3.6 in controls) and the fraction of the liver volume occupied by GST-P$^+$ foci (21.2 ± 5.3 versus 50.7 ± 17.3 in controls) (Astorg *et al.*, 1997).

In a study of similar design, all rats were injected intraperitoneally on days 13 and 19 with 1 mg/kg bw aflatoxin B$_1$ in 50% dimethylsulfoxide in water; 50 mg/kg 2-AAF were added to the diet on days 42–56; all rats were subjected to a two-thirds hepatectomy on day 49; and the rats received unsupplemented diet on days 56–63 (end of the study). The β-carotene content of the livers of rats receiving the compound was still 9.2 ± 1.4 μg/g liver at the time of partial hepatectomy, i.e. four weeks after cessation of β-carotene feeding. β-Caro-tene significantly inhibited the onset of liver preneoplastic foci; i.e. the number of GST-P$^+$ foci (318 ± 107 versus 773 ± 169 in controls), the mean volume (10^{-3} mm^3) of GST-P$^+$ foci (24.3 ± 4.3 versus 107.8 ± 46.8 in controls) and the fraction of the liver volume (mm^3/cm^3) occupied by GST-P$^+$ foci (9.5 ± 4.0 versus 55.4 ± 17.6 in controls) (Gradelet *et al.*, 1998).

(f)   Buccal pouch (Table 31)
Hamster: Buccal pouch tumours were induced in 30 randomly bred male Syrian hamsters [age

unspecified] by topical application of DMBA (as 620 μg/ml heavy mineral oil), three times a week for 22 weeks; 15 hamsters were not treated with the carcinogen. The day after the last treatment with DMBA, the tumours of two groups of 10 hamsters were painted with 250 μg/ml β-carotene [unspecified source] in mineral oil or mineral oil alone twice a week for four weeks, while the other group of DMBA-treated animals received no further treatment; 10 of the controls were treated with β-carotene and the other five with mineral oil. At the end of treatment with β-carotene, buccal pouch tumours were found in 2/10 hamsters that received the carotenoid and in all animals treated with DMBA or DMBA plus mineral oil. The mean numbers of tumours per animal were 1.50 ± 0.53 in the group given DMBA, 0.25 ± 0.46 in those given DMBA plus β-carotene ($p <$ 0.001; Student's t test) and 1.50 ± 0.37 in those given DMBA plus mineral oil. No tumours were found in hamsters treated with β-carotene or mineral oil only (Schwartz *et al.*, 1986).

Groups of 10 male randomly bred Syrian hamsters, 60–90 days old and weighing 96–120 g, were painted on the left buccal pouch with a 0.25% solution of DMBA in heavy mineral oil (about 0.6 mg DMBA on the pouch surface) three times per week, treated similarly with DMBA and also painted with a 2.5% solution of β-carotene in mineral oil (about 0.62 mg β-carotene on the pouch surface) three times per week on alternate days to DMBA, painted with β-carotene alone or untreated. All of the hamsters were killed 22 weeks after the start of the study. All of the DMBA-induced buccal pouch tumours were moderately to well-differentiated epidermoid carcinomas. β-Carotene reduced the tumour incidence from 9/10 to 4/10 ($p < 0.001$; χ^2 test), the total number of tumours from 20 to 12 ($p <$ 0.001; Student's t test), their mean diameter from 2.87 ± 1.5 mm to 0.98 ± 0.86 mm ($p <$ 0.001; Student's t test) and the tumour burden (total number of buccal pouch tumours x mean volume of tumours) from 242 to 6 mm^3 ($p < 0.001$; Student's t test). Moreover, the carcinomas in the β-carotene-treated animals were less pleomorphic, better differentiated, less invasive and formed more keratin than those in the animals treated with DMBA only. No buccal pouch tumours were

Table 31. Effects of β-carotene on buccal pouch tumorigenesis in male hamsters

No. of animals/ group	Carcinogen (dose, route)	β-Carotene (dose, route)	Treatment relative to carcinogen	Preventive efficacy	Reference
5–10	DMBA, 620 µg/ml; painting	250 µg/µl; painted onto tumours	After	Regression tumour incidence: 80% [SU] Tumour multiplicity: 83% ($p < 0.001$)	Schwartz et al. (1986)
10	0.25% DMBA in oil ± 0.6 mg, painting	2.5% in oil; ± 0.62 mg; painted three times/ week	During	Tumour incidence: 56% ($p < 0.001$) Tumour burden: 74% ($p < 0.001$)	Suda et al. (1986)
10	0.1% DMBA in oil ± 0.24 mg; painting	190 ng/ml oil; painted three times/week	During and after	Tumour incidence: 60–80% ($p < 0.001$) Tumour burden: 93–97% ($p < 0.001$)	Suda et al. (1986)
10	0.25% DMBA; 25 mg/kg bw, 3 times/week	0.025% solution (25 mg/kg bw) painted on buccal pouch	During	Carcinomas Incidence: 56% ($p < 0.001$) Burden: 51% ($p < 0.001$)	Suda et al. (1987)
20	0.5% DMBA; 3 times/ week	250 µg, injected into cheek pouch three times/week	After	Epidermoid carcinomas; regression Complete: 20% [SU] Partial: 80% [SU]	Schwartz & Shklar (1987)
10	0.5% DMBA; 0.4 mg/painting	250 µg/injection into pouches	After	Carcinoma burden: 98% [SU]	Schwartz & Shklar (1988)
20	0.5% DMBA; 0.6 mg/painting; 3 times/week	0.19 mg injected into buccal pouch 3 times/week	After	Carcinomas; regression Burden: 93% [SU]	Shklar & Schwartz (1988)
20	0.1% DMBA; painting 3 times/week for 28 weeks	0.14 mg/ painting (1.5 mg/kg bw) 3 times/week	During	Carcinomas Incidence (gross tumours): 45% [SU] Multiplicity: 45–49% [SU] Burden: 40–55% ($p < 0.001$)	Schwartz et al. (1988)
20	0.5% DMBA; 0.6 mg/painting	400 µg animal/day; by mouth	After	Carcinomas: none [SU]	Shklar et al. (1989)
20	0.15% DMBA; 0.4 mg/painting	1.4 mg/kg bw, gavage	During	Carcinoma incidence: 45% (NS) Carcinoma burden: 98% ($p < 0.001$) Carcinoma onset: 25% (NS)	Schwartz et al. (1989)

Table 31 (contd)

No. of animals/group	Carcinogen (dose)	Beta-carotene, dose, route	Treatment relative to carcinogen	Preventive efficacy	Reference
20	0.25% DMBA; painting 3 times/week	2.5%; painting 3 times/week	During	Tumours Incidence: 50% at one time ($p < 0.05$) During: Incidence, 70% ($p < 0.001$) Burden: 97% ($p < 0.001$) After: Incidence: 60% ($p < 0.001$) Burden: 91% ($p < 0.001$) During promotion: Incidence: 80% ($p < 0.001$) Burden: 96% ($p < 0.001$)	Hibino et al. (1990)
15–20	0.125 mg DMBA/application	250 mg/topical application	After	Cheek pouch and forestomach tumours: 100% [SU]	Gijare et al. (1990)
10	0.5% DMBA; 0.6 mg/painting	3.8 µg in liposomes/submucosal injection	After	Regression of carcinoma burden: 99.7% ($p < 0.05$)	Schwartz et al. (1991)
10	0.5% DMBA; 0.6 mg/painting	4 µg/submucosal injection	After	Regression carcinoma burden: 59% [SU]	Schwartz et al. (1991)
15	AcO-NDMA; 2 mg/kg bw/painting; twice weekly; 6 months	5.8 nmol/IL in drinking-water	Before, during and after	Tumours Incidence: 92% ($p < 0.001$) Burden: 100% ($p < 0.001$) Latency: 33% [SU]	Azuine & Bhide (1992)
10	0.5% DMBA; painting 3 times/week	50 µg/topical application	During	Tumour burden: 85% ($p < 0.001$)	Shklar et al. (1993)
10	DMBA; 0.6 mg/painting; 3 times/week; 14 weeks	10 mg/kg bw; painting; 3 times/week; 14 weeks	During	Carcinomas Incidence: 10% [SU] Number: 53% [SU] Burden: 18% (NS)	Schwartz & Shklar (1997)

DMBA, 7,12-dimethylbenz[a]anthracene; SU, statistics unspecified; NS, not significant; AcO-NDMA, N-nitroso(acetoxymethyl)methylamine found in animals treated with β-carotene alone or in untreated controls (Suda *et al.*, 1986).

Groups of 10 hamsters similar to those used above were painted on the left buccal pouch with a 0.1% DMBA solution in oil [dose unspecified] for 10 weeks followed by no treatment for the next six weeks and then painted with a 40% benzoyl peroxide solution in acetone for the next nine weeks; painted on the left buccal pouch as in group 1 but also painted during the first 10 weeks with 190 ng/ml β-carotene in mineral oil three times per week on alternate days to DMBA; painted on the left buccal pouch as in group 1 but also treated with β-carotene three times per week during the six weeks of no DMBA treatment; painted on the left buccal pouch as in group 1 but also painted with β-carotene three times per week on alternate days to benzoyl peroxide during the last nine weeks; painted on the left buccal pouch as in group 1 but also painted with mineral oil three times per week on alternate days to DMBA during the first 10 weeks; painted on the left buccal pouch as in group 1 but also painted with mineral oil three times per week during the six weeks of no DMBA treatment; painted on the left buccal pouch as in group 1 but also with mineral oil three times per week on alternate days to benzoyl peroxide during the last nine weeks; or were untreated. All animals were killed at 28 weeks. β-Carotene, whether applied simultaneously with DMBA, immediately after DMBA or simultaneously with benzoyl peroxide, significantly reduced the incidence of buccal pouch epidermoid carcinomas, the total number of these tumours, their mean diameter and the tumour burden (Table 32). Moreover, the tumours found in the β-carotene-treated animals were generally smaller and tended to be less invasive than those in the DMBA-treated animals not painted with β-carotene (Suda *et al.*, 1986).

Groups of 10 male Syrian hamsters [age unspecified] were painted on the left buccal pouch with a 0.25% solution of DMBA in heavy mineral oil three times per week for 22 weeks, similarly treated with DMBA and also painted with a 0.25% solution of β-carotene in mineral oil (0.25 mg/ml; 25 mg/kg bw) three times per week on alternate days to DMBA, painted with β-carotene or untreated. All animals were killed at 22 weeks. No buccal pouch tumours were found in untreated controls or animals treated with β-carotene only. β-Carotene reduced the number of animals with well- to moderately differentiated epidermoid carcinomas of the buccal pouch, from 9/10 to 4/10 ($p < 0.001$; χ^2

Table 32. Incidence, total number, diameter and total burden of buccal pouch tumours in groups of 10 male Syrian hamsters after repeated topical painting with 7,12-dimethylbenz[*a*]anthracene (DMBA) alone or combined with β-carotene (BC)

Treatment during			Tumour response of the buccal pouch			
First ten weeks	Next six weeks	Next nine weeks[a]	Incidence	Total no.	Mean diameter (mm)	Total burden (mm^3)
DMBA	–	BeP	10/10	34	3.2 ± 1.4	582.1
DMBA + BC	–	BeP	3/10[c]	3[d]	2.1 ± 0.78[d]	15.3 [d]
DMBA	BC	BeP	4/10[c]	7[d]	2.4 ± 0.41[d]	50.4 [d]
DMBA	–	BeP + BC	2/1 [c]	5[d]	2.3 ± 0.26[d]	32 [d]
DMBA + oil	–	BeP	8/10	28	ND	ND
DMBA	Oil	BeP	10/10	31	ND	ND
DMBA	–	BeP + oil	9/10	26	ND	ND
–	–	–	0/10	0	0	0

From Suda *et al.* (1986); ND, not determined

[a] Benzoyl peroxide (BeP) used as promoter

[b] Total number of tumours x mean tumour volume

[c] χ^2; $p < 0.001$ in comparison with first group

[d] Student's *t* test; $p < 0.001$ in comparison with first group

test) and the mean tumour burden from 2.88 ± 1.49 to 1.40 ± 0.76 ($p < 0.001$; Student's t test). The tumours in β-carotene-treated animals were generally less invasive, better differentiated, less pleomorphic and had more keratin than the tumours in animals treated only with DMBA (Suda *et al.*, 1987)

Epidermoid carcinomas were produced in the right buccal pouches of three groups of 20 adult male Syrian golden hamsters [age not further specified] by painting with a 0.5% solution of DMBA in heavy mineral oil three times per week for 13 weeks. Then, the right buccal pouches were injected with 0.1 ml of a solution of about 250 μg β-carotene in solvent added to minimal essential medium or with 0.1 ml the medium alone (sham-injected controls); 20 hamsters were not further treated. The experiment was terminated at 17 weeks. The body weights of the sham-injected DMBA controls (about 85 g) were consistently lower than those given β-carotene (120 g) and the uninjected animals (100 g). No tumour regression was seen in sham-injected or uninjected hamsters, all of which had multiple, large cheek-pouch tumours; two uninjected controls and one sham-injected animal died intercurrently with very large tumours and infection. β-Carotene caused complete gross tumour regression in 4/20 hamsters and partial regression in 16/20. In general, regression of large and multiple tumours tended to be incomplete, whereas total regression was usually seen of small or moderate tumours. The tumours in regression showed degeneration and infiltration of lymphocytes and macrophages, which often contained tumour necrosis factor. Stratified squamous epithelium adjacent to carcinomas with severe destruction was relatively unaffected and appeared essentially normal (Schwartz & Shklar, 1987).

Sixty randomly bred male Syrian hamsters, two to three months old, were painted on the right buccal pouch with a 0.5% solution of DMBA in heavy mineral oil (about 0.4 mg DMBA per painting) three times per week for 14 weeks, when each hamster appeared to have well-to-moderately differentiated epidermoid carcinomas of the buccal pouch. Then, the animals were divided randomly into three groups of 20 animals each: the tumour-bearing pouch

was injected twice weekly with 0 or 250 μg β-carotene in 0.1 ml minimal essential medium or was not injected. After four weeks, all of the hamsters were killed, and the numbers and sizes of the buccal pouch tumours were recorded. There was no significant difference in body weight between the groups. β-Carotene reduced the buccal pouch tumour burden (average tumour volume x number of tumours) from 2258.9 ± 5.6 mm³ (sham controls) or 2150.4 ± 5.0 mm³ (uninjected controls) to 42.7 ± 1.2 mm³ [number and size of tumours unspecified; no information on statistical analysis]. In the β-carotene-treated hamsters but not the controls, many buccal pouch tumours showed cellular degeneration and dense infiltration of lymphocytes and macrophages (Schwartz & Shklar, 1988).

The right buccal pouches of 60 male Syrian hamsters, 60–90 days old and weighing 95–125 g were painted with a 0.5% solution of DMBA in heavy mineral oil (about 0.6 mg DMBA per painting) three times a week for 14 weeks, when all hamsters had obvious, gross cheek pouch tumours of variable size and number. They were then were divided into three groups of 20 animals each, which were either not further treated or received injections into the right cheek pouch of 0.1 ml solvent plus minimal essential medium alone or containing 0.19 mg β-carotene, three times per week for four weeks. β-Carotene reduced the total burden of the moderate papillary epidermoid carcinomas from 1400 mm³ in the hamsters given DMBA or sham-injected with DMBA to 100 mm³ in those given β-carotene [no information on statistics]. In addition, a clearly elevated number of tumour necrosis factor-α-positive macrophages was found in the tumours and adjacent to regressing tumours in hamsters treated with β-carotene (Shklar & Schwartz, 1988).

Sixty non-inbred adult male hamsters, 60–90 days old and weighing 96–120 g were fed standard laboratory pellets, and their right buccal pouches were painted with a 0.1% solution of DMBA in heavy mineral oil three times per week for 28 weeks. The animals were divided into three groups of 20 hamsters each and were given either 0.14 mg β-carotene (1.5 mg/kg bw) in 0.4 ml mineral oil three times per week on alternate days to DMBA, mineral oil only or no further treatment. All hamsters were killed after 28 weeks, when obvious moderately large buccal pouch tumours were seen in untreated controls. There was no significant difference in body weight between the groups. All control hamsters and most of those given β-carotene had cheek pouch tumours, but the latter group had fewer, smaller tumours than the controls: numbers of animals with gross tumours, 20/20, 20/20 and 11/20 in the untreated control, the vehicle control and the β-carotene groups, respectively; mean numbers of tumours per animal, 3.5, 3.7 and 1.8; mean tumour burden, 85.5, 114.9 and 51.7 ($p < 0.001$; Student's t test). The control animals had proliferative epidermoid carcinomas that invaded the underlying connective tissue, numerous foci of hyperkeratosis with dysplasia and carcinoma *in situ* and lymphocyte infiltration into areas of tumour infiltration and carcinoma *in situ*. The tumours in β-carotene-treated animals resembled those in controls but were smaller and somewhat less invasive, and lymphocyte infiltration was more pronounced (Schwartz *et al.*, 1988).

The mucosa of the right buccal pouches of 60 male Syrian hamsters, 60–90 days old and weighing 95–125 g, were painted three times a week with a 0.5% solution of DMBA in heavy mineral oil (about 0.6 mg DMBA per painting) for 14 weeks, when all animals had moderate-size tumours. They were then divided into three groups of 20 animals each and received either no further treatment or daily oral injections of 0.2 ml vegetable oil with or without 400 μg β-carotene. Observations at 16, 18 and 20 weeks showed a gradual increase in the tumour burden in all groups. At 22 weeks, when most of the animals were weak and cachectic, all survivors were killed. Oral β-carotene administration did not appear to cause regression of these epidermoid carcinomas, the total tumour burden at 22 weeks being about 3700, 4000 and 4200 mm^3 in β-carotene-treated animals, vehicle controls and untreated controls, respectively [statistics unspecified] (Shklar *et al.*, 1989).

The mucosa of the right cheek pouch of three groups of 20 male Syrian hamsters [age unspecified], fed a normal hamster diet containing 22% protein and the required concentrations of vitamin A and E, was painted with 0.1% DMBA in heavy mineral oil (0.4 mg DMBA per painting) three times a week for 28 weeks. One group received no further treatment; the other two groups were given 0.4 ml of heavy mineral oil containing 0 or 1.4 mg/kg bw β-carotene (crystalline form, type IV), by gavage three times a week on alternate days to DMBA, for 28 weeks. A fourth group served as untreated controls. There was no significant difference in body weight between the groups, and there was no intercurrent mortality. Ingestion of β-carotene significantly inhibited the formation of buccal pouch squamous-cell carcinomas, as shown by the later onset of tumours (month 5 versus month 4 in both DMBA control groups), fewer tumour-bearing hamsters (11 versus 20 in both DMBA control groups), fewer tumours (50 versus 135 in the DMBA/vehicle control and 150 in the DMBA control group) and a significant decrease in the tumour burden after six months of treatment (66 mm^3 versus 3675 mm^3 in the DMBA/vehicle control and and 2450 mm^3 in the DMBA control group; $p < 0.001$, Student's t test). At the end of the treatment period, the average number of areas of cheek pouch with epithelial dysplasia was 3 in the group given β-carotene and 6 in both DMBA-treated groups. No buccal pouch tumours or sites of epithelial dysplasia were found in untreated controls. β-Carotene ingestion resulted in a histologically unique picture not seen in DMBA-treated controls: a dense, mixed, inflammatory infiltrate consisting predominantly of cytotoxic lymphocytes and macrophages producing tumour necrosis factor-α and localized areas of mast cells in the deep dermis adjacent to areas of dysplasia, carcinoma *in situ* and small foci of squamous-cell carcinoma (Schwartz *et al.*, 1989).

The left buccal pouches of three groups of 20 adult male Syrian golden hamsters, eight weeks old and weighing 90–100 g, were painted three times per week with a 0.25% solution of DMBA and on alternate days with a 2.5% solution of β-carotene (α-carotene-free) in heavy mineral oil or with DMBA or β-carotene alone [doses and treatment period unspecified]. At the time of autopsy, the body weights of animals treated with DMBA only were significantly lower than those in the other groups. Buccal pouch tumours were seen grossly in 6/20 hamsters treated with DMBA alone at 10 weeks, in 10/20 animals at 11 weeks and in 20/20 animals at 12.5 weeks. In contrast, buccal pouch tumours were seen in the group treated with both DMBA and β-carotene in 3/20 animals at 10 weeks, 5/20 animals at 11 weeks, 10/20 animals at 12.5 weeks, 14/20 animals at 14 weeks and 20/20 animals at 15 weeks. At 12.5 weeks, the difference in tumour incidence between the two groups was statistically significant ($p < 0.05$; Student's t test) (Hibino *et al.*, 1990).

The mucosa of the cheek pouches of 35 randomly bred male Syrian golden hamsters, four to six weeks of age and weighing 90–100 g, was painted with 50 μl of a 0.25% solution of DMBA in liquid paraffin (0.125 mg DMBA per application) twice weekly for one month. Fifteen days after the last DMBA treatment, a dose of 250 mg β-carotene suspended in liquid paraffin was applied to the cheek pouch of 20 hamsters in volumes of 50 μl, twice a week for 4.5 months. An additional group of 20 hamsters received only β-carotene, and another group of 15 hamsters served as untreated controls. At six months, immediately after the last β-carotene application, all hamsters were killed and examined grossly for the presence of cheek pouch tumours and forestomach papillomas. No tumours were found in hamsters treated with DMBA and β-carotene, whereas 10/15 hamsters treated only with DMBA had cheek pouch tumours and 15/15 had forestomach tumours [statistics unspecified]. No tumours were found in untreated controls or in hamsters treated with β-carotene only (Gijare *et al.*, 1990).

Oral squamous-cell carcinomas were induced in four groups of 10 young adult male Syrian hamsters [age not further specified] by painting the mucosa of the right cheek pouch with 0.5% DMBA in heavy mineral oil (0.6 mg DMBA per painting) three times per week for 16 weeks. Four groups of 10 hamsters were untreated. After 16 weeks, the tumour burden in the cheek pouches was determined, and the tumours of one group of DMBA-treated animals and one group of untreated controls were injected submucosally with 3.8 μg β-carotene encapsulated in 0.2-ml liposomes (large unilamellar vesicles composed of L-α-phosphatidyl-L-serine, L-α-phosphatidyl-ethanolamine and L-α-phosphatidylcholine in a ratio of 1:1:1), 0.2-ml liposomes not containing β-carotene, 4 μg β-carotene suspended in 0.2 ml phosphate-buffered saline containing 0.1% ethanol or 0.2 ml phosphate-buffered saline, three times per week for five weeks. There was no differences in body weight between the groups. The mean cheek pouch tumour burden in the four DMBA-treated groups at week 16, when the β-carotene treatment was started, was 2327.5 mm^3 (range, 2304–2600 mm^3), with 8.0 ± 1.0 tumours per pouch. β-Carotene in liposomes reduced the tumour burden significantly ($p < 0.05$; Student's t test), the average tumour burden being 48.1 and 7.6 mm^3 after four and five weeks of β-carotene treatment, respectively. β-Carotene suspended in saline also reduced the tumour burden but to a lesser extent than in liposomes, the average tumour burden being 1250.6 and 958.6 mm^3 after four and five weeks of treatment with β-carotene, respectively. Treatment with liposomes alone did not consistently reduce the tumour burden, and saline injection resulted in a gradual progression of the tumour burden (average, 8858.6 mm^3 after four weeks). No buccal pouch tumours were found in untreated controls. Treatment with β-carotene in liposomes was associated with cellular destruction of carcinomas, seen ultrastructurally as liposome accumulation, disorganization and clumping of tonofilaments, swelling of mitochondria, loss of Golgi apparatus, lysosomal rupture and degeneration of nuclei. Liposome administration alone resulted in accumulation of lipid debris in endocytic vesicles and in organelle disruption, but to a lesser degree than after administration of β-carotene-containing liposomes. Normal cheek pouch mucosal cells were not affected by the liposome injections (Schwartz *et al.*, 1991).

Two groups of 15 female inbred Syrian hamsters, eight weeks old, were given drinking-water with or without 5.8 μmol/L β-carotene (3.1 mg/d per animal) for 13 months. After two weeks, 2 mg/kg bw N-nitroso(acetoxymethyl)-methylamine (AcO-NDMA) were applied to the mucosa of the right cheek pouch, twice] for six months. Two additional groups of 15 hamsters received drinking-water alone or supplemented with β-carotene; no cheek pouch tumours were seen in these groups. β-Carotene increased the survival of the AcO-NDMA-treated hamsters, from 27 to about 67% [statistics unspecified], reduced the incidence of cheek pouch tumours from 14/15 to 1/15 ($p < 0.001$; χ^2 test), reduced the cheek pouch tumour burden from 600 ± 72 to 0.5 ± 0.0 mm^3 ($p < 0.001$; Student's t test) and lengthened the time to appearance of tumours from 5–10 to 8–12 months [statistics unspecified] (Azuine & Bhide, 1992).

The mucosa of the right buccal pouches of two groups of 10 male Syrian hamsters, 60–90 days old and weighing 92–123 g, was painted with a 0.5% solution of DMBA in heavy mineral oil three times per week for 12 or 14 weeks. One of the groups was not further treated, while the other received 50 µg β-carotene in 0.5 ml mineral oil by mouth [route not further specified] three times a week on alternate days to DMBA for 12 or 14 weeks. One-half of the animals in each group were killed after 12 weeks and the other half after 14 weeks. After both 12 and 14 weeks of treatment, β-carotene appeared to have significantly reduced the incidence of cheek pouch leukoplakia and also the incidence, area, volume and total burden of cheek pouch tumours, consisting of carcinomas *in situ* and early carcinomas, as exemplified by the tumour burdens of 2.89 ± 0.6 mm^3 for the DMBA controls and 0.434 ± 0.1 mm^3 for the β-carotene-treated group after 12 weeks ($p < 0.001$; Student's t test) (Shklar *et al.*, 1993).

The mucosa of the right buccal pouches of three groups of 10 male Syrian golden hamsters, 60–90 days old and weighing 95–125 g, was painted with a 0.5% solution of DMBA in heavy mineral oil (0.6 mg DMBA per painting) three times per week for 14 weeks. One of the groups also received oral applications of 10 mg/kg bw β-carotene in 0.5 ml mineral oil three times per week on alternate days to DMBA. Two other groups either were not further treated or were treated with mineral oil only. An additional group of 10 hamsters was treated with β-carotene only; no buccal pouch tumours were seen in these animals. β-Carotene reduced the number of animals with buccal pouch tumours,

which were well-to-moderately differentiated epidermoid carcinomas, from 10 in both control groups to 9, the total numbers of cheek-pouch tumours from 125 in controls and 130 in the vehicle controls to 60 [statistics unspecified] and the cheek pouch tumour burden from 174 200 mm^3 (mean of both control groups) to 142 300 mm^3 (not significant; Student's t test) (Schwartz & Shklar, 1997).

(g)　Stomach (Table 29)

Mouse: Groups of 20 inbred female Swiss mice, six to eight weeks old, and weighing 20–25 g, were given β-carotene (4.7 µmol/d per animal) in 0.1 ml palm oil by gavage or only palm oil for eight weeks. From week 3, a fourth group of 20 mice and 20 mice receiving β-carotene were given 1 mg benzo[*a*]pyrene in 0.1 ml palm oil by gavage twice a week for four weeks. After completion of treatment at eight weeks, the animals were observed for up to 180 days, when they were killed. The mean body-weight gain was similar in all groups. β-Carotene reduced the incidence of forestomach tumours from 20/20 to 3/20 ($p < 0.001$; χ^2 test) and the mean number of forestomach tumours per mouse from 7.0 ± 0.3 to 1.0 ± 0.0 ($p < 0.001$; Student's t test). No forestomach tumours were found in the groups treated with β-carotene or palm oil alone (Azuine *et al.*, 1992).

Rat: Two groups of 36 weanling male Wistar Crl rats, three weeks old and weighing about 50 g, were fed a powdered basic diet (NIH-07 containing 10 000 IU/kg vitamin A and 1.4 mg/kg carotene) supplemented with either 0.4% β-carotene from beadlets containing 10% β-carotene or placebo beadlets (4%) for two weeks; then the β-carotene and the placebo beadlet content of the diets was reduced to 0.2 and 2% in the respective diets, which were fed until termination of the study at 52 weeks. Starting at five weeks of age, all rats were given distilled water (pH 4) as drinking-water, containing 80 mg/L MNNG, to give daily intakes of 3.82 mg/kg bw for rats given β-carotene and 4.10 mg/kg bw for those on placebo. Two additional groups of 18 rats received drinking-water with no addition, and a group of eight rats served as untreated controls. There were no significant differences in body weight among the groups. β-Carotene did not affect MNNG-induced tumorigenesis, although the incidence of adenocarcinomas of the glandular stomach was slightly lower in animals given β-carotene (4/35) than in those treated with MNNG (7/36) (Jones et al., 1989).

(h)   Small intestine (Table 29)

Rat: Two groups of 28 weanling male Holtzman rats were fed regular chow supplemented with either 1% β-carotene (w/w) from beadlets containing 10% β-carotene or 10% placebo beadlets for 24 weeks. After four weeks, all rats received 16 weekly subcutaneous injections of 30 mg/kg bw symmetrical DMH dissolved in neutral sodium hydroxide-corrected phosphate-buffered saline, for a total dose of 480 mg/kg bw. At 24 weeks, the animals were killed. All rats had intestinal tumours, and β-carotene had no effect on the tumour response; e.g. small-bowel cancer occurred in 17/28 rats given β-carotene and 15/28 given placebo, and there were 1.29 small-bowel cancers per rat in those given β-carotene and 0.82 in those on placebo (not significant) (Colacchio & Memoli, 1986; Colacchio et al., 1989).

Thirty male Sprague-Dawley rats, five weeks old, were fed CE-2 basic diet for 26 weeks, and 20 were given the diet supplemented with 0.005% β-carotene (type III, from carrots, equivalent to 2.8 mg/kg bw) for 14 weeks followed by CE-2 basic diet for the final 12 weeks. From day 3, the rats were given weekly subcutaneous injections of 20 mg/kg bw DMH for 12 weeks. Twenty control rats were fed CE-2 basic diet for 26 weeks. At the end of week 26, the animals were killed and examined for the presence of small intestinal carcinomas. No significant difference in body weight was seen between the groups. β-Carotene did not reduce the incidence of small intestinal adenocarcinomas or mucinous adenocarcinomas, the rates being 6/30 in DMH-treated rats and 7/20 in those given β-carotene (Yamamoto et al., 1994).

(i)   Salivary glands (Table 33)

Rat: Two groups of young male Sprague-Dawley rats [age not further specified], weighing 130–160 g, received a single injection of 1 mg 7,12-dimethylbenz[a]anthracene (DMBA) dissolved in 20 ml olive oil into one of the submandibular salivary glands. The contralateral gland was injected with 20 ml olive oil alone. Immediately after injection, one of the groups (14 rats) was fed *ad libitum* a semisynthetic diet (AIN-76; 4000 IU/kg retinyl palmitate) supplemented with 100 mg/kg of diet β-carotene

Table 33. Effects of β-carotene on salivary gland tumorigenesis induced by injection of 1 mg 1,2-dimethylbenz[a]anthracene into the submandibular salivary gland of male Sprague-Dawley rats

No. of animals/ group	β-Carotene (dose, route)	Treatment relative to carcinogen	Preventive efficacy	Reference
9–14	100 ppm in diet	After	Carcinomas Incidence: 75% (NS)	Alam et al. (1984)
30	5, 25, 125 and 250 ppm in diet	Before, during and after	Gross tumours (three highest dose groups combined), 35% (p = 0.029) Carcinomas Incidence: none [SU]	Alam & Alam (1987)
30	250 ppm in diet	Before, during and after	Tumours Incidence: none (NS) Weight: 54% (NS)	Alam et al. (1988)

NS, not significant; SU, statistics unspecified

(*trans*-β-carotene, type I, synthetic crystalline; purity, > 95%), while the other group (nine rats) received the same diet without β-carotene. The animals were observed for 22 weeks, when all those remaining were necropsied. There was no appreciable difference in growth rate between the two groups. During the first 13 weeks, three rats given β-carotene died, probably as a result of vitamin K deficiency, and the vitamin K level in the diet was increased from 50 to 500 mg/kg from that time, with no further deaths. Well-differentiated squamous-cell carcinomas and poorly differentiated malignant salivary gland neoplasms resembling squamous-cell carcinomas [distribution over the groups unspecified] were found in 3/9 controls and in 1/11 animals given β-carotene, but the difference in tumour incidence was not statistically significant [method of statistical analysis unspecified]. In addition, 4/9 controls and 4/11 rats given β-carotene had salivary gland enlargement (designated as grossly observed tumours) due to fibrosis, inflammation, cysts and proliferation and metaplasia of the ductal epithelium (Alam *et al.*, 1984).

Five groups of 30 male weanling Sprague-Dawley rats were fed *ad libitum* a semi-purified diet supplemented with 0, 5, 25, 125 or 250 mg/kg of diet β-carotene (stabilized gelatin beadlets containing 10% all-*trans*-β-carotene). Placebo beadlets were added to the diet to compensate for the differences between doses. Uptake was demonstrated by measurement of significantly higher β-carotene levels in the liver at six weeks and at termination of the study. After six weeks, all rats received a single injection of 1 mg DMBA dissolved in 20 ml olive oil into one of the submandibular salivary glands, and the contralateral gland was injected with 20 ml olive oil alone. Rats were killed and necropsied 30–32 weeks after the start of the study and thus 24–26 weeks after the injection of DMBA. Body weight and survival were not affected by β-carotene administration. The β-carotene levels in serum and liver were significantly increased, in a dose-related manner, after both 6 and 32 weeks; e.g. the high dose resulted in a concentration of 1950 mg/g in the liver at 32 weeks, while none was detectable in con-

trols. Palpable salivary gland tumours appeared in rats fed diets supplemented with β-carotene two to three weeks after they appeared in controls [no further details given]. The incidences of submandibular salivary gland tumours observed grossly at autopsy were 17/29 in controls, 17/28 in rats given 5 mg/kg β-carotene, 10/25 in those given 25 mg/kg, 10/28 in those at 125 mg/kg and 11/26 in those at 250 mg/kg. The combined incidence of these tumours in the controls and rats at the low dose of β-carotene (34/57) was statistically significantly higher than that in the combined groups at higher doses of β-carotene (31/79) ($\chi^2 = 4.74$; $p = 0.029$). The incidences of malignant tumours in the submandibular salivary glands—partially to fully differentiated squamous-cell carcinomas, spindle-cell carcinomas and adenocarcinomas [distribution over the groups unspecified]—were 15/29, 14/28, 10/25, 12/28 and 11/26 in controls and rats at 5, 25, 125 and 250 mg/kg β-carotene, respectively [statistics and types of nonmalignant tumours unspecified]. The average weights of the submandibular salivary gland tumours were 32.6 ± 8.4, 25.4 ± 9.2, 18.0 ± 11.5, 19.2 ± 7.3 and 17.6 ± 10.9 g for the five groups, respectively. The incidences of tumours weighing 11 g or more were 9/29 in controls, 8/28 in animals at 5 mg/kg β-carotene and 10/79 in those at the combined higher doses, and the differences in incidence between the groups showed a statistically significant trend ($\chi^2 = 4.48$; $p = 0.034$) (Alam & Alam, 1987).

Two groups of 30 male weanling Sprague-Dawley rats, weighing 73 ± 1.0 g, were fed either basal AIN-76A diet (containing 4000 IU vitamin A) or basal diet supplemented with 250 mg/kg β-carotene (10% stabilized gelatin beadlets). Uptake was demonstrated by β-carotene measurement in the liver. After six weeks, one of the submandibular salivary glands of each rat was injected with 1 mg DMBA in 0.02 ml olive oil, while the contralateral gland was injected with 0.02 ml olive oil alone. Rats were killed 21–22 weeks after the DMBA injection, when more than 50% of the animals had developed submandibular salivary gland tumours, some of which were very large. There was no significant difference in body-weight gain between the two groups. The incidence of partially to fully differentiated squamous-cell carcinomas and undifferentiated spindle-cell submandibular salivary gland tumours was closely similar: all tumours: 20/28 in controls and 20/30 in rats given β-carotene; malignant tumours: 11/28 in controls and 16/30 (53%) in rats given β-carotene. The mean tumour weight was slightly lower in rats fed the β-carotene-supplemented diet (3.2 ± 0.8 g) than in rats fed the unsupplemented diet (7.0 ± 3.3 g). Two of 20 tumour-bearing control animals had submandibular salivary gland tumours weighing more than 40 g, whereas none of the rats given β-carotene had such large tumours. In addition, 4/20 tumour-bearing controls and 1/20 given β-carotene had tumours weighing more than 10 g (not significant; χ^2 test) (Alam *et al.*, 1988).

(j)   Pancreas *(Table 29)*

Rat: Eighty male weanling SPF albino Bor (WISW,Cpb) Wistar rats were fed standard laboratory chow and received two intraperitoneal injections of 30 mg/kg bw azaserine in 0.9% saline, one at 19 days and one at 26 days of age. One week after the second injection, the animals were switched to an AIN-76 diet with a high percentage of saturated fat (20% lard), with or without 60 mg/kg β-carotene added to the diet as water-dispersible beadlets containing 10% pure β-carotene [use of placebo beadlets unspecified]. Necropsy was performed 482–485 days after the second injection of azaserine. Food intake and body and pancreatic weights were similar in the two groups. β-Carotene significantly reduced the total number of atypical acinar-cell nodules in the pancreas that were 0.5–1.0 mm in diameter, with 338 in the control group and 194 in the group given β-carotene ($p < 0.05$; generalized linear regression, error is Poisson, link function is log); the number of atypical acinar-cell nodules with a diameter of 1.0–3.0 mm was also lower in the animals given β-carotene (146) than in controls (200), but the difference was not statistically significant. β-Carotene reduced the incidence of pancreatic tumours from 22/39 in controls to 9/37 and that of carcinomas from 15/39 in controls to 4/37 ($p < 0.05$ for both; regression analysis followed by χ^2 tests) (Appel *et al.*, 1991).

The effect of β-carotene on the initiation or early promotion and the late promotion phases of pancreatic carcinogenesis was studied in rats. A group of 16 female Wistar rats that had been mated one week earlier was maintained on a high-fat diet (25% fat, 25% casein, 0.37% DL-methionine, 36.79% wheat starch, 6.18% cellulose, 0.25% choline bitartrate, 4.32% AIN76 minerals, 1.24% AIN76 vitamins and 1.85% calcium phosphate), while the other 16 rats were divided into two groups and fed the high-fat diet supplemented with 100 or 1000 mg/kg β-carotene (added as a 30% solution in corn oil. When the pups were born, six groups of 20 male pups were formed and received the same diets as their mothers. At 14 and 21 days of age, pups received a subcutaneous injection of 30 mg/kg bw azaserine in saline, except for the pups in one group kept on unsupplemented diet which received subcutaneous injections of saline only. At five weeks of age, two of the three azaserine-treated groups fed the unsupplemented high-fat diet were switched to high-fat diet plus 100 or 1000 mg/kg β-carotene (to study the effects of β-carotene on the late promotion phase), while the third group was continued on the unsupplemented high-fat diet; two groups fed the high-fat diets with β-carotene were switched to the unsupplemented high-fat diet (to study the effects of β-carotene on the initiation or early promotion phase). The experiment was terminated when the rats were 29 weeks of age. Body and pancreatic weights were similar in all groups, and, as the animals consumed similar amounts of food, the calculated energy intake was also similar. β-Carotene inhibited azaserine-induced pancreatic carcinogenesis, the strongest effects occurring when β-carotene was administered during the late promotion phase (see Table 34). No (putative) preneoplastic or neoplastic lesions were seen in saline-treated rats (Appel & Woutersen, 1996).

Two groups of 20 male weanling albino Cbp:WU; Wistar random rats, 19 days old, received a single intraperitoneal injection of 30 mg/kg bw azaserine and were fed standard rodent diet. Twelve days later, they were given a high-fat diet (20% lard), either unsupplemented or supplemented with 56 mg/kg

Table 34. Putatively preneoplastic atypical acinar-cell nodules (AACN), carcinoma *in situ* and atypical acinar-cell foci (AACF) in the pancreas of azaserine-treated male Wistar rats at two phases of the carcinogenesis process

Diet	AACN					Carcinoma *in situ*		Multiplicity of
	No./cm^2	Area (mm^2)	No./cm^3	Mean diameter (μm)	Area as % pancreas	Incidence	Multiplicity	AACF > 1 mm
Initiation or early promotion phase								
HF	46.2	0.21	1521	409	9.5	3/15	7.0 ± 1.5	0.3 ± 0.2
HF/LBC	40.3	0.20	1281[a]	430	8.1	3/15	7.6 ± 1.6	0.2 ± 0.1
HF/HBC	30.7	0.18	1069[a]	405	5.5	4/15	4.8 ± 1.4	0.3 ± 0.2
Late promotion phase								
HF	46.2	0.21	1521	409	9.5	3/15	7.0 ± 1.5	0.3 ± 0.2
HF/LBC	29.8	0.18	1102[a]	389	5.3[a]	3/15	4.1 ± 1.6	0.2 ± 0.1
HF/HBC	33.9	0.20	1183[a]	408	6.7[a]	2/15	5.8 ± 1.4	0.1 ± 0.1

From Appel & Woutersen (1996); for details, see text

HF, high fat (25%); LBC, low β-carotene (100 mg/kg); HBC, high β-carotene (1000 mg/kg)

[a] $p < 0.05$; analysis of variance

β-carotene in the form of water-dispersible beadlets containing 10% pure β-carotene, for about four months [use of placebo beadlets not specified]. There were no significant differences in food intake, body weight or pancreatic weight between the two groups. β-Carotene did not significantly reduce the number of preneoplastic acidophilic foci per cm^2 (44.86 ± 5.51 versus 41.81 ± 5.01 in controls), their volume per cm^3 (2212 ± 248 versus 2034 ± 196 in controls), their transectional area (615 ± 57 mm^2 versus 648 ± 78 mm^2 in controls), their area as percentage of the pancreas (3.07 ± 0.51% versus 3.25 ± 0.79% in controls) or their diameter (237 ± 11 mm versus 241 ± 10 mm in controls), nor did it reduce the number of preneoplastic basophilic foci per cm^2 (12.07 ± 1.55 versus 13.41 ± 1.47 in controls), their volume per cm^3 (1261 ± 138 versus 1492 ± 167 in controls), their transectional area (137 ± 9 mm^2 versus 157 ± 15 mm^2 in controls), their area as percentage of the pancreas (0.17 ± 0.02% versus 0.20 ± 0.02% in controls) or their diameter (117 ± 4 μm versus 118 ± 6 μm in controls), except for the number of basophilic foci with a diameter > 192.5 μm, which appeared to be statistically significantly lower in animals on the β-carotene [number of foci and *p* value unspecified] (generalized linear model; error is Poisson, link function is log). No pancreatic tumours were reported (Woutersen & van Garderen-Hoetmer, 1988).

Hamster: Two groups of 40 male Syrian golden hamsters, five to six weeks old, fed a standard diet were injected subcutaneously with 20 mg/kg bw *N*-nitrosobis(2-oxopropyl)-amine (NBOPA [vehicle unspecified]) at six, seven and eight weeks of age. One week after the last NBOPA injection, all hamsters were fed a high-fat (20% lard) diet with or without 60 mg/kg β-carotene added to the diet as water-dispersible beadlets containing 10% pure β-carotene, for the rest of the experimental period [use of placebo beadlets unspecified]. The survivors were killed 364 or 365 days after the first injection of NBOPA. Hamsters fed the β-carotene-supplemented diet had lower body weights than the controls (*p* < 0.05; analysis of variance and Dunnett's test, two-sided). β-Carotene did not inhibit the development of (pre)neoplastic lesions in the pancreas, the incidences of advanced ductular lesions, carcinoma *in situ* and invasive carcinoma being 9/27, 5/27 and 12/27 in the controls and 11/34, 10/34 and 11/34 in the group fed the β-carotene-supplemented diet, respectively (χ^2 test) (Appel *et al.*, 1996).

Two groups of 20 male weanling Syrian golden hamsters fed standard diet were injected subcutaneously with 20 mg/kg bw NBOPA once weekly at five, six and seven weeks of age. Twelve days after the last NBOPA injection, the animals were fed a diet with a high percentage of saturated fat (20% lard), either unsupplemented or supplemented with 56 mg/kg β-carotene in the form of water-dispersible beadlets containing 10% pure β-carotene, for about four months [use of placebo beadlets unspecified]. There were no significant differences in food intake, body weight or pancreatic weight between the two groups. β-Carotene significantly reduced the total number of preneoplastic, large tubular ductal complexes in the pancreas, which are focal lesions composed of multiple lumina lined by cuboidal epithelial cells ($p < 0.05$; generalized linear model, one-tailed, error is Poisson, link function is log), the incidences being 14/19 in the unsupplemented group and 4/20 in the β-carotene-supplemented group. The numbers of preneoplastic tubular ductal complexes of intermediate size were also lower in the animals given β-carotene (33 in 20 animals) than in controls (49 in 19 animals), but the differences were not statistically significant. Two pancreatic carcinomas, one carcinoma *in situ* and one microcarcinoma were found in the controls and one microcarcinoma in the β-carotene supplemented group (Woutersen & van Garderen-Hoetmer, 1988).

(k)   Multiple organs (Table 29)
Rat: Two groups of 20 male Fischer 344/Du Crj rats, seven weeks old, received three subcutaneous injections of 40 mg/kg bw DMH dissolved in 0.9% saline during week 1 and then an intraperitoneal injection of 20 mg/kg bw MNU in citrate buffer twice per week during weeks 2 and 3. A group of 10 rats was similarly treated with the vehicles of DMH and MNU. At week 4, one carcinogen-treated group and the vehicle control group were placed on a diet supplemented with 0.2% β-carotene [not further specified]. At week 52, all survivors—15/20 carcinogen-treated, β-carotene-fed rats, 20/20 carcinogen-treated rats and 10/10 vehicle plus β-carotene-fed controls—

were killed and subjected to a complete autopsy. There was no significant difference in body weight between the groups. β-Carotene did not significantly reduce the development of organ-specific tumours, but the incidences of hyperplastic liver foci, colonic adenocarcinomas and nephroblastomas were lower in the carcinogen-treated group fed the β-carotene-supplemented diet than in the group treated with the carcinogens and fed unsupplemented basal diet: liver foci, 9/15 versus 16/22; colonic adenocarcinomas, 3/15 versus 9/20; nephroblastomas: 2/15 versus 6/20 (Imaida *et al.*, 1990).

(l)   Inoculated tumours (see Table 35)
Carotenoids have been reported to affect the growth and/or the rejection of tumours inoculated into recipient animals. While this effect is clearly therapeutic rather than preventive, since the target cells are established tumours, the Working Group decided to include these studies, primarily because intervention trials with carotenoids in high-risk groups like current smokers might include many individuals who are harbouring preclinical malignancies. The potential response of existing tumours to carotenoids is thus of interest.

C3HBA adenocarcinoma cells: Two groups of 10 female inbred C3H/HeJ mice, five weeks old, were fed a powdered diet containing 6190 IU/kg vitamin A palmitate and 4.3 mg/kg β-carotene, with or without the addition of 90 mg/kg β-carotene [formulation in the diet unspecified]. At day 4, all mice were inoculated subcutaneously with 10^4 C3HBA adenocarcinoma cells in the area above the right inguinal lymph node. β-Carotene reduced the tumour incidence and size, slightly increased the latency of the tumours and lengthened the survival time. Thus, the tumour incidences were 6/10 and 2/10 ($p < 0.05$; χ^2 test), the diameters of the tumours at day 46 were 13.5 ± 0.5 and 4.5 ± 0.3 mm ($p < 0.001$; Student's *t* test), the latency was 21.7 ± 3.2 and 26.5 ± 3.5 days (not significant) and the survival times were 70.2 ± 4.0 and 112.5 ± 5.5 days ($p < 0.06$; analysis of variance) in the unsupplemented and β-carotene-supplemented animals, respectively (Rettura *et al.*, 1982).

Table 35. Prevention or regression of tumour cell-inoculated or virus-induced tumours by β-carotene

Species, strain, sex	No. of animals/ group	Virus of tumour-cells (dose)	β-Carotene (dose, route)	Timing of treatment relative to virus or tumour-cell administration	Preventive efficacy	Reference
Inoculated tumour cells						
Mouse, C3H/HeJ, female	10	10^4 C3HBA cells	90 mg/kg diet	Before and during	Adenocarcinoma Incidence: 40% ($p < 0.05$); size: 67% ($p < 0.001$); latent period: 22% (NS); survival: 60% ($p < 0.06$)	Rettura et al. (1982)
Mouse, C3H/HeJ, female	10	2×10^5 C3HBA cells	90 mg/kg diet	After	Adenocarcinoma Survival: 59% ($p < 0.001$); size after 14 days: 52% [SU]	Rettura et al. (1982)
Mouse, CBA/J, male	10	2×10^5 C3HBA cells	90 mg/kg diet	After	Adenocarcinoma Survival: 49% ($p < 0.001$); size after 19 days: 34% [SU]	Rettura et al. (1982)
Mouse, C3H/HeJ, female	10	2×10^5 C3HBA cells	90 mg/kg diet	After	Adenocarcinoma Survival, 61% ($p < 0.001$); size after 12 days: 21% (SU)	Rettura et al. (1982)
Mouse, CBA/J, male	10–12	2×10^5 C3HBA cells	90 mg/kg diet	After	Adenocarcinoma Survival of mice, 49% ($p < 0.001$) Tumour growth: 75% [SU]	Seifter et al. (1983)
Mouse, CBA/J, male	10–12	2×10^5 C3HBA cells	90 mg/kg diet	After	Adenocarcinoma Survival of mice, 26% ($p < 0.001$) Tumour growth: 46% [SU]	Seifter et al. (1983)
Rat, Wistar, male	6	10^6 C-6 glioma cells	10 mg/kg bw, gavage (?)	Before and during	Gliomas Latency: 50% (SU) Weight: 67% ($p < 0.02$)	Wang et al. (1989)
Rat, Wistar, male	6	10^6 C-6 glioma cells	10 mg/kg bw, gavage (?)	After	Gliomas Incidence: 33% (SU) Weight: 55% (SU)	Wang et al. (1989)
Mouse, C3H, male	15	SCC-VII, 2×10^6 cells, single dose, s.c.	10 mg/kg bw; i.p., daily, 5 days	After	Carcinoma Growth: slightly delayed (NS)	Teicher et al. (1994)

Table 35 (contd)

Species, strain, sex	No. of animals/ group	Virus/tumour cells (dose)	β-carotene (dose, route)	Timing of treatment relative to virus or tumour-cell administration	Preventive efficacy	Reference
Mouse, C3H, male	15	SCC-VII, 2 x 10⁶ cells, single dose, s.c.	10 mg/kg bw; i.p., daily, 5 days	After	Carcinoma Growth: slightly delayed (NS)	Teicher *et al.* (1994)
Mouse, C3H, male	15	Fsall, 2 x 10⁶ cells, single dose, s.c.	10 mg/kg bw; i.p., 1, 3 or 5 doses	After	Fibrosarcoma Growth: One dose: slight (SU) Three doses: slight (SU) Five doses: moderate (SU)	Teicher *et al.* (1994)
Virus-induced tumours						
Mouse, CBA/J, male	10	M-MuSV, 0.1 ml of 10⁻¹ and 10⁻² g eq/ml	90 mg/kg diet	Before, during and after	Sarcoma *Low inoculum*: incidence, 35% (*p* < 0.005); latency, 43% (*p* < 0.005); persistence, 45% (*p* < 0.01); regression, 52% (*p* < 0.02); *High inoculum*: incidence, 47% (*p* < 0.009); latency, 48% (*p* < 0.008); persistence, 57% (*p* < 0.03); regression, 59% (*p* < 0.006)	Seifter *et al.* (1982)
Mouse, CBA/J, male	10	M-MuSV, 0.1 ml of 10⁻¹ and 10⁻² g eq/ml	120 mg/kg diet	Before, during and after	Sarcoma *Low inoculum*: incidence, 35% (*p* < 0.005); latency, 16% (*p* < 0.01); persistence, 46% (*p* < 0.03); regression, 54% *High inoculum*: incidence, 47% (*p* < 0.009); latency, 24% (*p* < 0.05); persistence, 35% (*p* < 0.1); regression, 45% (*p* < 0.01)	Seifter *et al.* (1982)
Mouse, CBA/J, male	10	M-MuSV, 0.2 ml of 10⁻¹ g eq/ml	[unspecified; probably 90 or 120 mg/kg diet]	After	Sarcoma regression: 100% [SU]	Seifter *et al.* (1982)

SU, statistics unspecified; NS, not significant; s.c., subcutaneously; i.p., intraperitoneally

Two groups of 10 female inbred C3H/HeJ mice, five weeks old, were fed a powdered basal diet containing 6190 IU/kg vitamin A palmitate and 4.3 mg/kg β-carotene for one week [formulation unspecified] and were then inoculated subcutaneously with 2 x 10^5 C3HBA adenocarcinoma cells in the area above the right inguinal lymph node. Several hours after inoculation, one of the groups was switched to basal diet supplemented with 90 mg/kg β-carotene, while the other group was maintained on basal diet for the remainder of the experiment. β-Carotene increased the average survival time of the mice from 34.9 ± 1.1 to 55.6 ± 3.0 days ($p < 0.001$; analysis of variance), and it slowed tumour growth but did not cause regression, the average tumour size being 6.5 and 2.5 mm five days after inoculation and 16.8 and 8.1 mm 14 days after inoculation in the unsupplemented and β-carotene-supplemented animals, respectively (Student's t test [p value unspecified]) (Rettura et al., 1982).

Two groups of 10 male CBA/J mice, five weeks old, were inoculated with 2 x 10^5 C3HBA adenocarcinoma cells in the outer aspect of the thigh and were maintained on powdered basal diet containing 15 000 IU/kg vitamin A and 6.5 mg/kg β-carotene [formulation unspecified]. After 13 days, when the tumours had reached a mean diameter of 6.2 ± 0.3 mm, one group of mice was switched to basal diet supplemented with 90 mg/kg β-carotene, while the other group was maintained on unsupplemented basal diet. β-Carotene increased the average survival time of the mice from 40.0 ± 2.8 to 59.5 ± 3.0 days ($p < 0.001$; analysis of variance); it slowed tumour growth but did not cause regression. After eight days on the β-carotene-supplemented diet, the average tumour diameter was 9.7 mm versus 14.7 mm in the unsupplemented animals, and after 19 days these values were 13.2 and 20.1 mm (Student's t test [p values unspecified]) (Rettura et al., 1982).

Two groups of 10 female C3H/HeJ mice, five weeks old, were inoculated subcutaneously with 2 x 10^5 C3HBA adenocarcinoma cells in the outer aspect of the thigh and were maintained on powdered basal diet containing 15 000 IU/kg vitamin A and 6.5 mg/kg β-carotene [no data on absorption]. When the

tumours reached an average diameter of 7.5 ± 0.2 mm, one group of mice was continued on the basal diet and the other was switched to basal diet supplemented with 90 mg/kg β-carotene. The average survival times were 36.3 ± 1.3 days for unsupplemented animals and 58.5 ± 3.5 days for the β-carotene-supplemented mice ($p < 0.001$; analysis of variance). β-Carotene reduced tumour growth: after 12 days of the β-carotene-supplemented diet, the average tumour diameter was about 17.1 mm, while that of the controls was about 21.7 mm (data presented as curves; Student's t test [p values unspecified]) (Rettura et al., 1982).

Twenty male CBA/J mice, six weeks old, were inoculated subcutaneously with 2 x 10^5 C3HBA adenocarcinoma cells in the outer aspect of the right thigh and were fed a basal diet containing 15 000 IU/kg vitamin A and 6.4 mg/kg β-carotene [formulation unspecified]. On day 13, when the mean diameter of the tumours was 6.2 ± 0.3 mm, the mice were randomly distributed into two groups, one of which was continued on unsupplemented basal diet and the other received basal diet supplemented with 90 mg/kg β-carotene. A similar experiment was begun nine weeks after the start of the first experiment, in which the mean tumour diameter on day 13 was 5.6 ± 0.2 mm. In neither study was there a significant difference in body weight between groups, and in both experiments β-carotene significantly increased the average survival time ($p < 0.001$ for both experiments; analysis of variance), from 41.2 to 61.2 days in experiment 1 and from 43.3 to 63.3 days in experiment 2. β-Carotene also slowed tumour growth considerably [statistics unspecified]: the average tumour diameter reached about 16.8 mm by weeks 12 and 21 in experiment 1 and by weeks 19 and 24 in experiment 2 in the unsupplemented and β-carotene-supplemented animals respectively (Seifter et al., 1983).

Rat C-6 glioma cells: Two groups of six male Wistar rats, three to four weeks old, were fed normal rodent chow and were given intraperitoneal injections of either 10 mg/kg bw β-carotene in 0.06% dimethylsulfoxide (v/v; 2 mg/ml) or dimethylsulfoxide alone on five consecutive days. Then, 10^6 C-6 glioma cells were inoculated subcutaneously into the right scapula. Eight to 10 weeks later, the animals were killed and the tumours were removed and weighed. In a second, similar experiment, β-carotene was administered intraperitoneally two weeks after tumour-cell inoculation. In the first experiment, β-carotene prolonged the time to 50% tumour incidence from 14 days in controls to 21 days in those given β-carotene [statistics unspecified]) and reduced the mean tumour weight from 67.0 ± 18.1 g in controls to 22.1 ± 24.4 g in animals given β-carotene ($p < 0.01$ [statistical test unspecified]). In the second experiment, β-carotene prolonged survival (at week 10, 3/6 controls and 5/6 animals given β-carotene were still alive), reduced the number of rats with tumours (6/6 in controls and 4/6 in those on β-carotene) and reduced the mean tumour weight from 147.1 ± 73.4 g in controls to 66.8 ± 44.3 g in those given β-carotene ($p < 0.05$ [statistical test unspecified]) (Wang et al., 1989).

SCC VII cells: Two groups of 15 male C3H mice, eight to ten weeks old, received subcutaneous implantations of 2 x 10^6 SCC-VII carcinoma cells into one leg. After seven days, one group of mice received intraperitoneal injections of 10 mg/kg bw β-carotene (soya-based emulsion) daily for five days, while the other group served as untreated controls. β-Carotene delayed the tumour growth, measured as the number of days required to reach a volume of 500 mm^3, by 0.3 ± 0.3 day [no further data presented; statistics unspecified] (Teicher et al., 1994).

FSaII cells: Three groups of 15 male C3H mice, eight to ten weeks old, received subcutaneous implantations of 2 x 10^6 FSaII fibrosarcoma cells into one leg. They then received intraperitoneal injections of 10 mg/kg bw β-carotene (soya-based emulsion) either once (on day 7), three times (on days 7, 9 and 11) or five times (on days 7–11). A fourth group of 15 male mice served as untreated controls. β-Carotene delayed tumour growth, measured as the number of days required to reach a volume of 500 mm^3, by 0.3 ± 0.3, 0.8 ± 0.3 and 1.2 ± 0.4 days after one, three and five injections, respectively [no further data presented; statistics unspecified] (Teicher et al., 1994).

(m)   Virus-induced tumours (Table 35)
Mouse: Two groups of 20 male inbred CBA/J mice, five weeks old, were fed powdered basal diet containing 6190 IU/kg vitamin A palmitate and 4.3 mg/kg β-carotene, with or without the addition of 90 mg/kg β-carotene, for life [formulation in the diet unspecified]. After three days, 10 mice of each group were inoculated intramuscularly with 0.1 ml of a suspension of Moloney murine sarcoma virus (M-MuSV; 10^{-1} g eq/ml), and the other 10 mice with 0.1 ml of the same viral suspension diluted 1:10 with buffer (10^{-2} g eq/ml) [study duration unspecified]. Several weeks later, a second experiment was conducted, in which the diet was supplemented with 120 instead of 90 mg/kg β-carotene. In a third experiment, 20 mice were fed the unsupplemented basal diet and were inoculated intramuscularly with a 0.2 ml M-MuSV suspension (10^{-1} g eq/ml) on day 1. By day 7, when the mice had a mean tumour score of 2 (on a scale of 1–4), 10 of the mice were fed the basal diet supplemented with β-carotene [concentration unspecified but probably 90 or 120 mg/kg], while the other 10 mice were continued on the unsupplemented basal diet for another 31 days, after which the experiment was terminated. Tumour incidence and persistence were reduced, the latency was increased, and tumour regression was accelerated in mice fed the β-carotene-supplemented diets before, during or after the inoculation of either the low or the high dose of M-MuSV. The tumour incidences were 20/20 and 13/20 ($p < 0.005$; χ^2 test) with the low inoculum and 17/20 and 9/20 ($p < 0.009$; χ^2 test) with the high inoculum in both unsupplemented and both β-carotene-supplemented groups, respectively. The tumour latencies were (Student's t test) 5.8 ± 0.3 and 8.3 ± 0.6 days ($p < 0.005$) with the low inoculum and 7.1 ± 0.4 and 10.5 ± 0.8 days ($p < 0.008$) with the high inoculum in the unsupplemented and 90 mg/kg β-carotene-supplemented diet groups, respectively, and 6.1 ± 0.2 and 7.1 ± 0.2 days ($p < 0.01$) with the low inoculum and 7.9 ± 0.3 and 9.8 ± 1.0 days ($p < 0.05$) with the high inoculum in the unsupplemented and 120 mg/kg β-carotene-supplemented diet groups, respectively. The average numbers of days of tumour persistence were (Student's t test) 12.9 ± 1.5 and 7.1 ± 1.1 ($p < 0.01$) with the low inoculum and 12.7

± 2.1 and 5.5 ± 1.0 ($p < 0.03$) with the high inoculum in the unsupplemented and 90 mg/kg β-carotene-supplemented groups, respectively, and 12.3 ± 1.5 and 6.6 ± 0.9 ($p < 0.03$) with the low inoculum and 8.5 ± 1.0 and 5.5 ± 1.0 ($p < 0.1$) with the high inoculum in the unsupplemented and 120 mg/kg β-carotene-supplemented diet groups, respectively. The average times of tumour regression (days from midpoint of maximum tumour size) were (Student's t test) 7.1 ± 1.1 and 3.4 ± 1.2 ($p < 0.02$) with the low inoculum and 6.8 ± 0.9 and 2.0 ± 0.0 ($p < 0.006$) with the high inoculum in the unsupplemented and 90 mg/kg β-carotene-supplemented diet groups, respectively, and 7.0 ± 0.9 and 3.2 ± 0.4 ($p < 0.005$) with the low inoculum and 5.1 ± 0.6 and 2.8 ± 0.5 with the high inoculum in the unsupplemented and 120 mg/kg β-carotene-supplemented diet group, respectively. When the β-carotene-supplemented diet was fed after the tumours had developed (third experiment), tumour regression was rapid (all tumours had disappeared by day 38), and none of the mice given the β-carotene supplement died, whereas 3/10 mice fed the unsupplemented diet died between days 28 and 30 and the tumours did not regress at all (Seifter et al., 1982).

4.2.1.2 β-Carotene with other potential inhibitors (Table 36)

(a) Skin

Four groups of 45 female hairless Crl:Skh1 (hr/hr) BR mice, 80 days old, were fed standard mouse chow either as such or fortified with 0.5% (w/w) β-carotene (type 1, all trans, synthetic, crystalline), 0.12% (w/w) vitamin E (D-α-tocopheryl succinate) or 0.5% β-carotene plus 0.12% vitamin E for 32 weeks. In week 11, all mice received a single application of 150 mg DMBA in acetone on the dorsal skin; one week later, 5 mg TPA in acetone were applied twice weekly for 11 weeks and once weekly for another nine weeks. There was no significant difference in body weight between the groups. In the groups fed diets containing β-carotene, its concentrations were significantly increased in liver and skin but remained near the detection limit in serum throughout the study. Skin tumours developed in 97.2% of the mice towards the

end of the study. In weeks 17 and 18, the incidence of skin tumours in mice given β-carotene or β-carotene plus vitamin E was statistically significantly lower than that in the controls ($p < 0.05$; Fisher's exact test [no further details given]). The first skin tumour appeared statistically significantly later in mice fed β-carotene than in controls, and the first to eighth tumours appeared significantly later in mice given β-carotene plus vitamin E than the first 10 tumours in controls ($p < 0.05$; Kruskal-Wallis test [no further details given]). The cumulative numbers of skin tumours in week 27 were 733 in the controls and 500, 551 and 579 in animals given β-carotene, vitamin E or β-carotene plus vitamin E, respectively [statistics unspecified]. Both the cumulative number of skin tumours and the time to their appearance were lower (analysis of variance) in the mice fed β-carotene ($p = 0.03$), vitamin E ($p = 0.06$) or β-carotene plus vitamin E ($p = 0.04$) than in the controls. Overall, the protective effect of dietary β-carotene was not affected by simultaneous administration of vitamin E (Lambert et al., 1994).

(b) Colon

Rat: Three groups of 20 male Fischer 344 rats, five weeks old, were maintained for five weeks on a semipurified diet containing 20% casein, 59% sucrose, 4% cellulose, 0.15% choline, 4% mineral mixture, 1% vitamin mixture and 12% olive oil (9.6% palmitic acid, 2.7% stearic acid, 80.6% oleic acid, 5.8% linoleic acid and 0.6% α-linolenic acid); 9% olive oil plus 3% perilla oil (6.2% palmitic acid, 2.0% stearic acid, 17.7% oleic acid, 15.2% linoleic acid and 56.0% α-linolenic acid) or 12% perilla oil. Three groups of rats fed one of these diets received 50 mg/kg bw per day β-carotene in distilled water orally for five weeks. At six, seven and eight weeks of age, 10 rats in each group were injected subcutaneously with 15 mg/kg bw azoxy-methane, and the other 10 animals in each group served as non-azoxymethane-treated controls. All rats were killed at 10 weeks of age (i.e. for the azoxymethane-treated rats, four weeks after the first administration of the carcinogen). The colons of five azoxymethane-treated rats and five non-azoxymethane-treated controls

Table 36. Effects of combinations of β-carotene and other chemicals or physical agents on tumorigenesis in experimental animals

Organ	Species, strain, sex	No. of animals/group	Carcinogen (dose, route)	β-Carotene (dose, route)	Other agent (dose, route)	Treatment relative to carcinogen	Preventive efficacy	Reference
Skin	Mouse, Crl:Slch2 (hr/hr) BR, female	45	DMBA, 150 mg; TPA, twice weekly, 11 weeks; once weekly, 9 weeks	0.5% in diet	0.12% vitamin E in diet	Before and during	Tumour incidence: β-Carotene: reduced ($p < 0.05$) Vitamin E: reduced ($p < 0.05$) β-Carotene + vitamin E: reduced ($p < 0.05$)	Lambert et al. (1994)
Colon	Rat, Fischer 344, male	5	Azoxymethane, 3 x 15 mg/kg bw, s.c.	50 mg/kg bw, orally in distilled water, daily	Perilla oil, 3 and 12% in diet	Before, during and after	Preneoplasia (aberrant crypt foci): β-Carotene (high dose): 26% ($p < 0.01$) Perilla oil (3%): 58% ($p < 0.01$) Perilla oil (12%): 82% ($p< 0.01$) Combination (3% perilla oil): 87% ($p < 0.01$) Combination (12% perilla oil): 91% ($p < 0.01$)	Komaki et al. (1996)
Colon	Rat, Fischer 344, male	20	Azoxymethane [dose and route unspecified]	1, 10 and 20 mg/kg diet	1 and 8% wheat bran in diet	During and after (?)	Aberrant crypt foci, multiplicity: 1% wheat bran + 20 mg β-carotene: 70% ($p < 0.05$) 8% wheat bran + 20 mg β-carotene: 80% ($p < 0.05$) Tumours, incidence: 1% wheat bran + 20 mg β-carotene: 73% ($p < 0.05$) 8% wheat bran + 20 mg β-carotene: 82% ($p < 0.05$)	Alabaster et al. (1996)
Lung	Mouse, A/J, female	24–28	NNK: total dose, 9.2 mg/mouse; drinking-water	2.14 g/kg diet	0.009 g/kg retinol in diet	Before, during and after	Tumours, combination: Incidence: none (NS) Multiplicity: 19% (NS)	Castonguay et al. (1991)
Respiratory tract	Hamster, male	20	NDEA; 17.8 mg/kg bw. s.c. twice weekly for 20 weeks	Injectable solution, 1.5 mg per injection, s.c., twice weekly for 20 weeks	Oltipraz; 300 mg/kg diet; 4-HPR; 98 mg/kg diet	Before, during and after	Carcinoma incidence: β-Carotene alone: 48% reduction (NS) β-Carotene + oltipraz: 90% reduction ($p < 0.005$) β-Carotene + oltipraz + 4 HPR: 100% reduction ($p < 0.001$)	Moon et al. (1994)

Table 36 (contd)

Organ	Species, strain, sex	No. of animals/ Group	Carcinogen (dose, route)	β-Carotene (dose, route)	Other agent (dose, route)	Treatment relative to carcinogen	Preventive efficacy	Reference
Buccal pouch	Hamster, male	20	0.5% DMBA (0.6 mg/ painting)	200 or 400 µg/ animal per day by mouth	200 or 400 µg α-tocopherol/animal per day	After	Carcinoma burden: β-carotene: none (SU) α-Tocopherol: none (SU) Combination: 87% (SU)	Shklar et al. (1989)
Buccal pouch	Hamster, male	10	0.5% DMBA, painted thrice weekly	50 µg/ animal, painted thrice weekly	12.5 µg β-carotene + 12.5 µg α-tocopherol + 12.5 µg glutathione + 12.5 µg ascorbic acid	During	Carcinoma burden: β-Carotene: 85% (p < 0.001) α-Tocopherol: 49% (p < 0.01) Glutathione: 85% (p < 0.01) Ascorbic acid: none (NS) Combination: 96% (p < 0.001)	Shklar et al. (1993)
Buccal pouch	Hamster, male	15	AcO-NDMA, 2 mg/kg bw/ painting; twice monthly, 6 months	5.8 µmol/L [?] in drinking-water	α-Tocopherol, 5.8 µmol/L [?] in drinking-water	Before, during and after	Tumour incidence: β-Carotene or α-tocopherol alone: 93% (p < 0.01) Combination: 100% (p < 0.01)	Azuine & Bhide (1992)
Pancreas	Rat, Bor(WISW, Cpb)Wistar, female	40	Azaserine, 30 mg/kg bw, i.p., two injections	60 mg/diet	10 g/kg vitamin C, 600 mg/kg vitamin E, 2.5 mg/kg selenium in diet	After	Carcinoma incidence: β-carotene: 71% (p < 0.05) Vitamin C: 42% (NS) Vitamin E: 37% (NS) Selenium: 53% (p < 0.05) Mixture: 71% (p < 0.05)	Appel et al. (1991)
Pancreas	Rats, Wistar, male	15?	Azaserine, 3 × 30 mg/kg bw, i.p.	100 and 1000 mg/kg diet	1 and 2.5 mg/kg selenium in diet	Before and during	Preneoplasia: β-Carotene (high dose): 42% (p < 0.05) Selenium (high dose): 23% (p < 0.05) Combination (high doses): 19% (p < 0.05) Combination (low doses): 36% (p < 0.05) Tumours Compounds alone and combined: none (NS)	Appel & Woutersen (1996)
Pancreas	Rats, Wistar, male	15?	Azaserine, 3 × 30 mg/kg bw, i.p.	100 and 1000 mg/kg diet	1 and 2.5 mg/kg selenium in diet	After	Preneoplasia β-Carotene (high dose): 29% (p < 0.05) Selenium (high dose): 36% (p < 0.01) Combination (high doses): 25% (p < 0.05) Combination (low dos): 24% (p < 0.05) Tumours Compounds alone and combined: none (NS)	Appel & Woutersen (1996)

Table 36 (contd)

Organ	Species, strain, sex	No. of animals/Group	Carcinogen (dose, route)	β-Carotene (dose, route)	Other agent (dose, route)	Treatment relative to carcinogen	Preventive efficacy	Reference
Pancreas	Hamster, male	40	NBOPA; 3 weekly doses of 20 mg; s.c.	60 mg/kg diet	10 kg/kg vitamin C in diet	After	Preneoplasia: none (NS) Carcinomas: none (NS)	Appel et al. (1996)
Fibrosarcoma	Mouse, C3H, male	15	FSaII, 2 x 10^6 cells, s.c	10 mg/kg bw; 3 doses, i.p.	150 mg/kg bw cyclophosphamide, 3 doses i.p. or 15 mg/kg carmustine, 3 doses i.p.	Before and during	Fibrosarcoma growth delay: β-Carotene + cyclophosphamide: 73% (SU) β-Carotene + carmustine: 112% (SU)	Teicher et al. (1994)
Fibrosarcoma	Mouse, C3H, male	15	FSaII, 2 x 10^6 cells, s.c.	10 mg/kg bw; 5 daily doses, i.p.	10 mg/kg bw melphalan, 3 doses i.p.; 40 mg/kg bw 5-fluorouracil, 5 doses, i.p.; 0.8 mg/kg bw methotrexate, 5 doses, i.p.; 150 mg/kg bw cyclophosphamide, 3 doses, i.p.	Before and during	Fibrosarcoma, growth delay: β-Carotene + melphalan: 333% (SU) β-Carotene + cyclophosphamide: 144% (SU) β-Carotene + methotrexate: none (SU) β-Carotene + 5-fluorouracil: none (rather, a significant decrease)	Teicher et al. (1994)
Fibrosarcoma	Mouse, C3H, male	15	FsaII, 2 x 10^6 cells, s.c.	10 mg/kg bw, 14 daily doses, s.c. plus 10 mg/kg bw minocycline, 14 daily doses, i.p.	10 mg/kw bw melphalan, single dose: i.p.; 10 mg/kg bw CDDP, single dose, i.p.; 150 mg/kg bw cyclophosphamide, 3 doses i.p.; 150 mg/kg bw ifosfamide, 3 doses, i.p.; 40 mg/kg bw 5-fluorouracil, 5 doses, i.p.; 15 mg/kg bw etopside, 5 doses, i.p.; 1.75 mg/kg bw adriamycin, 5 doses, i.p.	Before and during	Fibrosarcoma, growth delay: β-Carotene + minocycline + melphalan: 259% (SU) β-Carotene + minocycline + CDDP: 24% (SU) β-Carotene + minocycline + cyclophosphamide: 28% (SU) β-Carotene + minocycline + ifosfamide: 40% (SU) β-Carotene + minocycline + etopside: 243% (SU) β-Carotene + minocycline + adriamycin: 225% (SU) β-Carotene + minocycline + 5-fluorouracil: none (rather, a significant decrease)	Teicher et al. (1994)

Table 36 (contd)

Organ	Species, strain, sex	No. of animals/ Group	Carcinogen (dose, route)	β–Carotene, (dose, route)	Other agent (dose, route)	Treatment relative to carcinogen	Preventive efficacy	Reference
Fibro-sarcoma	Mouse, C3H, male	15	SCC VII, 2 × 10⁶ cells, s.c.	10 mg/kg bw, 5 daily doses, i.p.	10 mg/kg bw melphalan, single dose, i.p.; 10 mg/kg bw CDDP, single dose, i.p.; 150 mg/kg bw cyclophosphamide, 3 doses, i.p.; 15 mg/kg bw carmustine, 3 doses, i.p.; 40 mg/kg bw 5-fluorouracil, 5 doses, i.p.; 1.75 mg/kg bw adriamycin, 5 doses, i.p.	Before and during	Fibrosarcoma, growth delay β–Carotene + melphalan: 115% (SU) β–Carotene + cyclophos-phamide: 38% (SU) β–Carotene + CDDP or carmustine or 5-fluorouracil or adriamycin: none (SU)	Teicher et al. (1994)
Inoculated adeno-carcinoma cells	Mouse, CBA/J, male	10–12	2 × 10⁵ C3HBA cells	90 mg/kg diet	30 Gy X-rays	Ane fter	Adenocarcinoma β–Carotene: survival of mice, 49% (p < 0.001); tumour growth, 75% (SU) Irradiation: survival of mice, 105% (p < 0.001); tumour growth, partial regression (SU) Combination: complete tumour regression and no deaths (SU)	Seifter et al. (1983)
Inoculated adeno-carcinoma cells	Mouse, CBA/J, male	10–12	2 × 10⁵ C3HBA cells	90 mg/kg diet	30 Gy X-rays	After	Adenocarcinoma β–Carotene: survival of mice, 46% (p < 0.001); tumour growth, 26% Irradiation: survival of mice, 129% (p < 0.001); tumour growth, partial regression (SU) Combination: complete tumour regression and no deaths (SU)	Seifter et al. (1983)

i.p., intraperitoneally; NS, not significant; NBOPA, N-nitrosobis(oxopropyl)amine; s.c., subcutaneously; NDEA, N-nitrosodiethylamine; N-nitroso-methylamine; 4-HPR, N-(4-hydroxyphenyl)retinamide; DMBA, 7,12-dimethylbenz[a]anthracene; SU, statistics unspecified; AcO-NDMA, N-nitroso(acetoxymethyl)methylamine; NNK, 4-(N-nitrosomethylamino)-1-(3-pyridyl)-1-butanone; Fsall, fibrosarcoma cell line; CDDP, cis-diamminedichloroplatinum; SCC-VII, squamous-cell carcinoma cell line; C3HBA, adenocarcinoma cell line in each group were collected to establish the presence of colonic aberrant crypt foci and to count the number of aberrant crypts per colon and the number of aberrant crypts per focus. Mean food intake and mean body weights were not significantly affected by β-carotene or perilla oil. No neoplasms were found. Aberrant crypt foci were found only in the colons of rats treated with azoxymethane. β-Carotene and perilla oil alone and in combination significantly suppressed the development of these preneoplastic colonic changes (Table 37; Komaki et al., 1996).

The effects of β-carotene, incorporated at various concentrations into a high-fat diet with low or high levels of dietary fibre (wheat bran [formulation in the diet unspecified]), on the occurrence of aberrant crypt foci and tumours of the colon were investigated in four-week old male Fischer 344 rats given two subcutaneous injections of 15 mg/kg bw azoxymethane in saline in weeks 3 and 4. Six weeks after the last injection, five animals per group were killed and examined for the presence of aberrant crypt foci; the remaining animals were continued

on their respective diets for an additional 20 weeks. The results (Table 38) show a strong, dose-dependent protective effect of both β-carotene and wheat bran against colon carcinogenesis (Alabaster et al., 1995, 1996). [The Working Group noted discrepancies in the total number of aberrant crypt foci and the incidence of colonic adenomas between the two publications.]

(c) Lung
Mouse: Two groups of female A/J mice [initial number unspecified], six to seven weeks old, were fed powdered AIN-76A diet for 23 weeks; a third group received the same diet supplemented with 2.14 g/kg β-carotene (purity, 65%; 0.012 μmol/d per mouse [formulation in the diet unspecified]) plus 0.009 g/kg retinol (purity, 70%; 6 x 10^{-6} μmol/d per mouse) for 23 weeks. During weeks 2–9, all 24 mice given β-carotene plus retinol and 28 in one of the groups on the unsupplemented diet received 4-(N-nitrosomethylamino)-1-(3-pyridyl)-1-butanone (NNK) in the drinking-water, for a total dose of 9.2 mg per mouse. The body weights of mice given β-carotene plus retinol were slightly lower than

Table 37. Incidence and numbers of aberrant crypt foci in the colons of azoxymethane-treated male Fischer 344 rats fed diets containing perilla oil and β-carotene in distilled water

Dietary addition[a]	Incidence	No./colon	No.of aberrant crypts/colon	No. of aberrant crypts/focus
12% olive oil	5/5	217.4 ± 23.5	381 ± 38.1	1.76 ± 0.09
12% olive oil and 50 mg/kg bw β-carotene	5/5	159.8 ± 16.4[b]	267 ± 33.8[b]	1.67 ± 0.05
9% olive oil and 3% perilla oil	5/5	91.4 ± 15.5[b]	148.6 ± 29.4[b]	1.62 ± 0.08[c]
9% olive oil, 3% perilla oil and 50 mg/kg bw β-carotene	5/5	28.0 ± 8.3[b,d,e]	4.3 ± 11.3[b,d,e]	1.44 ± 0.09[b,d,f]
12% perilla oil	5/5	40.0 ± 16.5[b,e]	56.8 ± 15.0[b,e]	1.47 ± 0.18[b]
12% perilla oil and 50 mg/kg bw β-carotene	5/5	19.3 ± 11.0[b,d]	28.0 ± 16.5[b,d,g]	1.44 ± 0.03[b,d]

From Komaki et al. (1996); for further details, see text
[a] All rats received a subcutaneous injection of 15 mg/kg bw azoxymethane once a week for three weeks.
[b] Significantly different from group 1; $p < 0.01$: Dunnett's *t* test
[c] Significantly different from group 1; $p < 0.05$: Dunnett's *t* test
[d] Significantly different from group 2; $p < 0.01$: Dunnett's *t* test
[e] Significantly different from group 3; $p < 0.01$: Dunnett's *t* test
[f] Significantly different from group 3; $p < 0.05$: Dunnett's *t* test
[g] Significantly different from group 5; $p < 0.05$: Dunnett's *t* test

Table 38. Numbers of aberrant crypt foci (ACF) and incidence of tumours in the colon of azoxymethane-treated Fischer 344 rats fed a high-fat diet containing various concentrations of wheat bran and β-carotene

Group	Treatment Wheat bran (%)	β-Carotene (mg/kg)	No. of ACF/rat (n = 5)	Incidence of colon tumours (n = 15) Total	Adenoma	Carcinoma
1	1	0	44 ± 4.2	11/15	12/15[a]	6/15
2	1	1	$25^b \pm 3.3$	7/15	5/15	3/15
3	1	10	21 ± 0.7^c	3/15[e]	1/15	2/15
4	1	20	$13 \pm 2.9^{c,d}$	3/15[e]	2/15	1/15
5	8	0	21 ± 2.9^c	4/15[e]	2/15	2/15
6	8	1	16 ± 1.4^c	3/15[e]	1/15	2/15
7	8	10	$11 \pm 0.6^{c,d}$	2/15[e]	1/15	1.15
8	8	20	$9 \pm 0.6^{c,d}$	2/15[e]	1/15	1/15

From Alabaster *et al.* (1995, 1996), for further details, see text
[a] Given as 53% by Alabaster *et al.* (1995)
[b] Given as 35 by Alabaster *et al.* (1995)
[c] Statistically significantly different from group 1; $p < 0.05$; Student's *t* test
[d] Statistically significantly different from group 5; $p < 0.05$; Student's *t* test
[e] Statistically significantly different from group 1; $p < 0.05$; Student's *t* test

those of the untreated controls and comparable to those treated with NNK alone. Six of the 24 untreated controls developed lung tumours, with an average of 0.4 ± 0.1 tumours per surviving mouse. β-Carotene plus retinol did not reduce the incidence of tumours (24/24 versus 28/28 in the NNK-treated controls) or the number of tumours per surviving mouse (12.7 ± 3.1 versus 15.7 ± 2.7; not significant; Fisher's exact test) (Castonguay *et al.*, 1991).

Hamster: Male Syrian golden hamsters, five to six weeks of age were given subcutaneous injections twice weekly of 1.5 mg β-carotene (micellar form dispersed in an aqueous solution of 40 mg/ml), oltipraz at 300 mg/kg diet and N-(4-hydroxyphenyl)retinamide at 98 mg/kg diet, alone or in combination. After one week of the respective diets, groups of animals were given twice weekly subcutaneous injections of 17.8 mg/kg bw NDEA for 20 weeks; in the groups receiving β-carotene, NDEA was administered 24 h after the carotenoid injection. Vehicle controls received saline. At the termination of the study, after 25 weeks on the test diets, the entire respiratory tree was removed and the incidences of pulmonary carcinomas and tracheal papillomas were determined. None of agents significantly inhibited tumour formation when given alone, but β-carotene in combination with oltipraz synergistically decreased the incidence of carcinomas by 90% ($p < 0.005$), and β-carotene in combination with oltipraz and N-(4-hydroxyphenyl)retinamide resulted in a 100% reduction ($p < 0.001$) (Moon *et al.*, 1994).

(d)   Buccal pouch
Hamster: The mucosa of the right buccal pouches of 100 male Syrian hamsters, 60–90 days old and weighing 95–125 g, were painted three times per week with a 0.5% solution of DMBA in heavy mineral oil (about 0.6 mg DMBA per painting) for 14 weeks, when all animals had moderate-sized tumours in the right pouch. The animals were then divided into groups of 20 animals and received either no further treatment (controls), 0.2 ml vegetable oil daily by gavage (vehicle control) or the same volume of vegetable oil containing 400 µg β-carotene, 400

μg α-tocopherol or 200 μg β-carotene plus 200 μg α-tocopherol. At 22 weeks, the animals receiving β-carotene plus α-tocopherol were all alive and in good condition, and their treatment was extended to 28 weeks, whereas the animals in the other groups were weak and cachectic (four died and the others were killed for humane reasons), had significantly higher body weights (138 g) than the animals in the other groups (103 g), had a total buccal pouch tumour burden of about 500 mm³ as compared with about 3500–4200 mm³ in the other groups [data presented as diagrams only; no information on statistical analysis] and showed no metastases in the cervical lymph nodes, whereas metastatic spread to cervical lymph nodes was found in many other animals. β-Carotene treatment alone did not result in regression of these tumours, the total tumour burden at 22 weeks being about 3700 mm³ with β-carotene and 4000 mm³ in the vehicle controls. All of the tumours appeared to be epidermoid carcinomas, which underwent cellular degeneration only in animals treated with β-carotene plus α-tocopherol. At 28 weeks, no buccal pouch tumours were found grossly in several of the hamsters treated with β-carotene plus α-tocopherol, but some had tumours larger than those found at 14 weeks (Shklar et al., 1989).

The mucosa of the right buccal pouches of 60 male Syrian hamsters, 60–90 days old and weighing 92–123 g, was painted with a 0.5% DMBA solution in heavy mineral oil three times per week for 12 or 14 weeks. Groups of 10 animals received no further treatment (DMBA control group) or were given either a mixture of 12.5 μg β-carotene plus 12.5 μg DL-α-tocopherol acid succinate plus 12.5 μg reduced glutathione plus 12.5 μg L-ascorbic acid or 50 μg β-carotene, 50 μg reduced glutathione, 50 μg DL-α-tocopherol acid succinate or 50 μg L-ascorbic acid in a volume of 0.5 ml mineral oil by mouth [route of administration not further specified] three times per week on alternate days to DMBA, for 12 or 14 weeks. One-half of the animals in each group were killed after 12 weeks, and the other half after 14 weeks. At both times, treatment with the mixture, with β-carotene or with glutathione or α-tocopherol, but not ascorbic acid, appeared to have significantly reduced the incidence of cheek pouch leukoplakia and the incidence, area, volume and total burden of cheek pouch tumours (carcinomas in situ and early carcinomas), the mixture being significantly more effective than β-carotene, glutathione or α-tocopherol alone; e.g. the values for the tumour burden after 12 weeks were: 2.89 ± 0.6 mm³ for the DMBA control, 0.125 ± 0.01 mm³ for animals given the mixture ($p < 0.001$), 0.434 ± 0.1 mm³ for those given β-carotene ($p < 0.001$), 0.438 ± 0.1 mm³ for those given glutathione ($p < 0.01$), 1.47 ± 0.25 mm³ for those given α-tocopherol ($p < 0.01$) and 3.69 ± 0.62 mm³ for those given ascorbic acid (p value for difference between the mixture and β-carotene, < 0.01; between the mixture and glutathione,< 0.01 and and between the mixture and α-tocopherol, < 0.001; Student's t test) (Shklar et al., 1993).

Four groups of 15 female inbred Syrian hamsters, eight weeks old, were given drinking-water alone or with β-carotene at 5.8 nmol/L [formulation in the drinking-water unspecified], α-tocopherol at 5.8 nmol/L or β-carotene plus α-tocopherol for 13 months. After two weeks, 2 mg/kg bw AcO-NDMA were applied to the mucosa of the right cheek pouch twice monthly for six months; three additional groups of 15 hamsters were not treated with AcO-NDMA and did not develop cheek pouch tumours. Both β-carotene and α-tocopherol reduced the incidence of cheek pouch tumours induced by AcO-NDMA, from 14/15 to 1/15 ($p < 0.001$; χ^2 test), while no cheek pouch tumours were seen at death in hamsters given the combined treament ($p < 0.001$; χ^2 test). The time to appearance of tumours was 5–10 months in hamsters given AcO-NDMA alone, 8–12 months in those given β-carotene, 9 months in those given α-tocopherol and 6 months in those given β-carotene plus α-tocopherol [statistics unspecified] (Azuine & Bhide, 1992).

(e)   Pancreas

Rat: Groups of 40 male weanling SPF albino Bor (WISW,Cpb) Wistar rats were fed standard laboratory chow and received two intraperitoneal injections of 30 mg/kg bw azaserine in 0.9% saline, one at 19 days and one at 26 days of age. One week after the second injection, the animals were allocated randomly to one of eight groups. Each group was switched to an AIN-76 diet with a high concentration of saturated fat (20% lard) either as such (azaserine controls) [use of placebo beadlets unspecified] or supplemented with 60 mg/kg β-carotene (as water-dispersible beadlets containing 10% pure β-carotene), 10 g/kg vitamin C (as ascorbic acid), 60 mg/kg β-carotene plus 10 g/kg vitamin C, 600 mg/kg vitamin E (as 50% DL-α-tocopherol), 2.5 mg/kg selenium (as sodium selenite), 600 mg/kg vitamin E plus 2.5 mg/kg selenium, or 60 mg/kg β-carotene plus 10 g/kg vitamin C plus 600 mg/kg vitamin E plus 2.5 mg/kg selenium (mix). Autopsies were performed 482–485 days after the second injection of azaserine. Of the 27 animals in all groups that died or were killed before the final autopsy, 10 that died after day 380 were included in the final evaluation; five of these rats had pancreatic tumours, five had renal or hepatic failure, and one died with an unspecified head tumour. Food and energy intake were similar among the various groups, but food conversion efficiency was significantly lower in the groups fed diets supplemented with β-carotene plus vitamin C, selenium, selenium plus vitamin E or the mix. The body and pancreatic weights were similar, except that the mean body weight

of the group receiving the mix was significantly lower than that of the controls. β-Carotene, selenium and vitamin C, alone or in combination, reduced azaserine-induced pancreatic carcinogenesis (Table 39; Appel *et al.*, 1991).

The effect of β-carotene alone or in combination with selenium on the initiation or early promotion and late promotion phases of pancreatic carcinogenesis was studied in 96 azaserine-treated female Wistar rats which had been mated one week earlier. Half of the animals were maintained on a high-fat diet (25% fat, 25% casein, 0.37% DL-methionine, 36.79% wheat starch, 6.18% cellulose, 0.25% choline bitartrate, 4.32% AIN76 minerals supplying 0.13 mg selenium per kg diet, 1.24% AIN76 vitamins and 1.85% calcium phosphate); the other 48 rats were divided into six groups and were fed the high-fat diet supplemented with 100 or 1000 mg/kg β-carotene (added as a 30% suspension in corn oil), 1 or 2.5 mg/kg selenium (as sodium selenite), 100 mg/kg β-carotene plus 1 mg/kg selenium or 1000 mg/kg β-carotene plus 2.5 mg/kg selenium. When the pups were born, 14 groups of 20 males were formed and were fed the same diets as their mothers. At 14 and 21 days of age, the pups received a subcutaneous injection of 30 mg/kg bw azaserine in saline, except for those in one of the groups

Table 39. Atypical acinar-cell noduls (AACN) and tumours in the pancreas of azaserine-treated male Wistar rats maintained on a high-fat diet (HF) supplemented with β-carotene (BC), vitamin C (Vit C), vitamin E (Vit E) and/or selenium (Se) for 15 months

Diet	No. of animals	No. of AACN (diameter)		No. of tumour-bearing rats	No. of carcinoma-bearing rats	No. of adenoma-bearing rats
		0.5–1 mm	1–3 mm			
HF	39	338	200	22	15	7
HF + BC	37	194*	146	9*	4*	5
HF + Vit C	37	157**	104**	14	8	6
HF + BC + Vit C	38	128**	106**	14*	9	5
HF + Vit E	37	212	155	19	9	10
HF + Se	38	181***	97***	13**	7*	6
HF + Vit E + Se	39	150***	92***	9**	5*	4
HF + BC + Vit C + Vit E + Se	38	117***	56***	8**	4*	4

From Appel *et al.* (1991); for details, see text

* $p < 0.05$; ** $p < 0.01$; *** $p < 0.001$; generalized linear regression; error is Poisson, link function is log

kept on unsupplemented diet which received subcutaneous injections of saline only. At five weeks of age, six of the seven groups fed the unsupplemented diet were switched to one of the six supplemented diets to study the effects of the supplements on the late promotion phase; the seventh group was continued on the unsupplemented diet. Also at five weeks of age, the six groups fed the various supplemented diets were switched to unsupplemented diet to study the effects ofthe supplements on the initiation or early promotion phase. The experiment was terminated when the rats were 29 weeks of age. Body and pancreatic weights were similar in all groups, except that the group receiving 100 mg β-carotene and 1 mg/kg selenium had significantly higher body and absolute pancreatic weights [no further details given]. All animals consumed similar amounts of food, resulting in similar calculated energy intakes. β-Carotene and selenium inhibited azaserine-induced pancreatic carcinogenesis, the strongest effects occurring when selenium was given alone or in combination with β-carotene during the late promotion phase (see Table 40). No (putative) preneoplastic or neoplastic pancreatic lesions were found in saline-treated controls (Appel & Woutersen, 1996).

Hamster: Four groups of 40 male Syrian golden hamsters, five to six weeks old, were fed a standard diet and were injected subcutneously with 20 mg/kg bw NBOPA [vehicle unspecified] at six, seven and eight weeks of age. One week after the last injection, all hamsters were fed a high-fat diet (20% lard) either as such or supplemented with 60 mg/kg β-carotene (as waterdispersible beadlets containing 10% pure β-carotene), 10 g/kg vitamin C or 60 mg/kg β-carotene plus 10 g/kg vitamin C for the rest of the experiment [use of placebo beadlets unspecified]. Survivors were killed 364 or 365 days after the first injection of NBOPA. The body weights of the hamsters fed the diet supplemented with β-carotene were statistically significantly lower than those of the controls ($p < 0.05$; analysis of variance and Dunnett's t test, two-sided). The mean number of advanced ductular lesions in the pancreas was consistently lower in hamsters fed the diets supplemented with either vitamin C alone (1.9 ± 0.3) or

with vitamin C plus β-carotene (1.9 ± 0.3) than in controls (2.9 ± 0.5) or in the animals fed the diet supplemented only with β-carotene (2.9 ± 0.5), but the differences were not statistically significant (analysis of variance). Moreover, no statistically significant difference (χ^2 test) in the incidence or in the mean number of carcinomas *in situ* or invasive carcinomas was found between the various groups; e.g. the incidences of advanced ductular lesions were 9/27, 11/34, 16/35 and 19/35 in the controls and animals receiving β-carotene, vitamin C and β-carotene plus vitamin C, respectively, and those of invasive carcinomas were 12/27, 11/34, 11/35 and 9/35, respectively (Appel *et al.*, 1996).

(f)   Inoculated tumours

C3HBA adenocarcinoma cells: Groups of 10 female C3H/He mice, five weeks old, were inoculated subcutaneously with 2 x 10⁵ C3HBA adenocarcinoma cells in the outer aspect of the thigh and were maintained on powdered basal diet containing 15 000 IU/kg vitamin A and 6.5 mg/kg β-carotene. When the tumours reached an average diameter of 7.5 ± 0.2 mm, one group of mice was continued on the basal diet, one group was switched to basal diet supplemented with 90 mg/kg β-carotene, one group received basal diet supplemented with 5 mg/kg ascorbic acid, and one group received basal diet supplemented with both 90 mg/kg β-carotene and 5 mg/kg ascorbic acid. The average survival times of the mice were 36.3 ± 1.3 days without supplement, 58.5 ± 3.5 days with β-carotene (*p* < 0.001; analysis of variance), 38.1 ± 1.6 days with ascorbic acid and 56.7 ± 1.5 days with both supplements (*p* < 0.001; analysis of variance). β-Carotene, but not ascorbic acid alone or in combination with β-carotene, reduced tumour growth but did not cause tumour regression: after 12 days of feeding the various diets, the average tumour diameters were 21.7 mm without supplement, 17.1 mm with β-carotene, 21.5 mm with ascorbic acid and 17.4 mm with both supplements (Student's *t* test [*p* values unspecified]) (Rettura *et al.*, 1982).

Forty-four male CBA/J mice, six weeks old, were inoculated subcutaneously with 2 x 10⁵ C3HBA adenocarcinoma cells in the outer

Table 40. Putatively preneoplastic atypical acinar-cell nodules (AACN), carcinoma *in situ* and atypical acinar-cell foci (AACF) in the pancreas of azaserine-treated male Wistar rats fed a high-fat diet (HF) with β-carotene (BC) and/or selenium (Se) at two phases of the carcinogenesis process

Diet	AACN No./cm²	Area (mm²)	No./cm³	Mean diameter (mm)	Area as % pancreas	Carcinoma *in situ* Incidence	Multiplicity	Multiplicity of AACF > 1 mm
Initiation or early promotion phase								
HF	46.2	0.21	1521	409	9.5	3/15	7.0 ± 1.5	0.3 ± 0.2
HF + 100 mg/kg BC	40.3	0.20	1281*	430	8.1	3/15	7.6 + 1.6	0.2 ± 0.1
HF + 1000 mg/kg BC	30.7	0.18	1069*	405	5.5	4/27	4.8 ± 1.4	0.3 ± 0.2
HF + 1 mg/kg Se	36.2	0.18	1280*	384	6.5	5/11	3.1 ± 0.8	0.5 ± 0.2
HF + 2.5 mg/kg Se	35.8	0.18	1178*	407	6.4	2/15	5.0 ± 1.5	0.1 ± 0.1
HF + 100 mg/kg BC + 1 mg/kg Se	29.4	0.19	974*	412	5.5	5/15	6.8 ± 2.4	0.5 ± 0.2
HF + 1000 mg/kg BC + 2.5 mg/kg Se	37.4	0.18	1232*	416	6.9	4/15	6.0 ± 2.4	0.3 ± 0.2
Late promotion phase								
HF	46.2	0.21	1521	409	9.5	3/15	7.0 ± 1.5	0.3 ± 0.2
HF + 100 mg/kg BC	29.8	0.18	1102*	389	5.3*	3/15	4.1 ± 1.6	0.2 ± 0.1
HF + 1000 mg/kg BC	33.9	0.20	1183**	408	6.7*	2/15	5.8 ± 1.4	0.1 ± 0.1
HF + 1 mg/kg Se	25.5**	0.18	986*	392	4.6**	6/15	5.8 ± 1.3	0.4 ± 0.1
HF + 2.5 mg/kg Se	24.8**	0.17	973**	371	4.2**	5/15	2.7 ± 0.5	0.3 ± 0.1
HF + 100 mg/kg BC + 1 mg Se	31.2*	0.18*	1149**	382**	5.5**	3/15	4.7 ± 1.4	0.2 ± 0.1
HF + 1000 mg/kg BC + 2.5 mg/kg Se	26.5*	0.16*	1136**	357**	4.2**	3/15	4.0 ± 1.2	0.2 ± 0.1

From Appel & Woutersen (1996); for details, see text

* $p < 0.05$; ** $p < 0.01$; analysis of variance

aspect of the right thigh and were fed a basal diet containing 15 000 IU/kg vitamin A and 6.4 mg/kg β-carotene. On day 13, when the mean diameter of the tumours was 6.2 ± 0.3 mm, 20 mice were randomly selected and distributed into two groups of 10 animals, one of which was continued on unsupplemented basal diet and the other given basal diet supplemented with 90 mg/kg β-carotene. The tumours of the other 24 tumour-bearing mice received 3000 rad (30 Gy) X-irradiation, and the mice were divided randomly into two groups of 12, one of which was continued on unsupplemented diet, while the other received the supplement of β-carotene. One year after irradiation, five of the 10 surviving mice fed β-carotene were switched back to basal diet, while the other five animals were continued on the β-carotene-sup-plemented diet. A similar experiment was begun nine weeks after the first, in which the mean tumour diameter on day 13 was 5.6 ± 0.2 mm and the mice were switched back to basal diet 13.5 months after irradiation. In neither experiment was there a significant difference in body weight between groups. Unirradiated mice fed the unsupplemented diet had an aver-age survival time of 41.2 days in experiment 1 and 43.3 days in experiment 2. β-Carotene increased the average survival times to 61.2 and 63.3 days in experiments 1 and 2, respectively ($p < 0.001$ for each experiment; analysis of vari-ance), and slowed tumour growth considerably [statistics unspecified], an average tumour diameter of about 16.8 mm being reached in weeks 12 and 21 in experiment 1 and in weeks 19 and 24 in experiment 2 in the unsupple-mented and β-carotene-supplemented animals, respectively. Local irradiation alone increased the average survival time to 84.4 and 99.1 days in experiments 1 and 2, respectively ($p < 0.001$ for both experiments; analysis of variance), and caused partial tumour regression in nearly all mice (one mouse showed tumour regression to an impalpable level, indicating complete regression), but tumour growth resumed after 18 and 24 days in experiment 1 and 2, respec-tively. Local irradiation combined with feeding of β-carotene led to complete tumour regres-sion within 18 and 12 weeks in experiments 1 and 2, respectively. Twenty-two of the

24 irradiated mice fed the β-carotene-supple-mented diet survived for one year, whereas mice that were only irradiated or only fed β-carotene were all dead by three months. Of the six irradiated mice in experiment 1 that were switched back to unsupplemented basal diet after one year, two developed tumours after 133 and 275 days, whereas none of the five irradiated mice continued on the β-carotene-supplemented basal diet redeveloped tumours. In experiment 2, none of the 11 irradiated mice that were switched back to the unsupplemented basal diet after 13.5 months or continued on the β-carotene-supplemented basal diet redeveloped tumours (Seifter *et al.*, 1983).

SCC VII cells: Groups of 15 male C3H mice, eight to ten weeks old, were inoculated subcu-taneously with 2×10^6 SCC VII carcinoma cells into one leg; one of the groups served as untreated controls. Mice in seven of the groups received five daily intraperitoneal injections of 10 mg/kg bw β-carotene (soya-based emulsion) on days 7–11; one of these groups was not fur-ther treated, while the other six groups received either one intraperitoneal injection of 10 mg/kg bw melphalan or 10 mg/kg bw *cis*-diamminedichloroplatinum(II) (CDDP) on day 7, immediately after the β-carotene injection; three intraperitoneal injections of 150 mg/kg bw cyclophosphamide or 15 mg/kg bw carmus-tine on days 7, 9 and 11; or five intraperitoneal injections of 40 mg/kg bw 5-fluorouracil or 1.75 mg/kg bw adriamycin on days 7–11. Six groups that were not treated with β-carotene were similarly treated with melphalan, CDDP, cyclophosphamide, carmustine, 5-fluorouracil or adriamycin alone. Only a minimal delay in tumour growth (number of days required to reach a volume of 500 mm³), 0.3 ± 0.3 day, was seen with β-carotene alone. β-Carotene increased the delay in tumour growth caused by melpha-lan, from 2.7 ± 0.3 to 5.8 ± 0.6 days, and that due to cyclophosphamide from 13.5 ± 1.5 to 18.6 ± 1.7 days [statistics unspecified]. β-Carotene did not affect the delay in tumour growth caused by CDDP (6.7 ± 0.6 versus 6.8 ± 0.7 days), carmustine (3.2 ± 0.4 versus 3.4 ± 0.5 days), 5-fluorouracil (2.4 ± 0.3 versus 2.2 ± 0.3 days) or adriamycin (1.6 ± 0.3 versus

1.7 ± 0.3 days) [statistics unspecified] (Teicher *et al.*, 1994).

FSaII cells: Groups of 15 male C3H mice, eight to ten weeks old, were inoculated subcutaneously with 2 x 10⁶ FSaII fibrosarcoma cells into one leg. One of the groups served as untreated controls. Mice in four other groups received one intraperitoneal injection of 10 mg/kg bw β-carotene (soya-based emulsion) on day 7; one of these groups was not further treated, while the other three groups received one intraperitoneal injection of 10 mg/kg bw melphalan, 10 mg/kg bw CDDP or 150 mg/kg bw cyclophosphamide on day 7, immediately after the β-carotene injection. Three groups were similarly treated with melphalan, CDDP or cyclophosphamide alone. β-Carotene alone minimally delayed tumour growth, by 0.3 ± 0.3 day. It increased the delay in tumour growth caused by melphalan from 2.7 ± 0.4 to 3.7 ± 0.5 days, by CDDP from 7.5 ± 0.6 to 9.5 ± 1.1 days and by cyclophosphamide from 4.3 ± 0.5 to 8.0 ± 0.8 days [statistics unspecified]. Mice in three of the groups were injected intraperitoneally with 10 mg/kg bw β-carotene on days 7, 9 and 11; one of the groups was not treated further, while the two other groups received three intraperitoneal injections of 150 mg/kg bw cyclophosphamide or 15 mg/kg bw carmustine on days 7, 9 and 11. Two groups were similarly treated with cyclophosphamide or carmustine alone. β-Carotene delayed tumour growth slightly, by 0.8 ± 0.3 day, but it increased the delay in tumour growth caused by cyclophosphamide from 7.8 ± 0.7 to 13.5 ± 1.5 days and that by carmustine from 2.5 ± 0.4 to 5.3 ± 0.5 days [statistics unspecified]. Mice in five of the groups received an intraperitoneal injection of 10 mg/kg bw β-carotene on days 7–11; one of the groups was not treated further, while the four other groups received one intraperitoneal injection of 10 mg/kg bw melphalan on day 7, three intraperitoneal injections of 150 mg/kg bw cyclophosphamide on days 7, 9 and 11, or five intraperitoneal injections of 40 mg/kg bw 5-fluorouracil or 0.8 mg/kg bw methotrexate on days 7–11. Two groups were similarly treated with 5-fluorouracil or methotrexate alone. β-Carotene alone increased the delay in tumour growth by 1.2 ± 0.4 days [statistics unspecified]

and increased the delay in tumour growth due to melphalan from 2.7 ± 0.7 to 11.7 ± 0.9 days and that due to cyclophosphamide from 7.8 ± 0.7 to 19.0 ± 1.8 days [statistics unspecified]. It also decreased the delay in tumour growth caused by 5-fluorouracil from 7.6 ± 0.7 to 2.7 ± 0.5 days but did not affect the delay due to methotrexate (2.2 ± 0.4 versus 2.7 ± 0.5 days) (Teicher *et al.*, 1994).

Groups of five male C3H mice, eight to ten weeks old, were inoculated subcutaneously with 2 x 10⁶ FSaII fibrosarcoma cells into one leg. One of the groups served as an untreated control group, and eight groups received daily intraperitoneal injections of 10 mg/kg bw β-carotene (soya-based emulsion) plus 10 mg/kg bw minocycline on days 4–18. One of these groups was not further treated, while the other seven received one intraperitoneal injection of 10 mg/kg bw melphalan or CDDP on day 7, three intraperitoneal injections of 150 mg/kg bw cyclophosohamide or ifosfamide on days 7, 9 and 11 or five intraperitoneal injections of 40 mg/kg bw 5-fluorouracil, 15 mg/kg bw etopside or 1.75 mg/kg bw adriamycin on days 7–11. Seven groups were similarly treated with melphalan, CDDP, cyclophosphamide, ifosfamide, 5-fluorouracil, etopside or adriamycin alone. β-Carotene plus minocycline produced only a minimal delay in tumour growth, 0.3 ± 0.3 day [statistics unspecified], but increased the delay in tumour growth caused by melphalan from 2.7 ± 0.4 to 9.7 ± 0.9 days, by CDDP from 7.5 ± 0.6 to 9.3 ± 1.1 days, by cyclophosphamide from 7.8 ± 0.7 to 10 ± 1.2 days, by ifosfamide from 6.3 ± 0.7 to 8.8 ± 1.2 days, by etopside from 4.9 ± 0.7 to 16.8 ± 1.7 days and by adriamycin from 8.9 ± 1.0 to 28.9 ± 2.7 days [statistics unspecified]. β-Carotene alone decreased the growth delay caused by 5-fluorouracil from 7.6 ± 0.7 to 3.2 ± 0.4 days [statistics unspecified] (Teicher *et al.*, 1994).

4.2.1.3 Canthaxanthin (Table 41)

(a) Skin

Mouse: Four groups of 75 female Swiss albino 955 mice, nine to ten weeks old, were painted on a clipped, mid-dorsal area of the skin with 0.02 ml of a 0.5% solution of benzo[*a*]pyrene in acetone (0.1 mg benzo[*a*]pyrene per painting), twice a week for 60 weeks. Two of the four groups were kept in the dark except during treatment and observation; the other two groups were also kept in the dark but were exposed to long UV irradiation (300–400 nm; 5890 erg/cm^2 per s) for 2 h immediately after each skin painting. One of the groups kept in the dark and one of the groups subjected to UV irradiation were fed a normal rodent diet, while the other two groups were fed a diet containing 500 mg/kg canthaxanthin from 10% canthaxanthin-containing beadlets. After one month, the animals fed the canthaxanthin-supplemented diet received an additional dose of 100 mg/kg bw crystalline canthaxanthin as a 1% solution in arachis oil by stomach tube twice a week. Two additional groups of 75 mice fed a normal rodent diet and kept either continuously in the dark or subjected to UV irradiation for 2 h twice a week did not develop any skin tumours, and canthaxanthin had no consistent or significant effect on the incidence of benzo[a]pyrene-induced skin tumours in mice kept continuously in the dark during the final half of the experiment; however, during the final 20 weeks of the study, canthaxanthin significantly reduced the incidence of skin tumours in mice kept in the dark, from about 546 to 37% at 48 weeks and from about 67 to 47% at week 60 ($p < 0.01$ [statistics unspecified]). In comparison with benzo[a]pyrene alone, the combination with UV irradiation increased the skin tumour incidence by two- to sevenfold at various times. Canthaxanthin reduced the incidence of skin papillomas and epitheliomas induced by benzo[a]pyrene plus UV considerably, e.g. from about 12 to 3% at 20 weeks, from about 47 to 24% at 28 weeks, from about 61 to 38% at 38 weeks, from about 86 to 42% at 48 weeks and from about 96 to 43% at 60 weeks [statistics unspecified]. At the end of the study, the skin tumours in the various groups consisted of 10–20% papillomas and 80–90% squamous epitheliomas (Santamaria et al., 1981, 1983a,b, 1988).

Canthaxanthin (33 g/kg diet; 6.68 g/kg bw per day; from canthaxanthin-containing beadlets) was administered in the diet to three groups of 24 female hairless Philadelphia Skin and Cancer Hospital SKH/hr mice, five to eight weeks of age, for 30–32 weeks. Three groups of mice received placebo beadlets. After 10 weeks on the respective diets, skin tumours were induced by one of three methods, each being applied to one of the canthaxanthin-treated groups and to one of the placebo control groups. In the first method, the mice were irradiated with UV-B (7.2 kJ/m^2 of total energy, 54% of which was between 280 and 320 nm) three times a week for 22 weeks. In the second method, a 0.5% solution of DMBA in acetone was painted twice at an interval of two weeks onto the entire back of each mouse, followed—three weeks after the second DMBA treatment—by painting two drops of a 0.5% solution of croton oil in acetone on the entire back twice weekly for 16 weeks. In the third method, the DMBA treatment was followed two weeks later by UV-B irradiation (2.7 kJ/m^2 of total energy, 54% of which was between 280 and 320 nm) three times per week [period of treatment unspecified]. Representative skin tumours from about 30% of the mice were studied histologically. Each method of tumour induction resulted in both squamous-cell carcinomas and papillomas. Canthaxanthin significantly delayed the time to appearance, but not the yield, of skin tumours induced by UV-B irradiation alone, the first tumour > 1 mm^3 appearing in weeks 11 and 9 in the mice given canthaxanthin and in controls, respectively ($p < 0.01$; life-table analyses with χ^2 test). The time to appearance of the fifth tumour [unspecified] was also statistically significantly longer in the canthaxanthin-treated group than in those on placebo ($p < 0.05$; life-table analyses with χ^2 test). The yield of skin tumours induced by UV-B irradiation was also significantly reduced by canthaxanthin ($p < 0.005$; life-table analyses with χ^2 test), the average number of tumours per mouse being 0.5 and 1.59 after 11 weeks of treatment and 1.00 and 11.76 after 18 weeks of treatment in those fed canthaxanthin and those fed placebo, respectively. Canthaxanthin had no effect on the skin tumour response to DMBA plus croton oil [no further details given]. The onset of skin tumours induced by DMBA plus UV-B was significantly delayed by canthaxanthin, the first tumour appearing in the mice on placebo six weeks after the start of the treatment and

Table 41. Effects of canthaxanthin on tumorigenesis in experimental animals

Organ	Species, strain, sex	No. of animals/ group	Carcinogen (dose)	Canthaxanthin, dose, route	Treatment relative to carcinogen	Preventive efficacy	Reference
Skin	Mouse, Swiss, Albino, female	75	B[a]P, 0.1 mg/skin painting; UV (300–400 nm) 5890 erg/cm² per s	500 mg/kg diet + 100 mg/kg bw by gavage, twice/week	Before and during	Tumours, incidence B[a]P alone: 34% ($p < 0.01$) B[a]P/UV: 38% (SU)	Santamaria et al. (1981, 1983a,b,1988)
Skin	Mouse, SKH/hr, female	24	UV-B, (7.2 kJ/m²)	6.68 g/kg bw per day, diet	Before and during	Onset of skin tumours: 22% ($p < 025$) Tumour yield: 69% after 11 weeks ($p < 0.005$); 91% after 18 weeks ($p < 0.005$)	Mathews-Roth (1982)
Skin	Mouse, SKH/hr [sex unspecified]	[about 25]	UV-B, 8 x 10⁴ J/m², single fluence	33 g/kg diet	Before and after	Papillomas/carcinomas Incidence: 70% (NS) Number: none (NS)	Mathews-Roth (1983)
Skin	Mouse, SKH/hr [sex unspecified)	[about 25]	UV-B, 3.6 kJ/m², 3 times/week	33 g/kg diet	After	Papillomas/carcinomas Incidence After 7 weeks: 96% ($p < 0.02$) After 10 weeks: 95% ($p < 0.05$)	Mathews-Roth (1983)
Skin	Mouse, SKH:hr-1, female	24	UV-B, total dose, 10.8 J/cm²	0.001, 0.07, 3.3% to 2% in diet; beadlets	Before and during	Papillomas/carcinomas Incidence Low dose:none (NS) Mid dose: 39% ($p<0.025$) High dose: 64% ($p<0.05$) Multiplicity: Low and mid dose: none (NS) High dose: 49% ($p < 0.05$)	Mathews-Roth & Krinsky (1985)
Skin	Mouse, SKH'Hr-1, female	24	UV-B, one dose of 8 x 10⁴ J/m²	0.1% in diet; beadlets	Before or after, or before and after	Papillomas Incidence Before: 79% ($p < 0.0025$) After: 86% ($p < 0.00025$) Before and after: 50% ($p < 0.0025$)	Mathews-Roth & Krinsky (1987)
Skin	Mouse, C3H/HeN	50–120	UV-B; 30 min, 5 days/week; 24 weeks; 9.9 x 10⁵ J/m²	1% in diet; 18 weeks	During and after	Tumours Burden/mouse: 48% ($p = 0.008$) Tumour-free survival: none	Rybski et al. (1991)

Table 41 (contd)

Organ	Species, strain, sex	No. of animals/group	Carcinogen (dose)	Canthaxanthin, dose route	Treatment relative to carcinogen	Preventative efficacy	Reference
Skin	Mouse, C3H/HeNCrlBR, female	20–30	UV-B, 4.6 J/m² per s, total dose, 9.9 x 10⁵ J/m²	1% in diet	Before, during and after	Tumours Latency: none (SU) Incidence: none (NS) Burden: 45% (p= 0.0081)	Gensler et al. (1990)
Skin	Mouse, CD-1, female	10	DMBA [dose unspecified]; dermal application	200 mg/kg bw/day by oral gavage	After	Cumulative papilloma size, after 7 days: 15% (p < 0.01); after 14 days: 30% (p < 0.01)	Katsumura et al. (1996)
Colon	Rat, Fischer 344, male	28–30	Azoxymethane, 15 mg/kg bw, sc, 3 times	100 and 500 ppm in diet	After	High dose, incidence of adenocarcinoma: 67% (p < 0.05)	Tanaka et al. (1995b)
Colon, small bowel	Rat, Holtzman, male	27–28	DMH, 30 mg/kg bw, s.c., total dose, 480 mg/kg bw	1% in diet	Before, during and after	Tumours/cancers in colon and small bowel: none [rather, a clear increase]	Colacchio et al. (1989)
Urinary bladder	Mouse, ICR, male	31–36	250 ppm NBHBA in drinking-water	50 ppm in drinking-water	After	Carcinoma: 33% (NS) Preneoplasia: 25% (NS)	Tanaka et al. (1994)
Urinary bladder	Mouse, B6D2F₁	24	5 mg NBHBA, gavage, twice weekly	0.1% in diet	Before, during and after	Carcinoma incidence None (NS)	Mathews-Roth et al. (1991)
Liver	Rat, SPF-Wistar, male	9	2-Nitropropane, 6 x 100 mg/kg bw, i.p.	300 mg/kg diet	Before and during	Fraction of liver volume occupied by GST-P + foci: None	Astorg et al. (1996)
Liver	Rat, SPF-Wistar, male	9–10	NDEA, 100 mg/kg bw, i.p., single dose	300 mg/kg diet	Before and during	Fraction of liver volume occupied by GST-P + foci: 27% (NS)	Astorg et al. (1996)
Liver	Rat, SPF-Wistar, male	9–10	Aflatoxin B₁, 2 x 1 mg/kg bw, i.p.	300 mg/kg diet	Before and during	Fraction of liver volume occupied by GST-P⁺ foci: 92% (p < 0.05)	Gradelet et al. (1998)

Table 41 (contd)

Organ	Species, strain, sex	No. of animals/group	Carcinogen (dose)	Canthaxanthin, dose route	Treatment relative to carcinogen	Preventative efficacy	Reference
Buccal pouch	Hamster, male	20	0.5% DMBA; 3 times/week	250 µg in MEM, injected into cheek pouch twice weekly	After	Epidermoid carcinomas Regression Complete: 15% (SU) Partial: 85% (SU)	Schwartz & Shklar (1987)
Buccal pouch	Hamster, male	20	0.5% DMBA; 0.4 mg/painting	250 µg/ injection into pouch	After	Carcinoma burden: 94% (SU)	Schwartz & Shklar (1988)
Buccal pouch	Hamster, male	20	0.5% DMBA; 0.6 mg/painting, 3 times/week	0.19 mg in MEM injected into buccal pouch	After	Carcinoma burden: 71% (SU)	Shklar & Schwartz (1988)
Buccal pouch	Hamster, male	20	0.1% DMBA; painted 3 times/week	0.14 mg in mineral oil/painting (1.5 mg/kg bw)	During	Carcinoma: Incidence (gross tumours), 90% (SU) Multiplicity: 86% (SU) Burden: 99% (p < 0.001)	Schwartz et al. (1988)
Buccal pouch	Hamster, male	20	0.1% DMBA; 0.4 mg/painting	1.4 mg/kg bw; gavage	During	Carcinoma Incidence: 90% (SU) Burden: 99.6% (p < 0.001) Onset: 25% [SU]	Schwartz et al. (1989)
Mammary glands	Rat, Sprague-Dawley, female	10	MNU, 45 mg/kg bw; single dose, i.v.	1130, 3390 mg/kg in diet	After	Adenocarcinomas (p < 0.001) Incidence: none (NS) Multiplicity: none (NS) Latency: none (NS)	Grubbs et al. (1991)
Mammary glands	Rat, Sprague-Dawley, female	29–30	DMBA, 15 mg/rat, gavage	1130, 3390 mg/kg diet	Before	Adenocarcinoma Incidence: 28% (p < 0.05); Average number/rat: 58% (p < 0.05)	Grubbs et al. (1991)
Stomach	Mouse, Swiss, female	15–20	B[a]P: 1 mg, twice weekly, 4 weeks; gavage	4.7 µmol/animal per day, gavage	Before, during and after	Tumours Incidence: 80% (p < 0.001) Multiplicity: 86% (p < 0.001)	Azuine et al. (1992)
Small intestine	Rat, Holtzman, male	27–28	DMH; 30 mg/kg bw, s.c.; total dose, 480 mg/kg bw	1% in diet	Before, during and after	Tumours/cancer: none (rather, an increase)	Colacchio et al. (1989)

195

Table 41 (contd)

Organ	Species, strain, sex	No. of animals/group	Carcinogen (dose)	Canthaxanthin, dose route	Treatment relative to carcinogen	Preventative efficacy	Reference
Salivary gland	Rat, Sprague-Dawley, male	30	DMBA, 1 mg injected into submandibular salivary gland	250 ppm in diet	Before, during and after	Tumours Incidence: none (NS) Average weight: 75% (NS) Weight > 10 g: 100% ($p < 0.05$)	Alam et al. (1988)
Tongue	Rat, Fischer 344, male	17–24	20 ppm 4-NQO in drinking-water	0.01% in diet	Before and during	Carcinomas 100% ($p < 0.001$) Severe dysplasia: 90% ($p < 0.001$)	Tanaka et al. (1995a)
Tongue	Rat, Fischer 344, male	19–24	20 ppm 4-NQO in drinking-water	0.01% in diet	After	Carcinomas: 91% Severe dysplasia: 91% ($p < 0.001$)	Tanaka et al. (1995a)
–	Mouse, Balb/c, male and female	60	7×10^7 thymoma cells	7 or 14 mg/kg bw per day, gavage	Before, during and after	Tumour appearance Low dose: 70% ($p < 0.05$) High dose: 45% ($p < 0.05$) Survival Low dose: 30% ($p < 0.05$) High dose ($p < 0.05$)	Palozza et al. (1997)
–	Mouse, Balb/c, female	60	7×10^7 thymoma cells	14 mg/kg bw per day, gavage	After	Tumour appearance and survival: none	Palozza et al. (1997)

B[a]P, benzo[a]pyrene; UV, ultraviolet irradiation; SU, statistics unspecified; NS, not significant; DMBA, 7,12-dimethylbenz[a]anthracene; MNU, N-methyl-N-nitrosourea; i.v., intravenously; MEM, minimal essential medium; NBHA, N-nitrosobutyl(4-hydroxylbutylamine); 4-NQO, 4-nitroquinoline 1-oxide; s.c., subcutaneously; DMH, 1,2-dimethylhydrazine; GST-P*, placental glutathione S-transferase; NDEA, N-nitrosodiethylamine in the canthaxanthin-fed group after 13 weeks (appearance of first and tenth tumours, $p < 0.025$; life-table analyses with χ^2 test). Canthaxanthin also significantly reduced the yield of skin tumours induced by DMBA plus UV-B ($p < 0.05$; life-table analyses with χ^2 test), the average numbers of tumours per mouse being 0.25 and 0.85 after 13 weeks of treatment and 0.75 and 2.75 after 20 weeks of treatment in mice fed canthaxanthin and those fed placebo, respectively (Mathews-Roth, 1982).

An unspecified number of Philadelphia Skin and Cancer Hospital SKH/hr mice, five to eight weeks of age, were fed normal mouse chow and were irradiated with UV-B (3.6 kJ/m^2) for 20 min, three times per week for an unspecified period of time [at least 24 weeks]. As soon as a mouse developed a skin tumour ≥ 1 mm^3, it was allocated at random to a canthaxanthin-supplemented diet (33 g/kg diet from canthaxanthin-containing beadlets) or to placebo beadlet-supplemented control diet. Canthaxanthin significantly delayed the appearance of new skin papillomas and carcinomas ≥ 1 mm^3; e.g. the percentage of mice developing the seventh skin tumour after receiving the canthaxanthin-supplemented diet was 1% after seven weeks versus 26% in those on placebo ($p < 0.025$; life-table analysis) and 2% after 10 weeks versus 42% with placebo ($p < 0.05$; life-table analysis [incidences estimated from a figure]). Canthaxanthin also significantly delayed the development of skin tumours > 4 mm^3 (first subsequent tumour, $p < 0.05$; fifth tumour, $p < 0.001$; seventh tumour, $p < 0.01$; life-table analysis) and > 50 mm^3 (first tumour, $p < 0.001$; life-table analysis). In a second experiment, groups of mice received the canthaxanthin-supplemented diet (seven mice) or the placebo diet (nine mice) for 34 weeks. After 10 weeks on their respective diets, all mice were subjected to a large single fluence of UV-B irradiation (8×10^4 J/m^2) and were observed for 43 weeks [apparently, all mice were fed a normal diet during the last nine weeks of this period]. There was no intercurrent mortality. The first skin tumours were seen five weeks after exposure to UV-B, and no new skin tumours developed 21 weeks after exposure. Canthaxanthin did not

significantly reduce the incidence or total number of skin tumours > 1 mm^3 the incidences being 1/8 and 4/9 and the total numbers seven and five in the mice fed canthaxanthin and placebo, respectively (Mathews-Roth, 1983).

Six groups of 24 female hairless Philadelphia Skin and Cancer Hospital SKH/hr-1 mice, five to seven weeks old, were fed diets supplemented with canthaxanthin or placebo beadlets. Groups 1 and 2 were fed rodent chow supplemented with 3.3% canthaxanthin (3.3 g/kg diet) in beadlets or placebo beadlets for 16 weeks and then 2% canthaxanthin (2 g/kg diet) for another 22 weeks; groups 3 and 4 were fed a diet containing 0.07% canthaxanthin (700 mg/kg diet) or placebo beadlets for 30 weeks; groups 5 and 6 were fed diets containing 0.01% canthaxanthin (100 mg/kg diet) or placebo for 26 weeks and four days. All mice were subjected to UV-B irradiation (total dose, 10.8 J/m^2) for 16 weeks [schedule of irradiation unspecified], starting after 12 weeks on their diets for groups 1 and 2, after one month for groups 3 and 4 and after four days for groups 5 and 6. The animals were killed 10 weeks after irradiation. At the end of the study, the canthaxanthin content of the epidermis was found to be increased in a dose-related manner. Canthaxanthin at dietary concentrations of 3.3/2% and 0.07% prevented or delayed the appearance of UV-B-induced skin tumours; e.g. the percentages of mice with skin tumours 21 weeks after the start of the irradiation were 30% at the high dose and 84% with placebo ($p < 0.025$; Student's t test), 52% at the intermediate dose and 85% with placebo ($p < 0.0125$; Student's t test) and 52% at the low dose and 56% with placebo. The average numbers of tumours per mouse were also lower in animals at the intermediate and high doses than in those on placebo, but the difference was statistically significant only at the high dose; e.g. 21 weeks after the start of the irradiation, 1.34 at the high dose and 2.65 with the placebo ($p < 0.05$; Student's t test), 1.04 at the intermediate dose and 1.70 with the placebo and 1.58 at the low dose and 1.30 with the placebo (Mathews-Roth & Krinsky, 1985).

Groups of 24 female hairless Philadelphia Skin and Cancer Hospital SKH/hr-1 mice, five to seven weeks old, were fed a diet containing

0.1% canthaxanthin in beadlets, and two other groups received the same diet supplemented with placebo beadlets for six weeks. All mice then received a single exposure to 8×10^4 J/m^2 UV-B radiation for 220 min. Immediately after exposure, one of the groups on the canthaxanthin-supplemented diet was switched to the placebo diet and one of the placebo groups was switched to the canthaxanthin-supplemented diet, while the two other groups were continued on their respective diets. The animals were observed for 24 weeks after treatment. At the end of the study, canthaxanthin was detected in the skin even of animals that received the pigment before irradiation. There was no intercurrent mortality. The first tumours appeared five weeks after irradiation, some growing to 50 mm^3 but most measuring 1–4 mm^3. When canthaxanthin was fed before or after or only after exposure to UV-B, the incidences of skin tumours (mainly papillomas) were significantly (Fisher's exact test) reduced, being 14/24 for the group continuously fed the placebo diet, 2/24 for the group fed the canthaxanthin diet ($p < 0.00025$) and 3/24 ($p < 0.0025$) for the groups continuously fed the placebo or the canthaxanthin diet or fed the canthaxanthin-supplemented diet only after or only before exposure to UV-B (Mathews-Roth & Krinsky, 1987).

Specific pathogen-free, pigmented female C3H/HeN mice [exact number unspecified but > 105], five weeks old, were fed synthetic 76A basal diet either as such or supplemented with 1% (w/w) canthaxanthin for 18 weeks. The shaved back skin of 50 animals on unsupplemented basal diet and 55 on canthanxanthin-supplemented diet was then exposed to UV-B irradiation for 30 min/d on five days a week for 24 weeks (total dose, 9.9×10^5 J/m^2). No relevant difference in body weight was seen between the groups. By 27.5 weeks after the first UV-B irradiation, the average skin tumour burden per mouse given canthaxanthin was about 57 cm^2, whereas that in mice fed unsupplemented diet was 110 cm^2 ($p = 0.0081$; Wilcoxon rank sum test); however, the skin tumour-free survival rate was significantly lower in mice fed canthaxanthin (6/55) than in the group fed the unsupplemented diet (21/50; $p = 0.016$; Kaplan-Meyer with log-rank

method). None of the unirradiated mice developed skin tumours (Rybski et al., 1991).

Two groups of 20–30 female specific pathogen-free C3H/HeNCrlBR mice, six weeks old, were fed either basal diet (AIN 76A containing 4000 IU/kg retinyl palmitate) supplemented with 1% canthaxanthin from beadlets containing 10% canthaxanthin or basal diet supplemented with 10% placebo beadlets for at least 45.5 weeks [duration of study not further specified]. In weeks 18–42, the shaved back skin was exposed to UV-B irradiation (280–340 nm; 4.6 J/m^2 per s; total dose, 9.9×10^5 J/m^2) for 30 min/d on five days per week. No difference in body weight was seen between the two groups. Canthaxanthin did not affect the latency of skin tumours [no further details given] or reduce the incidence of skin tumours, the incidence at week 45 being 37% in the controls and 36% in those fed canthaxanthin. Canthaxanthin did, however, significantly reduce the mean skin tumour burden per mouse at 45 weeks, from about 105 mm^2 in the controls to about 58 mm^2 in the group fed the canthaxanthin-supplemented diet ($p = 0.0081$; analysis of variance) (Gensler et al., 1990).

Two groups of 75 female Swiss albino mice [age unspecified] were painted on a clipped area of the dorsal skin with 10 mg 8-methoxypsoralen in absolute ethanol twice a week for 80 weeks. One of the groups was fed a pelleted diet containing 100 mg/kg bw per day canthaxanthin for 80 weeks; after one month, these mice were given an additional 100 mg/kg bw canthaxanthin dissolved in arachis oil by gavage, twice weekly, 2 h before each painting with 8-methoxypsoralen. Both groups of mice were exposed to 1325×10^4 erg/cm^2 per s of long UV irradiation (300–400 nm) for 1 h/d for 80 weeks. Two comparable groups of mice similarly treated with 8-methoxypsoralen and canthaxanthin were not exposed to UV light and were kept in the dark. Eight other groups of mice served as vehicle, canthaxanthin and dark controls. Treatment with UV alone or combined with 8-methoxypsoralen resulted in malignant mammary gland tumours (types A, B and C adenocarcinomas, adenocanthomas and papillary carcinomas) and a few carcinomas of other skin appendages, with anaplastic small and large cells, actinotubular structures, polygonal sebaceous-like cells and carcinosarcomatous growth. Canthaxanthin reduced the incidence of the tumours induced by UV and 8-methoxypsoralen from 29/75 to 14/75 [statistics unspecified] and those induced by UV alone from 8/75 to 0 [statistics unspecified] (Santamaria et al., 1988; Santamaria & Bianchi, 1989).

Skin papillomas were induced in 20 female CD-1 mice, eight weeks old, by dermal application of DMBA for 60 days, until 10–20 papillomas had developed in each mouse. Two groups of 10 mice were then given 200 mg/kg bw per day canthaxanthin in 0.1 ml peanut oil or peanut oil alone. At day 14, the canthaxanthin concentrations were 0.011 μmol/L in serum, 1 nmol/g tissue in liver and 0.11 nmol/g tissue in skin papillomas, whereas no canthaxanthin was detected in controls. Mean food intake and mean body weights were not affected by canthaxanthin. The cumulative skin papilloma size (number of papillomas x diameter of each papilloma) on day 7 in mice given canthaxanthin was 92.5 ± 4.9% of the size measured at the start of treatment with canthaxanthin treatment and 81.6 ± 8.0% on day 14, the respective sizes in the control group being 109 ± 5.4% and 117.2 ± 10.9% ($p < 0.01$ at both times; Dunnett's t test) (Katsumura et al., 1996).

(b)   Colon
Rat: Three groups of 28 or 30 male Fischer 344 rats, four weeks old, were injected subcutaneously with 15 mg/kg bw azoxymethane once a week for three weeks. One group received no further treatment and was fed powdered basal diet CE-2 throughout the study (37 weeks). Starting one week after the last injection of azoxymethane, two further groups were fed the basal diet supplemented with 100 or 500 mg/kg canthaxanthin for 34 weeks, and two additional groups of 15 rats were fed either the unsupplemented basal diet or basal diet supplemented with 500 ppm canthaxanthin throughout the study. The body weights of azoxymethane-treated rats fed the diets containing canthaxanthin were slightly but statistically significantly lower than those of rats treated only with azoxymethane ($p < 0.05$ for the low dose and $p < 0.001$ for the high dose; Student's t test). Food

intake was not significantly affected by canthaxanthin supplementation. Canthaxanthin reduced both the incidence and multiplicity of azoxymethane-induced colon tubular adenomas and adenocarcinomas, the incidence and multiplicity of the adenocarcinomas being 4/28 ($p < 0.05$; Fisher's exact test) and 0.14 ± 0.35 at the high dose ($p < 0.05$; Student's t test) and 9/29 and 0.31 ± 0.46 at the low dose, in comparison with 13/30 and 0.53 ± 0.72 in the animals given azoxymethane alone. Canthaxanthin reduced the number of aberrant crypt foci per colon: 129 ± 63 at the high dose; $p < 0.05$; Student's t test; 169 ± 55 at the low dose, with 193 ± 55 in animals given azoxymethane alone. No tumours of the large intestine or aberrant crypt foci were found in rats fed the canthaxanthin-supplemented diet or in untreated controls (Tanaka et al., 1995b).

Two groups of 28 weanling male Holtzman rats were fed regular chow supplemented with either 1% canthaxanthin (w/w) from beadlets containing 10% canthaxanthin or 10% placebo beadlets for 24 weeks. After four weeks, all rats received 16 weekly subcutaneous injections of 30 mg/kg bw symmetrical DMH dissolved in neutral sodium hydroxide-corrected phosphate-buffered saline, for a total dose of 480 mg/kg bw. At 24 weeks, the animals were killed. All rats had colon tumours, and canthaxanthin clearly increased the numbers; e.g. the number of intestinal tumours was increased from 3.21 in those given placebo to 4.67 ($p < 0.0176$; Student's t test) and the number of colon cancers from 2.96 to 4.44 ($p < 0.0145$; Student's t test) (Colacchio et al., 1989).

(c)   Urinary bladder
Mouse: A group of 67 male ICR mice, six weeks old, were given 250 ppm NBHBA in their drinking-water for 20 weeks; 36 were then given tap water for 21 weeks, while the other 31 mice received tap water for one week and then tap water containing 50 mg/kg canthaxanthin for 20 weeks. A group of 15 mice was untreated, and a further 15 received 50 ppm canthaxanthin in dimethylsulfoxide in their drinking-water for 20 weeks, starting at week 21. Canthaxanthin did not affect the body weights of the mice. The incidence of transitional-cell

and squamous-cell carcinomas of the urinary bladder was slightly lower in the mice receiving NBHBA and canthaxanthin (10/31) than in those given NBHBA alone (15/36; not significant; χ^2 test). Similarly, the incidence of pre-neoplastic changes (simple and papillary or nodular hyperplasia) was 20/36 in the mice given NBHBA alone and 13/31 in those given NBHBA and canthaxanthin. The incidences of benign transitional-cell papillomas were comparable in the two groups: 2/36 with NBHBA and 3/31 with NBHBA and canthaxanthin. No (pre)neoplastic changes were observed in the urinary bladders of untreated or canthaxanthin-treated controls (Tanaka et al., 1994).

Two groups of 24 male B6D2F$_1$ mice, five to seven weeks old, were fed powdered rodent chow supplemented with either 10% canthax-anthin-containing beadlets (0.1% canthaxan-thin in the diet) or the same amount of placebo beadlets, for about seven months. After five weeks, all mice received 5 mg NBHBA in saline (total dose, 90 mg) by gastric tube twice weekly for nine weeks. The mice were killed six months after the first instillation of NBHBA. In a comparable study, the urinary bladder was found to contain canthaxanthin at 542 µg/100 g (range, 133–1000 µg/100 g). Canthaxanthin did not affect body weights and did not reduce the incidence of carcinoma in situ or transitional-cell carcinoma, the incidences in both groups being 15/24 (Mathews-Roth et al., 1991).

(d)   Liver
Rat: Two groups of 10 male SPF Wistar rats, 24–27 days old, were fed a semiliquid purified diet containing 10% corn oil and 6000 IU/kg vitamin A and supplemented with 300 mg/kg canthaxanthin from a 10% dispersible powder or the same diet supplemented with placebo powder for 21 days, followed by the same diet with no supplement for 21 days. On day 15, all rats were injected intraperitoneally with 200 mg/kg bw NDEA in 0.9% saline. 2-AAF was added to the diet at 50 mg/kg on days 42–56. On day 49, all rats were subjected to a two-thirds hepatectomy. From day 56 to the end of the experiment (day 70), the diets were supplemented with 500 ppm phenobarbital. There was no significant difference in body

weight between the two groups. Canthaxanthin accumulated in the liver (478 ± 148 µg/g liver on day 15), and its concentration was still high on day 49 (82 ± 14 µg/g liver) and at the end of the experiment (13 ± 2 µg/g liver). Canthaxanthin did not significantly (one-sided Dunnett's test and one-sided t test) inhibit the number of GGT$^+$ liver foci (24.4 ± 2.5 versus 28.4 ± 2.3 in controls), the number of GST-P$^+$ foci (60.2 ± 3.8 versus 51.4 ± 7.6 in controls), the mean area of GGT$^+$ foci (0.131 ± 0.01 mm^2 versus 0.145 ± 0.017 mm^2 in controls), the area occupied by GGT$^+$ foci (3.39 ± 0.43% versus 4.39 ± 0.82% in controls) or the area occupied by GST-P$^+$ foci (6.59 ± 0.69% versus 7.49 ± 1.45% in controls) (Astorg et al., 1996).

Wistar rats, 24–27 days old, were fed either a semiliquid purified diet containing 10% corn oil and 6000 IU/kg vitamin A supplemented with 300 mg/kg canthaxanthin from a 10% dispersible powder or the same diet supplemented with placebo powder for 28 days, followed by the same diet with no supplement for 21 days. On days 14, 16, 18, 21, 23 and 25, all rats were injected intraperitoneally with 100 mg/kw bw 2-nitropropane in 2% Tween 20. 2-AAF was added to the diet at 50 mg/kg on days 49–63. On day 56, all rats were subjected to a two-thirds hepatectomy. From day 63 to the end of the experiment (day 70), the rats received unsupplemented diet. The canthaxan-thin content of the livers of rats fed this carotenoid was still 26.2 ± 4.7 µg/g liver at the time of partial hepatectomy, i.e four weeks after cessation of canthaxanthin feeding. Canthaxanthin did not significantly inhibit the onset of preneoplastic foci in the liver, as seen from the number of GGT$^+$ foci per cm^3 liver (424 ± 74 versus 371 ± 53 in controls), the number of GST-P$^+$ foci (926 ± 144 versus 703 ± 120 in controls), the mean volume (10^{-3} mm^3) of GGT$^+$ foci (57.3 ± 14.3 versus 62.4 ± 20.6 in controls), the mean volume of GST-P$^+$ foci (89.7 ± 37.3 versus 59.9 ± 13.5 in controls), the fraction of the liver volume (mm^3/cm^3) occupied by GGT$^+$ foci (17.4 ± 5.1 versus 15.7 ± 5.5 in controls) or the fraction of the liver volume occupied by GST$^+$ foci (49.8 ± 13.9 versus 33.4 ± 8.6 in controls (Astorg et al., 1996).

In a similar study, the animals were fed the same diets for 21 days, followed by the diet with no supplement for 21 days. On day 14, all rats were injected intraperitoneally with 100 mg/kw bw NDEA in 0.9% saline; 2-AAF was added to the diet at 50 mg/kg on days 42–56; all rats were subjected to a two-thirds hepatectomy on day 49; and the rats received unsupplemented diet from day 56 to the end of the experiment on day 63. Canthaxanthin did not significantly inhibit the number of GGT$^+$ foci/cm^3 liver (224 ± 29 versus 205 ± 40 in controls), the number of GST-P$^+$ foci (2632 ± 222 versus 1853 ± 327 in controls), the mean volume (10^{-3} mm^3) of GGT$^+$ foci (66.1 ± 17.9 versus 61.0 ± 14.1 in controls), the mean volume of GST$^+$ foci (15.0 ± 2.2 versus 27.1 ± 8.4 in controls), the fraction of the liver volume (mm^3/cm^3) occupied by GGT$^+$ foci (9.6 ± 2.0 versus 10.8 ± 3.6 in controls) or the fraction of the liver volume occupied by GST-P$^+$ foci (36.8 ± 6.5 versus 50.7 ± 17.3 in controls) (Astorg *et al.*, 1996).

In a further study of similar design, all rats were injected intraperitoneally on days 13 and 19 with 1 mg/kg bw aflatoxin B$_1$ in 50% dimethylsulfoxide in water; 50 mg/kg 2-AAF were added to the diet on days 42–56; all rats were subjected to a two-thirds hepatectomy on day 49; and the rats received unsupplemented diet on days 56–63 (end of the study). The canthaxanthin content of the livers of rats receiving the compound was still 20.0 ± 4.4 µg/g liver at the time of partial hepatectomy, i.e. four weeks after cessation of canthaxanthin feeding. Canthaxanthin significantly inhibited the onset of liver preneoplastic foci, i.e. the number of GST-P$^+$ foci (275 ± 49 versus 773 ± 169 in controls), the mean volume (10^{-3} mm^3) of GST-P$^+$ foci (13.3 ± 2.1 versus 107.8 ± 46.8 in controls) and the fraction of the liver volume (mm^3/cm^3) occupied by GST-P$^+$ foci (4.2 ± 1.2 versus 55.4 ± 17.6 in controls) (Gradelet *et al.*, 1998).

(e) Buccal pouch

Hamster: Epidermoid carcinomas were produced in the right buccal pouches of three groups of 20 adult male Syrian golden hamsters [age not further specified] by painting with a 0.5% solution of DMBA in heavy mineral oil three times per week for 13 weeks. Then, the right buccal pouches were injected with 0.1 ml of a solution of about 250 µg canthaxanthin in solvent added to minimal essential medium or with 0.1 ml the medium alone (sham-injected controls); 20 hamsters were not further treated. The experiment was terminated at 17 weeks. No tumour regression was seen in sham-injected or uninjected hamsters, all of which had multiple, large cheek pouch tumours; two uninjected controls and one sham-injected animal died intercurrently with very large tumours and infection. Canthaxanthin caused complete gross tumour regression in 3/20 hamsters and partial regression in 17/20. In general, the regression of large and multiple tumours tended to be incomplete, whereas total regression was usually seen for small or moderate tumours. The tumours in regression showed degeneration and infiltration of lymphocytes and macrophages, which often contained tumour necrosis factor. Stratified squamous epithelium adjacent to the carcinomas with severe destruction was relatively unaffected and appeared essentially normal (Schwartz & Shklar, 1987).

Sixty randomly bred male Syrian hamsters, two to three months old, were painted on the right buccal pouch with a 0.5% solution of DMBA in heavy mineral oil (about 0.4 mg DMBA per painting) three times per week for 14 weeks, when each hamster appeared to have well-to-moderately differentiated epidermoid carcinomas of the buccal pouch. Then, the animals were divided randomly into three groups of 20 animals each; the tumour-bearing pouch was injected twice weekly with 0 or 250 µg canthaxanthin in 0.1 ml minimal essential medium or was not injected. After four weeks, all of the hamsters were killed, and the numbers and sizes of the buccal pouch tumours were recorded. There was no significant difference in body weight between the groups. Canthaxanthin reduced the buccal pouch tumour burden (average tumour volume x number of tumours) from 2258.9 ± 5.6 mm^3 (sham controls) or 2150.4 ± 5.0 mm^3 (uninjected controls) to 136.4 ± 1.4 mm^3 [number and size of tumours unspecified; no information on statistical analysis]. In the canthaxanthin-treated hamsters but not the controls, many buccal pouch tumours showed cellular degeneration and dense infiltration of lymphocytes and macrophages (Schwartz & Shklar, 1988).

The right buccal pouches of 60 male Syrian hamsters, 60–90 days old and weighing 95–125 g, were painted with a 0.5% solution of DMBA in heavy mineral oil (about 0.6 mg DMBA per painting) three times a week for 14 weeks, when all hamsters had obvious gross cheek pouch tumours of variable size and number. They were then were divided into three groups of 20 animals each, which were either not further treated or received injections into the right cheek pouch of 0.1 ml solvent plus minimal essential medium alone or containing 0.19 mg canthaxanthin, three times per week for four weeks. Canthaxanthin reduced the total burden of the moderate papillary epidermoid carcinomas from 1400 mm^3 in the hamsters given DMBA or sham-injected with DMBA to 100 mm^3 in those given canthaxanthin [no information on statistics]. In addition, a clearly elevated number of tumour necrosis factor-α-positive macrophages was found in the tumours and adjacent to regressing tumours in hamsters treated with canthaxanthin (Shklar & Schwartz, 1988).

Sixty non-inbred adult male hamsters, 60–90 days old and weighing 96–120 g, were fed standard laboratory pellets, and their right buccal pouches were painted with a 0.1% solution of DMBA in heavy mineral oil three times per week for 28 weeks. The animals were divided into three groups of 20 hamsters each and were given either 0.14 mg canthaxanthin (1.5 mg/kg bw) in 0.4 ml mineral oil three times per week on alternate days to DMBA, mineral oil only or no further treatment. All hamsters were killed after 28 weeks, when obvious, moderately large buccal pouch tumours were seen in untreated controls. There was no significant difference in body weight between the groups. All control hamsters and a few of those given canthaxanthin had gross cheek pouch tumours: 20/20, 20/20 and 2/20 in the untreated control, the vehicle control and the canthaxanthin groups, respectively; mean

numbers of tumours per animal: 3.5, 3.7 and 0.5; mean tumour burden: 85.5, 114.9 and 1.5 ($p < 0.001$; Student's t test). The control animals had proliferative epidermoid carcinomas that invaded the underlying connective tissue, numerous foci of hyperkeratosis with dysplasia and carcinoma *in situ* and lymphocyte infiltration into areas of tumour infiltration and carcinoma *in situ*. Canthaxanthin-treated animals had no carcinomas; however, scattered foci of dysplasia and carcinoma *in situ* undergoing degeneration and cellular destruction were seen, with dense accumulations of lymphocytes and histiocytes in the underlying connective tissue, often close to areas of dysplasia and sometimes so dense that the area resembled lymphoid tissue (Schwartz *et al.*, 1988).

The mucosa of the right buccal pouch of three groups of 20 male Syrian hamsters [age unspecified], fed a normal hamster diet containing 22% protein and the required concentrations of vitamin A and E, was painted with 0.1% DMBA in heavy mineral oil (0.4 mg DMBA per painting) three times a week for 28 weeks. One group received no further treatment; the other two groups were given 0.4 ml of heavy mineral oil containing 0 or 1.4 mg/kg bw canthaxanthin (crystalline form, type IV) by gavage three times a week on alternate days to DMBA, for 28 weeks. A fourth group served as untreated controls. There was no significant difference in body weight between the groups, and there was no intercurrent mortality. Ingestion of canthaxanthin significantly inhibited the formation of buccal pouch squamous-cell carcinomas, as shown by the later onset of tumours (month 5 versus month 4 in both DMBA control groups), fewer tumour-bearing hamsters (2 versus 20 in both DMBA control groups), fewer tumours (30 versus 135 in the DMBA/vehicle control and 150 in the DMBA control group) and a significant decrease in the tumour burden after six months of treatment (14 mm^3 versus 3675 mm^3 in the DMBA/vehicle control and 2450 mm^3 in the DMBA control group; $p < 0.001$, Student's t test). At the end of the treatment period, the average number of areas of cheek pouch with epithelial dysplasia was 3 in the group given canthaxanthin and 6 in both DMBA-treated groups. No buccal pouch tumours or sites of epithelial dysplasia were found in untreated controls. Canthaxanthin ingestion resulted in an inflammatory reaction of the cheek pouches not seen in DMBA-treated or DMBA/vehicle controls: a dense mixed inflammatory infiltrate consisting predominantly of cytotoxic lymphocytes and macrophages containing tumour necrosis factor-α and localized areas of mast cells in the deep dermis adjacent to areas of dysplasia, carcinomas *in situ* and small foci of squamous-cell carcinoma (Schwartz *et al.*, 1989).

The mucosa of the right buccal pouches of three groups of 10 male Syrian golden hamsters, 60–90 days old and weighing 95–125 g, was painted with a 0.5% solution of DMBA in heavy mineral oil (0.6 mg DMBA per painting) three times per week for 14 weeks. One of the groups also received oral applications of 10 mg/kg bw canthaxanthin in 0.5 ml mineral oil three times per week on alternate days to DMBA. Two other groups either were not further treated or were treated with mineral oil only. An additional group of 10 hamsters was treated with canthaxanthin only; no buccal pouch tumours were seen in these animals. Canthaxanthin reduced the number of animals with buccal pouch tumours, which were well-to-moderately differentiated epidermoid carcinomas, from 10 in both control groups to 8, the total numbers of cheek pouch tumours from 125 in controls and 130 in the vehicle controls to 30 [statistics unspecified] and the cheek pouch tumour burden from 174 200 mm^3 (mean of the two control groups) to 116 100 mm^3 ($p < 0.001$; Student's t test) (Schwartz & Shklar, 1997).

(f) Mammary gland

Rat: One group of 60 and two groups of 45 female Sprague-Dawley rats, 34 days of age, were fed rodent diet supplemented with 0 (placebo beadlets), 1130 or 3390 mg/kg canthaxanthin (in the form of beadlets) for 21 days. At 55 days of age, one day after dietary canthaxanthin supplementation was stopped, groups of 30 rats were each given 15 mg DMBA in sesame oil by gavage. The study was terminated 180 days after DMBA treatment. Only one rat receiving sesame oil alone died, after three weeks. After three weeks, the concentration of canthaxanthin in the liver was much higher (high dose, 610 µg/g; low dose, 416 µg/g) than in the mammary glands (high dose, 3.5 µg/g; low dose, 2.5 µg/g); it was not detected in either organ in vehicle controls. The incidences of mammary gland adenocarcinomas were [27/29] in the controls, [24/30] in rats given the low dose of canthaxanthrin and [20/30] in those given the high dose ($p < 0.05$; Fisher's exact test), and the average numbers of adenocarcinomas per rat in the respective groups were 5.4, 2.0 ($p < 0.05$) and 1.9 ($p < 0.05$; Wilcoxon's rank sum test). Canthaxanthin had no effect on the latency of the mammary gland carcinomas [not further specified]. The incidences of benign mammary tumours (fibromas, adenomas and fibroadenomas; 28–40% in the groups treated with DMBA) were not affected by canthaxanthin pretreatment. Two rats treated with the high dose of canthaxanthin but not with DMBA had benign mammary tumours (Grubbs *et al.*, 1991).

Four groups of 10 female Sprague-Dawley rats, 50 days of age, received an intravenous injection of 45 mg/kg bw MNU in saline (adjusted to pH 5.0 with 3% acetic acid), and two days later their diet was supplemented with 0 (placebo beadlets), 1130 or 3390 mg/kg canthaxanthin as beadlets or with 328 mg/kg retinyl acetate (positive control group). The study was terminated 90 days after MNU administration. After three months, the concentrations of canthaxanthin in the liver (high dose, 1690 µg/g; low dose, 1040 µg/g) were much higher than those in the mammary gland (high dose, 16 µg/g; low dose, 11 µg/g), but none was detected in either organ in vehicle controls. The incidences of mammary gland adenocarcinomas were 100% in the controls, 100% in rats at the low dose of canthaxanthrin, 90% in those at the high dose and 80% in the positive controls; and the average numbers of carcinomas per rat were 2.7, 2.0, 2.3 and 0.8, respectively ($p < 0.05$; Wilcoxon's rank sum test). The latency of the mammary carcinomas was not affected by canthaxanthin. No benign mammary gland tumours were found (Grubbs *et al.*, 1991).

(g)   Stomach

Mouse: Groups of 20 inbred female Swiss mice, six to eight weeks old, and weighing 20–25 g, were given canthaxanthin (4.7 µmol/d per animal) in 0.1 ml palm oil by gavage or only palm oil for eight weeks (15 animals). From week 3, a fourth group of 20 mice and 20 mice receiving canthaxanthin were given 1 mg benzo[*a*] pyrene in 0.1 ml palm oil by gavage twice a week for four weeks. After completion of treatment at eight weeks, the animals were observed up to 180 days, when they were killed. The mean body-weight gain was similar in all groups. Canthaxanthin reduced the incidence of gross forestomach tumours from 20/20 to 4/20 ($p < 0.001$; χ^2 test) and the mean number of forestomach tumours per mouse from 7.0 ± 0.3 to 1.0 ± 0.0 ($p < 0.001$; Student's *t* test). No forestomach tumours were found in the groups treated with canthaxanthin or palm oil alone (Azuine *et al.*, 1992).

(h)   Small intestine

Rat: Two groups of 28 weanling male Holtzman rats were fed regular chow supplemented with either 1% canthaxanthin (w/w) from beadlets containing 10% canthaxanthin or 10% placebo beadlets for 24 weeks. After four weeks, all rats received 16 weekly subcutaneous injections of 30 mg/kg bw symmetrical DMH dissolved in neutral sodium hydroxide-corrected phosphate-buffered saline, for a total dose of 480 mg/kg bw. At 24 weeks, the animals were killed. All rats had intestinal tumours. Canthaxanthin slightly enhanced small-bowel carcinogenesis; e.g. the incidence was increased from 15/28 in rats on placebo to 20/28 in those given canthaxanthin ($p < 0.0352$; χ^2 test), and the number of tumours of the small intestines per rat was 0.75 in rats on placebo and 1.22 in those fed canthaxanthin (not significant; Student's *t* test) (Colacchio *et al.*, 1989).

(i)   Salivary glands

Rat: Two groups of 30 male weanling Sprague-Dawley rats, weighing 73 ± 1.0 g, were fed either basal diet AIN-76A (containing 4000 IU vitamin A) or basal diet supplemented with 250 mg/kg of diet canthaxanthin (10% stabilized gelatin beadlets). After six weeks, one of the submandibular salivary glands of each rat was injected with 1 mg DMBA in 0.02 ml olive oil, while the contralateral gland was injected with 0.02 ml olive oil alone. Rats were killed 21–22 weeks after the DMBA injection, when more than 50% of the animals had developed submandibular salivary gland tumours, some of which were very large. There was no significant difference in body-weight gain between the two groups. The incidence of partially to fully differentiated squamous-cell carcinomas and undifferentiated spindle-cell submandibular salivary gland tumours was closely similar: all tumours, 20/28 in controls and 21/30 in rats given canthaxanthin; malignant tumours, 11/28 in controls and 14/30 in rats given canthaxanthin. The mean tumour weight was slightly lower in rats fed the canthaxanthin-supplemented diet (1.8 ± 0.5 g) than in rats fed the unsupplemented diet (7.0 ± 3.3 g). Two of 20 tumour-bearing control animals had submandibular salivary gland tumours weighing more than 40 g, whereas none of the rats given canthaxanthin had such large tumours. In addition, 4/20 tumour-bearing controls and 0/21 given canthaxanthin had tumours weighing more than 10 g ($p < 0.05$; χ^2 test) (Alam *et al.*, 1988).

(j)   Tongue

Rat: Three groups of 17–24 male Fischer 344 rats, four weeks old, received 20 ppm 4-NQO in their drinking-water for eight weeks. A group of 24 rats received no further treatment and was fed powdered basal diet CE-2 throughout the study; the two other groups were fed the basal diet supplemented with 0.01% canthaxanthin for 10 weeks starting just before the 4-NQO treatment (17 rats) or for 22 weeks starting one week after cessation of the 4-NQO treatment (19 rats). An additional group of 11 rats was fed the basal diet supplemented with 0.01% canthaxanthin throughout the study (32 weeks), and 12 rats served as untreated controls. Drinking-water containing 4-NQO was freshly prepared every two days, and diets containing canthaxanthin were prepared every week or every two weeks in a dark room and were stored in a dark, cold room (< 4 °C) until use. No relevant differences in body weight were seen between the groups. Canthaxanthin significantly reduced the incidence of tongue neoplasms ($p < 0.001$ or $p < 0.005$; Fisher's exact test): no squamous-cell carcinomas or papillomas of the tongue were found in the group fed canthaxanthin before and during treatment with 4-NQO, while 1/19 animals fed this diet after 4-NQO treatment had a squamous-cell carcinoma and 1/19 had a squamous-cell papilloma, whereas 13/24 squamous-cell carcinomas and 4/19 squamous-cell papillomas were seen in the group treated with 4-NQO only. Canthaxanthin also significantly reduced the incidence of squamous-cell hyperplasia and dysplasia of the tongue epithelium (Fisher's exact test): the incidences of hyperplasia were 24/24 , 8/17 ($p < 0.05$) and 12/19 ($p < 0.005$) and those of severe dysplasia, 14/24, 1/17 ($p < 0.001$) and 1/19 ($p < 0.001$) in the animals treated with 4-NQO, those fed canthaxanthin before and during 4-NQO treatment and those fed canthaxanthin after 4-NQO treament, respectively. No such lesions were seen in untreated controls or in rats fed the canthaxanthin-supplemented diet (Tanaka et al., 1995a).

(k)   Inoculated tumours

Mouse: Four groups of 60 female inbred Balb/c mice, six weeks old and weighing 22.5 ± 1.0 g, were fed an unpurified commercial diet and received olive oil alone, 7 or 14 mg/kg bw canthaxanthin in olive oil throughout the study or 14 mg/kg bw canthaxanthin in olive oil daily by gavage from day 15 of the study. Two groups of 60 male mice of the same strain and age and weighing 23.3 ± 2.0 g were kept on the same diet and received olive oil alone or 14 mg/kg bw canthaxanthin in olive oil daily by gavage throughout the study. At day 15, all mice were inoculated with 7×10^7 malignant Balb/c mouse thymoma cells of lymphatic origin. On days 15, 20 and 22, 10 mice from each group were killed for interim observations. No significant difference in food intake or body weight was observed between the groups. The weight of the thymus in the group receiving 14 mg/kg bw canthaxanthin throughout the study was higher than in the other groups. After 15 days of treatment, the concentrations of canthaxanthin in the livers of mice fed this carotenoid were

300 µg/g in females at the high dose, 150 µg/g in females at the low dose and 175 µg/g in the males, whereas no canthaxanthin was found in the livers of the controls. Treatment with canthaxanthin throughout the study delayed the appearance of macroscopic ascites and prolonged survival, the effects being dose-dependent and more pronounced in females than in males. The differences from controls in the appearance of ascites and in survival, expressed as percents [no further details given] were statistically significant ($p < 0.05$; analysis of variance). Canthaxanthin had no protective effect when administered only after inoculation of tumour cells (Palozza et al., 1997).

4.2.1.4   Canthaxanthin with other potential inhibitors (Table 42)

Mouse: Four groups of 20–30 female specific pathogen-free C3H/HeNCrlBR mice, six weeks old, were fed basal diet (AIN 76A containing 4000 IU/kg retinyl palmitate) supplemented with 1% canthaxanthin (from beadlets containing 10% canthaxanthin), basal diet supplemented with 120 000 IU/kg retinyl palmitate plus 10% placebo beadlets, basal diet supplemented with 1% canthaxanthin plus 120 000 IU retinyl palmitate plus 10% placebo beadlets, or basal diet only supplemented with 10% placebo beadlets, for at least 45.5 weeks [duration of study not further specified]. During weeks 18–42, the shaven back skin of the animals was irradiated with UV-B (280–340 nm; 4.6 J/m^2 per s; total UVB dose, 9.9×10^5 J/m^2) for 30 min/d on five days per week. The only difference in body weight between the groups was seen in mice fed the diet supplemented with canthaxanthin plus retinyl palmitate, which was on average 1.5 g lower than those of the controls. Canthaxanthin accumulated in the skin (86 µg/g wet tissue), and this accumulation was not affected by the presence of retinyl plamitate in the diet. Canthaxanthin and retinyl palmitate separately or in combination did not affect the latency of skin tumours [no further details given] or reduce the skin tumour incidence, the incidences at week 45 being 37% in controls, 36% in mice fed canthaxanthin, 32% in those fed retinyl

Table 42. Effects of canthaxanthin and retinyl palmitate on tumorigenesis in mouse skin

Strain, sex	No. of animals/ group	Carcinogen (dose, route)	Canthaxanthin (dose, route)	Other chemical(s) (dose, route)	Treatment relative to carcinogen	Preventive efficacy	Reference
C3H/HeNcrlBR, female	20–30	UV-B; total dose, 9.9 x 10^5 J/m^2	1% in diet	12 000 IU retinyl palmitate in diet	Before, during and after	Tumours Incidence (NS) and latency (SU): none Burden/mouse: Canthaxanthin: 45% (p = 0.0081) Retinyl palmitate: 41% (p = 0.0081) Combination: 68% (significant [p value unspecified])	Gensler et al. (1990)
C3H/HeN, female	50–120	UV-B; 30 min, 5 days/week, 18 weeks 9.9 x 10^5 J/m^2	1% in diet,	120 IU retinyl palmitate in diet	During and after	Tumours Burden/mouse: Canthaxanthin alone: 48% (p = 0.008) Retinyl palmitate alone: 46% (p = 0.0135 Combination: 65% (SU) Tumour-free survival None (rather, some decrease for canthaxanthin alone + the combination)	Rybski et al. (1991)

UV-B, ultraviolet B radiation; NS, not significant; SU, statistics unspecified

palmitate and 31% in those given canthaxanthin plus retinyl palmitate. Canthaxanthin and retinyl palmitate alone and in combination did, however, significantly reduce the mean skin tumour burden per mouse (analysis of variance): at 45 weeks, the tumour burden was about 105 mm^2 in the controls, about 58 mm^2 in the mice given canthaxanthin (p = 0.0081), 62 mm^2 in those given retinyl palmitate (p = 0.0135) and 34 mm^2 in those given the combination [p value unspecified] (Gensler et al., 1990).

Specific pathogen-free, pigmented female C3H/HeN mice [exact number unspecified but > 220], five weeks old, were fed synthetic 76A basal diet either as such or supplemented with 1% (w/w) canthaxanthin, 120 IU/g retinyl palmitate or 1% canthaxanthin plus 120 IU/g retinyl palmitate. The shaven back skin of 50 animals on unsupplemented diet, 55 given canthaxanthin, 120 given retinyl palmitate and 60 given canthaxanthin plus retinyl palmi-

tate was exposed to UV-B irradiation for 30 min/d on five days a week for 24 weeks (total dose, 9.9 x 10^5 J/m^2). In comparison with irradiated controls, irradiated mice fed canthaxanthin plus retinyl palmitate had significantly lower body weights (average difference, 1.5 g; analysis of variance [p value unspecified]). None of the unirradiated mice [number unspecified] developed skin tumours. By 27.5 weeks after the first UV-B irradiation, the average skin tumour burden per mouse was about 110 cm^2 for animals on basal diet, 57 cm^2 for those on canthaxanthin (p = 0.0081; Wilcoxon rank-sum test), 59 cm^2 for those on retinyl palmitate (p = 0.0135; Wicoxon rank-sum test) and 38 cm^2 for those on canthaxanthin plus retinyl palmitate [p value unspecified]. Canthaxanthin significantly reduced the rate of survival without a skin tumour (6/55) in comparison with mice fed the unsupplemented diet (21/55; p = 0.016; Kaplan-Meyer with log-rank), while the skin tumour-free survival of animals fed can-thaxanthin plus retinyl palmitate was 14/60 (p = 0.231; Kaplan-Meyer with log-rank) [skin tumour-free survival of mice fed retinyl palmitate unspecified] (Rybski *et al.*, 1991).

4.2.1.5 Lycopene (Table 43)

(a) Colon

Rat: Twenty-four female Sprague-Dawley rats, seven weeks old, received three intrarectal instillations of 4 mg MNU in 0.5 ml distilled water in week 1 and were then divided into groups of six animals, which received 0.2 ml corn oil containing 0, 0.24, 1.2 or 6 mg lycopene by intragastric gavage daily during weeks 2 and 5. In week 6, all rats were killed and their colons were examined for aberrant crypt foci. The numbers of aberrant crypt foci per colon, in comparison with controls (62.7 ± 7.2), were similar in the rats at the high dose (63.5 ±10.4) and slightly, not significantly (Student's t test) lower in those at the intermediate (45.7 ± 7.5) and low doses (40.4 ± 8.2). A similar study was carried out in which two lower doses and one identical dose of lycopene were used: 0, 0.06, 0.12 and 0.24 mg. The numbers of aberrant crypt foci per colon, in comparison with controls (69.3 ± 6.2) were statistically significantly lower in the animals at the high (42.7 ± 5.3) and intermediate doses (34.3 ± 6.5) ($p < 0.05$; Student's t test), but not in those at the low dose (50.7 ± 6.3) (Narisawa *et al.*, 1996).

(b) Lung

Mouse: Groups of 16 male and 16 female B6C3F$_1$ mice received combined treatment with 10 mg/kg bw NDEA by intraperitoneal injection, 120 mg/kg MNU in the drinking-water for five weeks and 29 mg/kg bw DMH by subcutaneous injection twice weekly for five weeks from day 11 after birth to week 9, or the vehicles. One group on the combined treatment then received 25 or 50 mg/kg synthetic lycopene from tomatoes in drinking-water [formulation unspecified] for 21 weeks (weeks 11–32), the other group on the combined treatment received no further compounds, and the third group was given only lycopene. At week 32, the mice were killed and examined histologically.

The incidences and multiplicity of lung adenomas and carcinomas in male mice in the group receiving the combined carcinogens and 50 ppm lycopene were significantly lower than those in the group receiving only the carcinogens: 12/16 versus 3/16 ($p < 0.02$) and 0.94 ± 0.17 versus 0.25 ± 0.14 ($p < 0.001$), respectively; no such effect was observed in females (Kim *et al.*, 1997).

(c) Liver

Mouse: Two groups of C3H/H3 mice, six weeks old, were given drinking-water with or without 0.005% lycopene (93% pure, of natural origin, dispersed as an emulsion) for 40 weeks. Lycopene suppressed spontaneous liver carcinogenesis, with a 56% reduction in incidence ($p < 0.05$) and an 88% reduction in multiplicity ($p < 0.01$) (Nishino, 1998).

Rat: Groups of nine Wistar rats, 24–27 days old, were fed either a semiliquid purified diet containing 10% corn oil and 6000 IU/kg vitamin A supplemented with 300 mg/kg lycopene (from a 5% oleoresin from tomato in vegetable oil) or the same diet with no supplement for 28 days, both followed by the same diet with no supplement for 21 days. On days 14, 16, 18, 21, 23 and 25, all rats were injected intraperitoneally with 100 mg/kw bw 2-nitropropane in 2% Tween 20. 2-AAF was added to the diet at 50 mg/kg on days 49–63. On day 56, all rats were subjected to a two-thirds hepatectomy. From day 63 to the end of the experiment (day 70), the rats received unsupplemented diet. The lycopene content of the livers of rats fed this carotenoid was still 16.3 ± 1.9 µg/g liver at the time of partial hepatectomy, i.e four weeks after cessation of lycopene feeding. Lycopene did not significantly inhibit the onset of preneoplastic foci in the liver, as seen from the number of GGT$^+$ foci per cm^3 liver (185 ± 35 versus 371 ± 53 in controls), the number of GST-P$^+$ foci (814 ± 203 versus 703 ± 120 in controls), the mean volume (10^{-3} mm^3) of GGT$^+$ foci (44.7 ± 5.9 versus 62.4 ± 20.6 in controls), the mean volume of GST-P$^+$ foci (53.9 ± 17.7 versus 59.9 ± 13.5 in controls), the fraction of the liver volume (mm^3/cm^3) occupied by GGT$^+$ foci (6.2 ± 1.7 versus 15.7 ± 5.5 in controls) or the fraction of the liver volume occupied by GST$^+$ foci (24.1 ± 6.0 versus 33.4 ± 8.6 n controls (Astorg *et al.*, 1997).

In a similar study, the animals were fed the same diets for 21 days, followed by the diet with no supplement for 21 days. On day 14, all rats were injected intraperitoneally with 100 mg/kw bw NDEA in 0.9% saline; 2-AAF was added to the diet at 50 mg/kg on days 42–56; all rats were subjected to a two-thirds hepatectomy on day 49; and the rats received unsupplemented diet from day 56 to the end of the experiment on day 63. Lycopene did not significantly inhibit the number of GGT^+ foci/cm^3 liver (163 ± 71 versus 205 ± 40 in controls) or the number of $GST-P^+$ foci (1952 ± 303 versus 1853 ± 327 in controls); it significantly decreased the mean volume (10^{-3} mm^3) of GGT^+ foci (21.8 ± 7.3 versus 61.0 ± 14.1) in controls), the mean volume of GST^+ foci (7.8 ± 1.8 versus 27.1 ± 8.4 in controls), the fraction of the liver volume (mm^3/cm^3) occupied by GGT^+ foci (1.7 ± 0.6 versus 10.8 ± 3.6 in controls) and the fraction of the liver volume occupied by $GST-P^+$ foci (10.6 ± 2.2 versus 50.7 ± 17.3 in controls) (Astorg et al., 1997).

In a study of similar design, all rats were injected intraperitoneally on days 13 and 19 with 1 mg/kg bw aflatoxin B_1 in 50% dimethylsulfoxide in water; 50 mg/kg 2-AAF were added to the diet on days 42–56; all rats were subjected to a two-thirds hepatectomy on day 49; and the rats received unsupplemented diet on days 56–63 (end of the study). The lycopene content of the livers of rats receiving the compound was still significant at the time of partial hepatectomy, i.e. four weeks after cessation of lycopene feeding. Lycopene did not significantly inhibit the onset of liver preneoplastic foci; i.e. the number of $GST-P^+$ foci (711 ± 116 versus 773 ± 169 in controls), the mean volume (10^{-3} mm^3) of $GST-P^+$ foci (56.7 ± 25.8 versus 107.8 ± 46.8 in controls) or the fraction of the liver volume (mm^3/cm^3) occupied by GST-P+ foci (31.5 ± 10.6 versus 55.4 ± 17.6 in controls) (Gradelet et al., 1998).

(d)   Mammary gland
Mouse: Two groups of female SHN/Mei mice, 40 days old, received AIN-76 TM diet either as such (21 animals) or supplemented with 0.00005% lycopene (27 animals). After 10 months, 11 controls and 14 lycopene-fed mice that had not developed palpable mammary gland tumours were killed, while the remaining mice were observed for another four months. No significant difference in body weight was seen between the two groups. Lycopene significantly suppressed the development of spontaneous mammary gland tumours: the incidences after 10 months were 8% in the lycopene-fed group and 24% in the controls, and after 13 months, 46% in the lycopene-fed group 82% in the controls; the first mammary tumours occurred in the controls at seven months and in the lycopene-fed group and 82% in the controls; the first mammary tumours occurred in the controls at seven months and in the lycopene-fed group at nine months ($p < 0.01$, incidence and onset of tumours considered simultaneously; analysis of variance). The mean number of hyperplastic alveolar nodules in the mammary glands was, however, higher in the lycopene-fed group than in the controls: in mice bearing no palpable tumours at 10 months, 2.9 ± 1.2 in nine controls and 7.9 ± 2.2 in 14 lycopene-fed animals (not significant; analysis of variance); in mice bearing palpable mammary tumours at 8–13 months, 15.7 ± 3.7 in six controls and 28.6 ± 4.7 in five mice fed lycopene (p < 0.05; analysis of variance) (Nagasawa et al., 1995).

(e)   Inoculated tumours
Rat C-6 glioma cells: Two groups of six male Wistar rats, three to four weeks old, were fed normal rodent chow and were given intraperitoneal injections of either 10 mg/kg bw lycopene in 0.06% dimethylsulfoxide (v/v; 2 mg/ml) or dimethylsulfoxide alone on five consecutive days. Then, 10^6 C-6 glioma cells were inoculated subcutaneously into the right scapula. Eight to 10 weeks later, the animals were killed and the tumours were removed and weighed. In a second, similar experiment, lycopene was administered intraperitoneally two weeks after tumour-cell inoculation. In the first experiment, lycopene prolonged the time to 50% tumour incidence from 14 days in controls to 21 days in those given lycopene [statistics unspecified]) and reduced the mean tumour weight by 57%, from 67.0 ± 18.1 g in controls to 28.7 ± 26.9 g in animals given lycopene ($p < 0.02$ [statistical test unspecified]). In the second experiment,

Table 43. Effects of lycopene on tumorigenesis in experimental animals

Organ	Species, strain, sex	No. of animals	Carcinogen (dose, route)	Lycopene (dose, route)	Treatment relative to carcinogen	Preventive efficacy	Reference
Colon	Rat, Sprague-Dawley, female	6	MNU, 4 mg, 3 doses, intrarectally	0.24, 1.2 and 6 mg; gavage, daily for 2 weeks	After	Aberrant crypt foci number/colon: Low dose: 36% (NS) Mid dose: 27% (NS) High dose: none (NS)	Narisawa et al. (1996)
Colon	Rat, Sprague-Dawley, female	6	MNU, 4 mg, 3 doses intrarectally	0.06, 0.12 and 0.24 mg; gavage, daily for 2 weeks	After	Aberrant crypt foci number/colon: Low dose: 27% (NS) Mid dose: 51% ($p < 0.05$) High dose: 38% ($p < 0.05$)	Narisawa et al. (1996)
Lung	Mouse, B6C3F$_1$, male and female	16	NDEA, 10 mg/kg bw, i.p., two doses at days 11 and 32 after birth; MNU, 120 ppm in drinking-water, from weeks 4 to 9; DMH; 20 mg/kg bw, s.c., two doses a week, from weeks 4 to 9	25 or 50 ppm in drinking-water	After	Tumours (adenoma + carcinoma) Incidence: 75% ($p < 0.02$) Multiplicity: 73% ($p < 0.001$)	Kim et al. (1997)
Liver	Mouse C3H/He, male	17–18	Spontaneous liver tumours	0.05% in drinking-water	Throughout	Liver tumours Incidence: 56% reduction ($p < 0.05$) Multiplicity: 88% reduction ($p < 0.01$)	Nishino (1998)
Liver	Rat, SPF-Wistar, male	9	2-Nitropropane, 6 × 100 mg/kg bw, i.p.	300 mg/kg diet	Before and during	Fraction of liver volume occupied by GST-P$^+$ foci: 28% (NS)	Astorg et al. (1997)
Liver	Rat, SPF-Wistar, male	9	NDEA, 100 mg/kg bw, single dose, i.p.	300 mg/kg diet	Before and during	Fraction of liver volume occupied by GST-P$^+$ foci: 79% ($p < 0.05$)	Astorg et al. (1997)
Liver	Rat, SPF-Wistar, male	10	Aflatoxin B$_1$, 2 × 1 mg/kg bw, i.p.	300 mg/kg diet	Before and during	Fraction of liver volume occupied by GST-P$^+$ foci: 57% (NS)	Gradelet et al. (1998)

Table 43 (contd)

Organ	Species, strain, sex	No. of animals	Carcinogen (dose, route)	Lycopene (dose, route)	Treatment relative to tumour cells	Preventive efficacy	Reference
Mammary gland	Mouse, SHN/Mei	21–27	–	0.00005% in diet	–	Tumours Incidence: at 10 months, 67%; at 13 months, 44% Onset: 22% ($p < 0.01$; incidence and onset combined) Preneoplasia Number: none; rather, a significant increase	Nagasawa et al. (1995)
–	Rat, Wistar, male	6	10^6 C-6 glioma cells	10 mg/kg bw, i.p.	Before and during	Gliomas Latency: 29% [SU] Weight: 57% ($p < 0.02$)	Wang et al. (1989)
–	Rat, Wistar, male	6	10^6 C-glioma cells	10 mg/kg bw, i.p.	After	Gliomas Latency: 34% [SU] Weight: 30% ($p < 0.05$)	Wang et al. (1989)

MNU, N-methyl-N-nitrosourea; NS, not significant; NDEA, N-nitrosodiethylamine; GST-P⁺, placental glutathione S-transferase-positive; SPF, specific pathogen-free; DMH, 1,2-dimethylhydrazine; i.p., intraperitoneally; s.c., subcutaneously; SU, statistics unspecified lycopene prolonged survival (at week 10, 3/6 controls and 5/6 animals given lycopene were still alive), reduced the number of rats with tumours (6/6 in controls and 4/6 in those on lycopene) and reduced the mean tumour weight by 30%, from 147.1 ± 73.4 g in controls to 102.8 ± 61.0 g in those given lycopene ($p < 0.05$ [statistical test unspecified]) (Wang *et al.*, 1989).

4.2.1.6   Lutein (Table 44)
(a) Skin
Mouse: Female ICR mice were shaved at the age of six weeks. One week after initiation by topical application of 100 µg DMBA in 100 ml acetone, TPA at 10 nmol/100 ml of acetone was applied once and then mezerein at 3 nmol for 15 weeks and 6 nmol for the subsequent 15 weeks, in 100 ml of acetone, twice a week.

Table 44. Effects of lutein on tumorigenesis in experimental animals

Organ	Species, strain, sex	No. of animals/ group	Carcinogen (dose, route)	Lutein (dose, route)	Treatment relative to carcinogen	Preventive efficacy	Reference
Skin	Mouse, ICR, female	15	DMBA; 100 µg, topical application, once TPA, as first stage promoter 10 nmol, topical application once Mezerein as second-stage promotor, 3 nmol for 15 weeks and 6 nmol for subsequent 15 weeks, topical application twice weekly	Lutein, 1 mmol, in 100 ml acetone, topical application, twice (45 min before and 16 h after TPA application)	Before and after first-stage promoter application	Skin tumours Multiplicity; 65% reduction at week 30 of promotion ($p < 0.05$)	Nishino (1998)
Colon	Rat, Sprague-Dawley, female	6	MNU, 4 mg, 3 doses intra-rectally	0.24, 1.2 and 6 mg; gavage, daily for 2 weeks		No. of aberrant crypt foci/colon: Low dose: 42% ($p < 0.050$) Mid-dose; 25% ($p < 0.05$) High dose: 32% ($p < 0.05$)	Narisawa *et al.* (1996)
Mammary gland	Mouse, Balb/c, female	20	WAZ-2T (SA) cells, s.c.	0.1 and 0.4% in diet	After	Tumour incidence at 28 days: Low dose: 45% (NS) High dose: 40% (NS) Tumour weight Low dose: 2.6 ± 0.2 ($p < 0.01$) High dose: 2.2 ± 0.2 ($p < 0.01$)	Chew *et al.* (1996)

DMBA, 7,12-dimethylbenz[*a*]anthracene; TPA, 12-*O*-tetradecanoylphorbol 13-acetate

Lutein at 1 mmol/100 ml acetone (molar ratio to TPA, 100) was then applied twice, 45 min before and 16 h after TPA application. Lutein suppressed skin tumour promotion by 65% at week 30 of promotion ($p < 0.005$) (Nishino, 1998).

(b) Colon

Rat: Twenty-four female Sprague-Dawley rats, seven weeks old, received three intrarectal instillations of 4 mg MNU in 0.5 ml distilled water in week 1 and were then divided into groups of six animals, which received 0.2 ml corn oil containing 0, 0.24, 1.2 or 6 mg lutein, by intragastric gavage daily during weeks 2 and 5. In week 6, all rats were killed and their colons were examined for aberrant crypt foci. The numbers of aberrant crypt foci per colon were statistically significantly lower at all three doses of lutein: 40.2 ± 4.3 at the low dose, 52.2 ± 4.0 at the intermediate dose and 46.8 ± 5.6 at the high dose, in comparison with 69.3 ± 6.2 in controls ($p < 0.05$; Student's t test) (Narisawa *et al.*, 1996).

(c) Inoculated tumours

WAZ-2T (-SA) cells: Three groups of 20 female Balb/c mice, eight weeks old, were fed a semi-purified diet (AIN-76A) containing 0, 0.1 or 0.4% lutein from marigold extract (37% lutein esters, 0.5% zeaxanthin esters, 56% other marigold extractives, mainly fatty acid esters of high-molecular-mass alcohols; lutein mono-myristate) mixed with the oil portion of the diet, throughout the experiment. After three weeks, each mouse was injected with 10^6 WAZ-2T (SA) murine mammary tumour cells suspended in Dulbecco's modified Eagle's medium supplemented with 10% newborn bovine serum and 5% insulin, into the right inguinal mammary fat pad. All mice were sacrificed 45 days after inoculation. No significant difference in food intake or body-weight gain was seen between the groups. The concentrations of lutein in plasma were increased ($p < 0.01$; Student's t test) by dietary lutein, but mice fed 0.4% lutein had a lower plasma lutein concentration (about 1.2 µmol/L) than those fed 0.1% lutein (about 1.7 µmol/L). The tumour incidence was not significantly reduced by lutein, being 100% in each group at the end of the study and 13/20 in the controls, 9/20

at the low dose and 8/20 at the high dose 28 days after inoculation. The final tumour weight was lower, however, in the mice fed lutein: 2.6 ± 0.2 g at the low dose and 2.2 ± 0.2 g at the high dose ($p < 0.01$; split-plot model) than in the control group (3.4 ± 0.4 g; $p < 0.02$; split-plot model, t test); the tumour latency in mice at the high dose (32.1 ± 0.4) was longer than that in controls (30.1 ± 0.4 days), whereas that of mice at the low dose (30.5 ± 0.4 days) was comparable (Chew *et al.*, 1996).

4.2.1.7 α-Carotene (Table 45)

(a) Skin

Mouse: The backs of 48 ICR mice [sex unspecified], seven weeks old, were shaved, and two days later the animals received a single application of 0.1 mg DMBA [vehicle unspecified] on the shaven skin. One week later, 1 µg (1.62 nmol) TPA was applied twice weekly for 20 weeks. Groups of 16 animals received 200 or 400 nmol α-carotene in 0.2 ml acetone simultaneously with each application of TPA, and the third group was treated with the vehicle in acetone. There was no significant difference in body weight among the groups. The first skin tumour (a papilloma) appeared in a control within nine weeks after the start of TPA applications, whereas in both α-carotene-treated groups the first skin tumour was seen after 13 weeks of TPA application. At 20 weeks, the percentages of mice bearing skin papillomas were 69, 25 and 13 [statistics unspecified], and the average numbers of skin tumours were 3.73, 0.27 ($p < 0.01$; Student's t test) and 0.13 ($p < 0.01$ [method of statistical analysis and standard deviations unspecified]) in the controls and those at the low and high doses of α-carotene, respectively. The tumours in α-carotene-treated animals were smaller than those in the controls; e.g. the average numbers of tumours 1–2 mm in diameter per mouse were 2.20 in controls, 0.20 at the low dose and 0.13 at the high dose [standard deviations unspecified]; furthermore, there were no tumours > 3 mm in diameter in the α-carotene-treated mice but 0.46/mouse [standard deviation unspecified] in controls [statistics unspecified]. The study was repeated with almost the same results [no further details

Table 45. Effects of α-carotene on tumorigenesis in experimental animals

Organ	Species, strain, sex	No. of animals/ group	Carcinogen (dose, route)	α-Carotene, (dose, route)	Treatment relative to carcingen	Preventive efficacy	Reference
Skin	Mouse, ICR [sex unspecified]	16	DMBA, 100 µg, single application; TPA, 1 µg twice weekly	200 and 400 nmol, skin application, twice wekly	After	Papillomas Incidence: high dose, 81% (SU); low dose, 64% (SU) Multiplicity: high dose, 97% ($p < 0.01$); low dose 93% ($p < 0.01$) Latency: both doses, 44% (SU)	Murakoshi et al. (1992); Nishino (1995)
Colon	Rat, Sprague-Dawley, female	6	MNU, 4 mg, 3 doses intra-rectally	0.24, 1.2 and 6 mg; gavage, daily for 2 weeks	After	No. of aberrant crypt foci/colon Low dose: 7% (NS) Mid dose: 18% (NS) High dose: 32% ($p < 0.05$)	Narisawa et al. (1996)
Lung	Mouse, ddY, male	16	4-NQO, 10 mg/kg bw, single, s.c. Glycerol (10%) in drinking-water	0.05% in drinking-water (3.27 mg/ mouse per day)	During and after	Type II adenoma Incidence: 22% (NS) Multiplicity: 67% ($p < 0.001$)	Murakoshi et al. (1992); Nishino (1995)
Liver	Mouse, C3H/He male	17	–	0.005% or 0.05% in drinking-water (0.25, 2.41 mg/mouse per day)	–	Liver carcinomas Incidence: high dose, 6% (NS), low dose, none (NS) Multiplicity: high dose, 52% ($p < 0.001$); low dose, 20% (NS)	Murakoshi et al. (1992)

NS, not significant; DMBA, 7,12-dimethylbenz[a]anthracene; TPA, 12-O-tetradecanoylphorbol 13-acetate; SU, statistics unspecified; 4-NQO, 4-nitroquinoline 1-oxide; s.c., subcutaneously; MNU, N-methyl-N-nitrosourea presented] (Murakoshi *et al.*, 1992; Nishino, 1995).

(b)   Colon

Rat: Twenty-four female Sprague-Dawley rats, seven weeks old, received three intrarectal instillations of 4 mg MNU in 0.5 ml distilled water in week 1 and were then divided into groups of six animals which received 0.2 ml corn oil containing 0, 0.24, 1.2 or 6 mg α-carotene by intragastric gavage daily during weeks 2 and 5. In week 6, all rats were killed and their colons were examined for aberrant crypt foci. The numbers of aberrant crypt foci per colon were lower in the animals given α-carotene (58.4 ± 4.9 at the low dose, 55.9 ± 5.3 at the intermediate dose and 42.4 ± 2.4 at the high dose) than in the controls (62.7 ± 7.2), but the difference was statistically significant only for the high dose ($p < 0.005$; Student's *t* test) (Narisawa *et al.*, 1996).

(c)   Lung

Mouse: Two groups of 16 male, specific pathogen-free ddY mice, six weeks old, received drinking-water containing either 0.05% α-carotene (as an emulsion containing 0.5% sucrose ester P-1750, 1.0% Sansoft 8000, 0.2% L-ascorbyl stearate and 4% peanut oil; mean α-carotene intake, 3.27 mg/d per mouse) or the emulsion without α-carotene for four weeks. On the first day, all mice received a single sub-cutaneous injection of 10 mg/kg bw 4-NQO dissolved in a mixture of olive oil and cholesterol (20:1), providing about 0.3 mg 4-NQO per mouse. During weeks 5–25, the drinking-water of all mice was supplemented with 10% glycerol. The mice were killed at week 30. No significant difference in water intake or body weight was seen between the two groups. There was no significant difference in the number of mice with lung tumours (type II adenoma), 94 and 73%, but the mean number of lung tumours per mouse was significantly reduced, from 4.06 ± 0.18 in controls to 1.33 ± 0.08 in animals given α-carotene ($p < 0.001$; Student's *t* test). The lung tumours were of similar size [not further specified] in the two groups. The study was repeated with similar results [no further details presented] (Murakoshi *et al.*, 1992; Nishino, 1995).

(d)   Liver

Mouse: Groups of 17 eight-week-old male C3H/He mice, which have a high spontaneous incidence of liver tumours, received 0.005 or 0.05% α-carotene mixed with the drinking-water as an emulsion containing 0.5% sucrose ester P-1750, 1% Sansoft 8000, 0.2% L-ascorbyl stearate and 4% peanut oil, to give mean α-carotene intakes of 0.25 and 2.41 mg/d per mouse, or the emulsion without α-carotene for 40 weeks, at the end of which the mice were killed. There was no significant difference in body weight or water intake between the groups. The numbers of animals with liver tumours (well-differentiated hepatocellular carcinomas) were 16/16 in controls, 15/15 at the low dose and 16/17 at the high dose, but the mean numbers of liver tumours per mouse were decreased, from 6.31 ± 0.62 in the controls to 5.07 ± 0.49 at the low dose and 3.00 ± 0.36 at the high dose ($p < 0.001$; Student's *t* test). There were no differences among the groups in the size [not further specified] or histological appearance of the tumours (Murakoshi *et al.*, 1992).

4.2.1.8   Fucoxanthin (Table 46)

(a)   Skin

Mouse: Two groups of 15 female ICR mice [age unspecified] received a single application of 0.1 mg DMBA on their shaved backs. One week later, 1.62 nmol TPA were applied twice weekly for 20 weeks. One of the groups received an application of 0.6 μmol fucoxanthin (prepared from the brown algae *Hijikia fusiforme*, a common edible seaweed in Japan) in 0.2 ml acetone simultaneously with each application of TPA; the other group was treated with 0.2 ml acetone only. In the latter group, 8/15 animals developed skin tumours, with an average of 2.20 tumours per mouse, whereas no skin tumours were found in fuxocanthin-treated mice (Nishino, 1995).

(b)   Small intestine

Mouse: Thirty-eight male C57Bl/6 mice [age unspecified] were given drinking-water containing 0.01% *N*-ethyl-*N*'-nitro-*N*-nitroso-guanidine (ENNG) for four weeks. During weeks 5–20, 20 mice received drinking-water containing 0.005% fucoxanthin (prepared

Table 46. Effects of fucoxanthin on tumorigenesis in experimental animals

Organ	Species, Strain sex	No. of animals/ group	Carcinogen (dose, route)	Fucoxanthin, (dose, route)	Preventive efficacy	Reference
Skin	Mouse, ICR, female	15	DMBA, 0.1 mg; single application	0.6 mmol; twice weekly, 19 weeks	Tumours: 100% (SU)	Nishino (1995)
Small intestine	Mouse, C57Bl/6, male	18–20	ENNG, 0.01% in drinking-water, 4 weeks	0.005% in drinking-water, 11 weeks	Tumours Incidence: 61% ($p < 0.05$) Multiplicity: 57% ($p < 0.05$)	Okazumi et al. (1993); Nishino (1995)

DMBA, 7,12-dimethylbenz[a]anthracene; SU, statistics unspecified; ENNG, N-ethyl-N'-nitro-N-nitrosoguanidine

from *Hijikia fusiforme* and added as an emulsion [vehicle unspecified]), while the other 18 mice received drinking-water supplemented with the fucoxanthin vehicle only. The mice were killed at week 20. Fucoxanthin reduced the incidence of duodenal tumour-bearing mice [type of tumour unspecified] from 14/18 to 6/20 ($p < 0.005$ [method of statistical analysis unspecified]) and the mean number of duodenal tumours per mouse from 1.28 to 0.55 ($p < 0.05$ [method of statistical analysis unspecified]) (Okuzumi *et al.*, 1993; Nishino, 1995).

4.2.1.9 Astaxanthin
(a) Small intestine and colon
Rat: Azoxymethane was used to induce carcinogenesis in the small intestine and colon of male Fischer 344 rats by subcutaneous injection at a dose of 15 mg/kg bw once a week for three weeks. One week after the last dose, the diets of two group of rats were supplemented with 100 or 500 mg/kg astaxanthin for 34 weeks; another group received only azoxymethane; one received only 500 mg/kg astaxanthin for 37 weeks; and one served as untreated controls. The incidence of intestinal adenocarcinomas and signet ring-cell carcinomas was 50% with azoxymethane alone; the incidence was reduced to 34% after supplementation with 100 ppm astaxanthin and to 28% with 500 ppm. Controls and rats given astaxanthin alone had no tumours (Tanaka *et al.*, 1995a).

(b) Oral cavity
Rat: A total of 133 male Fischer 344 rats were given 4-NQO for eight weeks to induce oral tumours. One group was fed a diet containing 0.01% astaxanthin for 10 weeks before exposure to 4-NQO; one was fed a diet with 0.01% astaxanthin for 22 weeks starting one week after exposure to 4-NQO; one received only astaxanthin throughout the study (32 weeks); one received a normal rat diet after 4-NQO administration; and one served as untreated controls. 4-NQO alone induced squamous-cell papillomas and carcinomas of the tongue in 54% of the rats, but no oral neoplasms developed in the rats that received astaxanthin before, during or after exposure to 4-NQO (Tanaka *et al.*, 1995a).

(c) Urinary bladder
Mouse: Urinary bladder tumours were induced in 144 male ICR mice by giving them drinking-water containing NBHBA. One group of mice received NBHBA alone for 20 weeks and then tap water for 21 weeks; one group received 50 mg/kg astaxanthin (a xanthophyll present in crustaceae, fish, shellfish and some fruits and vegetables but lacking provitamin A activity) in tap water one week after the end of exposure to NBHBA for 20 weeks; one group received 50 mg/kg astaxanthin only for 20 weeks after drinking tap water for the first 21 weeks of the experiment; and one group served as untreated controls. The incidence of transitional or

squamous-cell carcinomas of the bladder was 42% with NBHBA alone and 0% with astaxanthin alone and in the controls. Astaxanthin reduced the incidence of transitional-cell carcinomas from 31% with NBHBA alone to 3%, but had no effect on the incidence of squamous-cell carcinomas (Tanaka *et al.*, 1994).

4.2.1.10 Crocetin
(a) Skin
The skin of groups of 15 female CD-1 mice was treated topically with benzo[*a*]pyrene once a week for 10 weeks; after a one-week pause, mice were treated topically with 15 nmol TPA alone or in combination with 0.2 or 1.0 μmol crocetin (a carotenoid with no provitamin A activity which is present in *Gardenia fructus* and is widely used in Chinese herbal medicine) twice weekly for 20 weeks. Crocetin inhibited the number of tumours per mouse by 69% and reduced the proportion of mice with tumours by 81% (Wang, C.-J. *et al.*, 1996).

(b) Inoculated tumours
Rat C-6 glioma cells: Crocetin was given by intraperitoneal injection at 0 or 10 mg/kg bw to Wistar rats for five consecutive days, and on the sixth day, C-6 glioma cells were inoculated subcutaneously. In comparison with treatment only with glioma cells, crocetin prolonged the latency to 50% tumour incidence and caused a 60% reduction in mean tumour weight, from 67.0 to 26.6 g. In another group of rats that received the same dose of crocetin two weeks after tumour-cell inoculation, a significant reduction in mean tumour weight was seen, from 147.1 to 94.6 g (Wang *et al.*, 1989).

4.2.1.11 Mixtures of carotenoids (see Table 47)
(a) Skin
Mouse: Forty female ICR mice [age unspecified] received a single application of 0.1 mg DMBA on their shaven backs, and one week later received applications of 0.81 nmol TPA twice weekly for 16 weeks. Ten of the mice received simultaneous applications of 162 nmol palm-oil carotene (60% β-carotene, 30% α-carotene and 10% other natural carotenoids including γ-carotene and lycopene) in 0.2 ml acetone; the other 30 mice were similarly treated with 0.2 ml

acetone only. In these animals, the first tumour appeared within six weeks, and at the end of the experiment 29/30 of the mice in this group had developed skin tumours, with an average of 2.63 tumours per mouse. Palm-oil carotene treatment completely suppressed the skin tumour formation (Nishino, 1995).

(b) Colon
Rat: Twelve female Sprague-Dawley rats, seven weeks old, received three intrarectal instillations of 4 mg MNU in 0.5 ml distilled water in week 1 and were then divided into groups of six animals which received 0.2 ml corn oil containing 0 or 6 mg palm-oil carotene (an oleoresin from natural palm oil which consisted of a mixture of α-carotene, β-carotene and lycopene) by intragastric gavage, daily during weeks 2 and 5. In week 6, all rats were killed and their colons were examined for aberrant crypt foci. The number of foci per colon was 69.3 ± 6.2 in the controls and 51.3 ± 8.3 in the animals given palm-oil carotene, but the difference was not significant (Student's *t* test) (Narisawa *et al.*, 1996).

(c) Respiratory tract
Mouse: Twenty-six male ddY mice [age unspecified] received a single subcutaneous injection of 10 μg/kg bw 4NQO dissolved in a 20:1 mixture of olive oil and cholesterol. During weeks 5–30, 12 of these mice received drinking-water containing 10% glycerol plus 0.005% palm-oil carotene (60% β-carotene, 30% α-carotene and 10% other natural carotenoids including γ-carotene and lycopene, added as an emulsion [vehicle unspecified]), while the other 14 mice received drinking-water containing 10% glycerol plus the palm-oil carotene vehicle. Palm-oil carotene reduced the lung tumour incidence [tumour type unspecified] from [14/14] to [4/12] (*p* < 0.05 [method of analysis unspecified]) and the mean number of lung tumours per mouse from 3.06 to 0.58 (*p* < 0.001 [standard deviation and method of statistical analysis unspecified]) (Nishino, 1995).

(d) Liver
Mouse: Groups of 17 eight-week-old male C3H/He mice, which have a high spontaneous incidence of liver tumours, received drinking-

water containing 0.005 or 0.05% palm oil carotene (30% α-carotene, 60% β-carotene and 3% γ-carotene, 4% lycopene and 3% other [unspecified] carotenes, as an emulsion containing 0.5% sucrose ester P-1750, 1.0% Sansoft 8000, 0.2% L-ascorbyl stearate and 4% peanut oil), to give mean intakes of palm-oil carotene of 0.25 and 2.57 mg/d per mouse, or the emulsion without palm-oil carotene for 40 weeks, when the mice were killed. There was no significant difference in body weight or water intake between the groups. The numbers of animals with liver tumours (well-differentiated hepatocellular carcinomas) were 16/16 in controls, 15/15 at the low dose and 13/16 at the high dose, and the mean numbers of liver tumours per mouse were 6.31 ± 0.62 in the controls, 3.60 ± 0.40 at the low dose ($p < 0.001$; Student's t test) and 2.06 ± 0.37 at the high dose ($p < 0.001$; Student's t test). There was no difference among the groups in the size [not further specified] or histological appearance of the tumours (Murakoshi *et al.*, 1992; Nishino, 1995).

(e)   Buccal pouch
Hamster: Epidermoid carcinomas were produced in the right buccal pouches of three groups of 20 adult male Syrian golden hamsters [age not further specified] by painting the pouches with a 0.5% solution of DMBA in heavy mineral oil three times per week for 13 weeks. The pouches were then injected with 0.1 ml of minimal essential medium containing about 250 μg phycotene extracted from *Spirulina* and *Dunaliella* algae (chemical composition, 7% water, 9% ash, 71% proteins, 0.9% crude fibre, 1.8 g/kg xanthophylls, 1.9 g/kg carotene, chlorophylls a and b, α-carotene, neoxanthin and other xanthophylls [not further specified]) or with 0.1 ml of the medium (sham-injected controls); 20 hamsters were not further treated. The experiment was terminated at 17 weeks. The body weights of the sham-injected DMBA controls (about 85 g) were consistently lower than those of hamsters given phycotene (140 g) and the uninjected animals (100 g). No tumour regression was seen in sham-injected or uninjected hamsters, all of which had multiple, large cheek pouch tumours; two uninjected controls and one

sham-injected animal died intercurrently with very large tumours and infection. Phycotene caused complete gross tumour regression in 6/20 hamsters and partial regression in 14/20. In general, regression of the large and multiple tumours tended to be incomplete, whereas total regression was usually seen for small or moderate tumours. The tumours in regression showed degeneration and infiltration of lymphocytes and macrophages, which often contained tumour necrosis factor. Stratified squamous epithelium adjacent to the carcinomas with severe destruction was relatively unaffected and appeared essentially normal (Schwartz & Shklar, 1987).

Sixty male Syrian hamsters, two to three months old and weighing 95–125 g, were painted on the right buccal pouch with a 0.5% solution of DMBA in heavy mineral oil (about 0.6 mg DMBA per painting) three times per week for 14 weeks, when each hamster had obvious gross tumours of various sizes and numbers. Then, the animals were divided into groups of 20, and the tumour-bearing pouch was injected twice weekly with 0.1 ml minimal essential medium, alone or containing 0.19 mg of an extract of *Spirulina* and *Dunaliella* algae, three times weekly for four weeks. The algae extract reduced the total burden of cheek pouch tumours (moderately sized papillary epidermoid carcinomas) from 1400 mm^3 in the DMBA and sham-injected DMBA control groups to about 20 mm^3 in the animals given the algal extract [no information on statistics]. Both degeneration and a clearly increased number of tumour necrosis factor-α-positive macrophages were found in the tumours and adjacent to the regressing tumours in hamsters treated with the algal extract (Shklar & Schwartz, 1988).

Sixty non-inbred adult male hamsters, 60–90 days old and weighing 96–120 g, were fed standard laboratory pellets, and their right buccal pouches were painted with a 0.1% solution of DMBA in heavy mineral oil three times per week for 28 weeks. The animals were divided into three groups of 20 hamsters each and were given either 0.14 mg of an extract of *Spirulina* and *Dunaliella* algae (containing 20–25% zeaxanthin, 10–15% myxoanthophyll,

15–30% β-carotene, 10–15% echinenone, 20–25% β-cryptoxanthin and at least 10 other carotenoids; 1.5 mg/kg bw) in 0.4 ml mineral oil three times per week on alternate days to DMBA, mineral oil only or no further treatment. All hamsters were killed after 28 weeks, when obvious, moderately large buccal pouch tumours were seen in untreated controls. The body weights of the hamsters treated with the algal extract were higher (192 ± 38 g) than those of untreated controls (143 ± 20.0 g) or vehicle controls (152 ± 21 g). All control hamsters but none of those given the algal extract had cheek-pouch tumours ($p < 0.001$; Student's t test). The control animals had proliferative epidermoid carcinomas that invaded the underlying connective tissue, numerous foci of hyperkeratosis with dysplasia and carcinoma *in situ* and lymphocytic infiltration into areas of tumour infiltration and carcinoma *in situ*. The animals given the algal extract had no frank carcinomas, but scattered foci of dysplasia and carcinoma *in situ* undergoing degeneration and cellular destruction were seen. There were also dense accumulations of lymphocytes and histiocytes in the underlying connective tissue, often close to the areas of dysplasia and sometimes so dense that they resembled lymphoid tissue. When the lymphocyte infiltrate was light, it often had a perivascular distribution (Schwartz *et al.*, 1988).

The mucosa of the right cheek pouch of three groups of 20 male Syrian hamsters [age unspecified] fed a normal hamster diet containing 22% protein and the required concentrations of vitamin A and E, was painted with 0.1% DMBA in heavy mineral oil (0.4 mg DMBA per painting) three times a week for 28 weeks. One group received no further treatment; the other two groups were given 0.4 ml of heavy mineral oil containing 0 or 1.4 mg/kg bw of a mixture of at least 15 carotenoids (the main ones were zeaxanthin, 25–35%; myxoxanthophyl, 13–17%; β-carotene, 10–15%; echinenone, 11–13%; and β-cryptoxanthin, 6–23%), by gavage three times a week on alternate days to DMBA, for 28 weeks. A fourth group served as untreated controls. The mean body weight of the DMBA controls (85 g) was lower than that of the animals receiving the carotenoid mixture (125 g). Ingestion of the mixture prevented the formation of buccal pouch squamous-cell carcinomas completely, whereas all DMBA-treated controls had already developed such tumours after four months of treatment. At the end of treatment, the average number of areas of cheek pouch with epithelial dysplasia was 3 in the group given the carotenoid mixture and 6 in both DMBA-treated groups. No buccal pouch tumours or sites of dysplasia were found in untreated controls. Ingestion of the the carotenoid mixture resulted in a histologically unique picture not seen in DMBA-treated controls: a dense, mixed, inflammatory infiltrate consisting predominantly of cytotoxic lymphocytes and macrophages producing tumour necrosis factor-α and localized areas of mast cells in the deep dermis adjacent to areas of epithelial dysplasia (Schwartz *et al.*, 1989).

(f) Mammary gland
Mouse: Three groups of 15 litter-mate SHN/Mci mice, about two months old, were fed AIN-76TM diet containing 0.00022% retinyl palmitate or vitamin A-deficient AIN-76TM diet supplemented with either spray-dried *Dunaliella bardawil* powder, in which the β-carotene content of 0.000051% was increased to 0.03% after eight months, or an oily solution of an extract of *D. salina* Teod. (β-carotene content, 0.03%). These mice were were designated 'breeders'. The female litters of these mice, designated 'virgins', were fed the same diets as their mothers, with 27 controls, 33 on the *D. bardawil* diet and 29 on the *D. salina* diet. All three groups of breeders developed the first mammary tumour [not further specified] at six months of age and showed the same incidence of mammary tumours (about 50%) at eight months of age; however, the incidence and age at onset of tumours in groups fed the *Dunaliella*-supplemented diets was slightly but statistically significantly lower than in the controls ($p < 0.05$; analysis of variance [no further details given]). Among the virgins, the first mammary tumours appeared at five months of age in controls, one month later in the group given *D. bardawil* and two months later in the group given *D. salina*. Moreover, the incidence of mammary tumours among virgins given *Dunaliella* supplements

was lower than that in controls at 6, 7, 8, 9, 10 and 11 months of age ($p < 0.05$; analysis of variance). No significant difference in mammary tumorigenesis was found between the groups given *D. bardawil* and *D. salina*. *Dunaliella* had no significant effect on the normal growth of the mammary glands, preneoplastic growth (number and size of hyperplastic alveolar nodules) or neoplastic growth (number of tumours per mouse; growth rate per tumour) (Nagasawa *et al.*, 1989).

(g)   Forestomach

Mouse: Groups of 15 female Haffkine Swiss mice, six to eight weeks old and weighing 20–25 g, were maintained on standard diet, on standard diet without 0.75% (w/w) sesame oil or on sesame oil-free standard diet supplemented with 0.75 or 1.5% (w/w) palm oil. From week 3, all mice on the standard diet and all mice in one of two groups receiving sesame oil-free diet or diets supplemented with palm oil were given 1 mg benzo[*a*]pyrene in 0.1 ml peanut oil by gavage, twice a week for four weeks. At eight weeks, the animals were kept under observation, and all were killed at the age of 180 days. The mean body-weight gain was increased by 21% in mice on the 1.5% palm-oil diet [probably due to the higher oil content of this diet] but was similar in the other groups. Forestomach tumours developed in 13/15 mice on standard diet and treated with benzo[*a*]pyrene and in none of the mice not treated with benzo[*a*]pyrene. Palm oil reduced the incidence of forestomach tumours from 12/15 in the oil control group to 4/15 in mice given the low dose ($p < 0.00/$; χ^2 test) and to 0/15 in those at the high dose [statistics unspecified], and the mean number of forestomach tumours per mouse from 1.7 ± 0.3 to 1.0 ± 0.0 at the low dose ($p < 0.001$; Student's t test) (Azuine *et al.*, 1992).

(h)   Small intestine

Mouse: Fifty male C57B1/6 mice [age unspecified] were given drinking-water containing 0.01% ENNG for four weeks. During weeks 5–20, 28 mice received drinking-water containing 0.05% palm-oil carotene (60% β-carotene, 30% α-carotene and 10% other natural carotenoids including γ-carotene and lycopene, added as an emulsion [vehicle unspecified]), while the other 27 mice received drinking-water supplemented with the palm-oil carotene vehicle only. All surviving animals were killed at week 20. Palm-oil carotene decreased the incidence of duodenal tumours [type unspecified] from [18/27] to [13/28] ($p < 0.05$ [method of analysis unspecified]) and the mean number of duodenal tumours per mouse from 0.93 to 0.64 (not significant) (Nishino, 1995).

4.2.1.12 Other end-points

Various biological activities other than the end-points described above may be used as markers for the anticarcinogenic activity of carotenoids, including immuno-potentiating activity, modification of enzymatic activities and alterations in markers of differentiation and proliferation. Although these activities are mechanistic aspects of anticarcinogenesis, they are discussed in this section because surrogate end-points are needed for rapid evaluation of the anticarcinogenic activity of carotenoids.

(a)   Modulation of the immune system

The ability of carotenoids to modulate the immune system may play an important role in cancer prevention (reviewed by Bendich, 1989, 1990a,b,c). For example, they have been shown to enhance the responses of splenocytes to lymphocyte mitogens, modulate radiation-induced thymic involution and augment tumour immunity.

Dietary β-carotene and canthaxanthin enhanced the proliferative responses of T and B lymphocytes in male weanling Wistar Kyoto rats given diets supplemented with beadlets containing these carotenoids at a dose of 0.2% (w/w), as determined by the immune responses of splenocytes to the T-lymphocyte mitogens concanavalin A and phytohaemagglutinin and the B-lymphocyte mitogen lipopolysaccharide *in vitro*. The lymphocyte responses were consistently enhanced in groups fed β-carotene or canthaxanthin, although the only significant difference was seen in the response to concanavalin A after β-carotene administration and in the response to lipopolysaccharide after

Table 47. Effects of mixtures of carotenoids on tumorigenesis in experimental animals

Organ	Species, strain, sex	No. of animals/group	Carcinogen (dose, route)	Mixture of carotenoids	Treatment relative to carcinogen	Preventive efficacy	Reference
Skin	Mouse, ICR, female	10–30	DMBA, 0.1 mg; single application	Palm carotene; 162 nmol, twice weekly, 15 weeks	After	Tumours: 100% (SU)	Nishino (1995)
Colon	Rat, Sprague-Dawley, female	6	MNU, 4 mg, 3 doses intrarectally	Palm carotene; 6 mg, gavage, daily for 2 weeks	After	No. of aberrant crypt foci/colon: 26% (NS)	Narisawa et al. (1996)
Lung	Mouse, ddY, male	12–14	4-NQO, 10 mg; single, s.c.; 10% glycerol in drinking-water	Palm carotene; 0.005% in drinking-water	After	Tumours Incidence: 67% (p < 0.05)	Nishino (1995)
Liver	Mouse, C3H/He, male	17	–	Palm-oil carotene; 0.25 and 2.57 mg/mouse per day in drinking-water	–	Carcinomas Incidence: high dose, 19% (NS) Multiplicity: high dose, 67% (p < 0.001)	Murakoshi et al. (1992); Nishino (1995)
Buccal pouch	Hamster, male	20	0.5% DMBA; 3 times/week	Phycotene, 250 µg, injected into cheek pouch 3 times/week	After	Epidermoid carcinomas, regression Complete: 30% (SU) Partial: 70% (SU)	Schwartz & Shklar (1987)
Buccal pouch	Hamster, male	20	0.5% DMBA; 0.6 mg/painting, 3 times/week	0.19 mg in Spirulina Dulaliella extracts injected into buccal pouch	After	Carcinoma, regression Burden: 99% (SU)	Shklar & Schwartz (1988)
Buccal pouch	Hamster, male	20	0.1% DMBA; painted 3 times/week	Spirulina–Dunaliella extract; 0.14 mg/painting, 3 times/week	During	Carcinomas Incidence (gross tumours): 100% (SU)	Schwartz et al. (1988)
Buccal pouch	Hamster, male	20	0.1% DMBA; 0.4 mg/painting	Phycotene: 1.4 mg/kg bw; gavage	During	Carcinomas Regression: 100% (SU)	Schwartz et al. (1989)

Table 47 (contd)

Organ	Species, strain sex	No. of animals/ group	Carcinogen (dose)	Mixture of carotenoids	Treatment relative to carcinogen	Preventive efficacy	Reference
Mammary gland	Mouse, SHN/Mci female	15 breeders 27–33 virgins	–	*Dunaliella bardawil* powder; *Dunaliella-Salina* Teod. extract	–	Tumours Breeders: Incidence + latency: slight ($p < 0.05$) Virgins: Latency *Bardawil* powder: 20% (SU) Saline extract: 40% (SU) Incidence Both preparations: slight (SU)	Nagasawa et al. (1989)
Stomach	Mouse, Haffkine Swiss, female	15	B[a]P; 1 mg, twice weekly, gavage, 4 weeks	Palm oil; 0.75 or 1.5% in diet; 8 weeks	Before, during and after	Tumours Incidence: low dose, 66% ($p < 0.001$); high dose, 100% (SU) Multiplicity: low dose, 41% ($p < 0.001$)	Azuine et al. (1992)
Small intestine	Mouse, C57Bl/6, male	27–28	ENNG; 0.01% in drinking-water, 16 weeks	Palm carotene; 0.05% in drinking-water	After	Tumours Incidence: 41% ($p < 0.05$) Multiplicity 69% (NS)	Nishino (1995)

DMBA, 7,12-dimethylbenz[a]anthracene; SU, statistics unspecified; NS, not significant; MNU, *N*-methyl-*N*-nitrosourea; 4-NQO, 4-nitroquinoline 1-oxide; ENNG, *N*-ethyl-*N'*-nitro-*N*-nitrosoguanidine; B[a]P, benzo[a]pyrene canthaxanthin administration at week 20 (Bendich & Shapiro, 1986).

β-Carotene delayed radiation-induced thymic involution, which is one sign of immune system suppression. Five-week-old male CBA mice were maintained on basal diet containing 15 000 IU/kg vitamin A and 6.4 mg/kg β-carotene for one week before testing [formulation of the diet unspecified] and then received total-body γ-irradiation (600 rad). Supplementation of the basal diet with β-carotene at a dose of 90 mg/kg moderated thymic involution, the weights being 35.2 ± 1.0 g in unirradiated control mice ($p < 0.001$), 24.2 ± 1.0 g in irradiated mice and 33.2 ± 0.8 g in β-carotene-supplemented irradiated mice ($p < 0.005$) (Seifter et al., 1984).

β-Carotene was reported to augment immunity to syngeneic tumours. Female Balb/c mice aged eight weeks were injected subcutaneously with 10^7 syngeneic Balb/c Meth A fibrosarcoma cells. Oral administration of β-carotene dissolved in ethanol and then diluted to a final concentration of 600 μg/ml with phosphate-buffered saline, given at a dose of 0.2 ml/d per mouse for nine days, led to a 47% reduction in the tumour response after rechallenge with Meth A fibrosarcoma cells implanted subcutaneously on day 10. The tumour response to Meth 1, another syngeneic tumour of Balb/c origin, was unaffected by β-carotene, however, suggesting that β-carotene specifically augments the rejection of tumours through tumour-specific antigens. The immune lymph node cells responsible for the augmented rejection of tumour growth were found to be Thy-1-positive, Lyt-1-negative and Lyt-2-positive lymphocytes, which are presumably cytotoxic T lymphocytes (Tomita et al., 1987).

Immune-enhancing activity of carotenoids was also reported by Temple and Basu (1987) and by Basu et al. (1988).

(b)   Alterations in cell differentiation and proliferation

Alterations in the pattern of expression of keratin, a differentiation-specific marker, might be used as an intermediate biomarker of the anti-carcinogenic activity of carotenoids in squamous epithelia. Loss of high-molecular-mass (> 60 kDa) keratins, which are specific for and characteristic of normal keratinized squamous epithelia, has been observed in adenocarcinomas and squamous-cell carcinomas. The loss of 67-kDa keratins and reductions in 66- and 63-kDa keratins induced by DMBA in hamster cheek pouches was reversed by treatment with β-carotene. This modulatory effect correlated with a preventive effect against DMBA-induced carcinogenesis (Gijare et al., 1990).

The levels of polyamine, the labelling index of bromodeoxyuridine and the number and area of silver-stained nucleolar organizer region proteins, which are markers of proliferation, may also be useful as intermediate biomarkers, as the chemopreventive effect of carotenoids against 4-NQO-induced oral carcinogenesis was associated with suppression of the expression of these markers (Tanaka et al., 1994, 1995a).

4.2.2   Cells

4.2.2.1 Mammalian cells in vitro

(a)   Carotenoid delivery methods

As most carotenoids of interest are highly lipophilic and are virtually insoluble in water, supplying these molecules in a bioavailable form has been a major problem. This has been achieved in several ways. Tetrahydrofuran has been widely used as a solvent since its introduction for this purpose in 1991 (Bertram et al., 1991). If suitable precautions are taken, this solvent is not toxic and produces a pseudo-emulsion with high bioavailability (Cooney et al., 1993). The second successful method of delivery involves incorporating carotenoids into liposomes. Here too, adequate uptake of carotenoids into cells has been demonstrated (Muto et al., 1995). [The Working Group noted that considerable caution must be employed in interpreting results obtained with carotenoids in solvents such as hexane and ethanol which, when added to an aqueous solution and then evaporated (hexane) or solubilized (ethanol), cause precipitation of the carotenoid, often on the sides of the culture dish. In such situations, physical effects due to carotenoid crystals may contribute to any observed effects.]

Two carotenoids, β-carotene and canthaxanthin, are available commercially in the form of beadlets composed of a protein and carbohydrate matrix containing micro-dispersed carotenoid in oil. Control beadlets are also available, containing all of the packaging but no carotenoid. [The Working Group noted that the principal disadvantage of these beadlets, apart from the restriction to only the two carotenoids, is that they contain 90% packaging material that includes antioxidants.] This formulation has been successfully used both *in vitro* and *in vivo* (Pung *et al.*, 1988; Mayne & Parker, 1989). The concentrations of caro-tenoids reported in Tables 48–53 are those to which the cells were exposed. The concentrations that had biological effects were generally in the range 10^{-5}–10^{-7} mol/L, which are within those reported in human serum after and before supplementation, respectively (see Table 57).

(b)   *Effects on carcinogen-induced neoplastic transformation (see also Table 48)*
Neoplastically transformed foci can be produced in cultured C3H 10T/1/2 cells by application of methylcholanthrene or by exposure to ionizing radiation. Various carotenoids have been shown to reduce the incidence of such foci. Complete inhibition of transformation was achieved when carotenoids (10^{-5} mol/L) were applied seven days after removal of carcinogen and continued for four weeks, indicating that the activity did not affect metabolic activation of the carcinogen or repair of precarcinogenic lesions. Moreover, the inhibition was reversible upon withdrawal of the carotenoid, indicating that the activity was not due to direct cytotoxicity (Pung *et al.*, 1988). Dose–response relationships in the reduction in focus formation were seen in the range of 10^{-5} to 3×10^{-7} mol/L, and activity was observed with both provitamin A carotenoids, such as β-carotene, and non-provitamin A carotenoids, such as canthaxanthin and lycopene (Bertram *et al.*, 1991). β-Carotene and canthaxanthin were shown by the above protocol to be capable of inhibiting X-ray-induced transformation; however, only marginal inhibition was observed when the cultures were treated before, during and immediately after irradiation (Pung

et al., 1988). The studies indicate that carotenoids have little effect on initiation processes in cells. Cellular uptake and inhibition of transformation induced by β-carotene and canthaxanthin were comparable when they were applied in beadlets or as solutions in tetrahydrofuran. The chemopreventive activity of carotenoids did not correlate with their activity as antioxidants, as shown by decreases in thiobarbituric acid-reactive substances; methyl-bixin, the carotenoid with the highest antioxidant activity tested, was inactive as a chemopreventive agent (Zhang *et al.*, 1992). Of two synthetic carotenoids tested, a C_{22} compound was active whereas a C_{28} compound was not active in the 10T/1/2 assay system. Interestingly, the C_{28} compound had been reported to have greater antioxidant activity and was shown to achieve higher cellular levels than the C_{22} compound in this assay system (Pung *et al.*, 1993). When tested in the same system for their ability to inhibit benzo[*a*]pyrene-induced transformation, crocetin, a C_{20} diapocarotenoid, also prevented focus formation at concentrations between 10^{-4} and 3×10^{-5} mol/L. At the highest dose, it reduced focus formation by 75% in comparison with controls. Cells were treated with the carcinogen and the carotenoid simultaneously, and the carotenoid was maintained for an additional seven days followed by seven weeks with no treatment. Simultaneous treatment by a different protocol was shown to reduce the extent of covalent binding of benzo[*a*]pyrene to DNA (Chang *et al.*, 1996).

Treatment of normal mouse mammary cells with DMBA produces nodule-like alveolar lesions, which it has been suggested are premalignant (Table 49). β-Carotene at 10^{-6} mol/L in hexane reduced the incidence of these lesions by up to 60% (Som *et al.*, 1984). β-Carotene has also been shown to reduce the excess incidence of sister chromatid exchange produced in mouse mammary cells by exposure to DMBA or NDEA by up to 96%, when applied in hexane with simultaneous carcinogen treatment (Manoharan & Banerjee, 1985). For both end-points, the most effective reduction occurred when the

Table 48. Inhibition by carotenoids of carcinogen-induced neoplastic transformation

Cell line: end-point	Carcinogen (dose)	Treatment relative to carcinogen	Carotenoid (vehicle)[a]	Concentration (mol/L)	No. of foci/ no. of dishes	Preventive efficacy (% of vehicle control)		Comments	Reference
C3H 101/2: induction of neo-plastically trans-formed foci	MCA, 1 μg/ml, 24 h	7 days after then weekly	All-*trans* β-carotene (beadlets)	10^{-5}	0/24	0		β-Carotene less active than canthaxanthin across dose range 3×10^{-6}–10^{-6} mol/L ($p < 0.01$). Vehicle control (beadlets) did not differ from carcino-gen-only groups ($p = 0.78$)	Pung *et al.* (1988)
				3×10^{-6}	3/24	21.9	$p < 0.001$		
				10^{-6}	16/36	39.8	$p < 0.001$		
				3×10^{-7}	23/24	84.4	$p < 0.001$		
				10^{-7}	21/24	102.5			
				3×10^{-8}	22/24	103.0			
			Canthaxxthin (beadlets)	3×10^{-6}	0/21	0			
				10^{-6}	14/47	24.9	$p < 0.01$		
				3×10^{-7}	14/48	31.1	$p < 0.01$		
				10^{-7}	20/24	75.3	$p < 0.01$		
				3×10^{-8}	20/24	88.9			
				10^{-8}	21/24	100.2			
	No treatment			0	67/84				
					0/48				
C3H 10T1/2	X-ray 300 KPV 1.38 Gy/min	24 h prior and 1 h after radiation	All-*trans* β-carotene (beadlets)	10^{-5}	28/20	84	NS		Pung *et al.* (1988)
				10^{-6}	20/19	70	NS		
			Canthaxanthin (beadlets)	10^{-5}	26/20	72	NS		
				10^{-6}	22/20	58	NS		
				0	49/40				
C3H 10T1/2	X-ray, 6 Gy 300 KPV, 1.38 Gy/min	7 days after radiation then weekly	All-*trans* β-carotene (beadlets)	10^{-5}	4/20	6.0	$p < 0.01$	β–Carotene less active than cantha-xanthin at 3×10^{-6} mol/L ($p < 0.01$)	Pung *et al.* (1988)
				3×10^{-6}	23/20	40.0	$p < 0.01$		
				10^{-6}	35/20	64.0	$p < 0.03$		
			Canthaxanthin (beadlets)	3×10^{-6}	5/20	9.2	$p < 0.01$		
				10^{-6}	21/20	64.0	$p < 0.01$		
				3×10^{-7}	38/20	100			
	No treatment			0	223/80				
				0	4/20				

Table 48 (contd)

Cell line: end-point	Carcinogen (dose)	Treatment relative to carcinogen	Carotenoid (vehicle)[a]	Concentration (mol/L)	No. of foci/ no. of dishes	Preventive efficacy (% of vehicle control)		Comments	Reference
C3H 10T1/2	MCA, 3 μg/ml	7 days after MCA then weekly	Lycopene (solvent THF)	10^{-5}	16/24	45.3	$p < 0.01$		Bertram et al. (1991)
				3×10^{-6}	38/24	108.0	NS		
				10^{-6}	31/24	87.8			
				3×10^{-7}	64/24	181.2			
				0	108/72				
			α-Carotene (solvent THF)	10^{-5}	0/24	0	$p < 0.001$ for range		
				3×10^{-6}	19/24	53.8			
				10^{-6}	43/24	127.0			
				3×10^{-6}	44/24	124.0			
			Lutein (solvent THF)	10^{-5}	8.24	30	$p < 0.05$		
				3×10^{-6}	44/24	102			
				0	65/36				
C3H 10T1/2	Benzo[a]pyrene, 250 μg/ml	Simultaneously for 7 days	Crocetin (solvent DMSO)	10^{-4}	5/12			Dose–response increase in GST activity	Chang et al. (1996)
				5×10^{-5}	6/12				
				10^{-5}	15/12				
				0	21/12				

MCA, 3-methylcholanthrene; THF, tetrahydrofuran; DMSO, dimethylsulfoxide; NS, not significant; GST, glutathione S-transferase
[a] Beadlets: 10% carotenoid beadlets from Hoffmann-La Roche

Table 49. Inhibition by carotenoids of carcinogen-induced intermediate markers of response

Cell line: end-point	Carcinogen	Treatment relative to carcinogen	Carotenoid (vehicle)	Marker of response	Preventive efficacy	Reference
Mouse mammary cells: induction of nodule-like alveolar lesions	DMBA in DMSO, 7.8 μmol/L for 1 day on day 3–4 of culture		β-Carotene (solvent hexane), 10^{-6} mol/L	Lesions/glands	% reduction	Som et al. (1984)
		0–3 days		16/32	26	
		3–4 days		8/31	68	
		0–4 days		9/36	53	
		4–10 days		11/27		57
		0–10 days		10/33	26	
	DMSO			27/34	58	
				0/28	0	
Mouse mammary cells: induction of sister chromatid exchange	For 1 day on 3–4 of culture			Exchanges/chromosome	% reduction	Manoharan & Banerjee (1985)
	DMBA, 7.8 μmol/L	3–4 days	β-Carotene/hexane	0.25	96	
			Hexane control	0.55		
	NDEA, 14.6 μmol/L	3–4 days	β-Carotene/hexane	0.29	62	
			Hexane control	0.38		
	MNU, 1 μmol/L	3–4 days	β-Carotene/hexane	0.27	93	
			Hexane control	0.75		
	DMSO		No treatment	0.24		

carotenoids were added simultaneously with the carcinogen. [The Working Group noted that hexane was used as the solvent in both studies.]

(c) Effects on cell proliferation (see also Table 50)

Various carotenoids have been shown to reduce proliferation in a variety of cell lines. This action may be significant mechanistically in view of the role of proliferation in carcinogenesis and tumour progression (Ames *et al.*, 1993). β-Carotene and canthaxanthin caused small reductions in the logarithmic growth rates of mouse fibroblast 10T1/2 cells. Effective concentrations in transformation assays reduced the doubling time from 39 h in controls to 42 and 45 h in treated cell cultures, respectively. In carcinogen-initiated cells, these carotenoids caused 13 and 20% reductions in saturation density, respectively (Pung *et al.*, 1988). This reduction was not considered to contribute materially to the suppression of transformation. Reductions in proliferation have not been reported consistently: no effects were reported in normal or neoplastic mouse lung cells, whereas the same authors found decreased proliferation in 10T1/2 cells (Banoub *et al.*, 1996). In human cervical dysplastic and neoplastic cell lines, β-carotene at 10^{-5} mol/L caused an up to twofold increase in doubling time in dysplastic but not in cancer cells and reduced the expression of the epidermal growth factor receptor (Muto *et al.*, 1995). In human GOTO neuroblastoma cells, an interesting differential effect of α-carotene versus β-carotene was reported: while both compounds suppressed proliferation, α-carotene was about 10 times more active than the β-carotene and was cytostatic at 5×10^{-6} mol/L and cytotoxic at 10^{-5} mol/L. Cells were arrested in G_1 or G_0 and expressed less N-*myc* mRNA (Murakoshi *et al.*, 1989). Other carotenoids are also effective. Lycopene strongly inhibited proliferation of human endometrial (Ishikawa), mammary (MCF-7) and lung (NCI-H226) cancer cells, but α-carotene and β-carotene were far less effective. In contrast to cancer cells, normal human fibroblasts were less sensitive to lycopene (Levy *et al.*, 1995). The effects of β-carotene on human embryo fibroblasts was analysed by flow cytometry; a concentration of 2×10^{-5} mol/L for three days caused a 30% reduction in cell number and a 66% reduction in S-phase cells (Stivala *et al.*, 1996).

β-Carotene inhibited the growth of both nontumorigenic and tumorigenic human parotid acinar cells *in vitro*. The tumorigenic cells were clearly more sensitive to this effect, resulting in extensive morphological changes. Some dose–response relationship was seen (10 mg/ml versus 20 mg/ml). A mixture of β-carotene and α-tocopherol inhibited growth even more, but addition of vitamin C and/or retinoic acid did not increase the effect (Prasad & Kumar, 1996). In contrast, 1 μmol/L β-carotene stimulated the proliferation of mouse 3T3 cells, and the effect was more pronounced in the presence of higher serum concentrations; thus, at 10% serum, β-carotene almost doubled the incorporation of radiolabelled thymidine. The proliferative response to TPA was also statistically significantly increased ($p < 0.05$; Student's *t* test), and the levels of ornithine decarboxylase in β-carotene-treated cultures were increased (Okai *et al.*, 1996a). [The Working Group noted that the method of supplying the carotenoid to the cells was not described, and cellular uptake was not demonstrated.]

(d) Effects on tumour promotion (see also Table 50)

The ability of carotenoids to interfere with tumour promotion has been examined in two studies. In one, crocetin at 10^{-5} mol/L inhibited the translocation of protein kinase C from the cytoplasm to the membrane and reduced TPA-induced protein phosphorylation (Wang, C.-J. *et al.*, 1996). In a second study, β-carotene at 10^{-4}–10^{-5} mol/L inhibited protein phosphorylation induced by microcystin in mouse heptocytes and also suppressed the morphological changes (Matsushima-Nishiwaki *et al.*, 1995). The ability of a large series of carotenoids to inhibit the ability of TPA to activate Epstein-Barr virus in human Raji cells was examined. Simultaneous exposure of cells to TPA and carotenoids (at 16 μmol/L), both dissolved in dimethylsulfoxide, reduced activation of the

Table 50. Effects of carotenoids on cell proliferation, differentiation and tumour promotion

Cell line: end-point	Carotenoid (vehicle)	Concentration	Response	Comments	Reference
Human GOTO neuroblastoma cells: proliferation	α-Carotene	10^{-5} mol/L for 5 days 5×10^{-6} mol/L	Cytotoxic Cytostatic	Rapid cell loss	Murakoshi et al. (1989)
	β-Carotene (emulsion)	2×10^{-6} mol/L for 5 days 2×10^{-5} mol/L	Partial growth arrest Partial growth arrest	Comparable to 2×10^{-6} mol/L α-carotene	
Human embryonic fibroblasts: proliferation	β-Carotene (liposomes)	2.1×10^{-5} mol/L for 3 days	30% reduction in cell number, 66% reduction in S-phase cells	Decrease in S-phase cells	Stivala et al. (1996)
Human cervical cancer and dysplastic cell lines: proliferation; EGF receptor	β-Carotene (liposomes)	10^{-5} mol/L for 7 days	Reduction in growth rate for dysplastic but not cancer lines	Reduction in EGF binding and receptors in dysplastic lines	Muto et al. (1995)
Human normal keratinocytes, squamous-cell carcinoma, lung carcinoma lines: viability	β-Carotene or canthaxanthin (liposomes)	7×10^{-5} mol/L 3×10^{-4} mol/L for 5 h	Increased viability in normal cells, decreased in tumour cells (25%) versus controls	Little evidence for a dose–response relationship	Schwartz et al. (1990)
Human endometrial, mammary and lung cancer cell lines, normal human fibroblasts: proliferation	Lycopene, α- and β-carotene (THF)	$< 2 \times 10^{-6}$ mol/L for 1–4 days	Lycopene inhibited cell proliferation more effectively than α- or β-carotene	4–10 fold higher concentrations needed for α- and β-carotene effects	Levy et al. (1995)
Mouse normal and neoplastic lung cells C3H 10T/1/2 cells: proliferation	β-Carotene (dimethylformamide)	10^{-6}–10^{-5} mol/L for 1–5 days	No effect on proliferation Decreased proliferation	Bioavailability in dimethylformamide not assessed	Banoub et al. (1996)
F9 Embryonal cells: RAR-β reporter gene: differentiation; morphology; collagen expression	β-Carotene, canthaxanthin (THF)	10^{-5} mol/L for 5 days	Both carotenoids increased reporter gene expression and markers of differentiation	Carotenoids 10-fold less active than retinoic acid	Nikawa et al. (1995)

Table 50 (contd)

Cell line: end-point	Carotenoid (vehicle)	Concentration	Response	Comments	Reference
Human keratinocytes in organotypic culture: expression of markers of differentiation	β-Carotene, canthaxanthin (THF)	10^{-5} mol/L; 10^{-6} mol/L for 7 days	Both decreased expression of the 'mature' genes *keratin* 10 and *fillagrin*. No effect on basal keratin 14	Similar response seen with 10^{-6} mol/L retinoic acid	Bertram & Bortkiewicz (1995)
Mouse fibroblasts: induction of gap-junctional communication	Cathaxanthin, β-carotene lutein, α-carotene, lycopene (THF)	10^{-6}–10^{-5} mol/L	Increased communication	Activity in order listed: correlated with inhibition of carcinogenesis. Similar activity on *connexin* 43 expression	Zhang et al. (1992)
Human HL-60 cells: induction of markers of differentiation	β-Carotene, lutein (ethanol)	10^{-5} mol/L	Increased granulocyte differentiation	Equally active but much less active than retinoic acid	Gross et al. (1997)
Mouse Balb/c 3T3 cells: protein kinase C translocation	Crocetin (solvent not stated)	10^{-5} mol/L	Inhibited TPA-induced translocation and protein phosphorylation		Wang, C.-J. et al. (1996)
Mouse hepatocytes: inhibition of microcystin-induced protein phosphorylation	β-Carotene (liposomes)	10^{-5}–10^{-4} mol/L	Dose–response relationship in reduction in protein phosphorylation	Induction of morphological changes also suppressed	Matsushima-Nishiwaki et al. (1995)
Mouse Balb/c 3T3 cells: proliferation	β-Carotene (hexane)	10^{-6} mol/L	Increased cell numbers and TdR incorporation	Also increased ODC activity	Okai et al. (1996a)
Human Raji cells: expression of HPV antigen	β-Carotene (DMSO) α-Carotene Lutein Lycopene	16 μmol/L 16 μmol/L 16 μmol/L 16 μmol/L	25% reduction in expression 7.5% 11.8% 32.5%		Tsushima et al. (1995)

EGF, epidermal growth factor, THF, tetrahydrofuran; TPA, 12-O-tetradecanoylphorbol 13-acetate; ODC, ornithine decarboxylase; HPV, human papillomavirus; DMSO, dimethylsulfoxide virus by TPA, the order of potency being α-carotene (1.5%), β-carotene (25%), lycopene (32%) and canthaxanthin (47%), in comparison with TPA-treated controls (Tsushima *et al.*, 1995). [The Working Group noted that the effects on tumour promoters may be significant since carotenoids appear to inhibit post-initiation events.]

(e) Effects on cell differentiation (see also Table 50)

The human promyelocytic cell line HL-60 has been used widely in studies of differentiating agents. β-Carotene and lutein, supplied in ethanol at a concentration of 10^{-5} mol/L, have both been shown to induce granulocyte differentiation (Gross *et al.*, 1997). These compounds were, however, much less active than retinoic acid, which is now used clinically to induce differentiation in promyelocytic leukaemia. β-Carotene and canthaxanthin also modified the differentiation profile of human keratinocytes grown in organotypic culture. Concentrations of 10^{-6}–10^{-5} mol/L decreased the expression of mature *keratin 1* and increased the expression of the gap junction gene *connexin 43*, both expressed in suprabasal cells. Similar changes were produced by retinoic acid, but at lower concentrations. No effects were seen on basally expressed keratin (Bertram & Bortkiewicz, 1995). Thus, carotenoids appear to express many of the activities of retinoic acid but must be added at higher concentrations. Two studies have addressed the molecular basis of this activity by discerning whether conversion to retinoids is involved: in one, canthaxanthin was shown to up-regulate the expression of *connexin 43* but not *RAR-β*, a gene driven by a known retinoid-responsive element. In 10T1/2 and F9 cells, retinoic acid up-regulated the expression of both genes, which suggests that carotenoids act independently (Zhang *et al.*, 1992). Other investigators examined the ability of canthaxanthin to increase the expression of a reporter gene driven by the *RAR-β* promoter. The gene was activated, and an active retinoid (4-oxoretinoic acid) was shown chemically to be produced from canthaxanthin (Nikawa *et al.*, 1995).

(f) Protection from oxidative damage (see also Table 51)

An action shared by most, if not all, carotenoids, but to different degrees, is the ability to protect biological membranes from oxidative damage. In general, the ability of carotenoids to protect against exogenous free radical-initiated damage has been examined. This activity has been described for synthetic liposomes, in which β-carotene and canthaxanthin were equally active in preventing damage (Krinsky & Deneke, 1982); for lipid extracted from rat liver microsomes, in which the addition of β-carotene in hexane prevented damage (Palozza & Krinsky, 1991); and in rat liver microsomes themselves, in which addition of β-carotene in a chloroform–methanol solution prevented the formation of oxidation products. The activity of β-carotene appears to be synergistic with that of α-tocopherol (Palozza & Krinsky, 1992b).

Few investigators have examined the effects of carotenoids under more physiological conditions. In one study, feeding canthaxanthin as a beadlet formulation to vitamin E- and selenium-deficient chicks resulted in fewer oxidation products in liver membranes; however, this study was complicated by an increased concentration of α-tocopherol in the membranes which appeared to confer more protection than that afforded by canthaxanthin (Mayne & Parker, 1989). In a second study, conducted in cultured mouse fibroblasts, the addition of diverse carotenoids in tetrahydrofuran decreased the spontaneous production of membrane oxidation products, measured as thiobarbituric acid-reactive substances. While all carotenoids tested decreased production, the activity did not correlate with their ability to protect against neoplastic transformation or to increase the expression of *connexin 43* (Zhang *et al.*, 1991). In a clinical study, formation of thiobarbituric acid-reactive substances in plasma correlated negatively with total carotenoid serum concentrations; the effect was also found in cell cultures (Franke *et al.*, 1994).

(g) Effects on immune function in vitro (see also Table 52)

Carotenoids have been shown to enhance immune responsiveness. Incubation of human

Table 51. Effects of carotenoids on lipid oxidation *in vitro*

Test system	Carotenoid (solvent)	Concentration	Response	Comments	Reference
Synthetic liposomes: free radical-initiated damage	β-Carotene (lipid) Canthaxanthin (lipid)	5.5 mmol/mol 6.35 mmol/mol	Decreased oxidation products	Equal activity	Krinsky & Deneke (1982)
Rat liver microsome lipids: free radical-initiated damage	β-Carotene (hexane); cell-free	2–10 μmol/L	Decreased oxidation products	Additive with α-tocopherol	Palozza & Krinsky (1991)
Oxidation of methyl-linoleate: free radical-initiated damage	β-Carotene (chlorobenzene)	0.05–5 mmol/L	Decreased oxidation	More efficient at low pO_2	Burton & Ingold (1984)
Rat liver microsomes: free radical-initiated damage	β-Carotene (chloroform: methanol) cell-free	10 μmol/mg protein	Decreased oxidation products	Apparent synergy with α-tocopherol	Palozza & Krinsky (1992a)
Vitamin E- and selenium-deficient chicks: oxidation of liver membranes	Canthaxanthin (beadlets)	5 g/kg diet	Decreased oxidation products	Main protection due to increased vitamin E	Mayne & Parker (1989)
Mouse fibroblasts: membrane oxidation	β-Carotene (THF)	10^{-5} mol/L	Decreased oxidation products		Franke *et al.* (1994)
Mouse fibroblasts:membrane oxidation	Lutein, lycopene, methyl-bixin canthaxanthin, β-carotene, α-carotene (THF)	3×10^{-6} mol/L	Decreased oxidation products	Activity in order listed: not correlated with inhibition of carcinogenesis	Zhang *et al.* (1991)

THF, tetrahydrofuran

Table 52. Effects of carotenoids on immune function *in vitro*

Test system: end-point	Carotenoid	Concentration (mol/L)	Response	Magnitude	Comments	Reference
Expression of Fcγ receptors on human monocytes	β-Carotene	3×10^{-6}, 1 day	Inhibition of suppression induced by retinoic acid and by tumour extract	No increase in control expression of Fc receptors		Geisen et al. (1997)
Human T lympho-cytes: activation markers	Ethanol β-Carotene Canthaxanthin	10^{-8}	Increase in NK cells and cells with activation markers	5% 40% 60%	Response differed qualitatively from 13-cis-retinoic acid	Prabhala et al. (1989)
Mouse spleen cells: antibody production; cytokine secretion	Astaxanthin Zeaxanthin Lutein Lycopene Canthaxanthin Ethanol:hexane, 49:1	10^{-8}, 3 days	Increased reactivity No consistent response	2–3-fold increase over controls		Jyonouchi et al. (1996)
Mouse spleen cells: antibody production	Astaxanthin Lutein β-Carotene Ethanol:hexane, 49:1	10^{-8}	Increased reactivity Increased reactivity No consistent response	2–5-fold increase over controls		Lin et al. (1997)
Mouse spleen cells: response to antigen in vitro and in vivo	Astaxanthin β-Carotene Ethanol:hexane, 49:1	10^{-8} 10^{-8} 5 days	Astaxanthin but not β-carotene increased response to suboptimal antigen	2–5-fold increase over controls		Jyonouchi et al. (1995)
Human leukocytes: cytotoxic cytokine secretion	α-Carotene, β-carotene (ethanol)	10^{-9}–0.5×10^{-10}, 2 days	Increased secretion	60% decrease in proliferation		Abril et al. (1989)

peripheral blood mononuclear cells for 72 h with β-carotene or canthaxanthin at 10^{-8} mol/L in ethanol increased the number of cells expressing markers for natural killer cells, from about 5% to 40 and 60%, respectively, while the percentage of cells expressing the IL-2 receptor increased from about 5 to 20%. Similar changes were seen after exposure to retinoids (Prabhala *et al.*, 1989). Increased antibody production in response to challenge was reported in mouse spleen cells after treatment with carotenoids, including astaxanthin, lutein and β-carotene, all at 10^{-8} mol/L. This response appeared to depend upon T-lymphocyte activation. In the numerous assays evaluated, astaxanthin was generally the most potent carotenoid tested (Jyonouchi *et al.*, 1995, 1996; Lin *et al.*, 1997). [The Working Group noted that these authors used a methanol–hexane mixture to deliver the carotenoids to the cell cultures, and the bioavailability of the carotenoids was not determined.] Exposure of human mononuclear cells to β-carotene dissolved in methanol at 10^{-10} mol/L induced the secretion of a novel cytotoxic cytokine into the culture medium. This cytokine inhibited the growth of some human tumour cells but stimulated the growth of others. This activity was not seen with several retinoids that were tested (Abril *et al.*, 1989). [The Working Group noted that this effect, seen at an extremely low concentration, has not been replicated.] In other studies, β-carotene at 3×10^{-6} mol/L in chloroform inhibited the suppressive activity of retinoids on interferon secretion by human macrophages. Thus, in this system, carotenoids appear to antagonize the action of retinoids; no explanation was proposed for this unusual finding (Geisen *et al.*, 1997).

4.2.2.2 Antimutagenicity in short-term tests
Many studies have addressed the antimutagenic effects of carotenoids in short-term tests with prokaryotes and eukaryotes *in vitro*, and these have been reviewed (Krinsky, 1993a,b, 1994; Odin, 1997). Antimutagenicity profiles have been prepared for a limited number of assays of β-carotene (Waters *et al.*, 1990; Brockman *et al.*, 1992); these are shown graphically in Figure 7.

The results of studies with prokaryotes are summarized in Table 53.

umu C gene expression induced by the heterocyclic amine 3-amino-3,4-dimethyl-5*H*-pyrido[4,3-*b*]indole (Trp-P-1) in the TA1535/pSK strain 1002 of *Salmonella typhimurium* was inhibited by both β-carotene and canthaxanthin, with 50% inhibitory doses of 4.0×10^{-2} and 1.5×10^{-3} mmol/L, respectively. β-Carotene was ineffective when *umu* C expression was induced by the directly acting mutagens adriamycin and mitomycin C (Okai *et al.*, 1996b).

In Ames' *Salmonella*/microsome test, carotenoids appear in general to inhibit the mutagenicity of promutagens and to be ineffective against directly acting mutagens; however, conflicting data were generated in various laboratories with various mutagens. Thus, with regard to directly acting mutagens, β-carotene and canthaxanthin had no effect on the mutagenicity of MNNG in strains TA1535 and TA100 in one study (Santamaria *et al.*, 1988), whereas in another, β-carotene, canthaxanthin, 8'-apo-β-carotenal and 8'-apo-β-carotenoyl methyl-ester [The Working Group noted that the authors reported this carotenoid as '...carotene methylester'.] were found to inhibit the mutagenicity of the same compound in strain TA100, with dose-related effects (Azuine *et al.*, 1992). β-Carotene did not affect the direct mutagenicity of 4-NQO in strain TA100 (Camoirano *et al.*, 1994) and had a negligible or poor effect on the mutagenicity in TA100 of four directly acting complex mixtures, i.e. coal dust, diesel emission particles, tobacco snuff and airborne particles, with maximum inhibition of 11, 16, 16 and 39%, respectively (Ong *et al.*, 1989). β-Carotene did not affect the direct mutagenicity of 2-nitrofluorene in strain TA98, but decreased those of 1-nitropyrene and 3-nitrofluoranthene (Tang & Edenharder, 1997). The mutagenicity of 1-nitropyrene in strain YG1024 was also inhibited by lutein and by the xanthophylls (largely lutein) extracted from Aztec marigold (*Tagetes erecta*). Lutein had no effect on the DNA repair system of 1-nitropyrene-treated YG1024 (González de Mejía *et al.*, 1997a).

β-Carotene and canthaxanthin inhibited the mutagenicity induced in strain TA102 by 8-methoxypsoralen after UV-A irradiation in a

Figure 7. Antimutagenicity profile of β-carotene

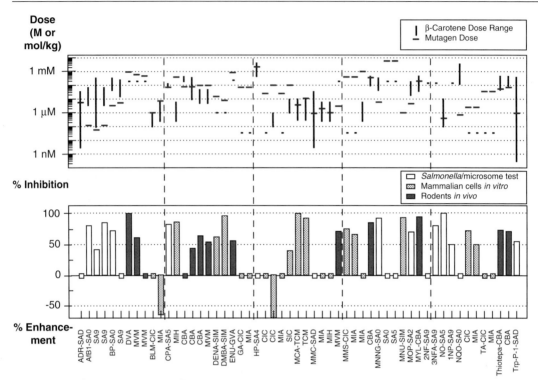

For definitions of test codes, see Appendix 2.
AFB₁, aflatoxin B₁; BP, benzo[a]pyrene; MNNG, N-methyl-N'-nitro-N-nitrosoguanidine; NDEA, N-nitrosodiethylamine; DMBA, 7,12-dimethylbenz[a]anthracene; MNU, N-methyl-N-nitrosourea; 4NQO, 4-nitroquinoline 1-oxide; BLM, bleomycin; GA, gallic acid; H₂O₂, hydrogen peroxide; MMC, mitomycin C; MMS, methylmethane sulfonate; TA, tannic acid; MCA, 3-methylcholanthrene; CPA, cyclophosphamide; ENU, N-ethyl-N-nitrosourea; Myl, myleran ; TT, thio-TEPA

normal atmosphere. In a nitrogen atmosphere, the photomutagenicity was decreased by 65%, and the two carotenoids had no protective effect (Santamaria *et al.*, 1988). β-Carotene, preincubated with bacterial broth cultures, inhibited the mutagenicity induced by nitric oxide or a mixture of nitric oxide plus nitrogen dioxide in strain TA1535 (Arroyo *et al.*, 1992). β-Carotene did not decrease the mutagenicity of hydrogen peroxide in strain TA104 (Han, 1992).

Most assays of promutagens in Ames' test showed protective effects of carotenoids. β-Carotene inhibited the mutagenicity of cyclophosphamide mediated by an exogenous metabolic system derived from a 9000 x *g* supernatant of rat liver (S9) in strain TA1535. Moreover, the mutagenicity of urine in the same strain was inhibited when the rats were treated simultaneously with cyclophosphamide and β-carotene, but not when β-carotene was added to the urine of cyclophosphamide-treated rats (Belisario *et al.*, 1985). The mutagenicity of aflatoxin B₁ in TA98 was decreased in the presence of β-carotene, with a maximum inhibition of 45% (Whong *et al.*, 1988), and by β-carotene, canthaxanthin, cryptoxanthin (extracted from orange juice) and a chloroform extract of carrot (51% β-carotene, 32% α-carotene and 17% other carotenoids). The doses of these compounds required to inhibit mutagenicity by 65% were 22, 37, 3 and 16 µg/plate in TA98, and 42, 44, 1 and 23 µg/plate in TA100, respectively. Inhibition by β-carotene and canthaxanthin was stronger during the metabolic

Table 53. Inhibition by carotenoids of standard mutagens in the *Salmonella*/microsome test

End-point	Code	Carotenoid (tested doses)[a]	Mutagen (tested doses)	S. typhimurium strain	Result[a]	S9 mix	LED/HID[b]	Reference
D	SAD	β-Carotene (0.0003–300 μmol/plate)	3-Amino-3,4-dimethyl-5H-pyrido[4,3-b]indole (Trp-P-1) (0.2 μg/ml)	TA1535/pSK1002	+	+	40 μmol/plate (ID_{50})	Okai et al. (1996b)
D	SAD	Canthaxanthin (0.0003–300 μmol/plate)	3-Amino-3,4-dimethyl-5H-pyrido[4,3-b]indole (Trp-P-1) (0.2 μg/ml)	TA1535/pSK1002	+	+	1.5 μmol/plate (ID_{80})	Okai et al. (1996b)
D	SAD	β-Carotene (0.003–30 μmol/plate)	Adriamycin (3 μg/ml)	TA1535/pSK1002	–	–	30 μmol/plate	Okai et al. (1996b)
D	SAD	β-Carotene (0.003–30 μmol/plate)	Mitomycin C (0.3 μg/ml)	TA1535/pSK1002	–	–	30 μmol/plate	Okai et al. (1996b)
G	SA5	β-Carotene (100–200 μg/plate)	Cyclophosphamide (50–300 μg/plate)	TA1535	+	+	200 μg/plate (ID_{74})	Belisario et al. (1985)
G	SA5	β-Carotene (0.1–10 μmol/plate)	Nitric oxide (10 ppm) or nitric oxide (8 ppm) plus nitrogen dioxide (5 ppm)	TA1535	+	–	1.0 μmol/plate	Arroyo et al. (1992)
G	SA9	β-Carotene (31.25–500 μg/plate)	Cigarette smoke condensate (0.01 cigarette equivalent/plate)	TA98	–	+	500 μg/plate	Terwel & van der Hoeven (1985)
G	SA9	β-Carotene (31.25–500 μg/plate)	Benzo[a]pyrene (5 μg/plate)	TA98	–	+	500 μg/plate	Terwel & van der Hoeven (1985)
G	SA2	β-Carotene (18.6 and 186 μmol/plate)	8-Methoxypsoralen (4.6 μmol/plate) + UV-A ($3–9 \times 10^3$ erg/cm²)	TA102	+	–	18.6 μmol/plate	Santamaria et al. (1988)
G	SA2	Canthaxanthin (dose unspecified)	8-Methoxypsoralen (4.6 μmol/plate) + UV-A ($3–9 \times 10^3$ ergs/cm²)	TA102	+	–	(dose unspecified)	Santamaria et al. (1988)
G	SA4	β-Carotene (1–10 μmol/plate)	Hydrogen peroxide (5 μmol/plate)	TA104	–	–	10 μmol/plate	Han (1992)

Table 53 (contd)

End-point	Code	Carotenoid (tested doses)[a]	Mutagen (tested doses)[a]	S. typhimurium strain	S9 mix	Result[b]	LED/HID[c]	Reference
G	SA9	β-Carotene (≤0.4 μmol/plate)	2-Nitrofluorene (dose unspecified)	TA98	–	–	0.4 μmol/plate	Tang & Edenharder (1997)
G	SA9	β-Carotene (≤0.4 μmol/plate)	1-Nitropyrene (dose unspecified)	TA98	–	+	0.4 μmol/plate (ID$_{80}$)	Tang & Edenharder (1997)
G	SA9	β-Carotene (≤0.4 μmol/plate)	3-Nitrofluoranthene (dose unspecified)	TA98	–	+	0.4 μmol/plate (ID$_{80}$)	Tang & Edenharder (1997)
G	SAS	Lutein (0.002–10 μg/plate)	1-Nitropyrene (0.06 μg/plate)	YG1024	–	+	0.2 μg/plate (ID$_{57}$)	Gonzáles de Mejia et al. (1997a)
G	SAS	Oleoresin (0.002–10 μg equivalents lutein/plate)	1-Nitropyrene (0.06 μg/plate)	YG1024	–	+	2 μg/plate (ID$_{83}$)	Gonzáles de Mejia et al. (1997a)
G	SAS	Xanthophyll (0.002–10 μg equivalents lutein/plate)	1-Nitropyrene (0.06 μg/plate)	YG1024	–	+	0.2 μg/plate (ID$_{52}$)	Gonzáles de Mejia et al. (1997a)
G	SA0	β-Carotene (186 μmol/plate)	N-Methyl-N'-nitro-N-nitrosoguanidine (3.4–13.6 μmol/plate)	TA100	–	–	186 μmol/plate	Santamaria et al. (1988)
G	SA5	β-Carotene (186 μmol/plate)	N-Methyl-N'-nitro-N-nitrosoguanidine (3.4–13.6 μmol/plate)	TA1535	–	–	186 μmol/plate	Santamaria et al. (1988)
G	SA0	Canthaxanthin (182 μmol/plate)	N-Methyl-N'-nitro-N-nitrosoguanidine (3.4–13.6 μmol/plate)	TA100	–	–	182 μmol/plate	Santamaria et al. (1988)
G	SA5	Canthaxanthin (182 μmol/plate)	N-Methyl-N'-nitro-N-nitrosoguanidine (3.4–13.6 μmol/plate)	TA1535	–	–	182 μmol/plate	Santamaria et al. (1988)
G	SA9	β-Carotene (type III) (0.00026–0.86 μmol/plate)	Aflatoxin B$_1$ (50 ng/plate)	TA98	+	+	0.86 μmol/plate (ID$_{42}$)	Whong et al. (1988)

Table 53 (contd)

End-point Code	Carotenoid (tested doses)[a]	Mutagen(tested doses)[a]	S. typhimurium strain	S9 mix	Result[b]	LED/HID[c]	Reference
G	SA9	β-Carotene (type III) (0.43–3.45 µmol/plate)	Fried beef (750 mg/plate)	TA98	+	–	3.45 µmol/plate	Ong et al. (1989)
G	SA9	β-Carotene (type III) (0.43–3.45 µmol/plate)	Coal dust (75 mg/plate)	TA98	–	–	3.45 µmol/plate	Ong et al. (1989)
G	SA9	β-Carotene (type III) (0.43–3.45 µmol/plate)	Diesel emission particles (2 mg/plate)	TA98	–	–	3.45 µmol/plate	Ong et al. (1989)
G	SA9	β-Carotene (type III) (0.43–3.45 µmol/plate)	Tobacco snuff (85 mg/plate)	TA98	–	–	3.45 µmol/plate	Ong et al. (1989)
G	SA9	β-Carotene (type III) (0.43–3.45 µmol/plate)	Airborne particles (4 mg/plate)	TA98	–	(+)	3.45 µmol/plate (ID$_{39}$)	Ong et al. (1989)
G	SA0	β-Carotene (5–100 µg/plate)	Aflatoxin B$_1$ (100 ng/plate)	TA100	+	+	42 µg/plate (ID$_{65}$)	He & Campbell (1990)
G	SA9	β-Carotene (5–100 µg/plate)	Aflatoxin B$_1$ (100 ng/plate)	TA98	+	+	22 µg/plate (ID$_{65}$)	He & Campbell (1990)
G	SA0	Canthaxanthin (5–100 µg/plate)	Aflatoxin B$_1$ (100 ng/plate)	TA100	+	+	44 µg/plate (ID$_{65}$)	He & Campbell (1990)
G	SA9	Canthaxanthin (5–100 µg/plate)	Aflatoxin B$_1$ (100 ng/plate)	TA98	+	+	37 µg/plate (ID$_{65}$)	He & Campbell (1990)
G	SA0	Cryptoxanthin (extracted from orange juice) (5–100 µg/plate)	Aflatoxin B$_1$ (100 ng/plate)	TA100	+	+	1 µg/plate (ID$_{65}$)	He & Campbell (1990)
G	SA9	Cryptoxanthin (extracted from orange juice) (5–100 µg/plate)	Aflatoxin B$_1$ (100 ng/plate)	TA98	+	+	3 µg/plate (ID$_{65}$)	He & Campbell (1990)
G	SA0	Carrot carotenoids (51% β-carotene, 32% β-carotene, 17% other carotenoids) (5–100 µg/plate)	Aflatoxin B$_1$ (100 ng/plate)	TA100	+	+	23 µg/plate (ID$_{65}$)	He & Campbell (1990)

Table 53 (contd)

End–point Code		Carotenoid (tested doses)[a]	Mutagen (tested doses)[a]	S. typhimurium strain	S9 mix	Result[b]	LED/HID[c]	Reference
G	SA9	Carrot carotenoids (51% β-carotene, 32% β-carotene, 17% other carotenoids) (5–100 µg/plate)	Aflatoxin B_1 (100 ng/plate)	TA98	+	+	16 µg/plate (ID_{65})	He & Campbell (1990)
G	SA0	Lycopene (extracted from tomato paste) (5–100 µg/plate)	Aflatoxin B_1 (100 ng/plate)	TA100	+	–	100 µg/plate	He & Campbell (1990)
G	SA9	Lycopene (extracted from tomato paste) (5–100 µg/plate)	Aflatoxin B_1 (100 ng/plate)	TA98	+	–	100 µg/plate	He & Campbell (1990)
G	SAS	Lutein (0.002–10 µg/plate)	Aflatoxin B_1 (0.5 µg/plate)	YG1024	+	+	10 µg/plate (ID_{49})	Gonzáles de Mejia et al. (1997b)
G	SAS	Oleoresin (0.002–10 µg equivalents lutein/plate)	Aflatoxin B_1 (0.5 µg/plate)	YG1024	+	+	2 µg/plate (ID_{66})	Gonzáles de Mejia et al. (1997b)
G	SAS	Xanthophyll plus (0.002–2 µg equivalents lutein/plate)	Aflatoxin B_1 (0.5 µg/plate)	YG1024	+	+	0.002 µg/plate (ID_{52})	Gonzáles de Mejia et al. (1997b)
G	SA0	β-Carotene (50–800 nmol/plate [?])[c]	1-Methyl-3-nitro-1-nitrosoguanidine (13.6 nmol/plate [?])	TA100	–	+	50 nmol/plate [?]	Azuine et al. (1992)
G	SA0	Canthaxanthin (50–800 nmol/plate [?])	1-Methyl-3-nitro-1-nitrosoguanidine (13.6 nmol/plate [?])	TA100	–	+	50 nmol/plate [?]	Azuine et al. (1992)
G	SA0	8'-Apo-β-carotenal (50–800 nmol/plate [?])	1-Methyl-3-nitro-1-nitrosoguanidine (13.6 nmol/plate [?])	TA100	–	+	50 nmol/plate [?]	Azuine et al. (1992)

Table 53 (contd)

End-point Code	Carotenoid (tested doses)[a]	Mutagen (tested doses)[a]	S. typhimurium strain	S9 mix	Result[b]	LED/HID[c]	Reference
G	SA0	8′-Apo-β-carotenoyl methylester (50–800 nmol/plate [?])	1-Methyl-3-nitro-1-nitrosoguanidine (13.6 nmol/plate [?])	TA100	–	+	50 nmol/plate [?]	Azuine et al. (1992)
G	SA0	β-Carotene (50–800 nmol/plate [?])	Benzo[a]pyrene (7.6 nmol/plate [?])	TA100	+	+	50 nmol/plate [?]	Azuine et al. (1992)
G	SA0	Canthaxanthin (50–800 nmol/plate [?])	Benzo[a]pyrene (7.6 nmol/plate [?])	TA100	+	+	50 nmol/plate [?]	Azuine et al. (1992)
G	SA0	8′-Apo-β-carotenal (50–800 nmol/plate [?])	Benzo[a]pyrene (7.6 nmol/plate [?])	TA100	+	+	50 nmol/plate [?]	Azuine et al. (1992)
G	SA0	8′-Apo-β-carotenoyl methylester (50–800 nmol/plate [?])	Benzo[a]pyrene (7.6 nmol/plate [?])	TA100	+	+	50 nmol/plate [?]	Azuine et al. (1992)
G	SA0	trans-β-Carotene (0.33–10 µmol/plate)	4-Nitroquinoline 1-oxide (2 nmol/plate)	TA100	–	–	10 µmol/plate	Camoirano et al. (1994)
G	SA9	trans-β-Carotene (0.33–10 µmol/plate)	Cigarette smoke (0.5 cigarettes smoked in a 20-L chamber)	TA98	+	+	4.3 µmol/plate (ID$_{50}$)	Camoirano et al. (1994)
G	SA0	β-Carotene (62–2000 µg/plate)	Cigarette smoke condensate (0.4 mg/plate)	TA100	+	–	2000 µg/plate	Romert et al. (1994)
G	SA9	β-Carotene (62–2000 µg/plate)	Cigarette smoke condensate (0.4 mg/plate)	TA98	+	–	2000 µg/plate	Romert et al. (1994)

S9 mix, 9000 x g microsomal fraction used as exogenous metabolic system; UV, ultraviolet radiation; [?] The Working Group noted a probable mistake in the unit of concentration.
[a] +, inhibition of genotoxicity; (+), weak inhibition of genotoxicity; –, no inhibition of genotoxicity
[b] LED, lowest effective (inhibitory) dose; HID, highest ineffective dose; ID$_x$, dose inhibiting the mutagenicity by x%, as indicated by the authors
[c] Reported as '8'-Apo-β-carotene methylester'

activation phase, whereas cryptoxanthin was more effective during the subsequent phenotypic expression phase. In the same study, lycopene extracted from tomato paste did not affect the mutagenicity of aflatoxin B_1 (He & Campbell, 1990). The S9-mediated mutagenicity of aflatoxin B_1 in strain YG1024 was inhibited by lutein and marigold extract. Lutein had a modest effect on the DNA repair system of aflatoxin B_1-pretreated YG1024 (González de Mejía et al., 1997b). Azuine et al. (1992) reported dose-dependent inhibition of the mutagenicity of benzo[a]pyrene in TA100 by β-carotene, canthaxanthin, 8'-apo-β-carotenal and 8'-apo-β-carotenoyl methylester [reported as '...carotene methylester']. In contrast, Terwel and van der Hoeven (1985) found no inhibition of the mutagenicity of benzo[a]pyrene in TA98 by β-carotene.

No effect of β-carotene was found on the S9-mediated mutagenicity of a cigarette-smoke condensate in strain TA98 (Terwel & van der Hoeven, 1985), but dose-related inhibition of the mutagenicity of mainstream cigarette smoke was reported, the dose that inhibited 50% of mutagenicity being 4.3 μmol/plate (Camoirano et al., 1994). β-Carotene decreased the mutagenicity of a cigarette-smoke condensate in strain TA98 but was ineffective and even enhanced mutagenicity in strain TA100 (Romert et al., 1994). It had no effect on the S9-mediated mutagenicity of a fried beef extract (Ong et al., 1989).

The results of studies on cultured mammalian cells are summarized in Table 54. A few studies were conducted on the anticlastogenic properties of carotenoids in animal cells by evaluating inhibition of sister chromatid exchange, micronuclei or chromosomal aberrations. β-Carotene inhibited the induction of sister chromatid exchange in Chinese hamster ovary cells subjected to oxidative stress. Reactive oxygen species were generated either by reaction of hypoxanthine with xanthine oxidase or by stimulating human leukocytes with TPA (Weitberg et al., 1985). In the same cells, β-carotene inhibited the induction of sister chromatid exchange by hydrogen peroxide but increased the frequency of chromosomal aberrations induced by the same oxidizing agent and did not affect the frequency of bleomycin-induced chromosomal aberrations

(Cozzi et al., 1997). β-Carotene also inhibited sister chromatid exchange induced by DMBA, NDEA or MNU in cultured Balb/c mouse mammary glands (Manoharan & Banerjee, 1985). Chinese hamster ovary cells were pretreated with β-carotene and, before challenge with clastogens, were washed in such a way that protection could occur only at the cell membrane or within the cells. Under these conditions, β-carotene significantly decreased the frequency of micronuclei and chromosomal aberrations induced by either methyl methanesulfonate or 4-NQO but had no protective effect against hydrogen peroxide, tannic acid or gallic acid. β-Carotene also failed to modulate the chromosomal aberrations induced by an extract of areca (betel) nut (Stich & Dunn, 1986). Both β-carotene and canthaxanthin inhibited the intrinsic chromosome instability, measured in terms of frequency of chromatid bridges and fragments, in strains of C127 mouse cells that had been transformed by bovine papillomavirus DNA and carried 20–165 copies of viral DNA per cell (Stich et al., 1990b). The effect of β-carotene on the frequency of chemically induced micronuclei in cytochalasin-blocked binucleate Chinese hamster ovary cells was evaluated with four different procedures for combining β-carotene and clastogens—pretreatment, simultaneous treatment, pretreatment plus simultaneous treatment or post-treatment. Irrespective of the procedure used, β-carotene did not significantly affect the frequency of micronuclei induced by the alkylating agents methyl methanesulfonate and mitomycin C. In the case of the radiomimetic agent bleo-mycin, β-carotene even enhanced the frequency of micronuclei when assayed by all of the procedures except after treatment (Salvadori et al., 1994) .

Both β-carotene and canthaxanthin, added one week after removal of the transforming agent, inhibited the development of transformed foci induced by 3-methylcholanthrene in C3H 10T1/2 mouse fibroblasts. Neither carotenoid inhibited X-ray-induced transformation when the cells were treated before and during irradiation, but they inhibited the subsequent development of transformed foci when the drugs were added one week after X-irradiation (Pung et al., 1988). These results were confirmed and expanded by the same group (Bertram *et al.*, 1991), who showed that, when carotenoids were continuously administered to methylcholanthrene-treated fibroblasts one week after removal of the carcinogen, some inhibited the production of transformed foci in a dose-dependent manner. In order of potency, this effect was produced by canthaxanthin, β-carotene, α-carotene and lycopene. Lutein was inhibitory at one dose only; renierapurpurin and bixin were inactive. Treatment of mammary epithelial cells from whole female Balb/c mouse mammary glands cultivated in a hormone-supplemented medium with DMBA resulted in the appearance of nodule-like alveolar lesions, which were assumed to be morphological markers of preneoplasia. β-Carotene caused a 68% inhibition of these lesions when added during exposure to the carcinogen and a 49% inhibition when added after exposure. The authors interpreted these data as suggesting an effect of β-carotene at both the initiation and the promotion stages (Som *et al.*, 1984).

β-Carotene induced morphological differentiation in mouse B-16 melanoma cells, as shown by the enlargement of cells with two or more cytoplasmic processes, growth inhibition and reduced survival of cells. Although less effective than β-carotene, α-carotene significantly reduced the growth of melanoma cells (Hazuka *et al.*, 1990).

Several carotenoids have been shown to enhance gap-junctional intercellular communication and to up-regulate the expression of *connexin 43*, a gene that encodes a major gap-junction protein. β-Carotene, α-carotene, canthaxanthin, lutein and lycopene increased gap-junctional intercellular communication in C3H 10T1/2 mouse fibroblasts; only methyl-bixin was ineffective. All of the carotenoids inhibited lipid peroxidation; however, this did not correlate with their ability to inhibit transport (Zhang *et al.*, 1991). A significant correlation was found between enhancement of junctional communication and inhibition of the development of 3-methylcholanthrene-induced transformed foci (Bertram *et al.*, 1991). The same group showed that β-carotene, canthaxanthin and lycopene up-regulate *connexin 43* expression at the mRNA and protein levels in the

same cellular system; again methyl-bixin was ineffective. Canthaxanthin did not induce the vitamin A-inducible gene *RAR-β*, indicating that the effect of carotenoids on *connexin 43* is independent of their classical provitamin A role (Zhang *et al.*, 1992). Whether canthaxanthin acts *per se* or via the formation of breakdown products such as 4-oxoretinoic acid is still unclear. β-Carotene and canthaxin also increased *connexin 43* expression in cultured human fibroblasts (Zhang *et al.*, 1992). The effects of β-carotene on C3H 10T1/2 cells and *connexin 43* expression have been confirmed, but no such effect was observed in non-transformed (C10) or neoplastic (E9 and 82-132) murine lung epithelial cells (Banoub *et al.*, 1996). In a study of 12 carotenoids on gap-junctional intercellular communication in C3H 10T1/2 mouse fibroblasts, all of the carotenoids containing a six-membered β ring, i.e. β-carotene, echinenone, canthaxanthin, 4-hydroxy-β-carotene, β-cryptoxanthin and retrodehydro-β-carotene, increased intercellular communication, whereas those with a five-membered-ring end group, namely dinor-canthaxanthin and violerythrin, had a weak effect, and capsorubin had none. Acyclic carotenedials of different chain lengths, i.e. crocetindial (C_{20}), 4,4'-diapocarotene-4,4'-diol (C_{30}) and 3,4,3',4'-tetradehydro-ψ,ψ-carotene-16,16'-dial (C_{40}), also had no effect (Stahl *et al.*, 1997). The effect of carotenoids on gap-junctional intercellular communication was independent of their ability to quench singlet oxygen. [The Working Group noted that increased gap-junctional communication may be mechanistically significant, since transfection of *connexin 43*, leading to its overexpression, has been reported to suppress the neoplastic phenotype in transformed human and mouse cells (Zhu *et al.*, 1991; Rose *et al.*, 1993).]

[3]H-Aflatoxin B$_1$ was found to bind the DNA of cultured C3H 10T1/2 mouse cells in the presence of S9 fractions from Aroclor-pretreated Sprague-Dawley rats. Binding of aflatoxin B$_1$ to DNA was inhibited by crocetin (Table 54). In parallel, an increase was observed in cytosolic reduced glutathione and in the activities of glutathione *S*-transferase and glutathione peroxidase. In the same study, crocetin inhibited the

Table 54. Inhibition by carotenoids of genetic and related effects in cultured mammalian cells

End-point	Code	Carotenoid (tested doses)[a]	Genotoxic agent (tested doses)[a]	Cells	Investigated effect	Result[a]	LED/HID[b]	Reference
Animal cells								
S	SIC	β-Carotene (0.1 μmol/plate)	Hypoxanthine (7 μg/ml) + xanthine oxidase (15 μg/ml)	Chinese hamster ovary cells	Sister chromatid exchange	+	0.1 μmol/plate	Weitberg et al. (1985)
S	SIC	β-Carotene (5–10 μmol/plate)	Human white blood cells (10⁷ cells) + 12-O-tetra-decanoylphorbol 13-acetate (0.1 μg/ml)	Chinese hamster ovarycells	Sister chromatid exchange	+	5 μmol/plate	Weitberg et al. (1985)
S	SIC	β-Carotene (1–10 μmol/plate)	Hydrogen peroxide (100 μmol/plate)	Chinese hamster ovary cells	Sister chromatid exchange	+	1 μmol/plate	Cozzi et al. (1997)
S	SIM	β-Carotene (1 μmol/plate)	7,12-Dimethylbenz[a]-anthracene (7.8 μmol/plate)	BALB/c mouse mammary organ cultures	Sister chromatid exchange	+	1 μmol/plate	Manoharan & Banerjee (1985)
S	SIM	β-Carotene (1 μmol/plate)	N-Nitrosodiethylamine (14.6 μ/plate)	BALB/c mouse mammary organ cultures	Sister chromatid exchange	+	1 μmol/plate	Manoharan & Banerjee (1985)
S	SIM	β-Carotene (1 μmol/plate)	N-Methyl-N-nitrosourea (1 μmol/plate)	BALB/c mouse mammary organ cultures	Sister chromatid exchange	+	1 μmol/plate	Manoharan & Banerjee (1985)
M	MIA	β-Carotene (0.035 μmol/plate)	Methyl methanesulfonate (400 μmol/plate)	Chinese hamster ovary cells	Micronuclei	+	0.035 μmol/plate	Stich & Dunn (1986)
M	MIA	β-Carotene (0.035 μmol/plate)	4-Nitroquinoline 1-oxide (2.5 μmol/plate)	Chinese hamster ovary cells	Micronuclei	+	0.035 μmol/plate	Stich & Dunn (1986)
M	MIA	β-Carotene (0.035 μmol/plate)	Hydrogen peroxide (25 μmol/plate)	Chinese hamster ovary cells	Micronuclei	–	0.035 μmol/plate	Stich & Dunn (1986)
M	MIA	β-Carotene (0.035 μmol/plate)	Tannic acid (60 μg/mL)	Chinese hamster ovary cells	Micronuclei	–	0.035 μmol/plate	Stich & Dunn (1986)
M	MIA	β-Carotene (0.035 μmol/plate)	Gallic acid (12 μg/mL)	Chinese hamster ovary cells	Micronuclei	–	0.035 μmol/plate	Stich & Dunn (1986)
C	CIC	β-Carotene (0.035 μmol/plate)	Methyl methanesulfonate (400 μmol/plate)	Chinese hamster ovary cells	Chromosomal aberrations	+	0.035 μmol/plate	Stich & Dunn (1986)

Table 54 (contd)

End-point	Code	Carotenoid (tested doses)[a]	Genotoxic agent (tested doses)[a]	Cells	Investigated effect	Result[a]	LED/HID[b]	Reference
C	CIC	β-Carotene (0.035 µmol/plate)	4-Nitroquinoline 1-oxide (2.5 µmol/plate)	Chinese hamster ovary cells	Chromosomal aberrations	+	0.035 µmol/plate	Stich & Dunn (1986)
C	CIC	β-Carotene (0.035 µmol/plate)	Hydrogen peroxide (25 µmol/plate)	Chinese hamster ovary cells	Chromosomal aberrations	–	0.035 µmol/plate	Stich & Dunn (1986)
C	CIC	β-Carotene (0.035 µmol/plate)	Tannic acid (60 µg/mL)	Chinese hamster ovary cells	Chromosomal aberrations	–	0.035 µmol/plate	Stich & Dunn (1986)
C	CIC	β-Carotene (0.035 µmol/plate)	Gallic acid (12 µg/mL)	Chinese hamster ovary cells	Chromosomal aberrations	–	0.035 µmol/plate	Stich & Dunn (1986)
C	CIC	β-Carotene (0.035 µmol/plate)	Areca nut (8 µg/ml/plate)	Chinese hamster ovary cells	Chromosomal aberrations	–	0.035 µmol/plate	Stich & Dunn (1986)
C	CIC	β-Carotene (0.1–1 µmol/plate)	Hydrogen peroxide (100 µmol/plate)	Chinese hamster ovary cells	Chromosomal aberrations	#	0.1 µmol/plate	Cozzi et al. (1997)
C	CIC	β-Carotene (0.1–1 µmol/plate)	Bleomycin (1 µg/mL)	Chinese hamster ovary cells	Chromosomal aberrations	–	1 µmol/plate	Cozzi et al. (1997)
C	CIT	β-Carotene (0.5 µmol/plate)	None	C127 mouse cells transformed by bovine papillomavirus DNA	Chromosome instability (chromatid bridges and fragments)	+	0.5 µmol/plate	Stich et al. (1990b)
C	CIT	Canthaxanthin (0.5 µmol/plate)	None	C127 mouse cells transformed by bovine papillomavirus DNA	Chromosome instability (chromatid bridges and fragments)	+	0.5 µmol/plate	Stich et al. (1990b)
M	MIA	β-Carotene (0.25–6.0 µmol/plate)	Methylmethane sulfonate (1 µmol/plate)	Chinese hamster ovary cells	Micronuclei in binucleated cells	–	6.0 µmol/plate	Salvadori et al. (1994)
M	MIA	β-Carotene (0.25–6.0 µmol/plate)	Mitomycin C (0.75–2.0 µmol/plate)	Chinese hamster ovary cells	Micronuclei in binucleated cells	–	6.0 µmol/plate	Salvadori et al. (1994)

Table 54 (contd)

End-point	Code	Carotenoid (tested doses)[a]	Genotoxic agent (tested doses)[a]	Cells	Investigated effect	Result[a]	LED/HID[b]	Reference
M	MIA	β-Carotene (0.25–6.0 µmol/plate)	Bleomycin (10 µg/ml)	Chinese hamster ovary cells	Micronuclei in binucleated cells	#	4.0 µmol/plate	Salvadori et al. (1994)
T	TCM	β-Carotene (0.03–10 µmol/plate)	Pretreatment with 3-methylcholanthrene (1 µg/ml)	C3H 10T$_{1/2}$ mouse fibroblasts	Cell transformation	+	1 µmol/plate	Pung et al. (1988)
T	TCM	β-Carotene (0.1–3 µmol/plate)	Pre-irradiation with X-rays (600 rad)	C3H 10T$_{1/2}$ mouse fibroblasts	Cell transformation	+	1 µmol/plate	Pung et al. (1988)
T	TCM	Canthaxanthin (0.3–3 µmol/plate)	Pre-irradiation with X-rays (600 rad)	C3H 10T$_{1/2}$ mouse fibroblasts	Cell transformation	+	1 µmol/plate	Pung et al. (1988)
T	TCM	β-Carotene (0.3–10 µmol/plate)	Pretreatment with 3-methyl-cholanthrene(1 or 3 µg/ml)	C3H 10T$_{1/2}$ mouse fibroblasts	Cell transformation	+	1 µmol/plate	Bertram et al. (1991)
T	TCM	α-Carotene (0.3–10 µmol/plate)	Pretreatment with 3-methyl-cholanthrene (1 or 3 µg/ml)	C3H 10T$_{1/2}$ mouse fibroblasts	Cell transformation	+	3 µmol/plate	Bertram et al. (1991)
T	TCM	Canthaxanthin (0.3–10 µmol/plate)	Pretreatment with 3-methyl-cholanthrene (1 or 3 µg/ml)	C3H 10T$_{1/2}$ mouse fibroblasts	Cell transformation	+	1 µmol/plate	Bertram et al. (1991)
T	TCM	Lycopene (0.3–10 µmol/plate)	Pretreatment with 3-methyl-cholanthrene (1 or 3 µg/ml)	C3H 10T$_{1/2}$ mouse fibroblasts	Cell transformation	+	10 µmol/plate	Bertram et al. (1991)
T	TCM	Lutein (0.3–10 µmol/plate)	Pretreatment with 3-methyl-cholanthrene (1 or 3 µg/ml)	C3H 10T$_{1/2}$ mouse fibroblasts	Cell transformation	+	10 µmol/plate	Bertram et al. (1991)
T	TCM	Renierapurpurin (0.3–10 µmol/plate)	Pretreatment with 3-methyl-cholanthrene (1 or 3 µg/ml)	C3H 10T$_{1/2}$ mouse fibroblasts	Cell transformation	−	10 µmol/plate	Bertram et al. (1991)
T	TCM	Bixin (0.3–10 µmol/plate)	Pretreatment with 3-methyl-cholanthrene (1 or 3 µg/ml)	C3H 10T$_{1/2}$ mouse fibroblasts	Cell transformation	−	10 µmol/plate	Bertram et al. (1991)

Table 54 (contd)

End-point	Code	Carotenoid (tested doses)[a]	Genotoxic agent (tested doses)[a]	Cells	Investigated effect	Result[a]	LED/HID[b]	Reference
T	???	β-Carotene (1 μmol/plate)	7,12-Dimethylbenz[a]anthracene (7.8 μmol/plate)	Cultured mammary glands from Balb/c female mice	Appearance of nodule-like alveolar lesions in mammary glands	+	1 μmol/plate	Som et al. (1984)
?	???	α-Carotene (37.2 μ mol/plate)	None	B-16 mouse melanoma cells	Morphological differentiation	+	37.2 μmol/plate	Hazuka et al. (1990)
?	???	β-Carotene (18.6–37.2 μmol/plate)	None	B-16 mouse melanoma cells	Morphological differentiation	+	18.6 μmol/plate	Hazuka et al. (1990)
–		β-Carotene (1–10 μmol/plate)	None	Non-transformed C10 mouse lung epithelial cells	Intercellular communication	–	10 μmol/plate	Banoub et al. (1996)
–		β-Carotene (1–10 μmol/plate)	None	Transformed E9 and 82-132 mouse lung epithelial cells	Intercellular communication	–	10 μmol/plate	Banoub et al. (1996)
–		β-Carotene (1–10 μmol/plate)	None	Non-transformed C10 mouse lung epithelial cells	Expression of connexin 43	–	10 μmol/plate	Banoub et al. (1996)
–		β-Carotene (1–10 μmol/plate)	None	Transformed E9 and 82-132 mouse lung epithelial cells	Expression of connexin 43	–	10 μmol/plate	Banoub et al. (1996)
–		β-Carotene (1–10 μmol/plate)	None	C3H 10T1/2 mouse fibroblasts	Intercellular communication	#	1 μmol/plate	Banoub et al. (1996)
–		β-Carotene (1–10 μmol/plate)	None	C3H 10T1/2 mouse fibroblasts	Expression of connexin 43	#	1 μmol/plate	Banoub et al. (1996)
–		β-Carotene (0.5–10 μmol/plate)	None	C3H 10T1/2 mouse fibroblasts	Intercellular communication	#	1 μmol/plate	Zhang et al. (1991)
–		Canthaxanthin (0.5–10 μmol/plate)	None	C3H 10T1/2 mouse fibroblasts	Intercellular communication	#	1 μmol/plate	Zhang et al. (1991)

Table 54 (contd)

End-point	Code	Carotenoid (tested doses)[a]	Genotoxic agent (tested doses)[a]	Cells	Investigated effect	Result[a]	LED/HID[b]	Reference
I		Lutein (0.5–10 µmol/plate)	None	C3H 10T1/2 mouse fibroblasts	Intercellular communication	#	5 µmol/plate	Zhang et al. (1991)
I		Lycopene (0.5–10 µmol/plate)	None	C3H 10T1/2 mouse fibroblasts	Intercellular communication	#	1 µmol/plate	Zhang et al. (1991)
I		Methyl-bixin (0.5–10 µmol/plate)	None	C3H 10T1/2 mouse fibroblasts	Enhancement of intercellular communication	–	10 µmol/plate	Zhang et al. (1991)
I		Methyl-bixin (10 µmol/plate)	None	C3H 10T1/2 mouse fibroblasts	Enhanced expression of connexin 43	–	10 µmol/plate	Zhang et al. (1992)
I		β-Carotene (10 µmol/plate)	None	C3H 10T1/2 mouse fibroblasts	Intercellular communication	+	10 µmol/plate	Stahl et al. (1997)
I		Echinenone (10 µmol/plate)	None	C3H 10T1/2 mouse fibroblasts	Intercellular communication	#	10 µmol/plate	Stahl et al. (1997)
I		Canthaxanthin (10 µmol/plate)	None	C3H 10T1/2 mouse fibroblasts	Intercellular communication	#	10 µmol/plate	Stahl et al. (1997)
I		4-Hydroxy-β-carotene (10 µmol/plate)	None	C3H 10T1/2 mouse fibroblasts	Intercellular communication	#	10 µmol/plate	Stahl et al. (1997)
I		β-Cryptoxanthin (10 µ mol/plate)	None	C3H 10T1/2 mouse fibroblasts	Intercellular communication	#	10 µmol/plate	Stahl et al. (1997)
I		Retrodehydro-β-carotene (10 µmol/plate)	None	C3H 10T1/2 mouse fibroblasts	Intercellular communication	#	10 µmol/plate	Stahl et al. (1997)
I		Capsorubicin (1 µmol/plate)	None	C3H 10T1/2 mouse fibroblasts	Intercellular communication	–	1 µmol/plate	Stahl et al. (1997)
I		Dinorcanthaxanthin (10 µmol/plate)	None	C3H 10T1/2 mouse fibroblasts	Intercellular communication	(#)	10 µmol/plate	Stahl et al. (1997)

Table 54 (contd)

End-point	Code	Carotenoid (tested doses)[a]	Genotoxic agent (tested doses)[a]	Cells	Investigated Effect	Result[a]	LED/HID[b]	Reference
I		Violerythrin (10 µmol/plate)	None	C3H 10T1/2 mouse fibroblasts	Intercellular communication	(#)	10 µmol/plate	Stahl et al. (1997)
I		C-20-Dialdehyde (10 µmol/plate)	None	C3H 10T1/2 mouse fibroblasts	Intercellular communication	–	10 µmol/plate	Stahl et al. (1997)
I		C-30-Dialdehyde (10 µmol/plate)	None	C3H 10T1/2 mouse fibroblasts	Intercellular communication	–	10 µmol/plate	Stahl et al. (1997)
I		C-40-Dialdehyde (10 µmol/plate)		C3H 10T1/2 mouse fibroblasts	Intercellular communication	–	10 µmol/plate	Stahl et al. (1997)
D	BID	β-Carotene (100–500 µmol/plate)	Aflatoxin B₁ (2 µmol/plate)	–	DNA adduct formation	+	100 µmol/plate	Bhattacharya et al. (1984)
D	BID	β-Carotene (10 µmol/plate)	Benzo[a]pyrene (10 µmol/plate)	Hamster tracheal epithelium	DNA adduct formation	+	10 µmol/plate	Wolterbeek et al. (1995b)
D	BID	Crocetin (10–100 µmol/plate)	3H–Aflatoxin B₁ (0.32 µg/ml)	C3H 10T1/2 mouse fibroblasts + S9 mix	Covalent binding to DNA	+	100 µmol/plate	Wang, C.-J et al. (1991a)
Human cells								
		Fucoxanthin (5-10 µg/mL)	None	Human neuroblastoma GOTO cells	Delay of cell cycle progession	+	10 µg/ml	Okuzumi et al. (1990)
		Fucoxanthin (5-10 µg/mL)	None	Human neuroblastoma GOTO cells	Decrease of N-myc expression	+	10 µg/ml	Okuzumi et al. (1990)
		β-Carotene (40 µmol/plate)	None	Human embryonic lung fibroblasts	Delay of cell cycle progession	+	40 µmol/plate	Stivala et al. (1996)
M	MIH	β-Carotene (0.25–6.0 µmol/plate)	Cyclophosphamide (400 µmol/plate)	Human hepatoma Hep G2 cells	Micronuclei	+	0.25 µmol/plate	Salvadori et al. (1993)
M	MIH	β-Carotene (0.25–6.0 µmol/plate)	Mitomycin C (1 µmol/plate)	Human hepatoma Hep G2 cells	Micronuclei	–	6.0 µmol/plate	Salvadori et al. (1993)

[a] +, inhibition of the investigated end-point; (+), weak inhibition of the investigated end-point; #, enhancement of the investigated end-point; (#), weak enhancement of the investigated end-point; –, no effect on the investigated end-point
[b] LED, lowest effective dose that inhibits or enhances the investigated effect; HID, highest ineffective dose

binding of metabolically activated aflatoxin B_1 *in vitro* to DNA extracted from the same cells (Wang, C.-J. *et al.*, 1991a). Binding of ^{3}H-aflatoxin B1 to calf thymus DNA, activated with liver microsomes from phenobarbital-induced Wistar rats, was significantly inhibited by β-carotene, 8'-apo-β-carotenal, 10'-apo-β-carotenal, cryptoxanthin and lutein, and the effect was ascribed to an action of these carotenoids on the microsomal activation of aflatoxin B_1. The other carotenoids tested, 12'-apo-β–carotenal, astaxanthin, canthaxanthin and torularhodin, had no protective effect in this acellular test system (Goswami *et al.*, 1989).

A limited number of studies have addressed the protective effects of carotenoids in cultured human cells (Table 54). Fucoxanthin arrested human neuroblastoma cells (GOTO) in the G_0 or G_1 phase of the cell cycle and decreased N-*myc* expression (Okuzumi *et al.*, 1990). β-Carotene incorporated into dipalmitoylphosphatidylcholine liposomes delayed the cell cycle in the G_1 phase in human embryonic lung fibroblasts in primary culture. This effect was independent of conversion to known retinoids (Stivala *et al.*, 1996). In a metabolically active line of human hepatoma cells (Hep G2), β-carotene inhibited the frequency of micronuclei induced by the indirectly acting clastogen cyclophosphamide but failed to inhibit the clastogenicity of the directly acting mutagen mitomycin C (Salvadori *et al.*, 1993).

Studies have also been carried out *in vivo* to evaluate the ability of β-carotene and other carotenoids to inhibit a variety of end-points, including DNA damage, mutation, clastogenic damage and adduction to DNA in rodents, either untreated or treated with physical or chemical carcinogens (Table 55). In all these studies, the carotenoids were administered orally, in the diet, in drinking-water or by gavage, and in almost all studies the carotenoids had protective effects. In particular, ingestion of β-carotene inhibited the formation of single-strand breaks in the forestomach mucosa of mice receiving benzo[*a*]pyrene by gavage 4 h before sacrifice (Lahiri *et al.*, 1993). Canthaxanthin, astaxanthin and β-apo-8'-carotenal were reported to inhibit the induction of DNA single-strand breaks in the livers of mice treated

intraperitoneally with aflatoxin B_1, whereas β-carotene was ineffective (Gradelet *et al.*, 1997). [The Working Group noted that no quantitative data were provided.]

β-Carotene inhibited the induction of 6-thioguanine-resistant T lymphocyes in the spleens of rats receiving an intraperitoneal injection of *N*-ethyl-*N*-nitrosourea, although the inhibition was non-linear within the range of β-carotene doses used (Aidoo *et al.*, 1995).

The ability of β-carotene to inhibit the frequency of micronuclei in bone-marrow polychromatic erythrocytes or peripheral blood reticulocytes of mice was investigated in several studies. Administration of β-carotene by gavage or in a diet containing *Dunaliella* decreased the 'spontaneous' frequency of micronuclei in reticulocytes. Micronuclei induced by whole-body exposure of mice to X-radiation were inhibited weakly only by the administration of β-carotene by gavage and not by feeding mice with *Dunaliella* in the diet (Umegaki *et al.*, 1994a). β-Carotene inhibited micronucleus formation in bone-marrow polychromatic erythrocytes induced by whole-body exposure of mice to γ-radiation (Abraham *et al.*, 1993) or by treatment with cyclophosphamide (Mukherjee *et al.*, 1991), mitomycin C or benzo[*a*]pyrene (Raj & Katz, 1985). In another study, however, β-carotene failed to inhibit the clastogenicity of benzo[*a*]pyrene (Lahiri *et al.*, 1993).

β-Carotene can inhibit the induction of chromosomal aberrations by cyclophosphamide in mouse bone-marrow cells (Mukherjee *et al.*, 1991; Salvadori *et al.*, 1992a,b), but it did not affect the frequency of chromosomal aberrations in bone-marrow cells of Chinese hamsters treated with cyclophosphamide, although it was effective when thiotepa, methyl methanesulfonate and busulfan were used as the clastogenic agents (Renner, 1985).

Administration of crocetin weakly inhibited the formation of DNA adducts in the livers of rats given an intraperitoneal injection of ^{3}H-aflatoxin B_1 (Wang, C.-J. *et al.*, 1991b). β-Carotene at 1–15 μmol/L, supplied either in tetrahydrofuran or liposomes, increased the extent of binding of aflatoxin B_1 to woodchuck hepatocyte DNA by up to twofold; however, no dose–response relationship was observed (Yu *et al.*, 1994).

Table 55. Inhibition by carotenoids of genetic and related effects in rodents *in vivo*

End-point	Code	Carotenoid (tested doses and administration route)[a]	Carcinogen (tested doses and administration route)[a]	Result[b]	Animal strain and species	LED/HID[c]	Reference
D	DVA	β-Carotene (2.5 mg/animal per day in drinking-water for 15 days)	Benzo[a]pyrene (240 mg/kg bw by gavage)	+	Swiss mice	2.5 mg/animal/day in drinking-water for 15 days (ID$_{100}$)	Lahiri et al. (1993)
D	DVA	β-Carotene (300 ppm in the diet for 15 days)	Aflatoxin B$_1$ (2 mg/kg bw i.p.)	–	Wistar rats	300 ppm in the diet for 15 days	Gradelet et al. (1997)
D	DVA	Canthaxanthin (300 ppm in the diet for 15 days)	Aflatoxin B$_1$ (2 mg/kg bw i.p.)	+	Wistar rats	300 ppm in the diet for 15 days [no quantitative data provided]	Gradelet et al. (1997)
D	DVA	Astaxanthin (300 ppm in the diet for 15 days)	Aflatoxin B$_1$ (2 mg/kg bw i.p.)	+	Wistar rats	300 ppm in the diet for 15 days [no quantitative data provided]	Gradelet et al. (1997)
D	DVA	β-Apo-8'-carotenal (300 ppm in the diet for 15 days)	Aflatoxin B$_1$ (2 mg/kg bw i.p.)	+	Wistar rats	300 ppm in the diet for 15 days [no quantitative data provided]	Gradelet et al. (1997)
G	GVA	β-Carotene (0.05–0.25% in drinking-water for up to 9 weeks)	N-Ethyl-N-nitrosourea (100 mg/kg bw i.p.)	+	Fischer 344 rats	0.05% in drinking-water for 3 weeks (ID$_{52}$)	Aidoo et al. (1995)
M	MVM	β-Carotene (2.5 mg/animal per day in drinking-water for 15 days)	Benzo[a]pyrene (240 mg/kg bw by gavage)	–	Swiss mice	2.5 mg/animal per day in drinking-water for 15 days	Lahiri et al. (1993)
M	MVM	β-Carotene (100 mg/kg food for 1 week)	Benzo[a]pyrene (150 mg/kg bw i.p.)	+	B6C3F1 mice	100 mg/kg food for 1 week (ID$_{41-61}$)	Raj & Katz (1985)
M	MVM	β-Carotene (100 mg/kg food for 1 week)	Mitomycin C (1 mg/kg bw i.p.)	+	B6C3F1 mice	100 mg/kg food for 1 week (ID$_{44-71}$)	Raj & Katz (1985)
M	MVM	β-Carotene (2.7–27 mg/kg bw orally for 7 days)	Cyclophosphamide (25 mg/kg bw i.p.)	(+)	Swiss albino mice	2.7 mg/kg bw orally for 7 days (ID$_{29}$)	Mukherjee et al. (1991)
M	MVM	β-Carotene (0.1–2.5 mg/kg bw orally for 7 days)	γ-Radiation (1.15 Gy, whole-body exposure)	+	Swiss albino mice	0.1 mg/kg bw orally for 7 days (ID$_{55}$)	Abraham et al. (1993)

Table 55 (contd)

End-point	Code	Carotenoid (tested doses and administration route)[a]	Carcinogen (tested doses and administration route)[a]	Result[b]	LED/HID[c]	Animal strain and species	Reference
M	MVM	*Dunaliella bardawil* (diet containing 0.03–0.2% β-carotene for 4 weeks)	None ('spontaneous' frequency of micronuclei)	+	Diet containing 0.2% β-carotene for 4 weeks (ID_{70})	ICR mice	Umegaki *et al.* (1994a)
M	MVM	*Dunaliella bardawil* (diet containing 0.03–0.2% β-carotene for 4 weeks)	X-Radiation (0.3 Gy, whole-body exposure)	–	Diet containing 0.2% β-carotene for 4 weeks	ICR mice	Umegaki *et al.* (1994a)
M	MVM	β-Carotene (300 mg/kg bw by gavage for 7 days)	None ('spontaneous' frequency of micronuclei)	(+)	300 mg/kg bw by gavage for 7 days (ID_{40})	ICR mice	Umegaki *et al.* (1994a)
M	MVM	β-Carotene (300 mg/kg bw by gavage for 7 days)	X-Radiation (0.3 Gy, whole-body exposure)	(+)	300 mg/kg bw by gavage for 7 days (ID_{25})	ICR mice	Umegaki *et al.* (1994a)
C	CBA	β-Carotene (2.7–27 mg/kg bw orally for 7 days)	Cyclophosphamide (25 mg/kg bw i.p.)	+	2.7 mg/kg bw orally for 7 days (ID_{49})	Swiss albino mice	Mukherjee *et al.* (1991)
C	CBA	β-Carotene (0.5–200 mg/kg bw by gavage for 5 days)	Cyclophosphamide (20 mg/kg bw i.p.)	+	25 mg/kg bw by gavage for 5 days (ID_{50})	Balb/C mice	Salvadori *et al.* (1992a,b)
C	CBA	β-Carotene (50–250 mg/kg bw by single gavage administration)	Thio-TEPA (13 mg/kg bw) by gavage	+	50 mg/kg bw by gavage (ID_{54})	Chinese hamsters	Renner et al. (1990)
C	CBA	β-Carotene (25–250 mg/kg bw single oral administration)	Thio-TEPA (10 mg/kg bw, single oral administration)	+	50 mg/kg bw single oral administration (ID_{47})	Chinese hamsters	Renner (1985)
C	CBA	β-Carotene (50–250 mg/kg bw single oral administration)	Methyl methanesulfonate (50 mg/kg bw i.p.)	+	50 mg/kg bw single oral administration (ID_{54})	Chinese hamsters	Renner (1985)
C	CBA	β-Carotene (20–250 mg/kg bw single oral administration)	Myleran (50 mg/kg bw, single oral administration)	+	50 mg/kg bw single oral administration (ID_{64})	Chinese hamsters	Renner (1985)
C	CBA	β-Carotene (100–250 mg/kg bw single oral administration)	Cyclophosphamide (20 mg/kg bw, single oral administration)	–	250 mg/kg bw single oral administration	Chinese hamsters	Renner (1985)
D	BVD	Crocetin (6–10 mg/kg bw by gavage for 3 days)	Aflatoxin B$_1$ (6 µg/kg bw i.p.)	(+)	6 mg/kg bw by gavage for 3 days (ID_{18})	Wistar rats	Wang, C.-J. *et al.* (1991b)

i.p., intraperitoneally

[a]Doses of carotenoids and carcinogens, and routes of administration are as reported by the authors

[b]+, inhibition of the investigated end-point; (+), weak inhibition of the investigated end-point; –, no effect on the investigated end-point

[c]LED, lowest effective dose that inhibits or enhances the investigated effect; HID, highest ineffective dose; ID_x, dose inhibiting the investigated end-point by x%, as indicated by the authors or calculated from their data

4.3 Mechanisms of cancer prevention

Several mechanisms of action have been proposed or suspected to contribute to any cancer-preventive effects of carotenoids. It must be remembered that most of these mechanisms have been examined only *in vitro* and that more complex interactions among the many dietary components and more complex mechanistic pathways are likely to occur *in vivo*.

4.3.1 Antioxidant properties

The body is continuously exposed to reactive oxygen species, which can damage biologically relevant macromolecules such as DNA, proteins and lipids (Sies & Stahl, 1995). These reactions may well be involved in the pathobiology of several diseases, including cancer. Reactive oxygen species may also affect gene expression, e.g. by the NF-κB and AP-1 pathways (Sen & Packer, 1996; Müller *et al.*, 1997). A number of naturally occurring compounds can scavenge reactive oxygen species.

The antioxidant properties of carotenoids are related to their extended system of conjugated double bonds. *In vitro*, carotenoids efficiently quench excited molecules such as singlet oxygen and can scavenge peroxyl radicals; interactions with other radicals have also been reported. The efficiency with which caro-tenoids can quench singlet oxygen or triplet sensitizers that lead to singlet oxygen formation is very high (Section 1), but there is no evidence that carotenoids act in this way in carcinogenesis.

Carotenoids also interact with radicals, and efficient scavenging of peroxyl radicals has been proposed (Burton & Ingold, 1984). It has been suggested that the radical adds to the carotenoid molecule to form a less reactive intermediate. Radical scavenging appears to be more efficient at low oxygen tension. Prooxidant effects of carotenoids have been reported at higher oxygen levels (Terao, 1989; Liebler, 1993; Palozza *et al.*, 1995).

Many studies have been reported of the interactions of carotenoids with peroxy radicals generated from a series of azo compounds as radical sources, e.g. 2,2'-azobisisobutyrylnitrile, 2,2'-azobis(2-amidinopropane) hydrochloride and 2,2'-azinobis(3-ethylbenzothiazoline)-β-sulfonic acid, diammonium salt (Alabaster *et al.*, 1995; Tanaka *et al.*, 1995b; Komaki *et al.*, 1996; Tyurin *et al.*, 1997; Woodall *et al.*, 1997). In organic solvents and in phospholid liposomes, the carotenoids are destroyed by reactions with radicals but also generally inhibit or decrease the peroxidation of unsaturated lipids. In most cases, lycopene was the most reactive carotenoid studied, followed by β-carotene, but much variation has been reported in the order of reactivity of carotenoids and their ability to inhibit peroxidation.

Several other radicals have been shown to react with β-carotene, and particularly nitrogen dioxide, which is relevant to the exposure of humans to tobacco smoke and air pollutants. The genotoxicity of nitrogen oxide and reactive oxygen species has been shown to be inhibited by carotenoids in short-term tests (see section 4.2.2.2). Supplementation with β-carotene resulted in a significant decrease in inducible nitric oxide synthase in patients with nonatrophic gastritis (Mannick *et al.*, 1996). Exposure to nitrogen dioxide may result in the interaction of radical cations on carotenoids with other cellular components. Glutathione enhances nitrogen dioxide-induced lipid peroxidation, possibly by the formation of thiyl radicals. Thus, β-carotene may give rise to a carotenoid adduct radical, which could lead to formation of a glutathione sulfoxide radical, a species that can have damaging effects *in vivo* (Everett *et al.*, 1996). This may be relevant to heavy exposure to nitrogen dioxide, as in tobacco smoke, and to the increased efficiency of glutathione in proliferating cells (Burdon, 1995).

Two measures have been used to investigate processes *in vivo*: circulating levels or excreted oxidation products and the response of blood consituents to oxidative stress *in vitro*. The use and interpretation of these measures is difficult, and in some studies it is not clear which has been used (Gutteridge, 1986; Halliwell & Chirico, 1993). The direct measurements include plasma phosphatidylcholine hydroperoxides and peroxide derivatives measured as serum thiobarbituric acid-reactive substances, urinary excretion of thioethers and 8-oxo-7,8-dihydro-2'-deoxyguanosine and excretion of pentane and ethane peroxidation products of ω-

3 and ω-6 fatty acids, respectively, in exhaled air. Higher levels of each purportedly indicate more oxidative stress and less antioxidant activity. Measures of oxidation *in vitro* include oxidation products induced by exposure to copper, 2,2'-azobis(2-amidinopropane) dihydrochloride, hydrogen peroixide, xanthine oxidase, hyoxanthine, horseradish peroxidase or activated phagocytes. Low-density lipoprotein cholesterol, total serum lipids and erythrocytes have been used as substrates. The measured outcomes in these studies include conjugated dienes (UV absorbance at 230–230 nm), lipid hydroperoxides (chemiluminescence), thiobarbituric acid-reactive substances and reduction in ferricytochrome C. The techniques involve assessment of the production of oxidized metabolites; like the direct measures, high levels indicate more marked oxidative stress. In contrast, the lag time for oxidation *in vitro* is a measure of resistance to oxidation, so that higher values are thought to indicate less oxidative stress or more effective antioxidant intervention.

The antioxidant actions of β-carotene have been investigated in animals and humans with a variety of measures of antioxidative efficacy (Krinsky, 1993a; Omaye *et al.*, 1997). Indicators of lipid peroxidation have been used in investigations of the antioxidant effects of carotenoids *in vivo*. In pigs, injection of β-carotene in mineral oil significantly blocked the increased expiration of ethane and pentane seen after the development of ascorbate deficiency. In rats, however, supplementation of the diet with β-carotene exacerbated the increased levels of malondialdehyde and 15-lipoxygenase activity seen in the testes after maintenance on a diet deficient in α-tocopherol. Other studies have provided no evidence of antioxidant effects.

It has been suggested that β-carotene has an antioxidative effect in humans. In a short-term trial conducted among elderly women, 90 mg/d of supplemental β-carotene was associated with a significant reduction in the production of phospholipid hydroperoxides after treatment of plasma with a free-radical initiator (Meydani *et al.*, 1994). Daily supplementation of smokers with 20 mg β-carotene resulted in a significant reduction in the excretion of pentane in the breath, although no similar effect was seen among nonsmokers, in whom the breath concentrations of pentane were lower (Allard *et al.*, 1994). In an intervention study, healthy, nonsmoking men were subjected to a two-week depletion period [undefined] and were then fed 40 mg of tomato juice containing lycopene daily for two weeks, followed by carrot juice containing 22.3 mg β-carotene and 15.7 mg α-carotene for two weeks and then spinach powder containing 11.3 mg lutein and other compounds for two weeks. All of the diets decreased the endogenous levels of strand breaks in lymphocyte DNA. Oxidative DNA base damage (assayed by single-cell microgel electrophoresis and endonuclease III incubation) was significantly reduced only during the intervention with carrot juice. When the men were maintained on a carotenoid-free diet for two weeks and were then given 15 or 120 mg/d supplemental β-carotene, the serum lipid peroxide concentrations were decreased (Pool-Zobel *et al.*, 1997). In a study with no controls, children with cystic fibrosis had decreased serum malondialdehyde concentrations after twice daily supplementation with 4.42 mg β-carotene (Lepage *et al.*, 1996). In contrast, volunteers who received 533 mg α-tocopherol, 1 g ascorbic acid, and 10 mg β-carotene for one month showed no change in the excretion of 8-hydroydeoxyguanosine (Witt *et al.*, 1992). [The Working Group noted that these studies involved antioxidant assays of uncertain relevance to human carcinogenesis.]

The effects on these measures of supplementation with β-carotene have been studied in several randomized clinical trials. In the largest study conducted to date of the antioxidant effects of β-carotene, 163 healthy male smokers were randomized to 14 weeks of placebo or 14 weeks of β-carotene treatment (two weeks of 40 mg β-carotene daily followed by 12 weeks of 20 mg daily); 150 men completed the trial. Urinary excretion of thioethers and 8-oxo-7,8-dihydro-2'-deoxyguanosine was assessed in three overnight urine specimens taken before and after treatment, from 123 subjects and 122 subjects, respectively. β-Carotene had no effect on excretion of the deoxyguanosine (van Poppel *et al.*, 1995), but at the end of the trial the group receiving β-carotene had 15% less urinary excretion of thioethers than those given the placebo (p = 0.002) (Bos *et al.*, 1992).

Exhaled oxidation products were assessed in two studies. In one, 15 subjects were given a carotenoid-free liquid diet for two weeks and were then randomized to receive 15 or 120 mg β-carotene in the diet daily for four weeks. The concentration of pentane in breath decreased in both groups after supplementation, but the decrease in those receiving the low dose was 26% (not statistically significant) and that in subjects given the higher dose was 40% (p = 0.04) (Gottlieb *et al.*, 1993). In another study, 42 nonsmokers and 28 smokers were randomized to four weeks of placebo or 20 mg of β-carotene daily. β-Carotene appeared to reduce the excretion of ethane, as both smokers and nonsmokers receiving β-carotene had non-significant decreases in ethane output, while those given placebo had a nonsignificant increase. The evidence with respect to pentane was mixed: the concentration of pentane in the breath was unchanged in nonsmokers and in smokers given the placebo but showed a non-significant decrease in smokers given β-carotene (Allard *et al.*, 1994). [The Working Group noted that in neither study was there a statistical comparison of the differences between groups given β-carotene and placebo.]

In studies of oxidation products induced in vitro, 46 smokers were randomized to 40 mg of β-carotene daily for two weeks, followed by 12 weeks of 20 mg β-carotene daily, or to 14 weeks of placebo. No substantial difference in copper-induced low-density lipoprotein oxidation was seen between the two groups (Princen *et al.*, 1992). In a further study, 30 hypercholesterolaemic, postmenopausal women were randomized to 30 mg β-carotene daily or placebo for 10 weeks. During the treatment period, women in the two groups showed similarly increased resistance to low-density lipoprotein oxidation *in vitro*: supplementation had no effect on the lag time of copper-induced oxidation or on the production of lipid peroxides (Nenseter *et al.*, 1995). In an uncontrolled study, 16 subjects showed no benefit with regard to copper-induced low-density lipoprotein oxidation after supplementation with 50–100 mg β-carotene daily for four weeks. In

fact, in comparison with baseline values, the duration of the lag phase of copper- and 2',2-azobis(2-amidinopropane) dihydrochloride-induced lipid peroxidation was shortened (Gaziano *et al.*, 1995b). Another study without concurrent controls also showed that β-carotene did not improve measures of the susceptibility of low-density lipoproteins to oxidation *in vitro* (Reaven *et al.*, 1993). [The Working Group noted that the absence of concurrent controls limits the conclusions that can be drawn.]

Richards *et al.* (1990) assessed several oxidation end-points—activated phagocytes and a xanthine oxidase/hypoxanthine superoxide-generating system—in 40 asymptomatic cigarette smokers randomized to receive placebo or 40 mg β-carotene daily for six weeks. Statistically significant reductions in several of the measures were seen in the group receiving β-carotene but not among subjects randomized to placebo. Allard *et al.* (1994; see above) found no significant change in hydrogen peroxide-induced malondialdehyde release from the erythrocytes of smokers and nonsmokers randomized to β-carotene or placebo, and Mobarhan *et al.* (1990; see Gottlieb *et al.*, 1993, above) also found no difference in the capacity of stimulated neutrophils to reduce ferricy-tochrome C. [The Working Group noted that no statistical comparison was made of the differences between groups given β-carotene and placebo in these three studies.]

In another study, phosphatidylcholine hydroperoxide generated in plasma by 2',2-azobis(2-amidinopropane)dihydrochloride was used to assess the antioxidant capacity of plasma Twelve healthy postmenopausal women were randomized to 90 mg β-carotene daily or placebo for three weeks. The induction period and phosphatidylcholine hydroperoxide production were unchanged in women given the placebo but the induction period lengthened and phosphatidylcholine hydroperoxide production decreased in those receiving β-carotene (Meydani *et al.*, 1994). [The Working Group noted that no statistical comparison was made between the two treatment groups and that baseline differences in the maximal production of phosphatidylcholine hydroperoxide suggest that the two groups may have differed in ways related to the end-points studied.]

Thus, although some studies have provided findings consistent with an antioxidant effect of β-carotene in vivo, others have reported no substantial benefit. Interpretation of the findings is complicated by the small size of many of the studies and the difficulties in interpreting the measurements used. Randomized, placebo-controlled trials of β-carotene administration *in vivo* are needed in order to investigate antioxidation capacity.

4.3.2 Modulation of carcinogen metabolism

Most studies *in vitro* in which an exogenous metabolic system or metabolically competent cells were used showed that carotenoids inhibit the genotoxic activity of promutagens and procarcinogens (see section 4.2.2.2). Certain carotenoids, such as astaxanthin and canthaxanthin, induce some phase-I enzymes, including CYP1A1 and CYPA2, and phase-II enzymes like UDP glucuronyl transferase, UGT1A6 and DT-diaphorase, in rat liver and intestine (Gradelet *et al.*, 1996b). Other carotenoids, such as β-carotene, lutein and lycopene, do not have an effect. This difference may bear on the balance of metabolic activation and inactivation of chemical carcinogens. For instance, cytochrome P450 1A induction could increase the detoxification of aflatoxin B_1 through the formation of aflatoxin M_1, a less genotoxic metabolite, and decrease its carcinogenic effects in rats (Gradelet *et al.*, 1998).

4.3.3 Effects on cell transformation and differentiation

The results of clinical trials indicate that β-carotene supplements can reduce the rate of cell proliferation in rectal crypts (see section 4.1.2.3). In cell cultures, carotenoids can prevent carcinogen-induced transformation and induce cell differentiation, although the effects on transformation induced by X-rays were restricted to the promotional phases of carcinogenesis (Pung *et al.*, 1988).

The main ligands for retinoid-responsive nuclear receptors (RAR and RXR) are all-*trans*- and 9-*cis*-retinoic acid. β-Carotene and other provitamin A carotenoids may produce retinoic acid from the retinal formed by central cleavage of the carotenoid or indirectly by excentric cleavage (Lin *et al.*, 1997). Thus, β-apo-14'-carotenoic acid, like retinoic acid (Lotan *et al.*, 1995), induces the nuclear receptor RARβ (Wang *et al.*, 1997), either directly or by its conversion to retinoic acid. Because carotenoids are generally less potent inducers of cell differentiation than retinoids, their actions on cell differentiation may require intracellular metabolism.

4.3.4 Effects on cell-to-cell communication

Enhanced gap-junctional communication between tumour cells and normal growth-inhibited cells is associated with decreased tumour-cell proliferation. Carotenoids stimulate gap-junction formation between cells *in vitro*, allowing more cell-to-cell communication, an effect correlated with their ability to inhibit cell transformation. This effect is mediated through increased formation of connexin 43, a transmembrane protein (Zhang *et al.*, 1991; see section 4.2.2).

4.3.5 Inhibition of cell proliferation and oncogene expression

Carotenoids delay cell cycle progression in cultured human cells. N-*myc* expression was also decreased in one study (see sections 4.1.2.5 and 4.2.2.2).

4.3.6 Effects on immune function

Enhancement of immune responses has been described in some experimental models. Beneficial effects of β-carotene have been demonstrated on T- and B-cell proliferation, numbers of T-helper cells and the cytotoxicity of natural killer cells (Bendich, 1991). The enhancement may be due to production of tumour-specific antigens (Tomita *et al.*, 1987; see also section 4.1.2.7).

4.3.7 Inhibition of endogenous formation of carcinogens

Highly carcinogenic N-nitrosamines are formed in the stomach by the reaction of secondary and tertiary amines with nitrosating agents. β-Carotene was shown in one study *in vitro* to inhibit the nitrosation of morpholine by nitrogen oxide and nitrogen dioxide (Arroyo *et al.*, 1992).

5.   Other Beneficial Effects

A number of carotenoids are being evaluated for health benefits other than cancer prevention. In this section, the scientific evidence in support of other potential health effects of carotenoids and the potential mechanisms involved is discussed.

5.1   Photosensitivity disorders

Carotenoids, including β-carotene and to a lesser extent canthaxanthin, have been used successfully in the treatment of certain photosensitivity diseases for more than 25 years. This clinical application derived from the recognition that carotenoids protect photosynthetic bacteria, algae and green plants against photosensitization (Mathews-Roth, 1987). As reviewed elsewhere (Mathews-Roth, 1993), most patients with the genetic disease, erythropoietic protoporphyria, benefit from high doses of supplementation with β-carotene and/or canthaxanthin. The recommended dose of β-carotene for adults with erythropoietic protoporphyria is about 180 mg/d—substantially higher than the doses investigated for cancer prevention (15–50 mg/d). Despite these relatively high doses, some patients with erythropoietic protoporphyria do not respond to carotenoid therapy, either because of poor absorption of the carotenoids or because of markedly elevated blood porphyrin concentrations. No serious side-effects of high doses of β-carotene supplements have been reported in such patients, and no long-term toxicity has been observed.

Erythropoietic protoporphyria is a disease of porphyrin metabolism, characterized by abnormally elevated concentrations of protoporphyrin (Mathews-Roth, 1987), which acts as an endogenous photosensitizer. As carotenoids can interact and quench photosensitizer triplet states and singlet oxygen, their efficacy in this disorder appears to be a consequence of the quenching of excited species.

Because of the therapeutic efficacy of β-carotene for erythropoietic protoporphyria, it has been evaluated for use in other photosensitivity diseases. For example, Kornhauser et al. (1990) evaluated the ability of β-carotene to protect against psoralen-induced phototoxicity in a murine model. β-Carotene reduced the prevalence of erythema in this model, despite relatively low dermal concentrations after its oral administration. High doses of β-carotene have also been evaluated for the prevention of sunlight-induced erythema, but the observed protective effects were too small for it to be recommended for the prevention of sunburn (Mathews-Roth et al., 1972; Garmyn et al., 1995).

5.2   Cardiovascular disease

The results of descriptive, cohort and case–control studies suggest that carotenoid- and/or β-carotene-rich diets may prevent cardiovascular disease, as reviewed elsewhere (Gaziano & Hennekens, 1993; Manson et al., 1993; Kohlmeier & Hastings, 1995). In a biochemical epidemiological study of plasma carotenoids (the vitamin substudy of the WHO/MONICA Project), plasma was obtained from about 100 healthy males at each of 16 study sites in Europe for analyses of antioxidant nutrients. The median antioxidant nutrient concentrations were then compared with the mortality rates from concurrent, age-specific ischaemic heart disease in the 16 study populations. The results showed a striking inverse correlation between those rates and plasma vitamin E concentrations ($r^2 = 0.63$). A similar comparison between the median plasma β-carotene concentrations and the rate of mortality from ischaemic heart disease revealed no association when all 16 study sites were considered ($r^2 = 0.04$), but a reasonably strong inverse association ($r^2 = 0.50$) when three study sites, all apparent outliers and all Finnish, were excluded from the analysis (Gey et al., 1993a).

In a prospective study in Basel, Switzerland, men who had low concentrations of β-carotene and vitamin C in their blood were at a significantly increased risk for subsequent ischaemic heart disease (RR, 1.96; $p = 0.022$) and stroke (RR, 4.17; $p = 0.002$) (Eichholzer et al., 1992; Gey et al., 1993b). Total serum carotenoids, measured at baseline in the placebo group of a trial on the primary prevention of coronary disease, were inversely related to subsequent coronary heart disease. Men in the highest quartile of total serum carotenoid concentrations had an adjusted relative risk of 0.64 (95% CI,

0.44–0.92); the relative risk among men who had never smoked was 0.28 (95% CI, 0.11–0.73) (Morris *et al.*, 1994). In a nested case–control study of serum antioxidant nutrients and subsequent myocardial infarct in a cohort study in Washington County, Maryland, USA, the risk for myocardial infarct was inversely associated with serum β-carotene concentration (*p* value for trend = 0.02). When the data were stratified by smoking status at the time blood was drawn, the excess risk associated with low serum concentrations of β-carotene, lycopene, lutein and zeaxanthin was confined to current smokers (Street *et al.*, 1994). Plasma carotene concentrations were significantly inversely related to the risk for angina pectoris, but the relationship was no longer statistically significant after adjustment for smoking (Riemersma *et al.*, 1991).

A different biochemical approach was used to quantify β-carotene status: β-carotene concentrations were measured in adipose tissue samples collected by needle aspiration from the buttocks of 683 people with myocardial infarct and 727 age-matched controls. The risk for myocardial infarct, adjusted for age, smoking and body mass index, in the lowest quintile of adipose β-carotene concentrations as compared with the highest was 1.78 (95% CI, 1.17-2.71); the risk was primarily confined to current smokers (odds ratio, 2.39; 95% CI, 1.35–4.25; versus an odds ratio of 1.07 for nonsmokers) (Kardinaal *et al.*, 1993). In a large, multicentre case–control study of acute myocardial infarct, trend analyses showed that the adipose tissue concentrations of β-carotene, α-carotene and lycopene were inversely associated with risk when modelled separately; however, the carotenoid concentrations were highly correlated, and when they were included simultaneously in the model, lycopene had the greatest protective effect (Kohlmeier *et al.*, 1997).

Of the studies in which diet was used to estimate β-carotene status, the study of US health professionals showed protective effects of dietary carotene, with a relative risk for coronary heart disease of 0.71 (95% CI, 0.55–0.92) for people in the top quintile of total carotene intake (> 19 034 IU/d) relative to the lowest quintile of intake. Smoking modified the effect:

the relative risk was 0.30 (95% CI, 0.11–0.82) among current smokers, 0.60 (95% CI, 0.38–0.94) among former smokers and 1.09 (95% CI, 0.66–1.79) among nonsmokers (Rimm *et al.*, 1993). Similar protective effects of dietary β-carotene were seen in the cohort of nurses, with a relative risk of 0.78 (95% CI, 0.59–1.03) for those in the top quintile of total β-carotene intake relative to those in the lowest quintile (Manson *et al.*, 1991). In contrast, a prospective cohort study of postmenopausal women showed that dietary intake of carotenoids was not associated with the risk for death from coronary heart disease in multivariate models (Kushi *et al.*, 1996). A study of the association between dietary carotenoid intake and coronary mortality in a Finnish cohort of men and women showed that dietary carotenoid (primarily β-carotene) intake was not associated with risk in men, and there was only a suggestion of an inverse association in women (Knekt *et al.*, 1994).

Epidemiological studies of cardiovascular disease, much like those of cancer, now often involve the use of intermediate end-points. One such end-point is the thickness of the intima media, which can be estimated by ultrasonography, as a measure of atherosclerosis. This method has been used to examine the relationship between atherosclerosis and antioxidant status. A progressive decrease in the thickness of the intima media on the common carotid arteries was found with increasing concentrations of total plasma carotenoids in both men and women. The association disappeared, however, after adjustment for potential confounders, most notably body mass index (Bonithon-Kopp *et al.*, 1997). In another study, progression of the thickness of the intima media was 92% greater in the lowest versus the highest quartile of plasma β-carotene concentrations (Salonen *et al.*, 1993).

The finding in numerous observational studies that increased intake of carotenoid-containing diets and higher blood concentrations of carotenoids are associated with reduced risks for cardiovascular disease cannot be interpreted as a specific protective effect of β-carotene or other carotenoids *per se*; that type of evidence can best be obtained by randomized trials.

Some of the first such studies were early analyses of 333 men enrolled in the Physicians' Health Study who were known to have stable angina or to have undergone coronary revascularization. In a preliminary report, subjects who received supplemental β-carotene (50 mg every other day) for five years had a 51% reduction in the risk for major coronary events and a 54% reduction in the risk for major vascular events (Gaziano, 1994). In a subsequent report on the same group of men, however, those assigned to β-carotene had a nonsignificant increase in the risk for death from cardiovascular disease (RR, 1.33; 95% CI, 0.78–2.26) (Gaziano et al., 1996; see also section 7.1).

In the full population of the Physicians' Health Study, 12 years of supplementation with β-carotene (50 mg every other day) had no significant effect on the risk for cardiovascular disease (Hennekens et al., 1996). In a trial for the prevention of oesophageal and gastric cancer in the general population in Linxian, China, the combination of β-carotene, vitamin E and selenium resulted in a 10% reduction in mortality due to cerebrovascular disease (RR, 0.90; 95% CI, 0.76–1.07), this disease accounting for about 25% of all deaths in this population (Blot et al., 1993). In people with oesophageal dysplasia, supplementation with a multivitamin–multimineral preparation plus 15 mg β-carotene reduced the rate of mortality from cerebrovascular disease by 37% (RR, 0.63; 95% CI, 0.37–1.07; Mark et al., 1996). The decrease was greater for men (RR, 0.42) than for women (RR, 0.93) (Li, J.-Y. et al., 1993).

The results of the ATBC and CARET trials with regard to cardiovascular disease suggest a possible harmful role of supplemental β-carotene and are considered elsewhere (see section 7.1). In the Skin Cancer Prevention Study, participants whose blood concentrations of β-carotene were highest when they were randomized had the lowest risk for death from cardiovascular disease in the succeeding 10 years (RR, 0.57; 95% CI, 0.34–0.95); however, there was no evidence that β-carotene supplementation had any effect on mortality from these diseases (RR, 1.16; 95% CI, 0.82–1.64) (Greenberg et al., 1996).

5.3 Age-related macular degeneration and cataract

Dietary carotenoids may be important in the prevention of two ocular conditions — age-related macular degeneration and senile cataract. The macula is a small, yellow region in the centre of the retina. Degeneration of the macula is the most common cause of irreversible blindness in people over the age of 65 (Seddon et al., 1994a; Snodderly, 1995). Cataracts are also problematic, cataract extraction being the most frequently performed surgical procedure among the elderly. While the causes of these conditions are not known, oxidative processes may play a role. Cataracts are thought to result from photo-oxidation of lens proteins, which results in protein damage, accumulation, aggregation and precipitation in the lens (Taylor, 1993). The cornea and lens filter out UV light, but visible blue light reaches the retina and may contribute to photic damage and other oxidative insults (Seddon et al., 1994a). Carotenoids might interfere with both processes.

The potential role of carotenoids in the prevention of age-related macular degeneration has been reviewed (Snodderly, 1995); this section is therefore not comprehensive but highlights key studies in this area. In a study of dietary intervention, an inverse association was found between the consumption of carotene-rich fruits and vegetables and the risk for age-related macular degeneration, on the basis of data from the first National Health and Nutrition Examination Survey in the USA (Goldberg et al., 1988). The association between carotenoid intake and advanced age-related macular degeneration was addressed in a large, multicentre case–control study involving 356 cases and 520 control subjects with other ocular conditions. Patients with this condition who were in the highest quintile of carotenoid intake had a 43% lower risk for macular degeneration than those in the lowest quintile (odds ratio, 0.57; 95% CI, 0.35–0.92). Intake of lutein and zeaxanthin (grouped in the carotenoid food composition database) was most strongly associated with the reduced risk. Increased consumption of spinach and collard greens, which are rich dietary sources of lutein and zeaxanthin, was also associated with a significant reduction in risk (Seddon *et al.*, 1994a). It is biologically plausible that lutein and zeaxanthin have protective effects against macular degeneration, as these carotenoids selectively accumulate in the macula (Bone *et al.*, 1988; Handelman *et al.*, 1988) and account for the yellow colour observed in this region of the retina. For unknown reasons, zeaxanthin is the dominant carotenoid at the centre of the fovea, whereas lutein dominates outside the foveal centre (Bone *et al.*, 1988). The specificity of incorporation of carotenoids into the macula may give some clues as to their role in the prevention of age-related macular degeneration.

Studies in which blood carotenoid concentrations were used as the measure of exposure also suggest protective effects against the risk for age-related macular degeneration. For example, in one case–control study, serum carotenoid concentrations were measured in 391 patients with neovascular age-related macular degeneration and 577 controls, and significant protective effects were reported for total carotenoids, β-carotene, α-carotene, cryptoxanthin and lutein/zeaxanthin, with odds ratios ranging from 0.3 to 0.5 for people in the 80th percentile or higher versus those in the 20th percentile or lower. Serum lycopene was not, however, protective in this study (odds ratio, 0.8; $p = 0.4$) (Eye Disease Case–Control Study Group, 1993). In contrast, an association was found only between the serum concentration of lycopene and age-related maculopathy in 167 case–control pairs drawn from a study in the USA, persons in the lowest quintile of lycopene concentration having a doubling in risk for maculopathy (Mares-Perlman *et al.*, 1994). In a study of ageing in Baltimore, USA, the relationship between plasma β-carotene concentration and age-related macular degeneration was studied in 226 patients. A nonsignificant inverse relationship was found (odds ratio for high quartile versus low, 0.62). Plasma lutein and zeaxanthin were not measured (West *et al.*, 1994). In a fourth study, no relationship was found between the plasma concentrations of α-carotene, β-carotene, β-cryptoxanthin, lutein and lycopene and the occurrence of age-related maculopathy; how-ever, the sample size was limited to 65 matched pairs (Sanders *et al.*, 1993).

New techniques are now available for measuring the optical density of retinal carotenoids (macular pigment) by noninvasive methods (see, e.g. Hammond & Fuld, 1992), which may provide a long-term measure of carotenoid status in this tissue, facilitating future epidemiological studies.

In the ATBC cancer prevention trial, a random sample of 990 participants were examined ophthalmologically at the end of the trial, and 66 cases of age-related macular degeneration were observed in the group receiving β-carotene versus 51 in those given placebo (difference not significant) (Teikari *et al.*, 1995).

The literature on antioxidant nutrients and cataract has also been reviewed (Taylor, 1993; Taylor *et al.*, 1995). Higher dietary intake of carotenoids or higher blood concentrations of carotenoids have been found to prevent various forms of cataract in some but not all studies. For example, subjects with low plasma carotenoid concentrations (< 20th percentile) had a 5.6-fold increased risk for any senile cataract and a 7.2-fold increased risk for cortical cataract when compared with subjects with high plasma carotenoid concentrations (> 80th percentile) (Jacques & Chylack, 1991). A cross-sectional analysis of serum α-carotene, β-carotene, lutein/zeaxanthin, lycopene and β-cryptoxanthin concentrations and the severity of nuclear and cortical opacities showed that higher concentrations of individual or total carotenoids were not associated overall, but higher serum β-carotene was protective in men and higher concentrations of α-carotene, β-cryptoxanthin and lutein were protective against nuclear sclerosis in men who smoked. In women, however, higher concentrations of carotenoids were associated with an increased severity of nuclear sclerosis (Mares-Perlman *et al.*, 1995).

Use of vitamin supplements and the risk for cataract were also evaluated in the Physicians' Health Study. Users of multivitamins, but not of vitamin C or E alone, resulted in a marginally significant decreased risk for cataracts in comparison with people who did not take these supplements (RR, 0.75; 95% CI, 0.55–1.01). The lower risk associated with β-carotene supplementation was seen in current and former smokers but not in people who had never smoked (Seddon *et al.*, 1994b).

[The Working Group noted that observational studies of cataracts, like those of most chronic diseases, are highly susceptible to confounding and must thus be interpreted cautiously. For example, markers of higher socio-economic status are consistently associated with a decreased risk for cataract (Sperduto *et al.*, 1990). Since higher socioeconomic status is also associated with a higher intake of micronutrients and with vitamin supplementation, any protective effects could well be due to confounding. Thus, evidence from trials is critical in evaluating potential health effects.]

The cancer prevention trials in Linxian, China, included ocular examinations for participants in the trial on dysplasia and for a subset of participants in the trial in the general population. The combination of β-carotene, α-tocopherol and selenium did not reduce the prevalence of cataract in the general population. In the dysplasia trial, however, there was a statistically significant, 36% reduction in the prevalence of nuclear cataract among persons aged 65–74 years who received supplements of multiple vitamins and minerals plus β-carotene (15 mg/d) for six years (Sperduto *et al.*, 1993).

There is currently no convincing evidence that supplementation with carotenoids can affect the development or progression of age-related cataracts or age-related macular degeneration. While supplemental lutein and zeaxanthin may be of value for the prevention of macular degeneration, extremely few data are available on the pharmacology, pharmacokinetics and toxicity of these supplements in humans or in animals.

5.4   Other effects

Antioxidants, including β-carotene and carotenoids, have been suggested to be of value in the prevention or management of a number of chronic conditions, including rheumatoid arthritis (Heliövaara *et al.*, 1994; Comstock *et al.*, 1997), impaired cognition in the elderly (Perrig *et al.*, 1997) and ageing (Cutler, 1991).

6.   Carcinogenicity

6.1   Humans

Two of the intervention trials described in section 4.1.1.3 suggest increased incidences of lung cancer. These are discussed below. Non-significant increases in the incidences of cancers at other sites in intervention trials and case–control studies are mentioned in the full descriptions of these studies in section 4.1.1.3.

6.1.1   ATBC Study

In the ATBC study (Alpha-Tocopherol, Beta Carotene Cancer Prevention Group, 1994a,b; Albanes *et al.*, 1996), involving 29 133 men who smoked at least five cigarettes daily at entry, with a median of 20 cigarettes per day and a median duration of smoking of 36 years, 894 cases of lung cancer were identified during the follow-up. The incidence of lung cancer was 16% higher among the men who received β-carotene than among those who did not (RR, 1.16; 95% CI, 1.02–1.33). The effect appeared to be stronger, but not significantly so, in participants who smoked at least 20 cigarettes daily at entry (RR, 1.25; 95% CI, 1.07–1.46) than in those who smoked 5–19 cigarettes daily (RR, 0.97; 95% CI, 0.76–1.23), and in those with higher alcohol intake (≥ 11 g of ethanol daily) (RR, 1.35; 95% CI, 1.01–1.81) than in those with a lower intake (RR, 1.03; 95% CI, 0.85–1.24). A 23% increase in the incidence of prostate cancer and a 25% increase of stomach cancer were also seen among men receiving β-carotene in comparison with those not receiving β-carotene, but these differences were not statistically significant; the incidences of cancers of the colon and rectum and urinary bladder were not affected by β-carotene.

6.1.2   CARET

The CARET (Omenn *et al.*, 1996a,b) involved 14 254 men and women 50–69 years of age who had at least 20 pack–years of cigarette smoking and either were currently smoking or had stopped smoking within the previous six years; 4060 men with substantial occupational exposure to asbestos were also included. Daily supplementation with β-carotene and retinyl palmitate was stopped 21 months early, after a median of 3.7 years of follow-up, because of clear evidence of no benefit and substantial evidence of possible harm. A total of 388 new cases of lung cancer were diagnosed during the follow-up. The actively treated group had a relative risk for lung cancer of 1.28 (95% CI, 1.04–1.57) as compared with those on placebo. This overall risk for lung cancer included relative risks of 1.40 (95% CI, 0.95–2.07) for workers exposed to asbestos, 1.42 (95% CI, 1.07–1.87) for heavy smokers who were smoking at the time of randomization and 0.80 (95% CI, 0.48–1.31) for previously heavy smokers who were no longer smoking at the time of randomization. In comparison with the group given placebo, those receiving the supplement in the highest quartile of alcohol intake had an increased risk for lung cancer (RR, 1.99; 95% CI, 1.28–3.09); a test for the heterogeneity of relative risks among quartiles of alcohol intake was statistically significant at the 0.01 level. Because of the lack of a consistent dose–response effect and the multiple tests performed, the authors considered this result to be only suggestive. There were no statistically significant differences in the risks for cancers at other sites.

6.1.3 Interpretation of trials suggesting carcinogenicity

The groups receiving β-carotene supplementation had an increased risk for lung cancer in both the ATBC Study and CARET (in which the group also received retinyl palmitate). No change in lung cancer risk was found in the Linxian or Physicians' Health studies, but their power to find a small change in lung cancer risk was limited by the relatively small number of cases of lung cancer. There was no statistically significant increase in the incidence of any other cancer in these studies. Thus, the question pertains to the possibility that β-carotene supplementation increased the risk for developing lung cancer.

Differences in the study populations and interventions may explain some of the results of the trials. In the ATBC Study and the PHS, all of the participants were men, whereas in the CARET and Linxian studies, half of the participants were women. Supplementation in the PHS was with β-carotene alone at 50 mg every

second day; in the ATBC study, β-carotene was given at 20 mg per day either alone or in combination with α-tocopherol; in the CARET, β-carotene was given at 30 mg per day in combination with vitamin A; and in Linxian, a combination of β-carotene at 15 mg per day, vitamin E and selenium was given. In the ATBC study, all of the participants were smokers, in the CARET, 60%, in the Linxian study, 30% and in PHS, only 11%. The CARET suggested increased risks for lung cancer among current smokers and asbestos-exposed workers but not among former smokers. In the ATBC study, the increased risk for lung cancer appeared to be confined to people smoking at least 20 cigarettes per day, and no effect on risk was found for those smoking 5–19 cigarettes per day (although the test for effect modification was not statistically significant). Years of cigarette smoking did not significantly modify the effect of β-carotene supplementation on lung cancer risk. These findings indicate that β-carotene supplementation accelerates the clinical appearance of lung cancer among current, heavy smokers. The ATBC study and CARET suggest that alcohol intake may modify the effect of β-carotene on lung cancer. The intake levels were, however, moderate: the median in the ATBC study was 11 g/day and that in the CARET, 3 g/day. In the ATBC study, the effect of β-carotene appeared to be stronger in men with a higher alcohol intake than in those with a lower intake; however, underestimation of alcohol intake is likely the higher the intake is. The CARET also suggested that the risk for lung cancer was greater in people with a high alcohol intake, but there was no consistent dose–response relationship. The separate effects of alcohol drinking and tobacco smoking are difficult to distinguish, as the two behaviours are correlated.

Other potentially important differences between the completed trials include baseline nutrient status and the population's response to the β-carotene intervention. As shown in Table 56, the population in the Linxian County study had notably low β-carotene concentrations at entry; in contrast, the physicians enrolled in the PHS had notably high β-carotene concentrations at entry. The study populations also varied in their plasma

Table 56. Serum concentrations of β-carotene before and after intervention in completed cancer prevention trials

Study	Serum β-carotene at entry (µg/dl)	Serum β-Carotene after intervention (µg/dl)	β-Carotene dose (manufacturer)
ATBC	[17][a]	[300][a]	20 mg/d (Roche)
CARET	[17][a,b]	[210][a]	30 mg/d (Roche)
PHS	[30][b,c]	[120][c]	50 mg on alternate days (BASF)
Linxian	6[c]	86[c]	15 mg/d (Roche)

ATBC, Alpha-Tocopherol Beta-Carotene; CARET, Beta-Carotene Retinol Efficacy Trial; PHS, Physicians' Health Study
[a] Median
[b] Level in placebo group after intervention
[c] Mean

responses to supplemental β-carotene. The participants in the two trials that provide evidence of potential harm (CARET and ATBC) also had the highest serum concentrations of β-carotene at the end of the intervention and those in the PHS and Linxian studies notably lower concentrations. The dose of β-carotene and the median serum β-carotene concentrations achieved in these studies exceeded by many times the dietary intake or serum concentration of β-carotene associated with a lowered risk for cancer in the epidemiological follow-up studies.

6.2   Experimental animals

Mouse: It was reported in an abridged paper that beadlets containing 11.5% β-carotene were incorporated into the diet of four groups of 100 male and 100 female CD-1 mice [age unspecified] at concentrations resulting in β-carotene doses of 100, 250, 500 or 1000 mg/kg bw per day [formulation in the diet unspecified]. Two groups of mice were fed either unsupplemented standard diet or standard diet supplemented with placebo beadlets. Administration of β-carotene for up to 105 weeks did not affect the spontaneous tumour profile [no further information was given on mortality or tumours] (Heywood *et al.*, 1985).
Rat: Two groups of 15 male and 15 female Wistar rats, 30–40 days old, were fed a 'synthetic' diet for 90 weeks followed by ground commercial laboratory chow pellets for another 20 weeks, either as such or supplemented with 0.1% β-carotene (96% all-*trans* isomer) [formulation in the diet unspecified]. After one year, four rats [sex unspecified] of each group were killed for interim observations. There was no significant difference in body weight between the two groups. At termination of the study at week 110, 7/26 controls [sex unspecified] and 13/26 rats fed β-carotene-fed [sex unspecified] were still alive. Extensive histopathological examination of the survivors revealed no treatment-related changes, except for storage of Sudan-positive material in the Kupffer cells of the livers of the rats fed β-carotene (Zbinden & Studer, 1958; Bagdon *et al.*, 1960) [The Working Group noted the small number of animals per group, the short treatment period, the absence of histopathological examination of the animals that died intercurrently and the lack of information on spontaneous tumours.]

It was reported in an abridged paper that beadlets containing about 11.5% β-carotene were incorporated into the diet of Sprague-Dawley rats at concentrations resulting in doses of 100, 250, 500 and 1000 mg/kg bw per day for life; other rats received either unsupplemented standard diet or standard diet supplemented with placebo beadlets. The F_{1a} pups were assigned to six groups of 60 males and 60 females, each receiving the same diet as their mothers. After 78 weeks, when the clotting times in all male rats appeared to be prolonged, 15 ppm heterazeen (a biologically active vitamin K analogue) was added to the diet of all rats. All survivors were killed when 20% of the controls on standard diet were still alive (week 116 for males and week 114 for females). The body-weight gain of animals at the three highest doses was lower than that of rats receiving placebo [no further details given; statistics unspecified]. β-Carotene did not affect the spontaneous tumour profile [no further information on mortality or tumours] (Heywood *et al.*, 1985).

No data were available to the Working Group on other carotenoids.

6.3   Mechanisms of carcinogenicity

Mechanisms to explain the excess incidence of lung cancers observed in persons receiving β-carotene supplements in the CARET and the ATBC study remain speculative. Possible mechanisms of effect to account for the observed excess, assuming that it is in fact real and attributable to β-carotene, are discussed below.

The results of the two trials strongly suggest that concurrent exposure to β-carotene and to a relatively high intensity of cigarette smoke is necessary for a harmful effect of β-carotene to occur. Moreover, the risk appears to be specific to lung cancer. The combination of tobacco smoke, which contains many free radicals and is strongly oxidative, and relatively high partial pressures of oxygen in the lung may trigger autooxidation of β-carotene and other carotenoids in the lung (discussed by Mayne *et al.*, 1996; see also Section 2). Under such conditions, the free radical of β-carotene may also serve as a propagator of free-radical formation. Transformed or damaged cells found in the lungs of long-term smokers might be particularly sensitive to either modulation of the oxidative state or the non-physiological concentrations of β-carotene present. This hypothesis is consistent with the work of Leo *et al.* (1992), which showed that ethanol-induced hepatotoxicity in a baboon model was exacerbated by a challenge of non-physiological doses of β-carotene. In this situation as well, damaged cells seem more susceptible to the adverse effects of β-carotene.

The amount of β-carotene that is autooxidized is known to be dose-dependent (see Table 56 for blood concentrations in this and other trials), and that might explain the lack of effect on lung cancer rates in the PHS. Similarly, as discussed elsewhere (Mayne *et al.*, 1996), asbestos fibres also produce an inflammatory response in lung, resulting in overproduction of reactive oxygen species.

The link between local oxidative stress in the lung and promoting effects of supplemental β-carotene is unclear; however, several critical regulatory pathways and signalling molecules are redox-regulated (e.g. NF-kB, and AP-1). Thus, it can be hypothesized that a pro-oxidant state in the lung, due to autooxidation of β-carotene and/or severe oxidative stress, might result in alterations in both cell proliferation and apoptosis. Liebler (1993), however, used in-vitro models of β-carotene and cigarette smoke to show that autooxidation of β-carotene occurs after exposure to tobacco but does not result in a prooxidant state except in models with β–carotene (Omaye *et al.*, 1997). This might suggest that oxidative metabolites of β-carotene, rather than a prooxidative state, are responsible for any effects observed.

Further considerations are the following:
• High concentrations of β-carotene present in the gastrointestinal tract at the same time as other carotenoids may inhibit the absorption of other protective phytochemicals, such as α-carotene and lutein. Although competitive interactions have been shown between various carotenoids when administered together in large amounts (Kostic *et al.*, 1995), large recurrent doses of β-carotene had little effect on other serum carotenoids in intervention trials (Albanes *et al.*, 1997; Mayne *et al.*, 1997).
• Cigarette smoke may activate leukocytes and macrophages to secrete oxidizing agents, with formation of carotenyl radical adducts by O_2^- (Trush & Kensler, 1991).

- β-Carotene may inhibit the apoptosis of preneoplastic or neoplastic cells, thus enhancing the survival of such cells. Supplements of β-carotene decreased apoptosis (Johnson *et al.*, 1996; Mannick *et al.*, 1996).
- β-Carotene may be an effective antioxidant in lung, thereby altering the redox state and potentially affecting redox-regulated aspects of cell proliferation and apoptosis. The lack of an effect (e.g. lung carcinogenicity) of vitamin E in the ATBC trial suggests, however, that this possibility is not likely.

These mechanisms are not mutually exclusive, and more than one may be involved.

7. Other Toxic Effects

7.1 Toxic and other adverse effects
7.1.1 Humans
Most of the available data on the safety of carotenoids concern β-carotene. Studies of toxicity in experimental animals have shown that β-carotene is not mutagenic or teratogenic. Doses of 20–180 mg/d β-carotene given for many years have been used to treat patients with erythropoietic protoporphyria, with no evidence of toxicity and without the development of abnormally elevated blood vitamin A concentrations (Mathews-Roth, 1986; Meyers *et al.*, 1996).

The conversion of β-carotene and other provitamin A carotenoids is regulated by the vitamin A status of individuals. Thus, high intakes of carotenoids do not lead to abnormally high vitamin A concentrations or symptoms of hypervitaminosis (Olson, 1994). Hyper-carotenaemia, or high serum concentrations of carotene, may occur when people take supplements containing 20 mg or more of β-carotene for extended periods. Hypercarotenaemia has also been seen in people who consume large quantities of food rich in β-carotene. People who take high concentrations of β-carotene supplements or who consume large quantities of carotene-rich foods may, in addition to having higher serum concentrations of β-carotene, develop yellow palms and soles, a condition technically known as hyper-carotenodermia. This condition can be clearly differentiated from jaundice because the whites of the eyes (sclera) are yellow only in patients with jaundice. The change disappears with discontinuation of increased intake (Lascari, 1981). Hyper-carotenaemia can also be caused by a rare genetic inability to convert β-carotene to vitamin A (McLaren & Zekian, 1971; Monk, 1982) and is sometimes seen in association with hypothyroidism, diabetes mellitus and hepatic and renal disease. The hypercarotenaemia is a secondary condition and is not the cause of these diseases (Meyers *et al.*, 1996).

In the ATBC study, 11% more total cardiovascular deaths, including deaths from ischaemic heart disease, all types of stroke and other cardiovascular disease, were seen in the men taking β-carotene (Alpha-Tocopherol Beta-Carotene Cancer Prevention Study Group, 1994b). When the analyses were restricted to the 1862 participants who had previously had a myocardial infarct, men who received β-carotene alone had relative risks of 1.75 (95% CI, 1.16–2.64) for fatal coronary heart disease and 3.44 (95% CI, 1.70–6.94) for fatal myocardial infarct (Rapola *et al.*, 1997). The corresponding relative risks for those who received β-carotene plus α-tocopherol were 1.58 (95% CI, 1.05–2.40) and 2.67 (95% CI, 1.30–5.46). Similarly, an increased number of deaths from cardiovascular disease was seen in the CARET among men taking supplemental β-carotene plus retinol: the relative risk was 1.26 (95% CI, 0.99–1.61; Omenn *et al.*, 1996b).

Limited data exist on the toxicity of other carotenoids. Canthaxanthin is an approved food colour additive, but it has been used without regulatory approval for attaining a skin colour similar to a suntan. Excessive intake produces discoloured plasma and faeces, which probably has no physiological significance; however, crystalline deposits occurred in the retinas of all subjects ingesting 60 mg, and a change in retinal function after long-term treatment was observed in a few persons with such deposits (Weber *et al.*, 1992). The changes in retinal function are relatively minor, however, and are corrected over a period of months or years as the canthaxanthin crystals disappear (Arden & Barker, 1991; Weber *et al.*, 1992). Similar canthaxanthin retinopathy induced in monkeys was not associated with retinol dysfunction or abnormal morphology (Goralczyk *et al.*, 1997).

In contrast, the retinas of patients with erythropoietic protoporphyria given high doses of β-carotene for up to 10 years showed no crystalline deposits. The dose of canthaxanthin required for this ocular response appears to be more than 30 mg/d (Köpcke *et al.*, 1995). The retinas of 26 patients with protoporphyria who received treatment with β-carotene (200 30-mg capsules per month for several months) for periods of 1–10 years were not found to have crystalline deposits; however, asymptomatic retinopathy, consisting of multiple, bright yellow, glistening crystalline deposits in and around the maculae, were observed in 6 of 50 patients who had ingested more than 200 30-mg doses of canthaxanthine as a photoprotectant and systemic skin colourant (Poh-Fitzpatrick & Barbera, 1984).

Lycopene is a more intensely coloured pigment than β-carotene. High lycopene intake also produces hypercarotenodermia; however, a deeper orange is usually observed than with β-carotene (Lascari, 1981).

There have been several other isolated reports of carotenoid-related toxicity; however, the findings are associated with very large intakes of foods containing β-carotene, among other constituents, or a genetic defect in the metabolism of carotenoids (Bendich, 1988; Ahmed *et al.*, 1994; Diplock, 1995; Olmedilla *et al.*, 1995; Svensson & Vahlquist, 1995).

7.1.2 *Experimental animals*

Few experimental studies of the toxicity of β-carotene *in vivo* have been reported. Many are quite dated and generally do not provide details of experimental outcomes. They are reviewed here as extensively as possible.

The toxicity of β-carotene, lycopene and bixin was studied in rats, rabbits and dogs given 7–1000 mg/d orally or intramuscularly by various schedules. No side-effects were reported; however, the number of animals was small and the histological examination rather simple (Zbinden & Studer, 1958). Similarly, in a multigeration study of rats receiving 0.1% β-carotene in the diet and in a study of toxicity in dogs receiving 0, 1, 10 or 100 mg/kg for five days per

week for 13 weeks, no side-effects were seen (Bagdon *et al.*, 1960).

The results of a two-year study in dogs, a study of toxicity and tumorigenicity in rats and a study of carcinogenicity in mice were reported in an abridged paper. The livers of treated dogs and mice had some histological changes, with vacuolated cells, but these were considered to be fat storage cells and of no major toxicological importance (Heywood *et al.*, 1985). [The Working Group did not have access to numerical results or statistical analyses.]

Certain beadlet formulations of β-carotene may potentiate the hepatotoxicity of alcohol. Rats were given vitamin A and β-carotene for two months, with or without beadlets or corresponding amounts of beadlets without β-carotene. Ethanol enhanced the concentrations of hepatic β-carotene in the presence of beadlets and to a lesser extent in their absence. As the configurations of the beadlets differed for the various β-carotene preparations, further studies may be needed (Leo *et al.*, 1997).

7.2 Reproductive and developmental effects

Exposure of many laboratory species and humans during pregnancy to high doses of preformed vitamin A induces a variety of malformations (reviewed by Schardein, 1993; Friedman & Polifka, 1994). In contrast, β-carotene consumption has not been associated with teratogenicity in humans (Anon., 1987; Pinnock & Alderman, 1992; Nau *et al.*, 1994).

7.2.1 *Humans*

In a review of reports of elevated β-carotene concentrations and adverse birth outcome, it was noted that no malformations were mentioned in one study of 149 infants delivered to women with exceptionally high concentrations of carotene in blood, and several other studies of hypercarotenaemic women did not mention malformations in the offspring or noted that the infants were themselves carotenaemic; a few showed reversible desquamation of the skin. The author concluded that no abnormalities in humans were attributable to the carotenoid molecule (Matthews-Roth, 1988). A similar conclusion was reached in a review of the literature on experimental animals and humans (Bendich, 1988) and in another, partial review of the same literature (Diplock, 1995).

No association was found between the β-carotene concentrations in the sera of women infected with the human immunodeficiency virus and vertical transmission of the virus to the fetus. The concentrations of β-carotene were 9.5 μg/dl in transmitters and 11.4 μg/dl in non-transmitters (Burger *et al.*, 1997).

The cryptoxanthin concentrations in the cord blood of human fetuses remained relatively constant, at 50 ng/ml, throughout gestation; however, the concentrations in cord blood were significantly higher in 18 infants with intrauterine growth retardation than in 65 with normal weight (Moji *et al.*, 1995).

No mention of any reproductive effects of lycopene in humans or experimental animals was included in recent reviews of the biochemistry and biophysics (Stahl & Sies, 1996) or potential human health effects (Gerster, 1997) of this carotenoid. No association was found between the lycopene concentrations in the sera of women infected with the human immunodeficiency virus and vertical transmission of the virus to the fetus. The concentrations of lycopene were 9.5 μg/dl in transmitters and 11.4 μg/dl in non-transmitters (Burger *et al.*, 1997)

7.2.2 *Experimental animals*

In one of the earliest studies of the toxicity of β-carotene, groups of 2–16 Wistar rats of each sex were exposed from 30–40 days of age to 0.1% in the diet for four generations. The offspring did not show signs of hypervitaminosis A syndrome (Bagdon *et al.*, 1960). [The Working Group noted the small sample sizes and the incomplete reporting of the results.]

In a review of studies of the effect of nutrient status on the reproductive efficiency of livestock, 12 studies of dairy cows supplemented with β-carotene showed positive effects, 10 studies showed no effect, and one study reported a detrimental effect (Hurley & Doane, 1989).

In a multigeneration test, groups of 15 male and 15 female rats were given β-carotene as 0.1% dietary mixture for 100 weeks. Three additional generations were produced; equal numbers of rats were maintained as controls. The sizes of the groups declined throughout the study due both to deaths unrelated to treatment and to sampling. No effects were observed on growth, food consumption, haematopoietic tissues or reproduction (Bagdon *et al.*, 1960).

β-Carotene was administered in beadlets (containing approximately 11.5%) in the diet of Sprague-Dawley rats through three generations. A total of 210 males and 420 females were assigned to one of six doses (0, 100, 250, 500 or 1000 mg/kg per day); one control group received the diet only and another received placebo beadlets. The dietary concentrations were reduced to 3.5% in nursing females from day 12 *post partum*, continuing through weaning, to avoid excess dosage of the growing young. The pregnancy rates, pregnancy performance, gestation periods and litter parameters were measured, and organ weights and the results of histopathological examinations were recorded for selected offspring of the F_{3b} pups on day 21. The authors stated that β-carotene had no effect on reproductive function (Heywood *et al.*, 1985). [The Working Group noted that the publication did not present actual data.] The same group reported that studies of teratogenicity in albino rabbits given daily oral doses of 0, 100, 200 or 400 mg/kg β-carotene by gavage on days 7–19 of gestation and in albino rats given daily doses of 0, 250, 500 or 1000 mg/kg on days 7–16 of gestation showed no evidence of embryotoxicity or teratogenicity in term fetuses. [The Working Group again noted the lack of data.]

β-Carotene was administered to groups of pregnant Sprague-Dawley rats as a 0.2% supplementation in the diet (about 125 mg/kg bw) in order to evaluate its potential to reduce the effects of of cigarette smoke (2 h per day throughout pregnancy) on fetal weight. Thus, rats underwent whole-body exposure to control air and to cigarette smoke, with or without β-carotene supplementation, although none received only β-carotene. The concentrations of retinol in the liver, but not in plasma, were higher in rats exposed to both smoke and β-carotene than in rats given placebo, and the plasma and liver concentrations of β-carotene were 0.46 μmol/L and 0.10 μmol/g, respectively; only trace concentrations were found in the other groups. β-Carotene did not prevent retardation of growth due to cigarette smoke, nor did it appear to accentuate the adverse effects on fetal development (Leichter & Dunn, 1992).

Canthaxanthin was microencapsulated in water-soluble beadlets and administered in the diet to four groups of rats during three generations at concentrations of 0, 250, 500 or 1000 mg/kg. No effects on reproductive function were reported, but reduced food consumption and growth and increased serum transaminase and alkaline phosphatase activity and increased cholesterol concentrations were seen in adult females at all doses. In the weanlings, the organ:body weight ratios were increased for the liver and decreased for the adrenals at all doses. At the two highest doses, some histopathological changes were evident in the livers of F_2 females (Mantovani, 1992). [The Working Group noted that experimental details and results were generally lacking from this brief report, which summarized a report from WHO (1990).]

7.3 Genetic and related effects
7.3.1 Humans
In a cross-sectional study, the concentrations of urinary aflatoxin B_1–DNA adducts in 85 healthy Taiwanese men were positively associated with their plasma concentrations of α- and β-carotene and inversely related to their plasma concentrations of lycopene (Yu et al., 1997).

7.3.2 Experimental systems
7.3.2.1 In vitro
Several studies have been reported on the mutagenicity of carotenoids in Ames' Salmonella/microsome test. As most of the results were generated in studies of the ability of these compounds to modulate the mutagenic response (see section 4.2.2.2), the results are limited to one or two strains of S. typhimurium. As shown in Table 57, all of the reported results are negative, with one exception. β-Carotene was not mutagenic in strains TA1535, TA1538, TA98 or TA100, either in the presence or absence of

exogenous metabolic activation, but significant enhancement of 'spontaneous' revertants in strain TA104 was reported in one study (Han, 1992). Canthaxanthin, 8'-apo-β-carotenal and 8'-apo-β-carotene methyl ester were not mutagenic in strain TA98 or TA100, either in the presence or absence of exogenous metabolic activation. Cryptoxanthin extracted from orange juice, carrot carotenoids containing 51% β-carotene, 32% α-carotene and 17% other carotenoids and lycopene extracted from tomato paste were not mutagenic in strain TA98 or TA100 in the presence of an exogenous metabolic system. β-Carotene also did not induce differential toxicity in Bacillus subtilis or Escherichia coli rec strains or reversion in strain W2P uvrA of E. coli, either in the absence of metabolic systems or in the presence of rat liver microsomes or caecal extracts.

In cultured mammalian cells, β-carotene did not affect the frequencies of sister chromatid exchange in cultured Balb/c mouse mammary glands, of sister chromatid exchange, chromosomal aberrations or micronucleus formation in Chinese hamster ovary cells or of micronuclei in metabolically competent Hep G2 human hepatoma cells.

7.3.2.2 In vivo
β-Carotene did not affect the frequency of 6-thioguanine-resistant T lymphocytes extracted from the spleens of Fischer 344 rats given 0.15% in drinking-water for two, four, six or eight weeks. Although at each time the frequency of these mutations was consistently higher than in untreated rats, the differences were not statistically significant (Aidoo et al., 1995). No significant variation was observed in the frequency of micronuclei in bone-marrow polychromatic erythrocytes of Swiss mice receiving 2.5 mg β-carotene in drinking-water daily for 15 days (Lahiri et al., 1993) or of hybrid $B6C3F_1$ mice receiving 100 mg/kg β-carotene in the diet for one week (Raj & Katz, 1985). β-Carotene also did not induce chromosomal aberrations in bone-marrow cells of Balb/c mice receiving β-carotene dissolved in corn oil by gavage at a concentration of 200 mg/kg bw for five days (Salvadori et al., 1992a,b). Two additional studies yielded

Table 57. Genetic and related effects of carotenoids in short-term tests in vitro and in vivo

End-point	Code	Test system	Result Without exogenous metabolic system	Result With exogenous metabolic system	HID[a]	Reference
β-Carotene						
D	BSD	Bacillus subtilis rec strains, differential toxicity	-	0	1 mg/ml	Kada et al. (1972)
D	ERD	Escherichia coli rec strains, differential toxicity	-	-	100 µg/ml	Haveland-Smith (1981)
G	ECW	Escherichia coli WP2 uvr A, reverse mutation	0	-	100 µg/ml	Haveland-Smith (1981)
G	SAO	Salmonella typhimurium TA100, reverse mutation	0	-	100 µg/plate	He & Campbell (1990)
G	SAO	Salmonella typhimurium TA100, reverse mutation	-	0	800 nmol/plate [?][c]	Azune et al. (1992)
G	SAO	Salmonella typhimurium TA100, reverse mutation	-	-	10 µmol/plate	Camoirano et al. (1994)
G	SA5	Salmonella typhimurium TA1535, reverse mutation	-	-	200 µg/plate	Belisario et al. (1985)
G	SA8	Salmonella typhimurium TA1538, reverse mutation	0	-	100 µg/ml	Haveland-Smith (1981)
G	SA9	Salmonella typhimurium TA98, reverse mutation	0	-	500 µg/plate	Terwel & van der Hoeven (1985)
G	SA9	Salmonella typhimurium TA98, reverse mutation	0	-	0.86 µmol/plate	Whong et al. (1988)
G	SA9	Salmonella typhimurium TA98, reverse mutation	-	-	3.45 µmol/plate	Ong et al. (1989)
G	SA9	Salmonella typhimurium TA98, reverse mutation	0	-	100 µg/plate	He & Campbell (1990)
G	SA9	Salmonella typhimurium TA98, reverse mutation	-	-	800 nmol/plate [?][c]	Azune et al. (1992)
G	SA9	Salmonella typhimurium TA98, reverse mutation	0	-	10 µmol/plate	Camoirano et al. (1994)
G	SAS	Salmonella typhimurium (other miscellaneous strains), reverse mutation	-	-	4151 µg/plate	Heywood et al. (1985)
G	SAS	Salmonella typhimurium (other miscellaneous strains), reverse mutation	-	0	10 µmol/L	Han (1994)
S	SIM	Sister chromatid exchanges, mouse cells in vitro	-	0	1 µmol/L	Manoharan & Banerjee (1985)
S	SIS	Sister chromatid exchange, Chinese hamster ovary cells in vitro	-	0	10 µmol/L	Cozzi et al. (1997)

Table 57 (contd)

End-point	Code	Test system	Result Without exogenous metabolic system	Result With exogenous metabolic system	HID[a]	Reference
β-Carotene (contd)						
M	MIA	Micronucleus induction, Chinese hamster ovary cells *in vitro*	–	0	6 µmol/L	Salvadori et al. (1994)
M	MIA	Micronucleus induction, Chinese hamster ovary cells *in vitro*	–	0	0.035 µmol/L	Stich & Dunn (1986)
C	CIS	Chromosomal aberrations, Chinese hamster ovary cells *in vitro*	–	0	0.035 µmol/L	Stich & Dunn (1986)
C	CIS	Chromosomal aberrations, Chinese hamster ovary cells *in vitro*	–	0	1 µmol/L	Cozzi et al. (1997)
M	MIH	Micronucleus induction, Hep G2 human hepatoma cells	–	0	6 µmol/L	Salvadori et al. (1993)
C	GVA	Gene mutation, rat T lymphocytes *in vivo*	0	–	0.15% in drinking-water for 8 weeks	Aidoo et al. (1995)
M	MVM	Micronucleus induction, mouse bone-marrow cells *in vivo*	0	–	100 mg/kg food for 1 week	Raj & Katz (1985)
M	MVM	*Micronucleus induction, mouse bone-marrow cells in vivo*	0	+	27 mg/kg bw orally for 7 days	Mukherjee et al. (1991)
M	MVM	Micronucleus induction, mouse bone-marrow cells *in vivo*	0	#	#	Umegaki et al. (1994a)
M	MVM	Micronucleus induction, mouse bone-marrow cells *in vivo*	0	–	2.5 mg/mouse in drinking-water for 15 days	Lahiri et al. (1993)
C	CBA	Chromosomal aberrations, mouse bone-marrow cells *in vivo*	0	+	27 mg/kg bw orally for 7 days	Mukherjee et al. (1991)
C	CBA	Chromosomal aberrrations, mouse bone-marrow cells *in vivo*	0	–	200 mg/kg bw by gavage for 5 days	Salvadori et al. (1992a,b)

Table 57 (contd)

End-point	Code	Test system	Result		HID[a]	Reference
			Without exogenous metabolic system	With exogenous metabolic system		
Canthaxanthin						
G	SA0	Salmonella typhimurium TA100, reverse mutation	0	–	100 µg/plate	He & Campbell (1990)
G	SAO	Salmonella typhimurium TA100, reverse mutation	–	–	800 nmol plate [?][c]	Azuine et al. (1992)
G	SA9	Salmonella typhimurium , TA98 reverse mutation	0	–	100 µg/plate	He & Campbell (1990)
G	SA9	Salmonella typhimurium TA98, reverse mutation	–	–	800 nmol plate[?]	Azuine et al. (1992)
8'-Apo-β-carotenal methylester						
G	SA0	Salmonella typhimurium TA100, reverse mutation	–	–	800 nmol/plate [?] [c]	Azuine et al. (1992)
G	SA9	Salmonella typhimurium TA98, reverse mutation	–	–	800 nmol/plate [?] [a]	Azuine et al. (1992)
Carrot carotenoids (51% β-carotene, 32% α–carotene, 17% other carotenoids)						
G	SA0	Salmonella typhimurium TA100, reverse mutation	–	–	800 nmol/plate [?] [c]	Azuine et al. (1992)
G	SA9	Salmonella typhimurium TA98, reverse mutation	–	–	800 nmol/plate [?] [c]	Azuine et al. (1992)
Cryptoxanthin (extracted from orange juice)						
G	SA0	Salmonella typhimurium TA100, reverse mutation	0	–	100 µg/plate	He & Campbell (1990)
G	SA9	Salmonella typhimurium TA98, reverse mutation	0	–	100 µg/plate	He & Campbell (1990)
G	SA0	Salmonella typhimurium TA100, reverse mutation	0	–	100 µg/plate	He & Campbell (1990)
G	SA9	Salmonella typhimurium TA98, reverse mutation	0	–	100 µg/plate	He & Campbell (1990)
Lycopene (extracted from tomato paste)						
G	SA0	Salmonella typhimurium TA100, reverse mutation	0	–	100 µg/plate	He & Campbell (1990)
G	SA9	Salmonella typhimurium TA98, reverse mutation	0	–	100 µg/plate	He & Campbell (1990)

[a] Result: + , positive; –, considered to be negative; 0, not tested; # 'spontaneous' frequency of micronuclei was decreased by either β-carotene or a diet containing β-carotene (see Table 55).

[b] Highest ineffective dose

[c] Presumably nmol/plate

conflicting results. In one study (Mukherjee *et al.*, 1991), oral administration of 27 mg/kg bw β-carotene significantly enhanced the frequencies of both micronuclei and chromosomal aberrations in bone-marrow cells of Swiss albino mice over that in controls receiving the solvent (olive oil) only. In contrast, another study (Umegaki *et al.*, 1994a) showed that β-carotene given by gavage or incorporated into a *Dunaliella bardawil* diet reduced the 'spontaneous' frequency of micronuclei in peripheral blood reticulocytes of ICR mice.

8. Summary of Data

8.1 Chemistry, occurrence and human exposure

The carotenoids are hydrophobic, lipophilic substances which, after ingestion, are absorbed with other lipids. The state in which the carotenoids occur in the food matrix, e.g. crystalline or not, their concentration, the availability of fat or oil and the presence of bile acids are major factors in determining their bioavailability. About 600 carotenoids have been isolated from natural sources, and some 100 or so of these are likely to be present in the human diet; however, of the carotenoids in serum, only six or seven have been studied in any depth, of which three are provitamin A carotenoids, i.e. β-carotene, α-carotene and β-cryptoxanthin. The main carotenoids that are addressed in this *Handbook* are found widely in fruits and vegetables and products derived from them; small amounts are also found in foods of animal origin such as some fish and crustaceans, egg yolk and dairy products. Some carotenoids, notably β-carotene, are used widely as food colourants and are produced synthetically or from biological sources for this purpose. Supplements of β-carotene, natural and synthetic, are widely available.

Fruits and green vegetables are the main sources of β-carotene and lutein in the human diet. Carrots are rich in β-carotene and are often the main source of α-carotene in temperate climates, depending on strain or variety. Tomatoes and tomato products are rich in lycopene. Yellow maize provides zeaxanthin and β-cryptoxanthin; various fruits such as oranges, peaches, apricots, mangoes and papayas, also contain β-cryptoxanthin. There is no major dietary source of canthaxanthin, although it is found in trout, crustaceans and sometimes in egg yolk after its use as an additive in feed. Canthaxanthin has been marketed in the past as an orally administered 'tanning' agent, but this use has been discontinued in several countries. A balanced diet provides a daily intake of a few milligrams of some of these compounds; the total might range from 4 to 10 mg/day. Much higher intakes can be achieved from certain foods such as carrots, red palm oil, mangos and concentrated tomato products. If supplements are taken, the intake increases accordingly. The daily intake of each of the other carotenoids listed, namely zeaxanthin, β-cryptoxanthin, canthaxanthin and α-carotene, is likely to be 1–5 mg.

In the body, all carotenoids are found in lipid environments, especially fatty tissues and membranes. Their presence in membranes may be important in relation to their biological actions.

The long system of conjugated double bonds that constitutes the light-absorbing chromophore of the carotenoids also makes these molecules rather unstable and very reactive towards oxidizing agents and free radicals. They can have antioxidant or pro-oxidant actions *in vitro*. Although antioxidant activity *in vivo* has not been proven, this has been proposed as a possible mechanism by which carotenoids could protect against cancer and other degenerative diseases.

Routine methods for the qualitative and quantitative analysis of carotenoids in foods and in blood and body tissues are usually based on reverse-phase high-performance liquid chromatography with the use of an in-line photodiode-array detector to generate ultraviolet or visible absorption spectra. Mass spectrometry and co-chromatography with authentic samples are required additionally for proper identification.

8.2 Metabolism and kinetics
8.2.1 Humans

In humans, carotenes and many xanthophylls are absorbed in the small intestine and appear in lipoproteins of the plasma. Although more than 20 carotenoids are found in plasma, the major components are lycopene, lutein, β-carotene, zeaxanthin, β-cryptoxanthin and α-carotene. The types and amounts of carotenoids in the plasma reflect those in the diet. Plasma carotenoids are taken up by essentially all tissues, the major repositories being the adipose tissue, liver and skin. The pattern of carotenoids in tissues reflects that in the plasma, with few exceptions.

Factors that influence serum carotenoid concentrations and presumably also those of tissues include the dietary intake of carotenoids, the fat content of the diet, the acidic fibre content of the diet, smoking, alcohol intake and food processing. The determinants of absorption and resulting blood and tissue concentrations are not well understood. In general, increased intake of both dietary and supplemental carotenoids leads to higher blood concentrations, but the bioavailability of purified or synthetic preparations is greater than than that of dietary components. Oral supplements of a given carotenoid markedly increase its concentrations in plasma and tissues. In vitamin A-sufficient subjects, carotenoid intake has little effect on the plasma concentrations of retinol.

The only known function of carotenoids in humans is as precursors of vitamin A. Only 50 of the approximately 600 carotenoids in nature, however, serve this role. The major pathway of enzymatic conversion is central cleavage of the carotenoid molecule, although asymmetric cleavage can also occur. Carotenoids can also be oxidized at other positions in the molecule, although such reactions have been little studied.

8.2.2 Experimental models

Distinct interspecies differences exist in the biokinetics of carotenoids and particularly in their intestinal absorption, their transport in plasma and, to a lesser extent, their metabolism in tissues. Most of the common laboratory animals are not suitable models for biokinetics in humans; however, two animal models have been developed to mimic the situation in humans: the ferret and the preruminant calf. Although both have some limitations, studies with these species have provided important information on carotenoid uptake and metabo-

lism. Use of non-human primates has provided promising results, but further evaluation of these models is needed. Other species, such as rats, chicks and pigs, may be considered for investigating specific aspects such as metabolism.

Carotenoids are metabolized differently in different species. The most marked difference is between vertebrates that efficiently absorb intact carotenoids, such as humans, other primates, cows and birds, and those that do not, such as most rodents and pigs. Because of these differences, research in humans is particularly important.

8.3 Cancer-preventive effects
8.3.1 Humans
The results of epidemiological studies, viewed in aggregate, do not support the notion that β-carotene has generalized cancer-preventive effects. The observational data suggesting cancer-preventive effects are most consistent for lung, oral and pharyngeal cancers, the incidences of which tend to be inversely related to β-carotene (or provitamin A carotenoid) intake or blood concentrations. One difficulty in interpreting these findings is that β-carotene may be only a marker of the intake of other beneficial substances in fruits and vegetables or perhaps other lifestyle habits. No clinical trial of β-carotene as a single agent, however, has shown a reduction in the risk for cancer at any specific site, and there is evidence of an increase in the risk for lung cancer among smokers and asbestos workers receiving β-carotene supplements at high doses, which resulted in blood concentrations an average of 10–15 times higher than normal. It is worth noting that the information from clinical trials reflects the first 12 years of intervention, and, at present, there are no data on the possible effects of longer intervention. There is virtually no information on β-carotene supplementation early in the carcinogenic process. Lastly, the doses used in the intervention trials greatly exceeded those consumed in normal diets. There is only limited, inconsistent information on carotenoids other than β-carotene.

Summarized below are the results of studies on β-carotene pertaining to specific cancers. The data for other cancer sites were generally less extensive and not indicative of either protection or harm.

Lung cancer

The most extensive results with regard to β-carotene pertain to cancers of the lung and bronchus. The vast majority of observational studies of dietary intake indicate a decreased risk with higher intake of carotene. There are also extensive, consistent findings that higher blood concentrations of β-carotene are associated with a decreased risk for lung cancer. In general, people with the highest intake or blood concentration have been found to have a 20–50% lower risk than those with the lowest values. In contrast, no clinical trial of β-carotene supplementation has shown a reduction in risk, and two of the three large trials found an increase in lung cancer occurrence among smokers; one also suggested an increase in asbestos workers.

Skin cancer

The results of epidemiological studies show no reduction in the risk for skin cancer associated with β-carotene intake or blood concentrations. One clinical trial indicated no reduction in the risk for basal- or squamous-cell skin cancer after supplementation for up to five years.

Oral and pharyngeal cancers

Some observational studies have shown inverse associations between dietary intake of β-carotene (or carotene), blood carotene concentrations and the risk for oral and pharyngeal cancers. Intervention trials of intermediate markers of oral carcinogenesis (oral leukoplakia or micronuclei) with supplemental β-carotene, alone and in combination with other agents, have shown regression. Many of these trials, however, have methodological limitations.

Oesophageal cancer

Observational studies of dietary intake of provitamin A carotenoids generally suggest inverse associations with the risk for oesophageal cancer. The results of two related intervention trials are available. In one trial, supplemental β-carotene given in combination with vitamin E and selenium had no effect on the rate of mortality from oesophageal cancer. In a related trial in the same population but restricted to persons with oesophageal dysplasia, supplemental β-carotene given with several other micronucrients was also of no benefit in preventing death from oesophageal cancer.

Gastric cancer

Some observational studies of either dietary or blood β-carotene concentrations showed inverse associations with gastric cancer or precancerous gastric lesions. The results of three intervention trials are available. In one trial, supplemental β-carotene given in combination with vitamin E and selenium showed a reduction of borderline significance in the risk for gastric cancer. The population studied was known to have several micronutrient deficiencies, and the relevance of these results for well-nourished populations is unclear. In a related trial in the same population but restricted to persons with oesophageal dysplasia, supplemental β-carotene given with several other micronutrients was of no benefit in preventing mortality from gastric cancer. In a third trial, no reduction in gastric cancer risk was observed.

Colorectal cancer and adenoma

Epidemiological studies show no clear pattern of reduced risk for either invasive cancer or adenoma in relation to β-carotene intake. Two clinical trials showed no reduction in the occurrence of adenoma after supplementation with β-carotene. None of the large trials of β-carotene supplementation suggests a decrease in the occurrence of colorectal cancer.

Cervical cancer

Some observational studies have shown inverse associations between dietary intake of various carotenoids or blood carotenoid concentrations and the risk for cervical neoplasia. One trial of low-dose β-carotene supplementation in women with cervical dysplasia in the Nether-lands gave no evidence of greater regression in this group.

8.3.2 Experimental systems
8.3.2.1 Cancer-preventive activity
β–Carotene

The cancer-preventive efficacy of β-carotene has been assessed in mouse, rat and hamster models, virus-induced tumour models and inoculated tumour cells.

In models of respiratory-tract carcinogenesis, β-carotene was ineffective in three studies in hamsters, and there were even indications of weak enhancement in two of these studies. In models of lung carcinogenesis in mice, β-carotene was ineffective in two studies.

The effects of β-carotene against skin carcinogenesis induced by various carcinogens were investigated in more than 20 studies in mice; β-carotene was effective in almost all. In the two studies in which it was ineffective, it was administered only before initiation or in the late stages of carcinogenesis. β-Carotene was effective in preventing buccal pouch carcinogenesis in hamsters in about 20 studies. It was ineffective in only one study when also given after tumour development. β-Carotene was also effective in preventing liver carcinogenesis in most of about 20 studies in male rats. In those studies involving administration of N-nitrosodiethylamine or 2-acetylaminofluorene, conflicting results were obtained. β-Carotene did not affect the incidence of liver tumours in a strain of mice with a high incidence of spontaneous tumours at this site. The cancer-preventive effects of β-carotene in models of colon carcinogenesis were investigated in one study in mice and in seven studies in rats. Conflicting results were found, and no pattern emerged to explain the differences. β-Carotene prevented pancreatic cancer in two of three studies in rats and in one of two studies in hamsters. No pattern emerged to explain the differences. The preventive effect of β-carotene on gastric carcinogenesis was demonstrated in one study in mice but not in one study in rats. β-Carotene prevented urinary bladder carcinogenesis in one of two studies in mice when given before, during and after carcinogen administration, but not in one study in rats. It was ineffective in models of small intestine carcinogenesis in two studies in rats. It showed some preventive effects against salivary gland carcinogenesis in one of three studies in rats.

In one model of multiorgan carcinogenesis in rats, β-carotene showed a tendency to decrease the incidences of preneoplastic liver foci, colon adenocarconomas and nephroblastomas.

β-Carotene was effective in three studies in models of malignant tumours induced in mice by Moloney murine sarcoma virus. In several studies in mice and rats inoculated with tumour cells, subsequent administration of β-carotene inhibited tumour growth, enhanced survival and in some cases resulted in tumour regression.

The cancer-preventive effects of β-carotene combined with other chemicals (vitamin C, vitamin E, retinol, glutathione, oltipraz, 4-hydroxyphenylretinamide, selenium, wheat bran or perilla oil) were investigated in three studies in rats and one study in hamsters with regard to pancreatic carcinogenesis, in three studies on buccal pouch cancer in hamsters, in two studies on colon carcinogenesis in rats, in one study on respiratory tract tumours in hamsters and in one study on lung tumours in mice. In all of these studies, the combinations were as effective or more effective than β-carotene alone, except for one study in hamsters in which β-carotene alone or combined with vitamin C was ineffective in preventing pancreatic carcinogenesis and one study in mice in which β-carotene alone or in combination with retinol was ineffective in preventing lung tumours.

β-Carotene inhibited neoplastic transformation in four studies. The effect required continuous treatment during the post-initiation phase of carcinogenesis and was reversible after withdrawal of treatment. β-Carotene inhibited the formation of aberrant lesions in mouse mammary cells in one study. Maximum inhibition was seen when treatment was simultaneous and continued for the duration of the experiment.

Canthaxanthin

The cancer-preventive efficacy of canthaxanthin was assessed in several mouse, rat and hamster models. It prevented skin carcinogenesis in eight studies in mice in which ultraviolet B irradiation was used as the carcinogen; conflicting results were obtained in two studies in which 7,12-dimethylbenz[a]anthracene was the carcinogen. Canthaxanthin was effective in all six studies in hamsters in which the buccal pouch was the target organ. It showed cancer-preventive effects in one of four studies of liver carcinogenesis in rats. The cancer-preventive efficacy of canthaxanthin was investigated in 10 studies in rats in models of cancers of the colon, mammary gland, tongue, small intestine, glandular stomach and salivary glands. In single studies, it was effective against cancers of the tongue and glandular stomach and ineffective against cancers of the salivary glands and small intestine. In studies of the colon and mammary gland, canthaxanthin was effective in one study and ineffective in another; the positive finding in mammary glands was associated with treatment before carcinogen administration. In two studies in mice, canthaxanthin had no preventive effect against urinary bladder cancer.

In one study in mice inoculated with malignant thymoma cells, canthaxanthin inhibited tumour growth when administered before and after tumour inoculation and appeared to be ineffective when given only after inoculation. It inhibited neoplastic transformation in cell cultures *in vitro*.

α-Carotene
In single studies in mice, α-carotene reduced the incidences of tumours of the liver, lung and skin, and in one study in rats it inhibited colon carcinogenesis. It inhibited neoplastic transformation *in vitro*.

Lycopene
A slight effect of lycopene was seen in two studies in rats in the aberrant crypt foci model of colon carcinogenesis. In models of liver carcinogenesis in rats, lycopene was ineffective in two studies and effective in one. In one study in mice, lycopene reduced the incidence of spontaneous mammary gland tumours but enhanced the development of preneoplastic mammary nodules. In another study, lycopene reduced the incidence of spontaneous liver tumours in mice. It was effective in one study of lung carcinogenesis in male but not female mice. It inhibited neoplastic transformation *in vitro*.

Lutein
In one study in rats, oral administration of lutein had preventive activity in the aberrant crypt foci model of colon carcinogenesis. In one study in mice, it was effective against skin carcinogenesis. In one study in mice inoculated with murine mammary tumour cells, lutein inhibited tumour growth. It inhibited neoplastic transformation *in vitro*.

Fucoxanthin
In single studies in mice, fucoxanthin applied to the skin was found to have preventive effects against skin tumours. Fucoxanthin in drinking-water inhibited the formation of tumours of the duodenum.

Mixtures
In four studies, *Spirulina–Dunaliella* extracts (containing 15–30% β-carotene, 20–25% xeaxanthin, 20–25% β-cryptoxanthin, 10–15% myxoxanthin, 10–15% echixenone and other carotenoids) were found to prevent cheek pouch carcinogenesis in hamsters. In one study in mice, diets supplemented with *Dunaliella* powder or *Dunaliella* extract (containing 0.03% β-carotene) reduced the incidence of spontanous mammary gland tumours. In single studies in mice, palm-oil carotene was effective in reducing the incidence of spontaneous liver cancer and of chemically induced carcinogenesis in the skin, lung, small intestine and stomach. In one study in rats, palm-oil carotene had no preventive effect in the aberrant crypt foci model of colon carcinogenesis.

8.3.2.2 Genetic and related effects
A number of carotenoids were evaluated for their ability to inhibit genetic and related effects *in vitro*. In most studies, carotenoids exerted protective effects against promutagens and mutagens that induce oxidative damage, whereas they did not affect the potency of directly acting mutagens. These findings were not always consistent, depending on the test compound and the laboratory that conducted the study. In addition to the usual limitations of in-vitro studies, resulting from the high concentrations of both genotoxic agents and modulators, the delivery system for carotenoids in these studies is very different from those *in vivo*.

In studies of the ability of orally administered carotenoids (mostly β-carotene) to inhibit genetic and related effects in mice, rats and hamsters treated with a variety of physical or chemical carcinogens, the end-points included production of single-strand breaks in the DNA of liver or forestomach mucosa, mutations in T lympocytes, micronucleus formation or chromosomal aberrations in bone-marrow cells and binding to liver DNA. The results of most of the studies were consistent with protective effects of carotenoids.

8.3.3 Mechanisms of cancer prevention

The following mechanisms of action have been proposed or suspected to contribute to any cancer-preventive effects of carotenoids. Most of these mechanisms have been studied only *in vitro*, and more complex interactions among dietary components and mechanistic pathways are likely to occur *in vivo*.

All of the carotenoids examined inhibited oxidative or free-radical-initiated damage to synthetic or biological membranes. Processes involving free radicals and reactive oxygen species may be important at various stages of the multistep carcinogenic process. Carotenoids can interact with reactive oxygen species, and they have also been shown to inhibit lipid peroxidation.

In experimental models, carotenoids have been shown to prevent malignant transformation of normal cells or to induce cell differentiation. Carotenoids can stimulate gap-junctional communication between cells *in vitro*, an effect postulated to reduce the aberrant proliferation of carcinogen-initiated cells. In five studies, β-carotene at concentrations that were not cytotoxic was reported to decrease proliferation. In one study, lycopene was reported to be more effective than α- or β-carotene. In two reports, effects were seen in normal and dysplastic cells but not in cancer cells. The prevention of both malignant transformation and proliferation may be due to the formation of biologically active molecules from carotenoids. In rats, some carotenoids can modulate the activities of carcinogen-metabolizing enzymes.

Carotenoids have immunomodulating effects that could enhance cellular defence systems, possibly involving tumour-specific anti-gens. In three studies, β-carotene was reported to increase various parameters of immune responsiveness. In two studies, no increases were observed, although responses were reported in response to astaxanthin. Canthaxanthin was reported to increase immune responsiveness in one study but not in another in which different effector cells and end-points were used.

Both β-carotene and canthaxanthin increased expression of a receptor gene driven by the *RAR-β* promoter, but this finding was not confirmed in another study in which expression of the endogenous gene was studied. In human keratinocytes grown in organotypic culture, β-carotene and canthaxanthin decreased expression of mature *keratin 10* and increased expression of *connexin 43*.

Thus, carotenoids, because they may act in several different biological processes, should be considered nutritional modulators and not solely antioxidant or pro-oxidant molecules. Various mechanisms account for the observed protective effects, including delay in cell-cycle progression, decreased expression of proto-oncogenes, enhancement of intercellular communication, inhibition of metabolic activation of promutagens, enhancement of detoxification of reactive metabolites and inhibition of mutagenicity related to oxidative damage. The similar effects of carotenoids with and without provitamin A activity indicate a direct protective role *in vitro*.

8.4   Other beneficial effects

Antioxidants, including β-carotene and carotenoids, have been suggested to be of value in the prevention of a number of chronic diseases. The only current therapeutic use of carotenoids is in the treatment of erythropoietic protoporphyria, a photosensitivity disease. Although the results of a number of observational studies suggest that carotenoids may be of value in the prevention of cardiovascular disease, the results of the intervention trials with β-carotene do not support this hypothesis. Lutein and zeaxanthin have been suggested to play specific roles in the prevention of age-related macular degeneration, but experimental data to support this hypothesis are not yet available. Senile cataract is another ocular condition potentially related to oxidation; carotenoids including β-carotene are being studied for a role in the prevention of this disorder, although the available results are somewhat inconsistent. Carotenoids have also been suggested to be of benefit for several other health outcomes including but not limited to ageing, impaired cognition, rheumatoid arthritis and cystic fibrosis; however, the data are scant.

8.5   Carcinogenic effects
8.5.1   Humans
The results of two intervention trials provide evidence suggesting that β-carotene increases the risk for lung cancer among current smokers. An increased risk for lung cancer was also seen in the trial that included workers who had been exposed to asbestos, most of whom were ex-smokers. Two other very large trials, which did not include large numbers of smokers or persons exposed to asbestos, did not show any increased risk for cancers at specific sites. The biological mechanism by which β-carotene at the doses used in the two trials may increase the risk for lung cancer in high-risk groups is not clear.

8.5.2   Experimental animals
β-Carotene was studied for carcinogenicity in one study in male and female rats and in one study in male and female mice, but the reports were available only in abridged form. Enhanced carcinogenesis was seen in isolated investigations of carotenoids administered in conjunction with carcinogens.

8.6   Other toxic effects
8.6.1   Humans
Hypercarotenodermia (discolouration of the skin) produced by intake of carotenoids at high doses is considered to be a reversible condition. Intake of high doses of supplemental β-carotene has been reported to increase the risk for death from cardiovascular disease in specific high-risk groups. Ingestion of canthaxanthin at high doses over long periods induces

reversible retinopathy characterized by macular deposits.

There is no evidence to suggest that β-carotene is toxic at the levels found in most diets.

8.6.2   Experimental systems
In some studies of the induction of genetic and related effects in vitro, carotenoids were used as controls, generally at one dose only. None of the carotenoids tested, i.e. β-carotene, canthaxanthin, 8′-apo-β-carotenal, 8′-apo-β-carotenoyl methyl ester, carrot extract, carotenoids, cryptoxanthin and lycopene, was genotoxic in bacteria. Moreover, β-carotene did not induce sister chromatid exchange, chromosomal aberration or micronuclei in cultured mammalian cells.

β-Carotene has not been found to induce adverse genetic or related effects in experimental studies in vivo. It did not induce micronuclei in bone-marrow cells of mice, and it was neither clastogenic in rodent bone-marrow cells nor mutagenic in rat spleen T lymphocytes, although some conflicting data have also been reported. β-Carotene has been reported to enhance the hepatotoxicity induced by a high intake of alcohol in animals. It was not toxic to either embryos or dams in studies of developmental toxicity in rats and rabbits.

9.   Recommendations for Research

(1) Intervention studies of various types
(2) Further investigations into food composition
(3) Better biomarkers
(4) Greater understanding of the metabolism of carotenoids
(5) Better animal models
(6) Greater understanding of the mechanisms of carcinogenesis

Research proposals should clearly address gaps in knowledge about carcinogenesis and should relate to issues in carotenoid research that would clearly help answer questions relating to carcinogenesis.

Experimental research has shown that carotenoids are powerful chemicals and in some situations can protect against cancer. As both provitamin A and non-provitamin A carotenoids have these properties, the mechanism(s) may not necessarily involve the formation of vitamin A and its biologically active metabolites. The mechanism(s) by which carotenoids inhibit carcinogenesis in experimental animals is not known.

Carotenoids can suppress cancer growth and development when they are applied to epithelial surfaces, when they are given orally and when injected into tissues. It is important to determine the uptake, transport and metabolism of the carotenoids in each case.

The natural site for carotenoids is membranes, where they affect the properties and those of associated processes and therefore potentially affect mechanisms of carcinogenesis. Research is required on caro-tenoid–cell membrane interactions in these situations and whether they are relevant to the prevention of cancer in humans.

Retinoids are clearly important in controlling cell differentiation and tissue growth. The morphogen, retinoic acid, can be formed directly from β-carotene in some circumstances. Central cleavage of carotenoids has been reported in many tissues, and there is evidence that the turnover of the provitamin A carotenoids β-carotene, α-carotene and β-cryptoxanthin is more rapid than that of the other major carotenoids in serum, suggesting conversion to retinol. Research should be conducted on the effects of carotenoids and carotenoid metabolites on events mediated by retinol receptors. This potential conversion could be studied by analysing endogenous responsive genes or by use of reporter constructs, which would allow the detection of activity ligands at levels as low as 10^{-10} mol/L.

Carotenoids are powerful quenchers of singlet oxygen and triplet sensitizers, a property that is relevant to the treatment of erythropoieticprotoporphyria. Furthermore, carotenoids can act as either antioxidants or pro-oxidants in chemical systems. The popular hypothesis that any biological activity of carotenoids can be attributed to an antioxidant or pro-oxidant role has not been proved. Research is required to evaluate critically the postulated antioxidant action of carotenoids *in vivo*, i.e. protection against oxidation mediated by free radicals. Interactions between carotenoids and vitamins E and C and other intracellular antioxidant defence mechanisms should also be studied.

There is accumulating evidence that metabolites of some of the common dietary carotenoids are produced oxidatively in biological fluids. Little is known about the basic mechanisms of oxidation of carotenoids or about reactions with free radicals. Research is required to understand the basic oxidative mechanisms that affect carotenoids *in vivo* in order to appreciate if and when carotenoids are influenced by such stresses.

Oxidative stress is a powerful signal (stimulator) of immune mechanisms. The operation of such mechanisms may be evident many years before clinical symptoms of disease appear; for example, a small depression in negative acute-phase proteins can be detected retrospectively 5–10 years before the appearance of clinical disease. Carotenoids are very sensitive to oxidation, and the presence of detectable oxidation products could be a useful marker of oxidative stress and of disease for use in epidemiological studies. Oxidation products of carotenoids may themselves have biological activity, and conversion within target tissues could explain much of their action. Research is needed to identify products of oxidation and metabolism and to examine their potential activity.

Major problems in assessing the cancer-preventive properties of carotenoids and in evaluating their adverse effects include the issues of antioxidant activity and their pro-oxidant role and the effects on lung cancer as related to cigarette smoking. The following research areas may be recommended:

- Development and application of suitable animal models for evaluating the oxidant and antioxidant properties of carotenoids *in vivo* and modulation of cigarette smoke-related biomarkers in the respiratory tract and cardiovascular system
- Implementation of phase-II trials to evaluate the oxidative and antioxidant effects of carotenoids and modulation of cigarette

smoke-related biomarkers in cells of the respiratory tract, e.g. pulmonary alveolarmacrophages.

Intervention studies with high doses of β-carotene provide evidence that people who are current smokers are at increased risk for lung cancer and cardiovascular disease when given supplements of β-carotene. Research is needed on the metabolic effects that smoking has on tissue metabolism and human physiology and on the effect of tobacco smoke on carotenoids *in vivo*.

Smoking is clearly associated with lower serum levels of some carotenoids. Research is required to determine whether this occurs through effects on the diet or on metabolism. Studies to determine the effects of tobacco smoke on carotenoids and of the interaction of carotenoids with smoke-exposed tissues should be conducted to better understand why β-carotene had the effect it did and whether this effect is unique or is common to all carotenoids.

Most of the observational studies were unable to distinguish the effects of individual carotenoids from those of substances in fruits and vegetables. Refinement of dietary databases, repetition of studies with adequate methods for evaluating diets and new biomarkers of intake should be pursued. Another approach is to capitalize on the fact that human populations differ in their intake of carotenoids. Research in regions where subpopulations have high intakes of specific carotenes deserves high priority.

10. Evaluation

10.1 Cancer-preventive activity
10.1.1 Humans
There is *evidence suggesting lack of cancer-preventive activity* for β-carotene when used as a supplement at high doses. There is *inadequate evidence* with regard to the cancer-preventive activity of β-carotene at the usual dietary levels. There is *inadequate evidence* with respect to the possible cancer-preventive activity of other individual carotenoids.

10.1.2 Experimental animals
There is *sufficient evidence for cancer-preventive activity* of β-carotene in experimental animals.

This evaluation is based on models of skin carcinogenesis in mice and buccal pouch carcinogenesis in hamsters. Findings in models of liver carcinogenesis in rats, colon carcinogenesis in rats and pancreatic carcinogenesis in rats and hamsters provide further support to this conclusion.

There is *sufficient evidence for cancer-preventive activity* of canthaxanthin in experimental animals. This evaluation is based on models of skin carcinogenesis in mice and buccal pouch carcinogenesis in hamsters. Findings in models of tongue cancer in rats and stomach carcinogenesis in mice provide additional support to this conclusion.

There is *limited evidence* that α-carotene has cancer-preventive activity from single studies of models of liver, lung, skin and colon carcinogenesis. There is *limited evidence* that lycopene has cancer-preventive activity from models of colon, liver, mammary gland and lung carcinogenesis. There is *limited evidence* that lutein has cancer-preventive activity from experimental models of colon and skin carcinogenesis. There is *limited evidence* that fucoxanthin has cancer-preventive activity from models of skin and duodenal carcinogenesis.

10.2 Overall evaluation
The results of studies in experimental animals and clinical studies in humans with regard to the cancer-preventive activity of β-carotene are conflicting. There is sufficient evidence that β-carotene has cancer-preventive activity against cancers of the skin and buccal pouch in experimental animals, supported by the results of studies in models of cancer of the liver, colon and pancreas. Moreover, there is considerable in-vitro and in-vivo evidence in animals that β-carotene inhibits the induction or expression of cancer-related events.

In observational epidemiological studies, β-carotene in blood or in the diet has been associated with reduced risks for cancers at many but not all sites. It is unclear, however, to what extent β-carotene itself is responsible for the decreased risks observed. Three large clinical trials indicate that supplementation with substantial doses of β-carotene does not prevent lung cancer and may actually increase the risk among individuals already at high risk (i.e. who are cigarette smokers or who have been occupationally exposed to asbestos). Although β-carotene is not known to be toxic in the short term, the intervention trials also suggest increased risks for cardiovascular death after supplementation. These trials do not provide clear evidence concerning cancers at specific sites other than the lung.

The discrepancies between the experimental and human observations and the findings from the intervention trials greatly complicate interpretation of the data on the effects of β-carotene. Understanding these discrepancies is an important aim of future research. Such investigation is also likely to provide insight into the process of carcinogenesis and increase knowledge about cancer prevention. Until such clarification is obtained, β-carotene supplements should not be recommended for use in cancer prevention in the general population and it should not be assumed that β-carotene is responsible for the cancer-protective effects of diets rich in carotenoid-containing fruits and vegetables.

Other carotenoids, canthaxanthin, α-carotene, lutein, lycopene and β-cryptoxanthin, have been investigated *in vitro* and in animal models, although not as extensively as β-carotene. There is *sufficient evidence* that canthaxanthin has cancer-preventive activity in animal models of cancers of the skin and buccal pouch, supported by the results of studies in models of cancers of the tongue and stomach. There is *limited evidence* that α-carotene, lycopene, lutein and fucoxanthin have cancer-preventive activity in a variety of animal models. Canthaxanthin inhibits the expression of cancer-related events *in vitro*.

The results of observational epidemiological for α-carotene, lycopene and lutein are much less extensive than those for β-carotene; no published results are available for canthaxanthin,. These carotenoids have not been studied in human trials for cancer prevention. Pending further research into their cancer-preventive activity, supplemental canthaxanthin, α-carotene, lutein and lycopene should not be recommended for use in cancer prevention in the general population, and it should not be assumed that the protective effects of diets rich in carotenoid-containing fruits and vegetables are due to any individual carotenoid.

References

Abraham, S.K., Sarma, L. & Kesavan, P.C. (1993) Protective effects of chlorogenic acid, curcumin and β-carotene against γ-radiation-induced in vivo chromosomal damage. *Mutat. Res.*, **303**, 109–112

Abril, E.R., Rybski, J.A., Scuderi, P. & Watson, R.R. (1989) Beta-carotene stimulates human leukocytes to secrete a novel cytokine. *J. Leukocyte Biol.*, **45**, 255–261

Adelekan, D.A., Thurnham, D.I. & Adekile, A.D. (1989) Reduced antioxidant capacity in paediatric patients with homozygous sickle cell disease. *Eur. J. clin. Nutr.*, **43**, 609–614

Ahmed, S., Lee, M.A. & Lieber, C.S. (1994) Interactions between alcohol and beta-carotene in patients with alcoholic liver disease. *Am. J. clin. Nutr.*, **60**, 430–436

Aidoo, A., Lyn-Cook, L.E., Lensing, S., Bishop, M.E. & Wamer, W. (1995) In vivo antimutagenic activity of β-carotene in rat spleen. *Carcinogenesis*, **16**, 2237–2241

Alabaster, O., Tang, Z., Frost, A. & Shivapurkar, N. (1995) Effect of beta-carotene and wheat bran on colonic aberrant crypt and tumor formation in rats exposed to azoxymethane and high dietary fat. *Carcinogenesis*, **16**, 127-132

Alabaster, O., Tang, Z. & Shivapurkar, N. (1996) Dietary fiber and the chemopreventive modulation of colon carcinogenesis. *Mutat. Res.*, **350**, 185–197

Alam, B.S. & Alam, S.Q. (1987) The effect of different levels of dietary beta-carotene on DMBA-induced salivary gland tumors. *Nutr. Cancer*, **9**, 93–101

Alam, B.S., Alam, S.Q., Weir, J.C., Jr & Gibson, W.A. (1984) Chemopreventive effects of beta-carotene and 13-*cis*-retinoic acid on salivary gland tumors. *Nutr. Cancer*, **6**, 4–12

Alam, B.S., Alam, S.Q. & Weir, J.C., Jr (1988) Effects of excess vitamin A and canthaxanthin on salivary gland tumors. *Nutr. Cancer*, **11**, 233–241

Alavanja, M.C.R., Brown, C.C., Swanson, C. & Brownson, R.C. (1993) Saturated fat intake and lung cancer risk among nonsmoking women in Missouri. *J. natl Cancer Inst.*, **85**, 1906–1916

Albanes, D., Heinonen, M., Pukkala, E. & Teppo, L. (1991) Dietary antioxidants and the risk of lung cancer. *Am. J. Epidemiol.*, **134**, 471–479

Albanes, D., Virtamo, J., Rautalahti, M., Haukka, J., Palmgren, J., Gref, C.-G. & Heinonen, O.P. (1992) Serum beta-carotene before and after beta-carotene supplementation. *Eur. J. clin. Nutr.*, **46**, 15–24

Albanes, D., Heinonen, O.P., Taylor, P. R., Virtamo, J., Edwards, B.K., Rautalahti, M., Hartman, A.M., Palmgren, J., Freedman, L.S., Haapakoski, J., Barret, M.J., Pietinen, P., Malila, N., Tala, E., Liippo, K., Salomaa, E.-R., Tangrea, J.A., Teppo, L., Askin, F., Taskinen, E., Erozan, Y., Greenwald, P. & Huttunen, J.K. (1996) α-Tocopherol and β-carotene supplements and lung cancer incidence in the Alpha-Tocopherol Beta-Carotene Cancer Prevention Study: Effects of base-line characteristics and study compliance. *J. natl Cancer Inst.*, **88**, 1560–1570

Albanes, D., Virtamo, J., Taylor, P.R., Rautalahti, M., Pietinen, P. & Heinonen, O.P. (1997) Effect of supplemental β-carotene, cigarette smoking and alcohol consumption on serum carotenoids in the Alpha-Tocopherol, Beta-Carotene Cancer Prevention Study. *Am. J. clin. Nutr.*, **66**, 366–372

Allard, J.P., Royall, D., Kurian, R., Muggli, R. & Jeejeebhoy, K.N. (1994) Effects of beta-carotene supplementation on lipid peroxidation in humans. *Am. J. clin. Nutr.*, **59**, 884–890

Alpha-Tocopherol Beta-Carotene Cancer Prevention Study Group (1994a) The Alpha-Toco-pherol Beta-Carotene Lung Cancer Prevention Study: Design, methods, participant characteristics and compliance. *Ann. Epidemiol.*, **4**, 1–10

Alpha-Tocopherol, Beta Carotene Cancer Prevention Study Group (1994b) The effect of vitamin E and beta carotene on the incidence of lung cancer and other cancers in male smokers. *New Engl. J. Med.*, **330**, 1029–1035

Ambrosone, C.B., Marshall, J.R., Vena, J.E., Laughlin, R., Graham, S., Nemoto, T. & Freudenheim, J.L. (1995) Interaction of family history of breast cancer and dietary antioxidants with breast cancer risk (New York, United States). *Cancer Causes Control*, **6**, 407–415

Ames, B.N., Shigenaga, M.K. & Gold, L.S. (1993) DNA lesions, inducible DNA repair, and cell division: Three key factors in mutagenesis and carcinogenesis. *Environ. Health Perspectives*, **101** (Suppl. 5), 35–44

Anon. (1987) Teratology Society position paper: Recommendations for vitamin A use during pregnancy. *Teratology*, **35**, 269–275

Appel, M.J. & Woutersen, R.A. (1996) Effects of dietary beta-carotene and selenium on initiation and promotion of pancreatic carcinogenesis in azaserine-treated rats. *Carcinogenesis*, **17**, 1411– 1416

Appel, M.J., Roverts, G. & Woutersen, R.A. (1991) Inhibitory effects of micronutrients on pancreatic carcinogenesis in azaserine-treated rats. *Carcinogenesis*, **12**, 2157–2161

Appel, M.J., Van Garderen-Hoetmer, A. & Woutersen, R.A. (1996) Lack of inhibitory effects of beta-carotene, vitamin C, vitamin E and selenium on development of ductular adenocarcinomas in exocrine pancreas of hamsters. *Cancer Lett.*, **103**, 157–162

Arden, G.B. & Barker, F.M. (1991) Canthaxanthin and the eye: A critical ocular toxicologic assessment. *J. Toxicol. cut. ocular Toxicol.*, **10**, 115–155

Arroyo, P.L., Hatch-Pigott, V., Mower, H.F. & Cooney, R.V. (1992) Mutagenicity of nitric oxide and its inhibition by antioxidants. *Mutat. Res.*, **281**, 193–202

Ascherio, A., Stampfer, M.J., Colditz, G.A., Rimm, E.B., Litin, L. & Willett, W.C. (1992) Correlations of vitamin A and E intakes with the plasma concentrations of carotenoids and tocopherols among American men and women. *J. Nutr.*, **122**, 1792–1801

Astorg, P., Gradelet, S., Leclerc, J., Canivenc, M.-C. & Siess, M.-H. (1994) Effects of β-carotene and canthaxanthin on liver xenobiotic-metabolizing enzymes in the rat. *Food Chem. Toxicol.*, **32**, 735– 742

Astorg, P, Gradelet, S. Bergès, R. & Suschetet, M. (1996) No evidence for an inhibitory effect of beta-carotene or of canthaxanthin on the initiation of liver preneoplastic foci by diethylnitrosamine in the rat. *Nutr. Cancer*, **25**, 27–34

Astorg, P. Gradelet, S., Bergès, R. & Suschetet, M. (1997) Dietary lycopene decreases the initiation of liver preneoplastic foci by diethylnitrosamine in the rat. *Nutr. Cancer*, **29**, 60–68

Azuine, M.A. & Bhide, S.V. (1992) Protective single/combined treatment with betel leaf and turmeric against methyl(acetoxymethyl)nitrosamine-induced hamster oral carcinogenesis. *Int. J. Cancer*, **51**, 412–415

Azuine, M.A., Amonkar, A.J. & Bhide, S.V. (1991) Chemopreventive efficacy of betel leaf extract and its constituents on 7,12-dimethylbenz(a)anthra-cene induced carcinogenesis and their effect on drug detoxification system in mouse skin. *Indian J. exp. Biol.*, **29**, 346–351

Azuine, M.A., Goswami, U.C., Kayal, J.J. & Bhide, S.V. (1992) Antimutagenic and anticarcinogenic effects of carotenoids and dietary palm oil. *Nutr. Cancer*, **17**, 287–295

Bagdon, R.E., Zbinden, G. & Studer, A (1960) Chronic toxicity studies of β-carotene. *Toxicol. appl. Toxicol.*, **2**, 225–236

Baghurst, P.A., McMichael, A.J., Slavotinek, A.H., Baghurst, K.I., Boyle, P. 7 Walker, A.M. (1991) A case–control study of diet and cancer of the pancreas. *Am. J. Epidemiol.*, **134**, 167–179

Bakker Schut, T.C., Puppels, G.J., Kraan, Y.M., Greve, J., van der Maas, L.L. & Figdor, C.G. (1997) Intracellular carotenoid levels measured by Raman microspectroscopy: Comparison of lymphocytes from lung cancer patients and healthy individuals. *Int. J. Cancer*, **74**, 20–25

Bandera, E.V., Freudenheim, J.L., Marshall, J.R., Zielezny, M., Priore, R., Brasure, J., Baptiste, M. & Graham, S. (1997) Diet and alcohol consumption and lung cancer risk in the New York State cohort (United States). *Cancer Causes Control*, **8**, 828–840

Banoub, R.W., Fernstrom, M. & Ruch, R.J. (1996) Lack of growth inhibition or enhancement of gap junctional intercellular communication and connexin43 expression by β-carotene in murine lung epithelial cells *in vitro*. *Cancer Lett.*, **108**, 35–40

Barbone, F., Austin, H. & Partridge, E.E. (1993) Diet and endometrial cancer: A case–control study. *Am. J. Epidemiol.*, **137**, 393–403

Barua, A.B., Kostic, D. & Olson, J.A. (1993) New simplified procedures for the extraction and simultaneous high-performance liquid chromatographic analysis of retinol, tocopherols and carotenoids in human serum. *J. Chromatogr.*, **617**, 257–264

Basu, T.K., Temple, N.J. & Hodgson, A.M. (1988) Vitamin A, beta-carotene and cancer. In: Tryfiades, G.P. & Prasad, K.N., eds, *Nutrition, Growth and Cancer*, New York, Alan R. Liss, pp. 217–228

Batieha, A.M., Armenian, H.K., Norkus, E.P., Morris, J.S., Spate, V.E. & Comstock, G.W. (1993) Serum micronutrients and the subsequent risk for cervical cancer in a population-based nested case control study. *Cancer Epidemiol. Biomarkers Prev.*, **2**, 335–339

Bauernfeind, J.C. (1972) Carotenoid vitamin A precursors and analogs in foods and feeds. *J. Agric. Food Chem.*, **20**, 456–473

Beems, R.B. (1987) The effect of beta-carotene on BP-induced respiratory tract tumors in hamsters. *Nutr. Cancer*, **10**, 197–204

Belisario, M.A., Pecce, R., Battista, C., Panza, N. & Pacilio, G. (1985) Inhibition of cyclophosphamide mutagenicity by β-carotene. *Biomed. Pharmacother.*, **39**, 445–448

Ben-Amotz, A., Mokady, S., Edelstein, S. & Avron, M. (1989) Bioavailability of a natural isomer mixture as compared with synthetic all-*trans*-β-carotene in rats and chicks. *J. Nutr.*, **119**, 1013–1019

Bendich, A. (1988) The safety of β-carotene. *Nutr. Cancer*, **11**, 207–214

Bendich, A. (1989) Carotenoids and the immune response. *J. Nutr.*, **119**, 112–115

Bendich, A. (1990a) Antioxidant micronutrients and immune responses. *Ann. N.Y. Acad. Sci.*, **587**, 168–180

Bendich, A. (1990b) Antioxidant vitamins and their functions in immune responses. *Adv. exp. Med. Biol.*, **262**, 35–55

Bendich, A. (1990c) Carotenoids and the immune system. In: Krinsky, N.I., Mathews-Roth, M.M. & Taylor, R.F., eds, *Carotenoids Chemistry and Biology*, New York, Plenum Press, pp. 323–335

Bendich, A. (1991) Beta-carotene and the immune response. *Proc. Nutr. Soc.*, **50**, 263–274

Bendich, A. & Olson, J.A. (1989) Biological actions of carotenoids. *FASEB J.*, **3**, 1927–1932

Bendich, A. & Shapiro, S.S. (1986) Effect of beta-carotene and canthaxanthin on the immune responses of the rat. *J. Nutr.*, **116**, 2254–2262

Berg, G., Kohlmeier, L. & Brenner, H. (1997) Use of oral contraceptives and serum beta-carotene. *Eur. J. clin. Nutr.*, **51**, 181–187

Bernhard, K. & Grosjean, M. (1995) Infrared spectroscopy. In: Britton, G., Liaaen-Jensen, S. & Pfander, H., eds, *Carotenoids*, Vol. 1B, *Spectroscopy*, Basel, Birkhaüser Verlag, pp. 117–134

Berset, D. & Pfander, H. (1985) Investigation of carotenoid composition in the petals of a garden hybrid Narcissus ccv 'Golden Harvest'. *Helv. chim. Acta*, **68**, 1149–1154

Bertram, J.S. & Bortkiewicz, H. (1995) Dietary carotenoids inhibit neoplastic transformation and modulate gene expression in mouse and human cells. *Am. J. clin. Nutr.*, **62**, 1327S–1336S

Bertram, J.S., Pung, A., Churley, M., Kappock, T.J., Wilkins, L.R. & Cooney, R.V. (1991) Diverse carotenoids protect against chemically induced neoplastic transformation. *Carcinogenesis*, **12**, 671–678

Bhattacharaya, R.K., Firozi, P.F. & Aboobaker, V.S. (1984) Factors modulating the formation of DNA adducts by aflatoxin B$_1$ *in vitro*. *Carcinogenesis*, **5**, 1359–1362

Bianchi-Santamaria, A., Dell'Orti, M., Frigoli, G., Gobbi, M., Arnaboldi, A. & Santamaria, L. (1994) Beta-carotene storage in rat organs following carrier mediated supplementation. *Int. J. Vit. Nutr. Res.*, **64**, 15–20

Bierer, T.L., Merchen, N.R., Nelson, D.R. & Erdman, J.W. (1993) Transport of newly-absorbed beta-carotene by the preruminant calf. *Ann. N.Y. Acad. Sci.*, **691**, 226–228

Bierer, T.L., Merchen, N.R. & Erdman, J.W. (1995) Comparative absorption and transport of five common carotenoids in preruminant calves. *J. Nutr.*, **125**, 1569–1577

Bingham, S.A., Gill, C., Welch, A., Day, K., Cassidy, A., Khaw, K.T., Sneyd, M.J., Key, T.J.A., Roe, L. & Day, N.E. (1994) Comparison of dietary assessment methods in nutritional epidemiology: Weighed records v. 24 h recalls, food-frequency questionnaires and estimated-diet records. *Br. J. Nutr.*, **72**, 619–643

Blaner, W.S. & Olson, J.A. (1994) Retinol and retinoic acid metabolism. In: Sporn, M.B., Roberts, A.B. & Goodman, D.S., eds, *The Retinoids: Biology, Chemistry, and Medicine*, 2nd Ed., New York, Raven Press, pp. 229–255

Blankenhorn, D.H. (1957) Carotenoids in man. IV. Carotenoid stores in normal adults. *J. biol. Chem.*, **229**, 809–816

Block, G., Coyle, L.M., Hartman, A.M. & Scoppa, S.M. (1994) Revision of dietary analysis software for the Health Habits and History Questionnaire. *Am. J. Epidemiol.*, **139**, 1190–1196

Blot, W.J., Li, J.Y., Taylor, P.R., Guo, W., Dawsey, S., Wang, G.-Q., Yang, C.S., Zheng, S.-F., Gail, M., Li, G.-Y., Yu, Y., Liu, B.-Q., Tangrea, J., Sun, Y.-H., Liu, F., Fraumeni, J.F., Jr, Zhang,, Y.-H. & Li, B. (1993) Nutrition intervention trials in Linxian, China: Supplementation with specific vitamin/mineral combinations, cancer incidence, and disease-specific mortality in the general population. *J. natl Cancer Inst.*, **85**, 1483–1492

Blot, W.J., Taylor, P.R., Li, J.Y. & Li, B. (1994) Lung cancer and vitamin supplementation (Letter). *New Engl. J. Med.*, **331**, 614

Blot, W.J., Li, J.Y., Taylor, P.R., Guo, W., Dawsey, S. & Li, B. (1995) The Linxian trials: Mortality rates by vitamin–mineral intervention group. *Am. J. clin. Nutr.*, **62** (Suppl.), 1424S–1426S

Boeing, H., Frentzel Beyme, R., Berger, M., Berndt, V., Gores, W., Korner, M., Lohmeier, R., Menarcher, A., Männl, H.F., Meinhardt, M., Müller, R., Ostermeier, H., Paul, F., Schwemmle, K., Wagner, K.H. & Wahrendorf, J. (1991) Case–control study on stomach cancer in Germany. *Int. J. Cancer,* **47**, 858–864

Bogden, J.D., Bendich, A., Kemp, F.W., Bruening, K.S., Shurnick, J.H., Denny, T., Baker, H. & Louria, D.B. (1994) Daily micronutrient supplements enhance delayed-hypersensitivity skin test responses in older people. *Am. J. clin. Nutr.*, **60**, 437–447

Bond, G.G., Thompson, F.E. & Cook, R.R. (1987) Dietary vitamin A and lung cancer: Results of a case–control study among chemical workers. *Nutr. Cancer*, **9**, 109–121

Bone, R.A., Landrum, J.T. & Tarsis, S.L. (1985) Preliminary identification of the human macular pigment. *Vision Res.*, **25**, 1531–1535

Bone, R.A., Landrum, J.T., Fernandez, L. & Tarsis, S.L. (1988) Analysis of the macular pigment by HPLC: Retinal distribution and age study. *Invest. Ophthalmol. vis. Sci.*, **29**, 843–849

Bone, R.A., Landrum, J.T., Hime, G.W., Cains, A. & Zamor, J. (1993) Stereochemistry of the human macular carotenoids. *Invest. Ophthalmol. vis. Sci.*, **34**, 2033–2040

Bone, R.A., Landrum, J.T., Friedes, L.M., Gomez, C.M., Kilburn, M.D., Menendez, E., Vidal, I. & Wang, W. (1997) Distribution of lutein and zeaxanthin stereoisomers in the human retina. *Exp. Eye Res.*, **64**, 211–218

Bonithon-Kopp, C., Coudray, C., Berr, C., Touboul, P.-J., Feve, J.M., Favier, A. & Ducimetiere, P. (1997) Combined effects of lipid peroxidation and antioxidant status on carotid atherosclerosis in a population aged 59–71 y. *Am. J. clin. Nutr.*, **65**, 121–127

Borenstein, B. & Bunnell, R.H. (1966) Carote-noids: Properties, occurrence, and utilization in foods. *Adv. Food Res.*, **15**, 195–276

Bos, R.P., van Poppel, G., Theuws, J.L.G. & Kok, F.J. (1992) Decreased excretion of thioethers in urine of smokers after the use of β-carotene. *Int. Arch. occup. environ. Health*, **64**, 189–193

Bostick, R.M., Potter, J.D., McKenzie, D.R., Sellers, T.A., Kushi, L.H., Steinmetz, K.A. & Folsom, A.R. (1993) Reduced risk of colon cancer with high intake of vitamin E: The Iowa women's health study. *Cancer Res.*, **53**, 4230–4237

Bowen, P.E., Mobarhan, S. & Smith, J.C., Jr (1993) Carotenoid absorption in humans. *Meth. Enzymol.*, **214**, 3–17

Brady, W.E., Mares-Perlman, J.A., Bowen, P. & Stacewicz-Sapuntzakis, M. (1996) Human serum carotenoid concentrations are related to physiologic and lifestyle factors. *J. Nutr.*, **126**, 129–137

Braga, C., La Vecchia, C., Negri, E., Franceschi, S. & Parpinel, M. (1997) Intake of selected foods and nutrients and breast cancer risk: An age- and menopause-specific analysis. *Nutr. Cancer*, **28**, 258–263

Breslow, R.A., Alberg, A.J., Helzlsouer, K.J., Bush, T.L., Norkus, E.P., Morris, J.S., Spate, V.E. & Comstock, G.W. (1995) Serological precursors of cancer: Malignant melanoma, basal and squamous cell skin cancer, and prediagnostic levels of retinol, β-carotene, lycopene, α-tocopherol and selenium. *Cancer Epidemiol. Biomarkers Prev.*, **4**, 837–842

Briefel, R., Sowell, A., Huff, D., Hodge, C., Koncikowski, S., Wright, J. & Gunter, E. (1996) The distribution of serum carotenoids in the US population, 1988–1994: Results from the Third National Health and Nutrition Examination Survey (NHANES III). *FASEB J.*, **10**, A813

Britton, G. (1995a) Structure and properties of carotenoids in relation to function. *FASEB J.*, **9**, 1551–1558

Britton, G. (1995b) UV/Visible spectroscopy. In: Britton, G., Liaaen-Jensen, S. & Pfander, H., eds, *Carotenoids*, Vol. 1B, *Spectroscopy*, Basel, Birkhaüser Verlag, pp. 13–62

Britton, G. (1995c) Example 1: Higher plants. In: Britton, G., Liaaen-Jensen, S. & Pfander, H., eds, *Cartenoids*, Vol. 1A, *Isolation and Analysis*, Basel, Birkhaüser Verlag, pp. 201–214

Britton, G., Liaaen-Jensen, S. & Pfander, H., eds (1995a) *Carotenoids*, Vol. 1A, *Isolation and Analysis*, Basel, Birkhaüser Verlag

Britton, G., Liaaen-Jensen, S. & Pfander, H., eds (1995b) *Carotenoids*, Vol. 1B, *Spectroscopy*, Basel, Birkhaüser Verlag

Brockman, H.E., Stack, H.F. & Waters, M.D. (1992) Antimutagenicity profiles of some natural substances. *Mutat. Res.*, **267**, 157–172

Brown, L.M., Blot, W.J., Schuman, S.H., Smith, V.M., Ershow, A.G., Marks, R.D. & Fraumeni, J.F. (1988) Environmental factors and high risk of esophageal cancer among men in coastal South Carolina. *J. Natl Cancer Inst.*, **80**, 1620–1625

Brown, E.D., Micozzi, M.S., Craft, N.E., Bieri, J.G., Beecher, G., Edwards, B.K., Rose, A., Taylor, P.R. & Smith, J.C., Jr (1989) Plasma carotenoids in normal men after a single ingestion of vegetables or purified β-carotene. *Am. J. clin. Nutr.*, **49**, 1258– 1265

Brubacher, G.B. & Weiser, H. (1985) The vitamin A activity of β-carotene. *Int. J. Vit. Nutr. Res.*, **55**, 5–15

Bruemmer, B., White, E., Vaughan, T.L. & Cheney, C.L. (1996) Nutrient intake in relation to bladder cancer among middle-aged men and women. *Am. J. Epidemiol.*, **144**, 485–495

Bueno de Mesquita, H.B., Maisonneuve, P., Runia, S. & Moerman, C.J. (1991) Intake of foods and nutrients and cancer of the exocrine pancreas: A population-based case–control study in the Netherlands. *Int. J. Cancer*, **48**, 540–549

Buiatti, E., Palli, D., Decarli, A., Amadori, D., Avellini, C., Bianchi, S., Bonaguri, C., Cipriani, F., Cocco, P., Giacosa, A., Marubini, E., Minacci, C., Puntoni, R., Russo, A., Vindigni, C., Fraumeni, J.F., Jr & Blot, W.J. (1990) A case–control study of gastric cancer and diet in Italy: II. Association with nutrients. *Int. J. Cancer*, **45**, 896–901

Bukin, Y.V., Zaridze, D.G., Draudin-Kryleno, V.A., Orlov, E.N., Sigacheva, N.A., Dawei, F., Kurtgzman, M.Ya., Schlenskaya, I.N., Gorbacheva, O.N., Nichipai, A.M., Kuvschinov, Yu.P., Poddubny, B.K. & Maximovitch, D.M. (1993) Effect of beta-carotene supplementation on the activity of ornithine decarboxylase (ODC) in stomach mucosa of patients with chronic atrophic gastritis. *Eur. J. Cance Prev.*, **2**, 61–68

Burdon, R.H. (1995) Superoxide and hydrogen peroxide in relation to mammalian cell proliferation. *Free Radical Med.*, **18**, 775–794

Burger, H., Kovacs, A., Weiser, B., Grimson, R., Nachman, S., Tropper, P., van Bennekim, A.M., Elie, M.C. & Blaner, W.S. (1997) Maternal serum vitamin A levels are not associated with mother–child transmission of HIV-1 in the United States. *J. acquir. immune Defic. Synd. hum. Retroviruses*, **14**, 321–326

Burney, P.G.J., Comstock, G.W. & Morris, J.S. (1989) Serologic precursors of cancer: Serum micronutrients and the subsequent risk for pancreatic cancer. *Am. J. clin. Nutr.*, **49**, 895–900

Burton G.W. & Ingold K.U. (1984) β-Carotene: An unusual type of lipid antioxidant. *Science*, **224**, 569–573

Bushway, R.J., Yang, A. & Yamani, A.M. (1986) Comparison of alpha- and beta-carotene content of supermarket vs roadside stand produce in Maine (Report 0734-9556). Orono, Maine, University of Maine

Byers, T., Marshall, J., Graham, S., Mettlin, C. & Swanson, M. (1983) A case–control study of dietary and nondietary factors in ovarian cancer. *J. natl Cancer Inst.*, **71**, 681–686

Byers, T.E., Graham, S., Haughey, B.P., Marshall, J.R. & Swanson, M.K. (1987) Diet and lung cancer risk: Findings from the Western New York Diet Study. *Am. J. Epidemiol.*, **125**, 351–363

Cahill, R.J., O'Sullivan, K.R., Mathias, P.M., Beattie, S., Hamilton, H. & O'Morain, C. (1993) Effects of vitamin antioxidant supplementation on cell kinetics of patients with adenomatous polyps. *Gut*, **34**, 963–967

Camoirano, A., Balansky, R.M., Bennicelli, C., Izzotti, A., D'Agostini, F. & De Flora, S. (1994) Experimental databases on inhibition of the bacterial mutagenicity of 4-nitroquinoline 1-oxide and cigarette smoke. *Mutat. Res.*, **317**, 89–109

Candelora, E.C., Stockwell, H.G., Armstrong, A.W. & Pinkham, P.A. (1992) Dietary intake and risk of lung cancer in women who never smoked. *Nutr. Cancer*, **17**, 263–270

Cantilena, L.R. & Nierenberg, D.W. (1989) Simultaneous analysis of five carotenoids in human plasma by five isocratic high performance liquid chromatography. *J. Micronutr. Anal.*, **6**, 181– 209

Cantilena, L.R., Stukel, T.A., Greenberg, E.R., Nann, S. & Nierenberg, D.W. (1992) Diurnal and seasonal variation of five carotenoids measured in human serum. *Am. J. clin. Nutr.*, **55**, 659–663

Castonguay, A., Pepin, P. & Stoner, G.D. (1991) Lung tumorigenicity of NNK given orally to A/J mice: Its application to chemopreventive efficacy studies. *Exp. Lung Res.*, **17**, 485–499

Chang, W.-C., Lin, Y.-L., Lee, M.-J., Shiow, S.-J. & Wang, C.-J. (1996) Inhibitory effect of crocetin on benzo(a)pyrene genotoxicity and neoplastic transformation in C3H 10T1/2 cells. *Anticancer Res.*, **16**, 3603–3608

Chen, L., Sly, L., Jones, C.S., Tarone, R. & De Luca, L.M. (1993) Differential effects of dietary beta-carotene on papilloma and carcinoma formation induced by an initiation–promotion protocol in SENCAR mouse skin. *Carcinogenesis*, **14**, 713–717

Chew, B.P., Wong, M.W. & Wong, T.S. (1996) Effects of lutein from marigold extract on immunity and growth of mammary tumors in mice. *Anticancer Res.*, **16**, 3689–3694

Chug-Ahuja, J.K., Holden, J.M., Forman, M.R., Mangels, A.R., Beecher, G.R. & Lanza, E. (1993) The development and application of carotenoid data-base for fruits, vegetables and related multicompo-nent foods. *J. Am. Diet Assoc.*, **93**, 318– 323

Chyou, P.-H, Nomura, M.Y.A., Hankin, J.H. & Stemmermann, G.N (1990) A case–cohort study of diet and stomach cancer. *Cancer Res.*, **50**, 7501– 7504

Clinton, S.K., Emenhiser, C., Schwartz, S.J., Bostwick, D.J., Williams, A.W., Moore, B.J. & Erdman, J.W.J. (1996) *cis–trans* Lycopene isomers, carotenoids and retinol in human prostate. *Cancer Epidemiol. Biomarkers Prev.*, **5**, 823–833

Colacchio, T.A. & Memoli, V. A. (1986) Chemoprevention of colorectal neoplasms. Ascor-bic acid and beta-carotene. *Arch. Surg.*, **121**, 1421–1424

Colacchio, T.A., Memoli, V.A. & Hildebrandt, L. (1989) Antioxidants vs carotenoids. *Arch. Surg.*, **124**, 217–221

Comstock, G.W., Helzlsouer, K.J. & Bush, T.L. (1991) Prediagnostic serum levels of carotenoids and vita-min E as related to subsequent cancer in Washington County, Maryland. *Am. J. clin. Nutr.*, **53**, 260S–264S

Comstock, G.W., Alberg, A.J. & Helzlsouer, K.J. (1993) Reported effects of long-term freezer storage on concentrations of retinol, β-carotene, and α-toco-pherol in serum or plasma summarized. *Clin. Chem.*, **39**, 1075–1078

Comstock, G.W., Alberg, A.J., Huang, H.Y., Wu, K., Burke, A.E., Hoffman, S.C., Norkus, E.P., Gross, M., Cutler, R.G., Morris, J.S., Spate, V.L. & Helzlsouer, K.J. (1997) The risk of developing lung cancer associated with antioxidants in the blood: Ascorbic acid, carotenoids, α-tocopherol, selenium, and total per-oxyl radical absorbing capacity. *Cancer Epidemiol. Biomarkers Prev.*, **6**, 907–916

Connett, J.E., Kuller, L.H., Kjelsberg, M.O., Polk, B.F., Collins, G., Rider, A. & Hulley, S.B. (1989) Relationship between carotenoids and cancer. The Multiple Risk Factor Intervention Trial (MRFIT) Study. *Cancer*, **64**, 126–134

Cooney, R.V., Kappock, T.J., Pung, A. & Bertram, J.S. (1993) Solubilization, cellular uptake, and activity of β-carotene and other carotenoids as inhibitors of neoplastic transformation in cultured cells. *Meth. Enzymol.*, **214**, 55–68

Cooney, R.V., Franke, A.A., Hankin, J.H., Custer, L.J., Wilkins, L.R., Harwood, P.J. & Le Marchand, L. (1995) Seasonal variations in plasma micronutrients and antioxidants. *Cancer Epidemiol. Biomarkers Prev.*, **4**, 207–215

Correa, P., Fontham, E., Pickle, L.W., Chen, V., Lin, Y.P. & Haenszel, W. (1985) Dietary determinants of gastric cancer in south Louisiana inhabitants. *J. natl Cancer Inst.*, **75**, 645–654

Cozzi, R., Ricordi R., Aglitti, T., Gatta, V., Perticone, P. & De Salvia, R. (1997) Ascorbic acid and β-carotene as modulators of oxidative damage. *Carcinogenesis*, **18**, 223–228

Craft, N.E. (1992) Carotenoid reversed-phase high-performance liquid chromatography methods: Reference compendium. *Meth. Enzymol.*, **213**, 185–205

Craft, N.E., Brown, E.D. & Smith, J.C., Jr (1988) Effects of storage and handling conditions on concentrations of individual carotenoids, retinol, and tocopherol in plasma. *Clin. Chem.*, **34**, 44–48

Cutler, R.G. (1991) Antioxidants and aging. *Am. J. clin. Nutr.*, **53**, 373S–379S

Daicker, B., Schiedt, K., Adnet, J.J. & Bermond, P. (1987) Canthaxanthin retinopathy. *Graefe's Arch. clin. exp. Ophthalmol.*, **225**, 189–197

Dartigues, J.-F, Dabis, F., Gros, N., Moise, A., Bois, G., Salamon, R., Dilhuydy, J.M. & Courty, G. (1990) Dietary vitamin A, beta carotene and risk of epidermoid lung cancer in south-western France. *Eur. J. Epidemiol.*, **6**, 261–265

Das, B.S., Thurnham, D.I. & Das, D.B. (1996) Plasma α-tocopherol, retinol and carotenoids in children with falciparum malaria. *Am. J. clin. Nutr.*, **64**, 94–100

Daudu, P.A., Kelley, D.S., Taylor, P.C., Burri, B.J. & Wu, M.M. (1994) Effect of a low beta-carotene diet on the immune functions of adult women. *Am. J. clin. Nutr.*, **60**, 969–972

Decarli, A., Liati, P., Negri, E., Franceschi, S. & La Vecchia, C. (1987) Vitamin A and other dietary factors in the etiology of esophageal cancer. *Nutr. Cancer*, **10**, 29–37

Devery, J. & Milborrow, B.V. (1994) β-Carotene-15,15'-dioxygenase (EC1.13.11.21) isolation reaction mechanism and an improved assay procedure. *Br. J. Nutr.*, **72**, 397–414

Dimenstein, R., Trugo, N.M., Donangelo, C.M., Trugo, L.C. & Anastacio, A.S. (1996) Effect of subadequate maternal vitamin-A status on placental transfer of retinol and beta-carotene to the human fetus. *Biol. Neonate*, **69**, 230–234

Dimitrov, N.V. & Ullrey, D.E. (1990) Bioavailability of carotenoids. In: Krinsky, N.I., Mathews-Roth, M.M. & Taylor, R.F., eds, *Carotenoids Chemistry and Biology*, New York, Plenum Press, pp. 269–277

Dimitrov, N.V., Meyer, C., Ullrey, D.E., Chenoweth, W., Michelakis, A., Malone, W., Boone, C. & Fink, G. (1988) Bioavailability of β-carotene in humans. *Am. J. clin. Nutr.*, **48**, 298–304

Diplock, A.T. (1995) Safety of antioxidant vitamins and beta-carotene. *Am. J. clin. Nutr.*, **62**, 1510S–1516S

Dorgan, J.F., Ziegler, R.G., Schoenberg, J.B., Hartge, P., McAdams, M.J., Falk, R.T., Wilcox, H.B. & Shaw, G.L. (1993) Race and sex differences in associations of vegetables, fruits, and carotenoids with lung cancer risk in New Jersey (United States). *Cancer Causes Control*, **4**, 273–281

Drewnowski, A., Rock, C.L., Henderson, S.A., Shore, A.B., Fischler, C., Galan, P., Preziosi, P. & Hercberg, S. (1997) Serum β-carotene and vitamin C as biomarkers of vegetable and fruit intakes in a community based sample of French adults. *Am. J. clin. Nutr.*, **65**, 1796–1802

Duszka, C., Grolier, P., Azim, E.-M., Alexandre-Gouabau, M.-C., Borel, P. & Azais-Braesco, V. (1996) Rat intestinal β-carotene dioxygenase activity is located primarily in the cytosol of mature jejunal enterocytes. *J. Nutr.*, **126**, 2550–2556

van Eewyk, J., Davis, F.G. & Bowen, P.E. (1991) Dietary and serum carotenoids and cervical intraepithelial neoplasia. *Int. J. Cancer*, **48**, 34–38

Eichholzer, M., Stahelin, H.B. & Gey, K.F. (1992) Inverse correlation between essential antioxidants in plasma and subsequent risk to develop cancer, ischemic heart disease and stroke respectively: 12-year follow-up of the Prospective Basel Study. In: Emerit, I. & Chance, B., eds, *Free Radicals and Aging*, Basel, Birkhauser Verlag, pp. 398–410

Eichholzer, M., Stähelin, H.B., Gey, K.F., Lüdin, E. & Bernasconi, F. (1996) Prediction of male cancer mortality by plasma levels of interacting vitamins: 17-year follow-up of the Prospective Basel Study. *Int. J. Cancer*, **66**, 145–150

Eiserich, J.P., van der Vliet, A., Handelman, G.J., Halliwell, B. & Cross, C.E. (1995) Dietary antioxidants and cigarette smoke-induced biomolecular damage: A complex interaction. *Am. J. clin. Nutr.*, **62**, 1490S–1500S

El-Gorab, M., Underwood, B.A. & Loerch, J.D. (1975) The role of bile salts in the uptake of β-carotene and retinol by rat everted gut sacs. *Biochim. biophys. Acta*, **401**, 265–277

Emenhiser, C., Sander, L.C. & Schwartz, S.J. (1995) Capability of a polymeric C30 stationary phase to resolve *cis–trans* carotenoid isomers in reversed-phase liquid chromatography. *J. Chromatogr. A*, **707**, 205–216

Enger, S.M., Longnecker, M.P., Chen, M.J., Harper, J.M., Lee, E.R., Frankl, H.D. & Haile, R.W. (1996) Dietary intake of specific carotenoids and vitamins A, C, and E, and prevalence of colorectal adenomas. *Cancer Epidemiol. Biomarkers. Prev.*, **5**, 147–153

Engle, A., Muscat, J.E. & Harris, R.E. (1991) Nutritional risk factors and ovarian cancer. *Nutr. Cancer*, **15**, 239–247

Englert, G. (1995) NMR spectroscopy. In: Britton, G., Liaaen-Jensen, S. & Pfander, H., eds, *Carotenoids*, Vol. 1B, *Spectroscopy*, Basel, Birkhäuser Verlag, pp. 147–260

Englert, G., Noack, K., Broger, E.A., Glinz, E., Vecchi, M. & Zell, R. (1992) Synthesis, isolation, and full spectroscopic characterization of eleven (*Z*)-isomers of (3*R*,3′*R*)-zeaxanthin. *Helv. chim. Acta*, **74**, 969–982

Epstein, J.H. (1977) Effects of beta-carotene on ultraviolet induced cancer formation in the hairless mouse skin. *Photochem. Photobiol.*, **25**, 211–213

Erdman, J.W., Bierer, T.L. & Gugger, E.T. (1993) Absorption and transport of carotenoids. *Ann. N.Y. Acad. Sci.*, **691**, 76–85

Ershov, Y.V., Bykhovsky, V.Y. & Dmitrovskii, A.A. (1994) Stabilization and competitive inhibition of β-carotene 15-15′-dioxygenase by carotenoids. *Biochem. mol. Biol. Int.*, **34**, 755–763

Estève, J., Riboli, E., Pequignot, G., Terracini, B., Merletti, F., Crosignani, P., Ascunce, N., Zubiri, L., Blanchet, F., Raymond, L., Repetto, F. & Tuyns, A.J. (1996) Diet and cancers of the larynx and hypopharynx: The IARC multi-center study in southwestern Europe. *Cancer Causes Control*, **7**, 240–252

Everett, S.A., Dennis, M.F., Patel, K.B., Maddix, S., Kundu, S.C. & Willson, R. (1996) Scavenging of nitrogen dioxide, thiyl, and sulfonyl free radicals by the nutritional antioxidant β-carotene. *J. biol. Chem.*, **271**, 3988–3994

Ewertz, M. & Gill, C. (1990) Dietary factors and breast-cancer risk in Denmark. *Int. J. Cancer*, **46**, 779–784

Eye Disease Case–Control Study Group (1993) Antioxidant status and neovascular age-related macular degeneration. *Arch. Ophthalmol.*, **111**, 104–109

Falk, R.T., Pickle, L.W., Fontham, E.T., Correa, P. & Fraumeni, J.F. (1988) Life-style risk factors for pancreatic cancer in Louisiana: A case–control study. *Am. J. Epidemiol.*, **128**, 324–336

Fernandez, E., La Vecchia, C., D'Avanzo, B., Negri, E. & Franceschi, S. (1997) Risk factors for colorectal cancer in subjects with family history of the disease. *Br. J. Cancer*, **75**, 1381–1384

Flores, M., Menchu, M.T., Lara, M.Y. & Arroyave, G. (1969) [Vitamin A content of foodstuffs included in the food composition tables used in Latin America.] *Arch. Latinoam. Nutr.*, **19**, 311–341 (in Spanish)

Fontham, E.T., Pickle, L.W., Haenszel, W., Correa, P., Lin, Y.P. & Falk, R.T. (1988) Dietary vitamins A and C and lung cancer risk in Louisiana. *Cancer*, **62**, 2267–2273

Fontham, E.T.H., Malcom, G.T., Sing, V.N., Ruiz, B., Schmidt, B. & Correa, P. (1995) Effect of β-carotene supplementation on serum α-tocopherol concentration. *Cancer Epidemiol. Biomarkers Prev.*, **4**, 801–803

Forman, M.R., Beecher, G., Muesing, R., Lanza, E., Olson, B., Campbell, W.S., McAdam, P., Schulman, J.D. & Graubard, B.I. (1996) The fluctuation of plasma carotenoid concentrations by phase of the menstrual cycle: A controlled diet study. *Am. J. clin. Nutr.*, **64**, 559–565

Franke, A.A., Harwood, P.J., Shimamoto, T., Lumeng, S., Zhang, L., Bertram, J.S., Wilkens, L.R., Le Marchand, L. & Cooney, R.V. (1994) Effects of micronutrients and antioxidants on lipid peroxidation in human plasma and in cell culture. *Cancer Lett.*, **79**, 17–26

Freudenheim, J.L., Graham, S., Marshall, J.R., Haughey, B.P., Cholewinski, S. & Wilkinson, G. (1991) Folate intake and carcinogenesis of the colon and rectum. *Int. J. Epidemiol.*, **20**, 368–374

Freudenheim, J.L., Graham, S., Byers, T.E., Marshall, J.R., Haughey, B.P., Swanson, M.K. & Wilkinson, G. (1992) Diet, smoking, and alcohol in cancer of the larynx: A case–control study. *Nutr. Cancer*, **17**, 33–45

Freudenheim, J.L., Marshall, J.R., Vena, J.E., Laughlin, R., Brasure, J.R., Swanson, M.K., Nemoto, T. & Graham, S. (1996) Premenopausal breast cancer risk and intake of vegetables, fruits, and related nutrients. *J. natl Cancer Inst.*, **88**, 340–348

Friedman, J.M. & Polifka, J.E. (1994) *Teratogenic Effects of Drugs: A Resource for Clinicians*, Baltimore, The Johns Hopkins University Press, pp. 654–655

Friedman, G.D., Blaner, W.S., Goodman, D.S., Vogelman, J.H., Brind, J.L., Hoover, R., Fireman, B.H. & Orentreich, N. (1986) Serum retinol-binding protein levels do not predict subsequent lung cancer. *Am. J. Epidemiol.*, **123**, 781–789

Frommel, T.O., Mobarhan, S., Doria, M., Halline, A.G., Luk, G.D., Bowen, P.E., Candel, A. & Liao, Y. (1995) Effect of beta-carotene supplementation on indices of colonic cell proliferation. *J. natl Cancer Inst.*, **87**, 1781–1787

Fukao, A., Tsubono, Y., Kawamura, M., Ido, T., Akazawa, N., Tsuji, I., Komatsu, S., Minami, Y. & Hisamichi, S. (1996) The independent association of smoking and drinking with serum beta-carotene levels among males in Miyagi, Japan. *Int. J. Epidemiol.*, **25**, 300–306

Fuller, C.J., Faulkner, H., Bendich, A., Parker, R.S. & Roe, D.A. (1992) Effect of beta-carotene supplementation on photosuppression of delayed-type hypersensitivity in normal young men. *Am. J. clin. Nutr.*, **56**, 684–690

Furr, H.C. & Clark, R.M. (1997) Intestinal absorption and tissue distribution of carotenoids. *J. nutr. Biochem.*, **8**, 364–377

Gao, Y.T., McLaughlin, J.K., Gridley, G., Blot, W.J., Ji, B.T., Dai, Q. & Fraumeni, J.F. (1994) Risk factors for esophageal cancer in Shanghai, China. II. Role of diet and nutrients. *Int. J. Cancer*, **58**, 197–202

Garewal, H. (1995) Antioxidants in oral cancer prevention. *Am. J. clin. Nutr.*, **62**, 1410S–1416S

Garewal, H.S., Meyskens, F.L., Jr, Killen, D., Reeves, D., Kiersch, T.A., Elletson, H., Strosberg, A., King, D. & Steinbronn, K. (1990) Response of oral leukoplakia to β-carotene. *J. clin. Oncol.*, **8**, 1715–1720

Garmyn, M., Ribaya Mercado, J.D., Russel, R.M., Bhawan, J. & Gilchrest, B.A. (1995) Effect of beta-carotene supplementation on the human sunburn reaction. *Exp. Dermatol.*, **4**, 104–111

Gärtner, C., Stahl, W. & Sies, H. (1996) Preferential increase in chylomicron levels of the xanthophylls lutein and zeaxanthin compared to β-carotene in the human. *Int. J. Vit. Nutr. Res.*, **66**, 119–125

Gärtner, C., Stahl, W. & Sies, H. (1997) Lycopene is more bioavailable from tomato paste than from fresh tomatoes. *Am. J. clin. Nutr.*, **66**, 116–122

Gaziano, J.M. (1994) Antioxidant vitamins and coronary artery disease risk. *Am. J. Med.*, **97** (Suppl. 3A), 18S–21S

Gaziano, J.M. & Hennekens, C.H. (1993) The role of beta-carotene in the prevention of cardiovascular disease. *Ann. N.Y. Acad. Sci.*, **691**, 148–155

Gaziano, J.M., Johnson, E.J., Russell, R.M., Manson, J.E., Stampfer, M.J., Ridker, P.M., Frei, B., Hennekens, C.H. & Krinsky, N.I. (1995a) Discrimination in absorption or transport of β-carotene isomers after oral supplementation with either all-*trans*- or 9-*cis*-β-carotene. *Am. J. clin. Nutr.*, **61**, 1248–1252

Gaziano, J.M., Hatta, A., Flynn, M., Johnson, E.J., Krinsky, N.I., Ridker, P.M., Hennekens, C.H. & Frei, B. (1995b) Supplementation of β-carotene in vivo and in vitro does not inhibit low density lipoprotein oxidation. *Atherosclerosis*, **112**, 187–195

Gaziano, J.M., Manson, J.E., Ridker, P.M., Buring, J.E. & Hennekens, C.H. (1996) Beta-carotene therapy for chronic stable angina. *Circulation*, **94**, 508

Geisen, C., Denk, C., Gremm, B., Baust, C., Karger, A., Bollag, W. & Schwarz, E. (1997) High-level expression of the retinoic acid receptor β gene in normal cells of the uterine cervix is regulated by the retinoic acid receptor α and is abnormally down-regulated in cervical carcinoma cells. *Cancer Res.*, **57**, 1460–1467

Gensler, H.L., Aickin, M. & Peng, Y.M. (1990) Cumulative reduction of primary skin tumor growth in UV-irradiated mice by the combination of retinyl palmitate and canthaxanthin. *Cancer Lett.*, **53**, 27–31

Gerber, M., Cavallo, F., Marubini, E., Richardson, S., Barbieri, A., Capitelli, E., Costa, A., Crastes de Paulet, A., Crastes de Paulet, P., Decarli, A., Pastorino, U. & Pujol, H. (1988) Liposoluble vitamins and lipid parameters in breast cancer. A joint study in northern Italy and southern France. *Int. J. Cancer*, **42**, 489–494

Gerster, H. (1997) The potential role of lycopene for human health. *J. Am. Coll. Nutr.*, **16**, 109–126

Gey, K.F., Stahelin, H.B. & Eichholzer, M. (1993a) Poor plasma status of carotene and vitamin C is associated with higher mortality from ischemic heart disease and stroke: Basel prospective study. *Clin. Invest.*, **71**, 3–6

Gey, K.F., Moser, U.K., Jordan P., Stähelin, H.B., Eichholzer, M. & Lüdin, E. (1993b) Increased risk of cardiovascular disease at suboptimal plasma concentrations of essential antioxidants: An epidemiological update with special attention to carotene and vitamin C. *Am. J. clin. Nutr.*, **57** (Suppl.), 787S–797S

Ghadirian, P., Simard, A., Baillargeon, J., Maisonneuve, P. & Boyle, P. (1991) Nutritional factors and pancreatic cancer in the Francophone community in Montreal, Canada. *Int. J. Cancer*, **47**, 1–6

Ghadirian, P., Lacroix, A., Maisonneuve, P., Perret, C., Potvin, C., Gravel, D., Bernard, D. & Boyle, P. (1997) Nutritional factors and colon carcinoma. A case–control study involving French Canadians in Montreal, Quebec, Canada. *Cancer*, **80**, 858–864

Gijare, P.S., Rao, K.V.K. & Bhide, S.V. (1990) Modulatory effects of snuff, retinoic acid, and beta-carotene on DMBA-induced hamster cheek pouch carcinogenesis in relation to keratin expression. *Nutr. Cancer*, **14**, 253–259

Giovannucci, E., Stampfer, M.J., Colditz, G.A., Rimm, E.B., Trichopoulos, D., Rosner, B.A., Speizer, F.E. & Willett, W.C. (1993) Folate, methionine, and alcohol intake and risk of colorectal adenoma. *J. natl Cancer Inst.*, **85**, 875–884

Giovannucci, E., Ascherio, A., Rimm, E.B., Stampfer, M.J., Colditz, G.A. & Willett, W.C. (1995) Intake of carotenoids and retinol in relation to risk of prostate cancer. *J. natl Cancer Inst.*, **87**, 1767–1776

Giuliano, A.R., Papenfuss, M., Nour, M., Canfield, L.M., Schneider, A. & Hatch, K. (1997) Antioxidant nutrients: Associations with persistent human papillomavirus infection. *Cancer Epidemiol. Biomarkers Prev.*, **6**, 917–923

Glover, J. (1960) The conversion of β-carotene into vitamin A. *Vit. Horm. (USA)*, **18**, 371–386

Goldberg, J., Flowerdew, G., Smith, E., Brody, J.A. & Tso, M.O.M. (1988) Factors associated with AMD: Analyses of data from the first NHANES. *Am. J. Epidemiol.*, **128**, 700–710

Gonzalez, C.A., Riboli, E., Badosa, J., Batiste, E., Cardona, T., Pita, S., Sanz, J.M., Torrent, M. & Agudo, A. (1994) Nutritional factors and gastric cancer in Spain. *Am. J. Epidemiol.*, **139**, 466–473

Gonzalez de Mejia, E., Loarca-Pina, G. & Ramos-

Gomez, M. (1997a) Antimutagenicity of xanthophylls present in Aztec marigold (*Tagetes erecta*) against 1-nitropyrene. *Mutat. Res.*, **389**, 219–226

Gonzalez de Mejia, E., Ramos-Gomez, M. & Loarca-Pina, G. (1997b) Antimutagenic activity of natural xanthophylls against aflatoxin B1 in *Salmonella typhimurium*. *Environ. mol. Mutag.*, **30**, 346–353

Goodman, D.S. & Huang, H.S. (1965) Biosynthesis of vitamin A with rat intestinal enzymes. *Science*, **149**, 879–880

Goodman, D.S., Blomstrand, R., Werner, B., Huang, H.S. & Shiratori, T. (1966a) The intestinal absorption and metabolism of vitamin A and β-carotene in man. *J. clin. Invest.*, **45**, 1615–1623

Goodman, D.S., Huang, H.S. & Shiratori, T. (1966b) Mechanism of the biosynthesis of vitamin A from β-carotene. *J. biol. Chem.*, **241**, 1929–1932

Goodman, G.E., Omenn, G.S. & CARET Co-investigators and Staff (1992) Carotene and retinol efficacy trial: Lung cancer chemoprevention trial in heavy cigarette smokers and asbestos-exposed workers. *Adv. exp. Med. Biol.*, **320**, 137–140

Goodman, G.E., Omenn, G.S., Thornquist, M.D., Lund, B., Metch, B. & Gylys-Colwell, I. (1993) The Carotene and Retinol Efficacy Trial (CARET) to prevent lung cancer in high risk populations: Pilot study with cigarette smokers. *Cancer Epidemiol. Biomarkers Prev.*, **2**, 389–396

Goodman, G.E., Metch, B.J. & Omenn, G.S. (1994) The effect of long-term β-carotene and vitamin A administration on serum concentrations of α-tocopherol. *Cancer Epidemiol. Biomarkers Prev.*, **3**, 429–432

Goodman, G.E., Thornquist, M.D., Kestin, M., Metch, B., Anderson, G., Omenn, G.S. & CARET Coinvestigators (1996) The association between participant characteristics and serum concentrations of β-carotene, retinol, retinyl palmitat and α-tocopherol among participants in the Carotene and Retinol Efficacy Trial (CARET) for prevention of lung cancer. *Cancer Epidemiol. Biomarkers Prev.*, **5**, 815–821

Goodwin, T.W., ed. (1976) *Chemistry and Biochemistry of Plant Pigments*, New York, Academic Press, pp. 225–261

Goodwin, T.W., ed. (1980) *The Biochemistry of the Carotenoids*, New York, Chapman & Hall, pp. 143–203

Goralczyk, R., Buser, S., Bausch, J., Bee, W., Zuklke, V. & Barker, F.M. (1997) Occurrence of birefringent retinal inclusions in cynomolgus monkeys after high doses of canthaxanthin. *Invest. ophthalmol. vis. Sci.*, **38**, 741–752

Goswami, U.C., Saloi, T.N., Firozi, P.F. & Bhattacharya, R.K. (1989) Modulation by some natural carotenoids of DNA adduct formation by aflatoxin B$_1$ *in vitro. Cancer Lett.*, **47**, 127–132

Gottlieb, K., Zarling, E.J., Mobarhan, S., Bowen, P. & Sugerman, S. (1993) β-Carotene decreases markers of lipid peroxidation in healthy volunteers. *Nutr. Cancer*, **19**, 207–212

Gradelet, S., Astorg, P., Leclerc, J., Chevalier, J., Vernevaut, M.F. & Siess, M.-H. (1996a) Effects of canthaxanthin, astaxanthin, lycopene and lutein on liver xenobiotic-metabolizing enzymes in the rat. *Xenobiotica*, **26**, 49–63

Gradelet, S., Leclerc, J., Siess, M.-H. & Astorg P.O. (1996b) β-Apo-8'-carotenal, but not β-carotene, is a strong inducer of liver cytochromes P4501A1 and 1A2 in rat. *Xenobiotica*, **26**, 909–919

Gradelet, S., Astorg, P., Pineau, T., Canivenc, M.C., Siess, M.H., Leclerc, J. & Lesca, P. (1997) Ah receptor-dependent CYP1A induction by two carotenoids, canthaxanthin and beta-apo-8'-carotenal, with no affinity for the TCDD binding site. *Biochem. Pharmacol.*, **54**, 307–315

Gradelet, S., Le Bon, A.-M., Bergès, R., Suschetet, M. & Astorg, P. (1998) Dietary carotenoids inhibit aflatoxin B$_1$-induced liver preneoplastic foci and DNA damage in the rat: Role of the modulation of aflatoxin B$_1$ metabolism. *Carcinogenesis*, **19**, 403–411

Graham, S., Marshall, J., Haughey, B., Brasure, J., Freudenheim, J., Zielezny, M., Wilkinson, G. & Nolan, J. (1990a) Nutritional epidemiology of cancer of the esophagus. *Am. J. Epidemiol.*, **131**, 454–467

Graham, S., Haughey, B., Marshall, J., Brasure, J., Zielezny, M., Freudenheim, J., West, D., Nolan, J. & Wilkinson, G. (1990b) Diet in the epidemiology of gastric cancer. *Nutr. Cancer*, **13**, 19–34

Graham, S., Hellmann, R., Marshall, J., Freudenheim, J., Vena, J., Swanson, M., Zielezny, M., Nemoto, T., Stubbe, N. & Raimondo, T. (1991) Nutritional epidemiology of postmenopausal breast cancer in western New York. *Am. J. Epidemiol.*, **134**, 552–566

Graham, S., Zielezny, M., Marshall, J., Priore, R., Freudenheim, J., Brasure, J., Haughey, B., Nasca, P. & Zdeb, M. (1992) Diet in the epidemiology of postmenopausal breast cancer in the New York State cohort. *Am. J. Epidemiol.*, **136**, 1327–1337

Granado, F., Olmedilla, B., Blanco, I. & Rojas-Hidalgo, E. (1992) Carotenoid composition of raw and cooked Spanish vegetables. *J. Agric. Food Chem.*, **40**, 2135–2140

Granado, F., Olmedilla, B., Blanco, I. & Rojas-Hidalgo, E. (1996) Major fruit and vegetable contributors to the main serum carotenoids in the Spanish diet. *Eur. J. clin. Nutr.*, **50**, 246–250

Greenberg, E.R., Baron, J.A., Stukel, T.A., Stevens, M.M., Mandel, J.S., Spencer, S.K., Elias, P.M., Lowe, N., Nierenberg, D.N., Bayrd, G., Vance, J.C., Freeman, D.H., Clendenning, W.E., Kwan, T. & the Skin Cancer Prevention Study Group (1990) A clinical trial of betacarotene to prevent basal-cell and squamous-cell cancers of the skin. *New Engl. J. Med.*, **323**, 789–795

Greenberg, E.R., Baron, J.A., Tosteson, T.D., Freeman, D.H., Beck, G.J., Bond, J.H., Colacchio, T.A., Coller, J.A., Frankl, H.D., Haile, R.W., Mandel, J.S., Nierenberg, D.W., Rothstein, R., Snover, D.C., Stevens, M.M., Summers, R.W. & van Stolk, R. (1994) A clinical trial of antioxidant vitamins to prevent colorectal adenoma. *New Engl. J. Med.*, **331**, 141–147

Greenberg, E.R., Baron, J.A., Karagas, M., Stukel, T.A., Nierenberg, D.N., Stevens, M.M., Mandel, J.S. & Haile, R.W. (1996) Mortality associated with low plasma concentration of beta carotene and the effect of oral supplementation. *J. Am. med. Assoc.*, **275**, 699–703

Gregory, J.R., Foster, K., Tyler, H. & Wiseman, M. (1990) *The Dietary and Nutritional Survey of British Adults*, London, Her Majesty's Stationery Office

Gridley, G., McLaughlin, J.K., Block, G., Blot, W.J., Winn, D.M., Greenberg, R.S., Schoenberg, J.B., Preston Martin, S., Austin, D.F. & Fraumeni, J.F. (1990) Diet and oral and pharyngeal cancer among blacks. *Nutr. Cancer*, **14**, 219–225

Grizzle, J., Omenn, G., Goodman, G.E., Thornquist, M.D., Rosenstock, L., Barnhart, S., Balmes, J., Cherniak, M., Cone, J., Cullen, M., Glass, A., Keogh, J. & Valanis, B. (1991) Design of the Beta-Carotene and Retinol Efficacy Trial (CARET) for chemoprevention of cancer in populations at high risk: Heavy smokers and asbestos-exposed workers. In: Pastorino, U. & Hong, W.K., eds, *Chemoimmuno Prevention of Cancer*, Stuttgart, Georg Thieme Verlag, pp. 167–172

Gross J. (1991) *Pigments in Vegetables, Chlorophylls and Carotenoids*, New York, Van Nostrand Reinhold, pp. 99–112

Gross, M.D., Bishop, T.D., Belcher, J.D. & Jacobs, D.R., Jr (1997) Induction of HL-60 cell differentiation by carotenoids. *Nutr. Cancer*, **27**, 169–173

Grubbs, C.J., Eto, I., Juliana, M.M & Whitaker, L.M. (1991) Effect of canthaxanthin on chemically induced mammary carcinogenesis. *Oncology*, **48**, 239–245

Gruszecki, W.I. & Sielewiesiuk, J. (1990) Orientation of xanthophylls in phosphatidyl choline multibilayers. *Biochim. biophys. Acta*, **1023**, 405–412

Gugger, E.T. & Erdman, J.W. (1996) Intracellular β-carotene transport in bovine liver and intestine is not mediated by cytosolic protein. *J. Nutr.*, **126**, 1470–1474

Gugger, E.T., Bierer, T.L., Henze, T.M., White, W.S. & Erdman, J.W. (1992) β-Carotene uptake and tissue distribution in ferrets (*Mustela putorius furo*). *J. Nutr.*, **122**, 115–119

Gunson, H.H., Merry, A.H., Britton, G. & Stratton, F. (1984) Detection of carotenoids in blood donors taking Orobronze: A cautionary note. *Clin. Lab. Haematol.*, **6**, 287–292

Gutteridge, J.M. (1986) Aspects to consider when detecting and measuring lipid peroxidation. *Free Radical Res. Commun.*, **1**, 173–184

Haenszel, W., Correa, P., Lopez, A., Cuello, C., Zarama, G., Zavala, D. & Fontham, E. (1985) Serum micronutrient levels in relation to gastric pathology. *Int. J. Cancer*, **36**, 43–48

Halliwell, B. & Chirico, S. (1993) Lipid peroxidation: Its mechanism, measurement, and significance. *Am. J. clin. Nutr.*, **57**, 715S–724S

Hammond, B.R. & Fuld, K. (1992) Interocular differences in macular pigment density. *Invest. Ophthalmol. vis. Sci.*, **33**, 350–355

Han, J.S. (1992) Effects of various chemical compounds on spontaneous and hydrogen peroxide-induced reversion in strain TA104 of *Salmonella typhimurium*. *Mutat. Res.*, **266**, 77–84

Handelman, G.J., Dratz, E.A., Reay, C.C. & van Kuijk, F.J.G.M. (1988) Carotenoids in the human macula and whole retina. *Invest. Ophthalmol. vis. Sci.*, **29**, 850–855

Handelman, G.J., Snodderly, D.M., Krinsky, N.I., Russett, M.D. & Adler, A.J. (1991) Biological control of the primate macular pigment. *Invest. Ophthalmol. vis. Sci.*, **32**, 257–267

Handelman, G.J., Snodderly, D.M., Adler, A.J., Russett, M.D. & Dratz, E.A. (1992) Measurement of carotenoids in human and monkey retinas. *Meth. Enzymol.*, **213**, 220–230

Handelman, G.J., Packer, L. & Cross, C.E. (1996) Destruction of tocopherols, carotenoids, and retinol in human plasma by cigarette smoke. *Am. J. clin. Nutr.*, **63**, 559–565

Hansen, S. & Maret, W. (1988) Retinal is not formed *in vitro* by enzymatic central cleavage of β-carotene. *Biochemistry*, **27**, 200–206

Hansson, L.-E., Nyren, O., Bergstrom, R., Wolk, A., Lindgren, A., Baron, J. & Adami, H.O. (1994) Nutrients and gastric cancer risk: A population-based case–control study in Sweden. *Int. J. Cancer*, **57**, 638–644

Harris, R.W., Forman, D., Doll, R., Vessey, M.P. & Wald, N.J. (1986) Cancer of the cervix uteri and vitamin A. *Br. J. Cancer*, **53**, 653–659

Harris, R.W.C., Key, T.J.A., Silcocks, P.B., Bull, D. & Wald, N.J. (1991) A case–control study of dietary carotene in men with lung cancer and in men with other epithelial cancers. *Nutr. Cancer*, **15**, 63–68

Hart, D.J. & Scott, K.J. (1995) Development and evaluation of an HPLC method for the analysis of carotenoids in foods, and the measurement of carotenoid content of vegetables and fruits commonly consumed in the UK. *Food Chem.*, **54**, 101–111

Hathcock, J.N., Hattan, D.G., Jenkins, M.Y., McDonald, J.T., Sundaresan, P.R. & Wilkening, V.L. (1990) Evaluation of vitamin A toxicity. *Am. J. clin. Nutr.*, **52**, 183–202

Haveland-Smith, R.B. (1981) Evaluation of genotoxicity of some natural food colors. *Mutat. Res.*, **91**, 285–290

Hayes, R.B., Bogdanovicz, J.F.A.T., Schroeder, F.H., de Bruijn, A., Raatgever, J.W., van der Maas, P.J., Oishi, K. & Yoshida, O. (1988) Serum retinol and prostate cancer. *Cancer*, **62**, 2021–2026

Hazuka, M.B., Edeards Prasad, J., Newman, F., Kinzie, J.J. & Prasad, K.N. (1990) Beta-carotene induces morphological differentiation and decreases adenylate cyclase activity in melanoma cells in culture. *J. Am. Coll. Nutr.*, **9**, 1443–1459

He, Y. & Campbell, C. (1990) Effects of carotenoids on aflatoxin B_1-induced mutagenesis in *S. typhimurium* TA100 and TA98. *Nutr. Cancer*, **13**, 243–253

He, Y., Root, M.M., Parker, R.S. & Campbell, T.C. (1997) Effects of carotenoid-rich food extracts on the development of preneoplastic lesions in rat liver and on in-vivo and in-vitro antioxidant status. *Nutr. Cancer*, **27**, 238–244

Hebert, J.R., Hurley, T.G., Hsieh, J., Rogers, E., Stoddard, A.M., Sorensen, G. & Nicolosi, R.J. (1994) Determinants of plasma vitamins and lipids: The Working Well Study. *Am. J. Epidemiol.*, **140**, 132–147

Hebuterne, X., Wang, X.-D., Johnson, E.J., Krinsky, N.I. & Russell, R.M. (1995) Intestinal absorption and metabolism of 9-*cis*-β-carotene *in vivo*: Biosynthesis of 9-*cis*-retinoic acid. *J. Lipid Res.*, **36**, 1264–1273

Hebuterne, X., Wang, X.-D., Tang, G.-W., Smith, D.E. & Russell, R.M. (1996) *In vivo* biosynthesis of retinoic acid from β-carotene involves an excentric cleavage pathway in ferret intestine. *J. Lipid Res.*, **37**, 482–492

Heilbrun, L.K, Nomura, A., Hankin, J.H. & Stemmermann, N.G. (1989) Diet and colorectal cancer with special reference to fiber intake. *Int. J. Cancer*, **44**, 1–6

Heinonen, M. (1990) Food groups as the source of vitamin A and beta-carotene in Finland. *Int. J. Vit. Nutr. Res.*, **61**, 3–9

Heinonen, M.I., Ollilainen, V., Linkola, E.K., Varo, P.T. & Koivistoinen, P.E. (1989) Carotenoids in Finnish foods: Vegetables, fruits, and berries. *J. Agric. Food Chem.*, **37**, 655–659

Heliövaara, M., Knekt, P., Aho, K., Aaran, R.K., Alfthan, G. & Aromaa, A. (1994) Serum antioxidants and risk of rheumatoid arthritis. *Ann. rheum. Dis.*, **53**, 51–53

Helzlsouer, K.J., Comstock, G.W. & Morris, J.S. (1989) Selenium, lycopene, α-tocopherol, β-carotene, retinol, and subsequent bladder cancer. *Cancer Res.*, **49**, 6144–6148

Helzlsouer, K.J., Alberg, A.J., Norkus, E.P., Morris, J.S., Hoffman, S.C. & Comstock, G.W. (1996) Prospective study of serum micronutrients and ovarian cancer. *J. natl Cancer Inst.*, **88**, 32–37

Hengartner, U., Bernhard, K., Meyer, K., Glinz, E. & Englert, G. (1992) Synthesis, isolation, and NMR-spectroscopic characterization of fourteen (Z)-isomers of lycopene and of some acetylenic didehydro- and tetradehydrolycopenes. *Helv. chim. Acta*, **75**, 1848–1865

Hennekens, C.H.& Eberlein, K. (1985) A randomised trial of aspirin and β-carotene among US physicians. *Prev. Med.*, **14**, 165–168

Hennekens, C.H., Buring, J.E. & Peto, R. (1994) Antioxidant vitamins: Benefits not yet proved (Editorial). *New Engl. J. Med.*, **330**, 1080–1081

Hennekens, C.H., Buring, J.E., Manson, J.E, Stampfer, M., Rosner, B., Cook, N.R., Belanger, C., LaMotte, F., Gaziano, J.M., Ridker, P.M., Willett, W. & Peto, R. (1996) Lack of long-term supplementation with beta carotene on the incidence of malignant neoplasms and cardiovascular disease. *New Engl. J. Med.*, **334**, 1145– 1149

Herrero, R., Potischman, N., Brinton. L.A., Reeves, W.C., Brenes, M.M., Tenorio, F., de Britton, R.C. & Gaitan, E. (1991) A case–control study of nutrient status and invasive cervical cancer. *Am. J. Epidemiol.*, **134**, 1335–1346

Heseker, H., Kohlmeier, M., Schneider, R., Speitling, A. & Kubler, W. (1991) [Vitamin supply to adults in the Federal Republic of Germany.] *Ernahrungs-wissenschaft*, **38**, 227–233 (in German)

Heywood, R., Palmer, A.K., Gregson, R.L. & Hummler, H. (1985) Toxicity of beta-carotene. *Toxicology*, **36**, 91–100

Hibino, T., Shimpo, K., Kawai, K., Chihara, T., Maruta, K., Arai, M., Nagatsu, T. & Fujita, K. (1990) Polyamine levels of urine and erythrocytes on inhibition of DMBA-induced oral carcinogenesis by topical beta-carotene. *Biogenic Amines*, 7, 209–216

Hicks, R.M., Turton, J.A., Tomlinson, C.N., Gwynne, J., Chrysostomou, E., Nandra, K. & Pedrick, M. (1984) No effect of β-carotene on the response of an inbred mouse strain to the bladder carcinogen N-butyl-N-(4-hydroxybutyl)nitrosamine (BBN). *Proc. Nutr. Soc.*, 43, 2A

High, E.G. & Day, H.G. (1951) Effects of different amounts of lutein, squalene, phytol and related substances on the utilization of carotene and vitamin A for storage and growth in the rat. *J. Nutr.*, 43, 245–250

Hinds, M.W., Kolonel, L.N., Hankin, J.H. & Lee, J. (1984) Dietary vitamin A, carotene, vitamin C and risk of lung cancer in Hawaii. *Am. J. Epidemiol.*, 119, 227–237

Hirose, M., Hasegawa, R., Kimura, J., Akagi, K., Yoshida, Y., Tanaka, H., Miki, T., Satoh, T., Wakabayashi, K., Ito, N. & Shirai, T. (1995) Inhibitory effects of 1-O-hexyl-2,3,5-trimethylhydroquinone (HTHQ), green tea catechins and other antioxidants on 2-amino-6-methyldipyrido[1,2-a:3',2'-d]imidazole (Glu-P-1)-induced rat hepatocarcinogenesis and dose-dependent inhibition by HTHQ of lesion induction by Glu-P-1 or 2-amino-3,8-dimethylimidazo[4,5-f]quinoxaline (MeIQx). *Carcinogenesis*, 16, 3049–3055

Ho, S.C., Donnan, S.P., Martin, C.W. & Tsao, S.Y. (1988) Dietary vitamin A, beta-carotene and risk of epidermoid lung cancer among Chinese males. *Singapore med. J.*, 29, 213–218

Holland, B., Welch, A.A., Unwin, I.D., Buss, D.H. Paul, A.A. & Southgate, D.A.T. (1991a) *McCance and Widdowson's The Composition of Foods*, 5th Ed., Cambridge, Royal Society of Chemistry

Holland, B., Unwin, I.D. & Buss, D.H. (1991b) *Vegetables, Herbs and Spices*, Fifth supplement to *McCance and Widdowson's The Composition of Foods*, 5th Ed., Cambridge, Royal Society of Chemistry

Hollander, D. & Ruble, P.E. (1978) β-Carotene intestinal absorption: Bile, fatty acid, pH, and flow rate effects on transport. *Am. J. Physiol.*, 235, E686–E691

Holmberg, L., Ohlander, E.M., Byers, T., Zack, M., Wolk, A., Bergström, R., Bergkvist, L., Thurfjell, E.,

Bruce, A.S. & Adami, H.O. (1994) Diet and breast cancer risk. *Arch. intern. Med.*, 154, 1805–1811

Hoppe, P.P. & Schoner, F.J. (1987) Application of carotenoids to animal nutrition and bioavailability of synthetic β-carotene in laboratory animals and calves (Abstract 53). In: *Proceedings of the 8th International Symposium on Carotenoids*, Boston, MA, 27–31 July 1987

Hoppe, P.P., Chew, B.P., Safer, A., Stegemann, I. & Biesalski, H.K. (1996) Dietary β-carotene elevates plasma steady-state and tissue concentrations of β-carotene and enhances vitamin A balance in preruminant calves. *J. Nutr.*, 126, 202–208

Howard, A.N., Williams, N.R., Palmer, C.R., Cambou, J.P., Evans, A.E., Foote, J.W., Marques-Vidal, P., McCrum, E.E., Ruidavets, J.B., Nigdikar, S.V., Rajput-Williams, J. & Thurnham, D.I. (1996) Do hydroxy carotenoids prevent coronary heart disease? A comparison between Belfast and Toulouse. *Int. J. Vit. Nutr. Res.*, 66, 113–118

Howe, G.R., Harrison, L. & Jain, M. (1986) A short diet history for assessing dietary exposure to N-nitrosamines in epidemiologic studies. *Am. J. Epidemiol.*, 124, 595–602

Howe, G.R., Hirohata, T., Hislop, T.G., Iscovich, J.M., Yuan, J.M., Katsouyanni, K., Lubin, F., Marubini, E., Modan, B., Rohan, T., Toniolo, P. & Yu, S.-Z. (1990) Dietary analysis and risk of breast cancer: Combined analysis of 12 case–control studies. *J. natl Cancer Inst.*, 82, 561–569

Howe, G.R., Ghadirian, P., Bueno de Mesquita, H.B., Zatonski, W.A., Baghurst, P.A., Miller, A.B., Simard, A., Baillargeon, J., De Waard, F., Pazewozniak, K., McMichael, A.J., Jain, M., Hsieh, C.C., Maisonneuve, P., Boyle, P. & Walker, A.M. (1992) A collaborative case–control study of nutrient intake and pancreatic cancer within the SEARCH programme. *Int. J. Cancer*, 51, 365–372

Hsing, A.W., Comstock, G.W., Abbey, H. & Polk, B.F. (1990) Serologic precursors of cancer. Retinol, carotenoids, and tocopherol and risk for prostate cancer. *J. natl Cancer Inst.*, 82, 941–946

Hu, J., Nyren, O., Wolk, A., Bergstrom, R., Yuen, J., Adami, H.O., Guo, L., Li, H., Huang, G., Xu, X., Zhao, F., Chen, Y., Wang, C., Qin, H., Hu, C. & Li, Y. (1994) Risk factors for oesophageal cancer in northeast China. *Int. J. Cancer*, 57, 38–46

Hu, J., Johnson, K.C., Mao, Y., Xu, T., Lin, Q., Wang, C., Zhao, F., Wang, G., Chen, Y. & Yang, Y. (1997) A case–control study of diet and lung cancer in northeast China. *Int. J. Cancer,* **71**, 924–931

Hughes, D.A., Wright, A.J.A., Finglas, P.M., Peerless, A.C.J., Bailey, A.L., Astley, S.B., Pinder, A.C. & Southon, S. (1997) Comparison of effects of beta-carotene and lycopene supplementation on the expression of functionally associated mole-cules on human monocytes. *Biochem. Soc. Trans.,* **25**, S206

Humble, C.G., Samet, J.M. & Skipper, B.E. (1987) Use of quantified and frequency indices of vitamin A intake in a case–control study of lung cancer. *Int. J. Epidemiol.,* **16**, 341–346

Hunter, D.J., Manson, J.E., Colditz, G.A., Stampfer, M.J., Rosner, B., Hennekens, C.H., Speizer, F.E. & Willett, W.C. (1993) A prospective study of the intake of vitamins C, E, and A and the risk of breast cancer. *New Engl. J. Med.,* **329**, 234–240

Hurley, W.L. & Doane, R.M. (1989) Recent developments in the roles of vitamins and minerals in reproduction. *J. Dairy Sci.,* **72**, 784

Imaida, K., Hirose, M., Yamaguchi, S. Takahashi, S. & Ito, N. (1990) Effects of naturally occurring antioxidants on combined 1,2-dimethylhydrazine- and 1-methyl-1-nitrosourea-initiated carcinogenesis in F344 rats. *Cancer Lett.,* **55**, 53–59

Ingram, D.M., Nottage, E. & Roberts, T. (1991) The role of diet in the development of breast cancer: A case–control study of patients with breast cancer, benign epithelial hyperplasia and fibrocystic disease of the breast. *Br. J. Cancer,* **64**, 187–191

Inhoffen, H.H., Pommer, H. & Bohlmann, F. (1950) [Synthesis of carotenoids. XIV. Total synthesis of β-carotene.] *Ann. Chem.,* **569**, 237–246 (in German)

Iscovich, J.M., Iscovich, R.B., Howe, G.R., Shiboski, S. & Kaldor, J.M. (1989) A case–control study of diet and breast cancer in Argentina. *Int. J. Cancer,* **44**, 770–776

Isler, O., Ruegg, R. & Schwieter, U. (1967) Carotenoids as food colorants. *Pure appl. Chem.,* **14**, 245–263

Ito, Y., Sasaki, R., Minohara, M., Otani, M. & Aoki, K. (1987) Quantitation of serum carotenoid concentrations in healthy inhabitants by high-performance liquid chromatography. *Clin. chim. Acta,* **169**, 197–208

Ito, Y., Suzuki, S., Yagyu, K., Sasaki, R., Suzuki, K. & Aoki, K. (1997) Relationship between serum carotenoid levels and cancer death rates in the residents, living in a rural area of Hokkaido, Japan. *J. Epidemiol.,* **7**, 1–8

IUPAC Commission on the Nomenclature of Organic Chemistry and IUPAC–IUB Commission on Biochemical Nomenclature (1975) Nomencla-ture of carotenoids. *Pure appl. Chem.,* **41**, 407–431

Jacques, P.F. & Chylack, L.T., Jr (1991) Epidemio-logic evidence of a role for the antioxidant vitamins and carotenoids in cataract prevention. *Am. J. clin. Nutr.,* **53**, 352S–355S

Jain, M., Howe, G.R., Johnson, K.C. & Miller, A.B. (1980a) Evaluation of a diet history questionnaire for epidemiologic studies. *Am. J. Epidemiol.,* **111**, 212–219

Jain, M., Cook, G.M., Davis, F.G., Grace, M.G., Howe, G.R. & Miller, A.B. (1980b) A case–control study of diet and colorectal cancer. *Int. J. Cancer,* **26**, 757–768

Jain, M., Burch, J.D., Howe, G.R., Risch, H.A. & Miller, A.B. (1990) Dietary factors and risk of lung cancer: Results from a case–control study, Toronto, 1981–1985. *Int. J. Cancer,* **45**, 287–293

Järvinen, R., Knekt, P., Seppanen, R. & Teppo, L. (1997) Diet and breast cancer risk in a cohort of Finnish women. *Cancer Lett.,* **114**, 251–253

Jinno, K., Okada, Y., Tanimizu, M., Hyodo, I., Kurimoto, H., Sunahara, S., Takenaka, H. & Moriwaki, S. (1994) Decreased serum levels of β-carotene in patients with hepatocellular carcinoma. *Int. Hepatol. Comm.,* **2**, 43–46

Johnson, E.J. & Russell, R.M. (1992) Distribution of orally administered β-carotene among lipoproteins in healthy men. *Am. J. clin. Nutr.,* **56**, 128–135

Johnson, E.J., Suter, P.M., Sahyoun, N., Ribaya-Mercado, J.D. & Russell, R.M. (1995) Relation between β-carotene intake and plasma and adipose tissue concentrations of carotenoids and retinoids. *Am. J. clin. Nutr.,* **62**, 598–603

Johnson, T.M., Yu, Z.X., Ferrans, V.J., Lowenstein, R.A. & Finkel, T. (1996) Reactive oxygen species are downstream mediators of p53-dependent apoptosis. *Proc. natl Acad. Sci. USA,* **93**, 11848–11852

Jones, R.C., Sugie, S., Braley, J. & Weisburger, J.H. (1989) Dietary beta-carotene in rat models of gastrointestinal cancer. *J. Nutr.*, **119**, 508–514

Jyonouchi, H., Sun, S.N., Tomita, Y. & Gross, M.D. (1995) Astaxanthin, a carotenoid without vitamin A activity, augments antibody responses in cultures including T-helper cell clones and suboptimal doses of antigen. *J. Nutr.*, **125**, 2483–2492

Jyonouchi, H., Sun, S., Mizokami, M. & Gross, M.D. (1996) Effects of various carotenoids on cloned, effector-stage T-helper cell activity. *Nutr. Cancer*, **26**, 313–324

Kaaks, R., Riboli, E. & Sinha, R. (1997) Biochemical markers of dietary intake. In: Toniolo, P., Boffetta, P., Shuker, D.E.G., Rothman, N., Hulka, B. & Pearce, N., eds, *Application of Biomarkers in Cancer Epidemiology* (IARC Scientific Publications No. 142), Lyon, IARC, pp. 103–126

Kada, T.K., Tulikawa, K. & Sadaie, Y. (1972) *In vitro* and host–mediated 'rec-assay' procedures for screening chemical mutagens, and phloxine, a mutagenic red dye detected. *Mutat. Res.*, **16**, 165–174

Kalandidi, A., Katsouyanni, K., Voropoulou, N., Bastas, G., Saracci, R. & Trichopoulos, D. (1990) Passive smoking and diet in the etiology of lung cancer among non-smokers. *Cancer Causes Control*, **1**, 15–21

Kaplan, L.A., Lau, J.M. & Stein, E.A. (1990) Carotenoid composition, concentrations and relationships in various human organs. *Clin. Physiol. Biochem.*, **8**, 1–10

Karagas, M.R., Greenberg, E.R., Nierenberg, D., Stukel, T.A., Morris, J.S., Stevens, M.M. & Baron, J.A. (1997) Risk of squamous cell carcinoma of the skin in relation to plasma selenium, α-tocopherol, β-carotene, and retinol: A nested case–control study. *Cancer Epidemiol. Biomarkers Prev.*, **6**, 25–29

Kardinaal, A.F.M., Kok, F.J., Ringstad, J., Gomez-Aracena, J., Mazaev, V.P., Kohlmeier, L., Martin, B.C., Aro, A., Kark, J.D., Delgado-Rodriguez, M., Riemersma, R.A., van't Veer, P., Huttunen, J.K. & Martin-Moreno, J.M. (1993) Antioxidants in adipose tissue and risk of myocardial infarction: The EURAMIC study. *Lancet*, **342**, 1379–1384

Karrer, P. & Eugster, C.H. (1950) [Synthesis of carotinoids. II. Total synthesis of β-carotenes.] *Helv. chim. Acta*, **33**, 1172–1174 (in German)

Katsouyanni, K., Willett, W., Trichopoulos, D., Boyle, P., Trichopoulou, A., Vasilaros, S., Papadiamantis, J. & MacMahon, B. (1988) Risk of breast cancer among Greek women in relation to nutrient intake. *Cancer*, **61**, 181–185

Katsumura, N., Okuno, M., Onogi, N., Moriwaki, H., Muto, Y & Kojima, S. (1996) Suppression of mouse skin papilloma by canthaxanthin and β-carotene *in vivo*: Possibility of the regression of tumorigenesis by carotenoids without conversion to retinoic acid. *Nutr. Cancer*, **26**, 203–208

Kaugars, G.E., Silverman, S., Jr, Lowas, J.G.L., Brandt, R.B., Riley, W.T., Dao, Q., Singh, V.N. & Gallo, J. (1994) A clinical trial of antioxidant supplements in the treatment of oral leukoplakia. *Oral Surg. oral Med. oral Pathol.*, **78**, 462–468

Kazi, N., Radvany, R., Oldham, T., Keshavarzian, A., Frommel, T.O., Libertin, C. & Mobarhan, S. (1997) Immunomodulatory effect of beta-carotene on T lymphocyte subsets in patients with resected colonic polyps and cancer. *Nutr. Cancer*, **28**, 140–145

Key, T.J.A., Silcocks, P.B., Davey, G.K., Appleby, P.N. & Bishop, D.T. (1997) A case–control study of diet and prostate cancer. *Br. J. Cancer*, **76**, 678–687

Khachik, F., Beecher, G.R. & Goli, M.B. (1991) Separation, identification, and quantification of carotenoids in fruits, vegetables and human plasma by high performance liquid chromatography. *Pure appl. Chem.*, **63**, 71–80

Khachik, F., Goli, M.B., Beecher, G.R., Holden, J.M., Lusby, W.R., Tenorio, M.D. & Barrera, M.R. (1992a) Effect of food preparation on qualitative and quantitative distribution of major carotenoid constituents of tomatoes and several green vegetables. *J. Agric. Food Chem.*, **40**, 390–398

Khachik, F., Beecher, G.R., Goli, M.B., Lusby, W.R. & Smith, J.C. (1992b) Separation and identification of carotenoids and their oxidation products in the extracts of human plasma. *Anal. Chem.*, **64**, 2111–2122

Khachik, F., Beecher, G.R. & Smith, J.C., Jr (1995) Lutein, lycopene, and their oxidative metabolites in chemoprevention of cancer. *J. cell. Biochem.*, **22**, 236–246

Khachik, F., Spangler, C.J., Smith, J.C., Canfield, L.M., Steck, A. & Pfander, H. (1997) Identification, quantification, and relative concentrations of carotenoids and their metabolites in human milk and serum. *Anal. Chem.*, **69**, 1873–1881

Kikendall, J.W., Burgess, M. & Bowen, P.E. (1990) Effect of oral beta carotene on recurrence of colonic adenomas (Abstract). *Gastroenterology*, **98**, A289

Kikendall, J.W., Mobarhan, S., Nelson, R., Burgess, M. & Bowen, P.E. (1991) Oral beta carotene does not reduce the recurrence of colorectal adenomas (Abstract). *Am. J. Gastroenterol.*, **36**, 1356

Kim, D.J., Takasuka, N., Kim, J.M., Sekine, K., Ota, T., Asamoto, M., Murakoshi, M., Nishino, H., Nir, Z. & Tsuda, H. (1997) Chemoprevention by lycopene of mouse lung neoplasia after combined initiation treatment with DEN, MNU and DMH. *Cancer Lett.*, **120**, 15–22

Kirkpatrick, C.S., White, E. & Lee, J.A.H. (1994) Case–control study of malignant melanoma in Washington State. II. Diet, alcohol, and obesity. *Am. J. Epidemiol.*, **139**, 869–880

Klepsch, E. & Baltas, A. (1994) European Parliament and Council Directive 94/36/EC of 30 June 1994 on colours for use in food stuffs. *Off. J. Eur. Community*, **L237**, 13–29

Kliewer, S.A., Umesono, K. & Evans, R.M. (1994) The retinoid X receptors. In: Blomhoff, R., ed., *Vitamin A in Health and Disease*, New York, Marcel Dekker, pp. 239–255

Knekt, P., Aromaa, A., Maatela, J., Aaran, R.-K., Nikkari, T., Hakama, M., Hakulinen, T., Peto, R. & Teppo, L. (1990) Serum vitamin A and subsequent risk of cancer: Cancer incidence follow-up of the Finnish Mobile Clinic Health Examination Survey. *Am. J. Epidemiol.*, **132**, 857–870

Knekt, P., Aromaa, A., Maatela, J., Alfthan, G., Aaran, R.-K., Nikkari, T., Hakama, M., Hakulinen, T. & Teppo, L. (1991) Serum micronutrients and risk of cancers of low incidence in Finland. *Am. J. Epidemiol.*, **134**, 356–361

Knekt, P., Reunanen, A., Jarvinen, R., Seppanen, R., Heliovaara, M. & Aromaa, A. (1994) Antioxidant vitamin intake and coronary mortality in a longitudinal population study. *Am. J. Epidemiol.*, **139**, 1180–1189

Kohlmeier, L. & Hastings, S.B. (1995) Epidemiologic evidence of a role of carotenoids in cardiovascular disease prevention. *Am. J. clin. Nutr.*, **62** (Suppl.), 1370S–1376S

Kohlmeier, L. & Kohlmeier, M. (1995) Adipose tissue as a medium for epidemiologic exposure assessment. *Environ. Health Perspectives*, **103** (Suppl. 3), 99–106

Kohlmeier, L., Kark, J.D., Gomez Gracia, E., Martin, B.C., Steck, S.E., Kardinaal, A.F., Ringstad, J., Thamm, M., Masaev, V., Riemersma, R., Martin Moreno, J.M., Huttunen, J.K. & Kok, F.J. (1997) Lycopene and myocardial infarction risk in the EURAMIC Study. *Am. J. Epidemiol.*, **146**, 618–626

Kolonel, L.N., Hankin, J.H. & Yoshizawa, C.N. (1987) Vitamin A and prostate cancer in elderly men: Enhancement of risk. *Cancer Res.*, **47**, 2982–2985

Kolonel, L.N., Yoshizawa, C.N. & Hankin, J.H. (1988) Diet and prostatic cancer: A case–control study in Hawaii. *Am. J. Epidemiol.*, **127**, 999–1012

Komaki, C., Okuno, M., Onogi, N., Moriwaki, H., Kawamori, T., Tanaka, T., Mori, H. & Muto, Y. (1996) Synergistic suppression of azoxymethane-induced foci of colonic aberrant crypts by the combination of beta-carotene and perilla oil in rats. *Carcinogenesis*, **17**, 1897–1901

Koo, L.C. (1988) Dietary habits and lung cancer risk among Chinese females in Hong Kong who never smoked. *Nutr. Cancer*, **11**, 155–172

Köpcke, W., Barker, F.M. & Schalch, W. (1995) Canthaxanthin deposition in the retina: A biostatistical evaluation of 411 patients. *J. Toxicol. cutaneous ocular Toxicol.*, **14**, 89–104

Kornhauser, A., Warner, W. & Lambert, L. (1990) β-Carotene protection against phototoxicity *in vivo*. In: Krinsky, N.I., Mathews-Roth, M.M. & Taylor, R.F., eds, *Carotenoids Chemistry and Biology*, New York, Plenum Press, pp. 301–312

Kostic, D., White, W.S. & Olson, J.A. (1995) Intestinal absorption, serum clearance and interactions between lutein and β-carotene when administered to human adults in separate or combined oral doses. *Am. J. clin. Nutr.*, **62**, 604–610

Krinsky, N.I. (1993a) Actions of carotenoids in biological systems. *Ann. Rev. Nutr.*, **13**, 561–587

Krinsky, N.I. (1993b) Micronutrients and their influence on mutagenicity and malignant transformation. *Ann. N.Y. Acad. Sci.*, **686**, 229–242

Krinsky, N.I. (1994) Carotenoids and cancer: Basic research studies. In: Frei, B., ed., *Natural Antioxidants in Human Health and Disease*, New York, Academic Press, pp. 239–261

Krinsky, N.I. & Deneke, S.M. (1982) Interaction of oxygen and oxy-radicals with carotenoids 1. *J. natl Cancer Inst.*, **69**, 205–210

Krinsky, N.I., Cornwell, D.G. & Oncley, J.L. (1958) The transport of vitamin A and carotenoids in human plasma. *Arch. Biochem. Biophys.*, **73**, 233–246

Krinsky, N.I., Russett, M.D., Handelman, G.J. & Snodderly, D.M. (1990a) Structural and geometrical isomers of carotenoids in human plasma. *J. Nutr.*, **120**, 1654–1662

Krinsky, N.I., Mathews-Roth, M.M., Welankiwar, S., Sehgal, P.K., Lausen, N.C.G. & Russett, M. (1990b) The metabolism of [^{14}-C]β-carotene and the presence of other carotenoids in rats and monkeys. *J. Nutr.*, **120**, 81–87

Kromhout, D. (1987) Essential micronutrients in relation to carcinogenesis. *Am. J. clin. Nutr.*, **45**, 1361–1367

Kull, D. & Pfander, H. (1995) List of new carotenoids. In: Britton, G., Liaaen-Jensen, S. & Pfander, H., eds, *Carotenoids*, Vol. 1A., Basel, Birkhäuser Verlag, pp. 295–317

Kune, S., Kune, G.A. & Watson, L.F. (1987) Case–control study of dietary etiological factors: The Melbourne colorectal cancer study. *Nutr. Cancer*, **9**, 21–42

Kune, G.A., Kune S., Watson, L.F., Pierce, R., Field, B., Vitetta, L., Merenstein, D., Hayes, A. & Irving, L. (1989) Serum levels of β-carotene, vitamin A, and zinc in male lung cancer cases and controls. *Nutr. Cancer*, **12**, 169–176

Kune, G.A., Bannerman, S., Field, B., Watson, L.F., Cleland, H., Merenstein, D. & Vitetta, L. (1992) Diet, alcohol, smoking, serum β-carotene, and vitamin A in male nonmelanocytic skin cancer patients and controls. *Nutr. Cancer*, **18**, 237–244

Kune, G.A., Kune, S., Field, B., Watson, L.F., Cleland, H., Merenstein, D. & Vitetta, L. (1993) Oral and pha-ryngeal cancer, diet, smoking, alcohol, and serum vitamin A and β-carotene levels: A case–control study in men. *Nutr. Cancer*, **20**, 61–70

Kushi, L.H., Folsom, A.R., Prineas, R.J., Mink, P.J., Wu, Y. & Bostick, R.M. (1996) Dietary antioxidant vitamins and death from coronary heart disease in post-menopausal women. *New Engl. J. Med.*, **334**, 1156–1162

Lahiri, M., Maru, G.B. & Bhide, S.V. (1993) Effect of plant phenols, β-carotene and α-tocopherol on benzo[a]pyrene-induced DNA damage in the mouse forestomach mucosa (target organ) and bone marrow polychromatic eryth-rocytes (non-target organ). *Mutat. Res.*, **303**, 97–100

Lakshman, M.R., Mychkovsky, I. & Attlesey, M. (1989) Enzymatic conversion of all-*trans*-β-carotene to retinal by a cytosolic enzyme from rabbit and rat intestinal mucosa. *Proc. natl Acad. Sci. USA*, **86**, 9124–9128

Lambert, L.A., Koch, W.H., Wamer, W.G. & Kornhauser, A. (1990) Antitumor activity in skin of Skh and Sencar mice by two dietary β-carotene formulations. *Nutr. Cancer*, **13**, 213– 221

Lambert, L.A., Wamer, W.G., Wei, R.R., Lavu, S., Chirtel, S.J. & Kornhause, R.A. (1994) The protective but nonsynergistic effect of dietary beta-carotene and vitamin E on skin tumorigenesis in Skh mice. *Nutr. Cancer*, **21**, 1–12

Landrum, J.T., Bone, R.A. & Kilburn, M.D. (1997) The macular pigment: A possible role in protection from age-related macular degeneration. *Adv. Pharmacol.*, **38**, 537–556

Lascari, A.D. (1981) Carotenemia. A review. *Clin. Pediatr.*, **20**, 25–29

La Vecchia, C., Decarli, A., Fasoli, M. & Gentile, A. (1986) Nutrition and diet in the etiology of endome-trial cancer. *Cancer*, **57**, 1248–1253

La Vecchia, C., Negri, E., Decarli, A., D'Avanzo, B. & Franceschi, S. (1987a) A case–control study of diet and gastric cancer in northern Italy. *Int. J. Cancer*, **40**, 484–489

La Vecchia, C., Decarli, A., Negri, E., Parazzini, F., Gentile, A., Cecchetti, G., Fasoli, M. & Franceschi, S. (1987b) Dietary factors and the risk of epithelial ovarian cancer. *J. natl Cancer Inst.*, **79**, 663– 669

La Vecchia, C., Negri, E., Decarli, A., D'Avanzo, B., Gallotti, L., Gentile, A. & Franceschi, S. (1988a) A case–control study of diet and colorectal cancer in northern Italy. *Int. J. Cancer*, **41**, 492–498

La Vecchia, C., Decarli, A., Fasoli, M., Parazzini, F., Franceschi, S., Gentile, A. & Negri, E. (1988b) Dietary vitamin A and the risk of intraepithelial and invasive cervical neoplasia. *Gynecol. Oncol.*, **30**, 187–195

La Vecchia, C., Negri, E., Decarli, A., D'Avanzo, B. & Franceschi, S. (1988c) Risk factors for hepatocellular carcinoma in northern Italy. *Int. J. Cancer*, **42**, 872–876

La Vecchia, C., Negri, E., Decarli, A., D'Avanzo, B., Liberati, C. & Franceschi, S. (1989) Dietary factors in the risk of bladder cancer. *Nutr. Cancer*, **12**, 93–101

La Vecchia, C., Ferraroni, M., D'Avanzo, B., Decarli, A. & Franceschi, S. (1994) Selected micronutrient intake and the risk of gastric cancer. *Cancer Epidemiol. Biomarkers Prev.*, **3**, 393–398

Lee, H.P., Gourley, L., Duffy, S.W., Estève, J., Lee, J. & Day, N.E. (1989) Colorectal cancer and diet in an Asian population: A case–control study among Singapore Chinese. *Int. J. Cancer*, **43**, 1007–1016

Lee, H.P., Gourley, L., Duffy, S.W., Estève, J., Lee, J. & Day, N.E. (1991) Dietary effects on breast cancer risk in Singapore. *Lancet*, **337**, 1197–1200

LeGardeur, B.Y., Lopez, S.A. & Johnson, W.D. (1990) A case–control study of serum vitamins A, E, and C in lung cancer patients. *Nutr. Cancer*, **14**, 133–140

Leichter, J. & Dunn, B.P. (1992) Effect of β-carotene supplementation on fetal growth of rats exposed to cigarette smoke during pregnancy. *Biochem. Arch.*, **8**, 97–204

Le Marchand, L., Yoshizawa, C.N., Kolonel, L.N., Hankin, J.H. & Goodman, M.T. (1989) Vegetable consumption and lung cancer risk: A population-based case–control study in Hawaii. *J. natl Cancer Inst.*, **81**, 1158–1164

Le Marchand, L., Hankin, J.H., Kolonel, L.N. & Wilkens, L.R. (1991) Vegetable and fruit consumption in relation to prostate cancer risk in Hawaii: A reevaluation of the effect of dietary beta-carotene. *Am. J. Epidemiol.*, **133**, 215–219

Le Marchand, L., Hankin, J.H., Kolonel, L.N., Beecher, G.B., Wilkens, L.R. & Zhao, L.P. (1993) Intake of specific carotenoids and lung cancer risk. *Cancer Epidemiol. Biomarkers Prev.*, **2**, 183– 187

Leo, M.A., Kim, C.-I., Lowe, N. & Lieber, C.S. (1992) Interaction of ethanol with β-carotene: Delayed blood clearance and enhanced hepatotoxicity. *Hepatology*, **15**, 883–891

Leo, M.A., Ahmed, S., Aleynik, S.I., Siegel, J.H., Kasmin, F. & Lieber, C.S. (1995) Carotenoids and tocopherols in various hepatobiliary conditions. *J. Hepatol.*, **23**, 550–556

Leo, M.A., Aleynik, S.I., Aleynik, M.K. & Lieber, C.S. (1997) Beta-carotene beadlets potentiate hepatotoxicity of alcohol. *Am. J. clin. Nutr.*, **66**, 1461–1469

Lepage, G., Champagne, J., Ronco, N., Lamarre, A., Osberg, I., Sokol, R.J. & Roy, C.C. (1996) Supplementation with carotenoids corrects increased lipid peroxidation in children with cystic fibrosis. *Am. J. clin. Nutr.*, **64**, 87–93

Levi, F., La Vecchia, C., Gulie, C. & Negri, E. (1993a) Dietary factors and breast cancer risk in Vaud, Switzerland. *Nutr. Cancer*, **19**, 327–335

Levi, F., Franceschi, S., Negri, E. & La Vecchia, C. (1993b) Dietary factors and the risk of endometrial cancer. *Cancer*, **71**, 3575–3581

Levy, J., Bosin, E., Feldman, B., Giat, Y., Miinster, A., Danilenko, M. & Sharoni, Y. (1995) Lycopene is a more potent inhibitor of human cancer cell proliferation than either alpha-carotene or beta-carotene. *Nutr. Cancer*, **24**, 257–266

Levy, L.W., Regalado, E., Navarrete, S. & Watkins, R.H. (1997) Bixin and norbixin in human plasma: Determination of the absorption of a single dose of annatto food color. *Analyst*, **122**, 977–980

Li, B., Taylor, P.R., Li, J.Y., Dawsey, S.M., Wang, W., Tangrea, J.A., Liu, B.Q., Ershow, A.G., Zheng, S.F., Fraumeni, J.F., Jr, Yang, Q., Yu, Y., Sun, Y., Li, G., Zhang, D., Greenwald, P., Lian, G.-T., Yang, C.S. & Blot, W.J. (1993) Linxian nutrition intervention trials: Design, methods, participant characteristics and compliance. *Ann. Epidemiol.*, **3**, 577–585

Li, J.-Y., Taylor, P.R., Li, B., Dawsey, S., Wang, G.-Q., Ershow, A.G., Guo, W., Liu, S.-F., Yang, C.S., Shen, Q., Wang, W., Mark, S.D., Zou, X.-N., Greenwald, P., Wu, Y.-P. & Blot, W.J. (1993) Nutrition intervention trials in Linxian, China: Multiple vitamin/mineral supplementation, cancer incidence, and disease-specific mortality among adults with esophageal dysplasia. *J. natl Cancer Inst.*, **85**, 1492–1498

Liebler, D.C. (1993) Antioxidant reactions of carotenoids. *Ann. N.Y. Acad. Sci.*, **669**, 20–31

Lin, B.C., Wong, C.W., Chen, H.W. & Privalsky, M.L. (1997) Plasticity of tetramer formation by retinoid X receptors: An alternative paradigm for DNA recognition. *J. biol. Chem.*, **272**, 9860–9867

Lipkin, M., Bhandari, M., Hakissian, M., Croll, W. & Wong, G. (1994) Surrogate endpoint biomarker assays in phase II chemoprevention clinical trials. *J. Cell Biochem.*, **19**, 47–54

London, S.J., Stein, E.A., Henderson, I.C., Stampfer, M.J., Wood, W.C., Remine, S., Dmochowski, J.R., Robert, N.J. & Willett, W.C. (1992) Carotenoids, retinol, and vitamin E and risk of proliferative benign breast disease and breast cancer. *Cancer Causes Control*, **3**, 503–512

Long, C., ed. (1961) *Handbook of Biochemistry*, Cleveland, Ohio, CRC Press, p. 639

Lotan, R., Xu, X.C., Lippman, S.M., Ro, J.Y., Lee, J.S., Lee, J.J. & Hong, W.K. (1995) Suppression of retinoic acid receptor-β in premalignant oral lesions and its up-regulation by isotretinoin. *New Engl. J. Med.*, **332**, 1405–1410

Mackerras, D., Buffler, P.A., Randall, D.E., Nichaman, M.Z., Pickle, L.W. & Mason, T.J. (1988) Carotene intake and the risk of laryngeal cancer in coastal Texas. *Am. J. Epidemiol.*, **128**, 980–988

MacLennan, R., Macrae, F., Bain, C., Battistutta, D., Chapuis, P., Gratten, H., Lambert, J., Newland, R.C., Ngu, M., Russell, A., Ward, M., Wahlqvist, M.L. & Australian Polyp Prevention Project (1995) Randomized trial of intake of fat, fiber, and beta carotene to prevent colorectal adenomas. *J. natl Cancer Inst.*, **87**, 1760–1766

Maclure, M. & Willett, W. (1990) A case–control study of diet and risk of renal adenocarcinoma. *Epidemiology,* **1**, 430–440

Macrae, F.A., Hughes, N.R., Bhathal, P.S., Tay, D., Selbie, L. & MacLennan, R. (1991) Dietary suppression of rectal epithelial cell proliferation (Abstract 383). *Gastroenterology*, **100**, 1991

Maiani, G., Mobarhan, S., Ceccanti, M., Ranaldi, L., Gettner, S., Bowen, P., Friedman, H., De Lorenzo, A. & Ferro-Luzzi, A. (1989) Beta-carotene serum response in young and elderly females. *Eur. J. clin. Nutr.*, **43**, 749–761

Maiani, G., Pappalardo, G., Ferro-Luzzi, A., Raguzzini, A., Azzini, E., Guadalaxara, A., Trifero, M., Frommel, T. & Mobarhan, S. (1995) Accumulation of β-carotene in normal colorectal mucosa and colonic neoplastic lesions in humans. *Nutr. Cancer*, **24**, 23–31

Malaker, K., Anderson, B.J., Beecroft, W.A. & Hodson, D.I. (1991). Management of oral mucosal dysplasia with beta-carotene retinoic acid: A pilot cross-over study. *Cancer Detect. Prev.*, **15**, 335–340

Malvy, D.J.-M., Burtschy, B., Arnaud, J., Sommelet, D., Leverger, G., Dostalova, L., Drucker, J., Amédée-Manesme, O. & the 'Cancer in Children and Antioxidant Micronutrients' French Study Group (1993) Serum beta-carotene and antioxidant micronutrients in children with cancer. *Int. J. Epidemiol.*, **22**, 761–771

Manetta, A., Schubbert, T., Chapman, J., Schell, M.J., Peng, Y.-M., Liao, S.Y. & Meyskens, F.J., Jr (1996) β-Carotene treatment of cervical intraepithelial neoplasia: A phase II study. *Cancer Epidemiol. Biomarkers Prev.*, **5**, 929–932

Mangels, A.R., Holden, J.M., Beecher, G.R., Forman, M.R. & Lanza, E. (1993) Carotenoid content of fruits and vegetables: An evaluation of analytic data. *J. Am. Diet. Assoc.*, **93**, 284–296

Mannick, E.E., Bravo, L.E., Zarama, G., Realpe, J.L., Zhang, X., Ruiz, B., Fontham, E.T., Mera, R., Miller, M.J. & Correa, P. (1996) Inducible nitric oxide synthase, nitrotyrosine, and apoptosis in *Helicobacter pylori* gastritis: Effect of antibiotics and antioxidants. *Cancer Res.*, **56**, 3238–3243

Manoharan, K. & Banerjee, M.R. (1985) Beta-carotene reduces sister chromatid exchanges induced by chemical carcinogens in mouse mammary cells in organ culture. *Cell Biol. int. Rep.*, **9**, 783–789

Manson, J.E., Stampfer, M., Willett, W.C., Colditz, G.A., Rosner, B., Speizer, F.E. & Hennekens, C.H. (1991) A prospective study of antioxidant vitamins and incidence of coronary heart disease in women (Abstract). *Circulation*, **84** (Suppl. II), 546

Manson, J.E., Gaziano, J.M., Jonas, M.A. & Hennekens, C.H. (1993) Antioxidants and cardiovascular disease: A review. *J. Am. Coll. Nutr.*, **12**, 426–432

Mantovani, A. (1992) The role of multigeneration studies in safety assessment of residues of veterinary drugs and additives. *Ann. Inst. super. Sanita*, **28**, 429–435

Mares-Perlman, J.A., Brady, W.E., Klein, R., Klein, B.E.K., Palta, M., Bowen, P. & Stacewicz-Sapuntzakis, M. (1994) Serum levels of carotenoids and tocopherols in people with age-related maculopathy (Abstract). *Invest. Ophthalmol. vis. Sci.*, **35**, 2004

Mares-Perlman, J.A., Brady, W.E., Klein, B.E.K., Klein, R., Palta, M., Bowen, P. & Stacewicz-Sapuntzakis, M. (1995) Serum carotenoids and tocopherols and severity of nuclear and cortical opacities. *Invest. Ophthalmol. vis. Sci.*, **36**, 276–288

Margetts, B.M. & Jackson, A.A. (1993) Interaction between people's diet and their smoking habits: The dietary and nutritional survey of British adults. *Br. med. J.*, **307**, 1381–1384

Margetts, B.M. & Jackson, A.A. (1996) The determinants of plasma β-carotene: Interaction between smoking and other lifestyle factors. *Eur. J. clin. Nutr.*, **50**, 236–238

Mark, S.D., Liu, F., Li, J., Gail, M., Shen, Q., Dawsey, S., Liu, F., Taylor, P.T., Li, B. & Blot, W.J. (1994) Effect of vitamin and mineral supplementation on esophageal cytology: Results from the Linxian Dysplasia Trial. *Int. J. Cancer*, **57**, 162–166

Mark, S.D., Wang, W., Fraumeni, J.F., Jr, Li, J.-Y., Taylor, P.R. Wang, G.Q., Wande, G., Dawsey, S.M., Li, B. & Blot, W.J. (1996) Lowered risks of hypertension and cerebrovascular disease after vitamin/mineral supplementation. *Am. J. Epidemiol.*, **143**, 658–664

Marshall, J.R., Graham, S., Byers, T., Swanson, M. & Brasure, J. (1983) Diet and smoking in the epidemiology of cancer of the cervix. *J. natl Cancer Inst.*, **70**, 847–851

Marubini, E., Decarli, A., Costa, A., Mazzoleni, C., Andreoli, C., Barbieri, A., Capitelli, E., Carlucci, M., Cavallo, F., Monferroni, N., Pastorino, U. & Salvini, S. (1988) The relationship of dietary intake and serum levels of retinol and beta-carotene with breast cancer. Results of a case–control study. *Cancer*, **61**, 173–180

Mathews-Roth, M.M. (1982) Antitumor activity of beta-carotene, canthaxanthin and phytoene. *Oncology*, **39**, 33–37

Mathews, Roth, M.M. (1983) Carotenoid pigment administration and delay in development of UV-B-induced tumors. *Photochem. Photobiol.*, **37**, 509–511

Mathews-Roth, M.M. (1986) β-Carotene therapy for erythropoietic protoporphyria and other photosensitivity diseases. *Biochemie*, **68**, 875–884

Mathews-Roth, M.M. (1987) Photoprotection by carotenoids. *Fed. Proc.*, **46**, 1890–1893

Mathews-Roth, M.M. (1988) Lack of genotoxicity with beta-carotene. *Toxicol. Lett.*, **41**, 185–191

Mathews-Roth, M.M. (1993) Carotenoids in erythropoietic protoporphyria and other photosensitivity diseases. *Ann. N.Y. Acad. Sci.*, **691**, 127–138

Mathews-Roth, M.M. & Gulbrandsen, C.L. (1974) Transport of beta-carotene in serum of individuals with carotenemia. *Clin. Chem.*, **20**, 1578–1579

Mathews-Roth, M.M. & Krinsky, N.I (1985) Carotenoid dose level and protection against UV-B induced skin tumours. *Photochem. Photobiol.*, **42**, 35–38

Mathews-Roth, M.M. & Krinsky, N.I. (1987) Carotenoids affect development of UV-B induced skin cancer. *Photochem Photobiol.*, **46**, 507–509

Mathews Roth, M.M., Pathak, M.A., Parrish, J., Fitzpatrick, T.B., Kass, E.H., Toda, K. & Clemens, W. (1972) A clinical trial of the effects of oral beta-carotene on the responses of human skin to solar radiation. *J. Invest. Dermatol.*, **59**, 349–353

Mathews-Roth, M.M., Pathak M.A., Fitzpatrick T.B., Harber L.C. & Kass E.H. (1977) Beta-carotene therapy for erythropoietic protoporphyria and other photosensitive diseases. *Arch. Dermatol.*, **113**, 1229–1232

Mathews-Roth, M.M., Welankiwar, S., Sehgal, P.K., Lausen, N.C.G., Russett, M. & Krinsky, N.I. (1990) Distribution of [^{14}-C]canthaxanthin and [^{14}-C]lycopene in rats and monkeys. *J. Nutr.*, **120**, 1205–1213

Mathews-Roth, M.M., Lausen, N., Drouin, G., Richter, A. & Krinsky, N. (1991) Effects of carotenoid administration on bladder cancer prevention. *Oncology*, **48**, 177–179

Matsushima-Nishiwaki, R., Shidoji, Y., Nishiwaki, S., Yamada, T., Moriwaki, H. & Muto, Y. (1995) Suppression by carotenoids of microcystin-induced morphological changes in mouse hepatocytes. *Lipids*, **30**, 1029–1034

Mayne, S.T. (1996) Beta-carotene, carotenoids, and disease prevention in humans. *FASEB J.*, **10**, 690–701

Mayne, S.T. & Parker, R.S. (1986) Subcellular distribution of dietary beta-carotene in chick liver. *Lipids*, **21**, 164–169

Mayne, S.T. & Parker, R.S. (1989) Antioxidant activity of dietary canthaxanthin. *Nutr. Cancer*, **12**, 225–236

Mayne, S.T., Janerich, D.T., Greenwald, P., Chorost, S., Tucci, C., Zaman, M.B., Melamed, M.R., Kiely, M. & McKneally, M.F. (1994) Dietary beta carotene and lung cancer risk in US nonsmokers. *J. natl Cancer Inst.*, **86**, 33–38

Mayne, S.T., Handelman, G.J. & Beecher, G. (1996) β-Carotene and lung cancer promotion in heavy smokers: A plausible relationship? (Editorial). *J. natl Cancer Inst.*, **88**, 1513–1515

Mayne, S., Cartmel, B., Silva, F., Fallon, B., Briskin, K., Baum, M., Shor-Posner, G. & Goodwin, W.J., Jr (1997) Effect of supplemental beta-carotene on plasma concentrations of carotenoids, retinol and alpha-tocopherol in humans (Abstract). *FASEB J.*, **11**, A448

McLaren, D.S. & Zekian, B. (1971) Failure of enzymic cleavage of β-carotene. The cause of vitamin A deficiency in a child. *Am. J. Dis. Child.*, **121**, 278–280

McLarty, J.W. (1995) Beta-carotene, vitamin A and lung cancer chemoprevention: Results of an intermediate endpoint study. *Am. J. clin. Nutr.*, **62**, 1431S–1438S

McLaughlin, J.K., Mandel, J.S., Blot, W.J., Schuman, L.M., Mehl, E.S. & Fraumeni, J.F. (1984) A population-based case–control study of renal cell carcinoma. *J. natl Cancer Inst.*, **72**, 275–284

McLaughlin, J.K., Gridley, G., Block, G., Winn, D.M., Preston Martin, S., Schoenberg, J.B., Greenberg, R.S., Stemhagen, A., Austin, D.F., Ershow, A.G., Blot, W.J. & Fraumeni, J.F., Jr (1988) Dietary factors in oral and pharyngeal cancer. *J. natl Cancer Inst.*, **80**, 1237–1243

Menkes, M.S., Comstock, G.W., Vuilleumier, J.P., Helsing, K.J., Rider, A.A. & Brookmeyer, R. (1986) Serum beta-carotene, vitamins A and E, selenium, and the risk of lung cancer. *New Engl. J. Med.*, **315**, 1250–1254

Mettlin, C. (1989) Milk drinking, other beverage habits, and lung cancer risk. *Int. J. Cancer*, **43**, 608–612

Mettlin, C., Selenskas, S., Natarajan, N. & Huben, R. (1989) Beta-carotene and animal fats and their relationship to prostate cancer risk. A case–control study. *Cancer*, **64**, 605–612

Meydani, M., Martin, A., Ribaya-Mercado, J.D., Gong, J., Blumberg, J.B. & Russell, R.M. (1994) Beta-carotene supplementation increases antioxidant capacity of plasma in older women. *J. Nutr.*, **124**, 2397–2403

Meyer, F. & White, E. (1993) Alcohol and nutrients in relation to colon cancer in middle-aged adults. *Am. J. Epidemiol.*, **138**, 225–236

Meyer, J.C., Grundmann, H.P., Seeger, B. & Schnyder, U.W. (1985) Plasma concentrations of beta-carotene and canthaxanthin during and after stopping intake of a combined preparation. *Dermatology*, **171**, 76–81

Meyers, D.G., Maloley, R.A. & Weeks, D. (1996) Safety of antioxidant vitamins. *Arch. intern. Med.*, **156**, 925–935

Meyskens, F.L., Jr & Manetta, A. (1995) Prevention of cervical intraepithelial neoplasia and cervical cancer. *Am. J. clin. Nutr.*, **62**, 1417S–1419S

Micozzi, M., Beecher, G.R., Taylor, P.R. & Khachlik, F. (1990) Carotenoid analyses of selected raw and cooked foods associated with a lower risk for cancer. *J. natl Cancer Inst.*, **82**, 282–285

Micozzi, M.S., Brown, E.D., Edwards, B.K., Bieri, J.G., Taylor, P.R., Khachik, F., Beecher, G.R. & Smith, Jr., J.C. (1992) Plasma carotenoid response to chronic intake of selected foods and β-carotene supplements in men. *Am. J. clin. Nutr.*, **55**, 1120–1125

Milas, N.A., Davis, P., Belic, I. & Fles, D.A. (1950) Synthesis of β-carotene. *J. Am. chem. Soc.*, **72**, 4844

Mobarhan, S., Bowen, P., Andersen, B., Evans, M., Stacewicz Sapuntzakis, M., Sugerman, S., Simms, P., Lucchesi, D. & Friedman, H. (1990) Effects of beta-carotene repletion on beta-carotene absorption, lipid peroxidation, and neutrophil superoxide formation in young men. *Nutr. Cancer*, **14**, 195–206

Mobarhan, S., Shiau, A., Grande, A., Srinivas, K., Stacewicz-Sapuntzakis, M., Oldham, T., Liao, Y., Bowen, P., Dyavanapalli, M., Kazi, N., McNeal, K. & Frommel, T. (1994) β-Carotene supplementation results in an increased serum and colonic mucosal concentration of β-carotene and a decrease in α-tocopherol concentration in patients with colonic neoplasia. *Cancer Epidemiol. Biomarkers Prev.*, **3**, 501–505

Moji, H., Murata, T., Morinobu, T., Manago, M., Tamai, H., Okamoto, R., Mino, M., Fujimura, M. & Takeuchi, T. (1995) Plasma levels of retinol, retinol-binding protein, all-*trans* beta-carotene and cryptox-anthin in low birth weight infants. *J. nutr. Sci. Vitaminol.*, **41**, 595–606

Mokady, S. & Ben-Amotz, A. (1991) Dietary lipid level and the availability of β-carotene of *Dunaliella-bardawil* in rats. *Nutr. Cancer*, **15**, 47–52

Mokady, S., Avron, M. & Ben-Amotz, A. (1990) Accumulation in chick livers of 9-*cis* versus all-*trans* β-carotene. *J. Nutr.*, **120**, 889–892

Monk, B.E. (1982) Metabolic carotenaemia. *Br. J. Dermatol.*, **106**, 485–488

Moon, R.C., Rao, K.V., Detrisac, C.J., Kelloff, G.J., Steele, V.E. & Doody, L.A. (1994) Chemoprevention of respiratory tract neoplasia in the hamster by oltipraz, alone and in combination. *Int. J. Oncol.*, **4**, 661–667

Moore, T., ed. (1957) *Vitamin A*, Amsterdam, Elsevier

Moreno, F.S., Rizzi, M.B.S.L., Dagli, M.L.Z. & Penteado, M.V.C. (1991) Inhibitory effects of beta-carotene on preneoplastic lesions induced in Wistar rats by the resistant hepatocyte model. *Carcinogenesis*, **12**, 1817–1822

Moreno, F.S., Wu, T.-S., Penteado, M.V.C., Rizzi, M.B.S.L., Jordão, A.A., Almeida-Muradian, L.B. & Dagli, M.L.Z. (1995) A comparison of beta-carotene and vitamin A effects on a hepatocarcinogenesis model. *Int. Vitam. Nutr. Res.*, **65**, 87–94

Morris, D.L., Kritchevsky, S.B. & Davis, C.E. (1994) Serum carotenoids and coronary heart disease. The Lipid Research Clinics Coronary Primary Prevention Trial and Follow-up Study. *J. Am med. Assoc.*, **272**, 1439–1441

Mukherjee, A., Agarwal, K., Aguilar, M.A. & Sharma, A. (1991) Anticlastogenic activity of beta-carotene against cyclophosphamide in mice in vivo. *Mutat. Res.*, **263**, 41–46

Müller, J.M., Rupec, R.A. & Baeuerle, P.A. (1997) Study of gene regulation by NK-kappa B and AP-1 in response to reactive oxygen intermediates. *Methods*, **11**, 301–312

Multiple Risk Factor Intervention Trial Research Group (1982) Multiple Risk Factor Intervention Trial. Risk factor changes and mortality results. *J. Am. med. Assoc.*, **248**, 1465–1477

Munoz, S.E., Ferraroni, M., La Vecchia, C. & Decarli, A. (1997) Gastric cancer risk factors in subjects with family history. *Cancer Epidemiol. Biomarkers Prev.*, **6**, 137–140

Murakoshi, M., Takayasu, J., Kimura, O., Kohmura, E., Nishino, H., Iwashima, A., Okuzumi, J., Sakai, T., Sugimoto, T., Imanishi, J. & Iwasaki, R. (1989) Inhibitory effects of α-carotene on proliferation of the human neuroblastoma cell line GOTO. *J. natl Cancer Inst.*, **81**, 1649–1652

Murakoshi, M., Nishino, H., Satomi, Y., Takayasu, J., Hasegawa, T., Tokuda, H., Iwashima, A., Okuzumi, J., Okabe, H., Kitano, H. & Iwasaki, R. (1992) Potent pre-ventive action of alpha-carotene against carcinogen-esis: spontaneous liver carcinogenesis and promoting stage of lung and skin carcinogenesis in mice are sup-pressed more effectively by alpha-carotene than by beta-carotene. *Cancer Res.*, **52**, 6583–6587

Murata, T., Tamai, H., Morinobu, T., Manago, M., Takenaka, H., Hayashi, K. & Mino, M. (1994) Effect of long-term administration of beta-carotene on lym-phocyte subsets in humans. *Am. J. clin. Nutr.*, **60**, 597–602

Muto, T., Shidoji, Y., Moriwaki, H., Kawaguchi, T. & Noda, T. (1995) Growth retardation in human cervi-cal dysplasia-derived cell lines by beta-carotene through down-regulation of epidermal growth factor receptor. *Am. J. clin. Nutr.*, **62**, 1535S–1540S

Nagao, A. & Olson, J.A. (1994) Enzymatic formation of 9-*cis*, 13-*cis*, and all-*trans* retinals from isomers of β-carotene. *FASEB J.*, **8**, 968–973

Nagao, A., During, A., Hoshino, C., Terao, J. & Olson, J.A. (1996) Stoichiometric conversion of all *trans* β-carotene to retinal by pig intestinal extract. *Arch. Biochem. Biophys.*, **328**, 57–63

Nagasawa, H., Konishi, R., Sensui, N., Yamamoto, K. & Ben-Amotz, A. (1989) Inhibition by beta-carotene-rich algae *Dunaliella* of spontaneous mammary tumourigenesis in mice. *Anticancer Res.*, **9**, 71–76

Nagasawa, H., Mitamura, T. Sakamoto, S. & Yamamoto, K. (1995) Effects of lycopene on sponta-neous mammary tumour development in SHN virgin mice. *Anticancer Res.*, **15**, 1173–1178

Nair, P.P., Lohani, A., Norkus, E.P., Feagins, H. & Bhagavan, H.N. (1996) Uptake and distribution of carotenoids, retinol, and tocopherols in human colonic epithelial cells *in vivo*. *Cancer Epidemiol. Biomarkers Prev.*, **5**, 913–916

Napoli, J.L. & Race, K.R. (1988) Biogenesis of retinoic acid from β-carotene. *J. biol. Chem.*, **263**, 17372–17377

Narisawa, T. Fukaura, Y., Hasebe, M., Ito, M., Aizawa, R., Murakoshi, M., Uemura, S., Khachik, F. & Nishino, H. (1996) Inhibitory effects of natural carotenoids, alpha-carotene, beta-carotene, lycopene and lutein, on colonic aberrant crypt foci formation in rats. *Cancer Lett.*, **107**, 137–142

Nathanail, L. & Powers, H.J. (1992) Vitamin A status of young Gambian children: Biochemical evaluation and conjunctival impression cytology. *Ann. trop. Paediatr.*, **12**, 67–73

Nau, H., Chahoud, I., Dencker, L., Lammer, E.J., & Scott, W.J. (1994) Teratogenicity of vitamin A and retinoids. In: Blomhoff, R., ed., *Vitamin A in Health and Disease*, New York, Marcel Dekker, pp. 615–663

Negri, E., La Vecchia, C., Franceschi, S., D'Avanzo, B., Talamini, R., Parpinel, M., Ferraroni, M., Filiberti, R., Montella, M., Falcini, F., Conti, E. & Decarli, A. (1996) Intake of selected micronutrients and the risk of breast cancer. *Int. J. Cancer,* **65**, 140–144

Nells, H.J.C.F. & De Leenheer, A.P. (1983) Isocratic nonaqueous reversed-phase liquid chromatography of carotenoids. *Anal. Chem.*, **55**, 270–275

Nenseter, M.S., Volden, V., Berg, T., Drevon, C.A., Ose, L. & Tonstad, S. (1995) No effect of beta-carotene supplementation on the susceptibility of low density lipoprotein to in vitro oxidation among hypercholesterolaemic, postmenopausal women. *Scand. J. clin. Lab. Invest.*, **55**, 477–485

Nierenberg, D.W. & Nann, S.L. (1992) A method for determining concentrations of retinol, tocopherol and five carotenoids in human plasma and tissue samples. *Am. J. clin. Nutr.*, 56, 417–426

Nierenberg, D.W., Stukel, T.A., Baron, J.A., Dain, B.J. & Greenberg, E.R. (1989) Determinants of plasma levels of beta-carotene and retinol. *Am. J. Epidemiol.*, **130**, 511–521

Nierenberg, D.W., Stukel, T.A., Mott, L.A. & Greenberg, E.R. (1994) Steady-state serum concentra-tion of alpha tocopherol not altered by supplemen-tation with oral beta carotene. *J. natl Cancer Inst.*, **86**, 117–120

Nikawa, T., Schulz, W.A., van den Brink, C.E., Hanusch, M., van der Saag, P., Stahl, W. & Sies, H. (1995) Efficacy of all-*trans*-β-carotene, canthaxan-thin, and all-*trans*-, 9-*cis*-, and 4-oxoretinoic acids in inducing differentiation of an F9 embryonal carcino-ma RARβ-lacZ reporter cell line. *Arch. Biochem. Biophys.*, **316**, 665–672

Nishino, H. (1995) Cancer chemoprevention by nat-ural carotenoids and their related compounds. *J. cell. Biochem.*, **22** (Suppl.), 231–235

Nishino, H. (1998) Cancer prevention by natural carotenoids. *J. cell. Biochem.* (in press)

Nomura, A.M.Y., Stemmermann, G.N., Heilbrun, L.K., Salkeld, R.M. & Vuilleumier, J.P. (1985) Serum vitamin levels and the risk of cancer of specific sites in men of Japanese ancestry in Hawaii. *Cancer Res.*, **45**, 2369–2372

Nomura, A.M.Y., Kolonel, L.N., Hankin, J.H. & Yoshizawa, C.N. (1991) Dietary factors in cancer of the lower urinary tract. *Int. J. Cancer*, **48**, 199–205

Nomura, A.M.Y., Stemmermann, G.N. & Chyou, P.-H. (1995) Gastric cancer among the Japanese in Hawaii. *Jpn. J. Cancer Res.*, **86**, 916–923

Nomura, A.M., Ziegler, R.G., Stemmermann, G.N., Chyou, P.H. & Craft, N.E. (1997) Serum micronutri-ents and upper aerodigestive tract cancer. *Cancer Epidemiol. Biomarkers Prev.*, **6**, 407–412

Nonomura, A.M. (1990) Industrial biosynthesis of carotenoids. In: Krinsky, N.I., Mathews-Roth, M.M. & Taylor, R.F., eds, *Carotenoids: Chemistry and Biology*, New York, Plenum Press, pp. 365–374

Norum, K.R. (1993) Acute myeloid leukaemia and retinoids. *Eur. J. clin. Nutr.*, **47**, 77–87

Novotny, J.A., Dueker, S.R., Zech, L.A. & Clifford, A.J. (1995) Compartmental analysis of the dynamics of β-carotene metabolism in an adult volunteer. *J. Lipid Res.*, **36**, 1825–1838

Novotny, J.A., Zech, L.A., Furr, H.C., Dueker, S.R. & Clifford, A.J. (1996) Mathematical modeling in nutri-tion: Constructing a physiologic compartmental model of the dynamics of β-carotene metabolism. *Adv. Food Nutr. Res.*, **40**, 25–54

Nyandieka, H.S., Wakhis, J. & Kilonzo, M.M. (1990) Association of reduction of AFB_1-induced liver tumours by antioxidants with increased activity of microsomal enzymes. *Indian J. Med. Res.*, **92**, 332–336

Ocké, M.C., Schrijver, J., Obermann-de Boer, G.L., Bloemberg, B.P.M., Haenen, G.R.M.M. & Kromhout, D. (1995) Stability of blood (pro)vitamins during four years of storage at –20 °C: Consequences for epidemiologic research. *J. clin. Epidemiol.*, **48**, 1077–1085

Ocké, M.C., Bueno de Mesquita, H.B., Feskens, E.J., van Staveren, W.A. & Kromhout, D. (1997) Repeated measurements of vegetables, fruits, beta-carotene, and vitamins C and E in relation to lung cancer. The Zutphen Study. *Am. J. Epidemiol.*, **145**, 358–365

Odin, A.P. (1997) Vitamins as antimutagens: Advantages and some possible mechanisms of antimutagenic action. *Mutat. Res.*, **386**, 39–67

O'Fallon, J. & Chew, B.P. (1984) The subcellular distribution of β-carotene in bovine corpus luteum. *Proc. Soc. exp. Biol. Med.*, **177**, 406–411

Ohno, Y., Yoshida, O., Oishi, K., Okada, K., Yanabe, H. & Schroeder, F.H. (1988) Dietary β-carotene and cancer of the prostate: A case–control study in Kyoto, Japan. *Cancer Res.*, **48**, 1331–1336

Oishi, K., Okada, K., Yoshida, O., Yanabe, H., Ohno, Y., Hayes, R.B. & Schroeder, F.H. (1988) A case–control study of prostatic cancer with reference to dietary habits. *Prostate*, **12**, 179–190

Okai, Y., Higashi-Okai, K., Yano, Y. & Otani, S. (1996a) All *trans* β-carotene enhances mitogenic responses and ornithine decarboxylase activity of BALB/c 3T3 fibroblast cells induced by tumor promotor and fetal bovine serum but suppresses mutagen dependent *umu C* gene expression in *Salmonella typhimurium* (TA 1535/pSK 1002). *Cancer Lett.*, **99**, 15–21

Okai, Y., Higashi-Okai, K., Nakamura, S.-I., Yano, Y. & Otani, S. (1996b) Suppressive effects of retinoids, carotenoids and antioxidant vitamins on heterocyclic amine-induced *umu C* gene expression in *Salmonella typhimurium* (TA1535/pSK 1002). *Mutat. Res.*, **368**, 133–140

Okuzumi, J., Nishino, H., Murakoshi, M., Iwashima, A., Tanaka, Y., Yamane, T., Fujita, Y. & Takahashi, T. (1990) Inhibitory effects of fucoxanthin, a natural carotenoid, on N-*myc* expression and cell cycle progression in human malignant tumor cells. *Cancer Lett.*, **55**, 75–81

Okuzumi, J., Takahashi, T., Yamana, T., Kiato, Y., Nagake, M., Ohya, K., Nishino, H. & Tanaka, Y. (1993) Inhibitory effects of flucoxanthin, a natural carotenoid on N-ethyl-N'-nitro-N-nitrosoguanidine induced mouse duodenal carcinogenesis. *Cancer Lett.*, **68**, 159–168

Olmedilla, B., Grando, F., Rojas-Hidalgo, E. & Blanco, I. (1990) A rapid separation of ten carotenoids, three retinoids, alpha-tocopherol, and d-alpha-tocopherol acetate by high performance liquid chromatography and its application to serum and vegetable samples. *J. liq. Chromatogr.*, **13**, 1455–1485

Olmedilla, B., Granado, F., Blanco, I. & Rojas-Hidalgo, E. (1994) Seasonal and sex-related variations in six serum carotenoids, retinol, and α-tocopherol. *Am. J. clin. Nutr.*, **60**, 106–110

Olmedilla, B., Granado, F. & Blanco, I. (1995) Hyper-beta-carotenemia unrelated to diet: A case of brain tumor. *Int. J. Vit. Nutr. Res.*, **65**, 21–23

Olsen, G.W., Mandel, J.S., Gibson, R.W., Wattenberg, L.W. & Schuman, L.M. (1991) Nutrients and pancreatic cancer: A population-based case–control study. *Cancer Causes Control*, **2**, 291–297

Olson, J.A. (1961) The conversion of radioactive β-carotene into vitamin A by the rat intestine *in vivo*. *J. biol. Chem.*, **236**, 349–356

Olson, J.A. (1983) Formation and function of vitamin A. In: Porter, J.W. & Spurgeon, D.L., eds, *Biosynthesis of Isoprenoid Compounds*, New York, John Wiley & Sons, pp. 371–412

Olson, J.A. (1984) Serum levels of vitamin A and carotenoids as reflectors of nutritional status. *J. natl Cancer Inst.*, **73**, 1439–1444

Olson, J.A. (1993) Molecular actions of carotenoids. *Ann. N.Y. Acad. Sci.*, **691**, 156–166

Olson, J.A. (1994) Absorption, transport and metabolism of carotenoids in humans. *Pure appl. Chem.*, **66**, 1011–1016

Olson, J.A. (1998) Carotenoids. In: Shils, M.E., Olson, J.A., Shike, M. & Ross, A.C., eds, *Modern Nutrition in Health and Disease,* 9th Ed., Baltimore, Williams & Wilkins (in press)

Olson, J.A. & Hayaishi, O. (1965) The enzymatic cleavage of β-carotene into vitamin A by soluble enzymes of rat liver and intestine. *Proc. natl Acad. Sci. USA*, **54**, 1364–1370

Omaye, S.T., Krinsky, N.I., Kagan, V.E., Mayne, S.T., Liebler, D.C. & Bidlack, W.R. (1997) Symposium overview: Beta-carotene: Friend or foe? *Fundam. appl. Toxicol.*, **40**, 163–174

Omenn, G.S. (1996) Micronutrients (vitamins and minerals) as cancer-preventive agents In: Stewart, B.W., McGregor, D. & Kleihues, P., eds, *Principles of Chemoprevention* (IARC Scientific Publication No. 139), Lyon, IARC, pp. 33–45

Omenn, G.S., Goodman, G.E., Grizzle, J., Thornquist, M.D., Rosenstock, L., Barnhart, S., Anderson, G., Balmes, J., Cherniak, M.G., Cone, J., Cullen, M., Glass A., Keogh, J., Mejskens, F., Jr & Valanis, B. (1991) CARET, the β-Carotene and Retinol Efficacy Trial to prevent lung cancer in asbestos-exposed workers and smokers. *Anti-cancer Drugs*, **2**, 79–86

Omenn, G.S. & CARET Coinvestigators (1993a) CARET, the Beta-Carotene and Retinol Efficacy Trial to prevent lung cancer in asbestos-exposed workers and in smokers. *Sourcebook on Asbestos Diseases: Medical, Legal, and Engineering Aspects*, **7**, 219–241

Omenn, G.S., Goodman, G.E., Thornquist, M.D., Rosenstock, L., Barnhart, S., Gylys-Colwell, I., Metch, B. & Lund, B. (1993b) The β-Carotene and Retinol Efficacy Trial (CARET) to prevent lung cancer in high risk populations: Pilot study with asbestos-exposed workers. *Cancer Epidemiol. Biomarkers Prev.*, **2**, 381–387

Omenn, G.S., Goodman, G.E., Thornquist, M.D., Grizzle, J., Rosenstock, L., Barnhart, S., Balmes, J., Cherniak, M.G., Cone, J., Cullen, M., Glass, A., Keogh, J., Mejskens, F., Jr, Valanis, B. & Williams, J., Jr (1994) The β-Carotene and Retinol Efficacy Trial (CARET) for chemoprevention of lung cancer in high risk populations: Smokers and asbestos-exposed workers. *Cancer Res.*, **54** (Suppl.), 2038S–2043S

Omenn, G.S., Goodman, G.E., Thornquist, M.D., Balmes, J., Cullen, M.R., Glass, A., Keogh, J.P., Meyskens, F.L., Jr, Valanis, B., Williams, J.H., Jr, Barnhart, S., Cherniack, M.G., Brodkin, C.A. & Hammar, S. (1996a) Risk factors for lung cancer and for intervention effects in CARET, the Beta-Carotene and Retinol Efficacy Trial. *J. natl Cancer Inst.*, **88**, 1550–1559

Omenn, G.S., Goodman, G.E., Thornquist, M.D., Balmes, J., Cullen, M.R., Glass, A., Keogh, J.P.,

Meyskens, F.L., Jr, Valanis, B., Williams, J.H., Jr, Barnhart, S. & Hammar, S. (1996b) Effects of a combination of beta carotene and vitamin A on lung cancer and cardiovascular disease. *New Engl. J. Med.*, **334**, 1150–1155

Omenn, G.S., Goodman, G.E., Thornquist, M.D., Barnhart, S., Balmes, J., Cherniak, M.G., Cullen, M., Glass, A., Keogh, J., Liu, D., Mejskens, F., Jr, Perloff, M., Valanis, B. & Williams, J., Jr (1996c) Chemoprevention of lung cancer: The β-Carotene and Retinol Efficacy Trial (CARET) in high risk smokers and asbestos-exposed workers. In: Hakama, M., Beral, V., Buiatti, E., Faivre, J. & Parkin, D.M., eds, *Chemoprevention in Cancer Control* (IARC Scientific Publication No. 136), Lyon, IARC, pp. 67–85

O'Neill, M.E. & Thurnham, D.I. (1998) Intestinal absorption of β-carotene, lycopene and lutein in men and women following a standard meal; response curves in the triglyceride-rich lipoprotein fraction. *Br. J. Nutr.*, **79**, 149–159

Ong, A.S.H. & Tee, E.S. (1992) Natural source of carotenoids from plants and oils. *Meth. Enzymol.*, **213**, 142–167

Ong, T., Whong, W.–Z., Stewart, J.D. & Brockman, H.E. (1989) Comparative antimutagenicity of 5 compounds against 5 mutagenic complex mixtures in *Salmonella typhimurium* strain TA98. *Mutat. Res.*, **222**, 19–25

Orentreich, N., Matias, J.R., Vogelman, J.H., Salkeld, R.M., Bhagavan, H. & Friedman, G.D. (1991) The predictive value of serum β-carotene for subsequent development of lung cancer. *Nutr. Cancer*, **16**, 167–169

Orr, J.W., Jr, Wilson, K., Bodiford, C., Cornwell, A., Soong, S.J., Honea, K.L., Hatch, K. & Shingleton, H.M. (1985) Nutritional status of patients with untreated cervical cancer. *Am. J. Obstet. Gynecol.*, **151**, 632–635

Oshima, S. Sakamoto, H., Ishiguro, Y. & Terao, J. (1997) Accumulation and clearance of capsanthin in blood plasma after the ingestion of paprika juice in men. *J. Nutr.*, **127**, 1475–1479

Palan, P.R., Romney, S.L., Mikhail, M., Basu, J. & Vermund, S.H. (1988) Decreased plasma β-carotene levels in women with uterine cervical dysplasias and cancer. *J. natl Cancer Inst.*, **6**, 454–455

Palan, P.R., Mikhail, M.S., Basu, J. & Romney, S.L. (1991) Plasma levels of antioxidant β-carotene and α-tocopherol in uterine cervix dysplasias and cancer. *Nutr. Cancer*, **15**, 13–20

Palan, P.R., Mikhail, M.S., Basu, J. & Romney, S.L. (1992) β-Carotene levels in exfoliated cervico-vaginal epithelial cells in cervical intraepithelial neoplasia and cervical cancer. *J. Obstet. Gynecol.*, **167**, 1899–1903

Palozza, P. & Krinsky, N.I. (1991) The inhibition of radical-initiated peroxidation of microsomal lipids by both α-tocopherol and β-carotene. *Free Radicals Biol. Med.*, **11**, 407–414

Palozza, P. & Krinksy, N.I. (1992a) Antioxidant effects of carotenoids *in vivo* and *in vitro*: An overview. *Meth. Enzymol.*, **213**, 402–420

Palozza, P. & Krinsky, N.I. (1992b) β-Carotene and α-tocopherol are synergistic antioxidants. *Arch. Biochem. Biophys.*, **297**, 184–187

Palozza, P., Calviello, G. & Bartoli, G.M. (1995) Prooxidant activity of β-carotene under 100% oxygen pressure in rat liver microsomes. *Free Radicals Biol. Med.*, **19**, 887–892

Palozza, P., Calviello, G., Serini, S., Moscato, P., Luberto, C. & Bartoli, G.M. (1997) Antitumor effect of an oral administration of canthaxanthin on BALB/c mice bearing thymoma cells. *Nutr. Cancer*, **28**, 199–205

Pamuk, E.R., Byers, T., Coates, R.J., Vann, J.W., Sowell, A.L., Gunter, E.W. & Glass, D. (1994) Effect of smoking on serum nutrient concentrations in African–American women. *Am. J. clin. Nutr.*, **59**, 891–895

Pan, W.-H., Wang, C.-Y., Huang, S.-M., Yeh, S.-Y., Lin, W.-G., Lin, D.-I. & Liaw, Y.-F. (1993) Vitamin A, vitamin E or beta-carotene status and hepatitis B-related hepatocellular carcinoma. *Ann. Epidemiol.*, **3**, 217–224

Parker, R.S. (1988) Carotenoid and tocopherol composition of human adipose tissue. *Am. J. clin. Nutr.*, **47**, 33–36

Parker, R.S. (1996) Absorption, metabolism, and transport of carotenoids. *FASEB J.*, **10**, 542–551

Parker, R.S. (1997) Bioavailability of carotenoids. *Eur. J. clin. Nutr.*, **51**, S86–S90

Pastorino, U., Pisani, P., Berrino, F., Andreoli, C., Barbieri, A., Costa, A., Mazzoleni, C., Gramegna, G. & Marubini, E. (1987) Vitamin A and female lung cancer: A case–control study on plasma and diet. *Nutr. Cancer*, **10**, 171–179

Paul, A.A. & Southgate, D.A.T. (1976) *McCance and Widdowson's The Composition of Foods*, 4th rev. Ed., London, Her Majesty's Stationery Office

Pedrick, M.S., Turton, J.A. & Hicks, R.M. (1990) The incidence of bladder cancer in carcinogen-treated rats is not substantially reduced by dietary β-carotene (Abstract). *Int. J. Vit. Nutr. Res.*, **60**, 189

de Pee, S. & West, C.E. (1996) Dietary carotenoids and their role in combating vitamin A deficiency: A review of the literature. *Eur. J. clin. Nutr.*, **50** (Suppl. 3), S38–S53

de Pee, S., West, C.E., Muhilal, Karyadi, D. & Hautvast, J.G.A.J. (1995) Lack of improvement in vitamin A status with increased consumption of dark-green leafy vegetables. *Lancet*, **346**, 75–81

Peng, Y.S., Peng, Y.M., McGee, D.L. & Alberts, D.S. (1994) Carotenoids, tocopherols, and retinoids in human buccal mucosal cells: Intra- and interindividual variability and storage stability. *Am. J. clin. Nutr.*, **59**, 636–643

Peng, Y.-M., Peng, Y.-S., Lin, Y., Moon, T., Roe, D.J. & Ritenbaugh, C. (1995) Concentration and plasma–tissue–diet relationships of carotenoids, retinoids and tocopherols in humans. *Nutr. Cancer*, **23**, 233–246

Perrig, W.J., Perrig, P. & Stahelin, H.B. (1997) The relation between antioxidants and memory performance in the old and very old. *J. Am. Geriatr. Soc.*, **45**, 718–724

Peters, R.K., Pike, M.C., Garabrant, D. & Mack, T.M. (1992) Diet and colon cancer in Los Angeles County, California. *Cancer Causes Control*, **3**, 457–473

Peters, J.C., Lawson, K.D., Middleton, S.J. & Triebwasser, K.C. (1997) Assessment of the nutritional effects of Olestra, a nonabsorbed fat replacement: Summary. *J. Nutr.*, **127** (Suppl. 8), 1719S–1728S

Pfander, H. (1987) *Key to Carotenoids*, Basel, Birkhäuser Verlag

Phillips, R.W., Kikendall, J.W., Luk, G.D., Willis, S.M., Murphy, J.R., Maydonovitch, C., Bowen, P.E., Stacewicz-Sapuntzakis, M. & Wong, R.K. (1993) Beta-carotene inhibits rectal mucosal ornithine decarboxylase activity in colon cancer patients. *Cancer Res.*, **53**, 3723–3275

Pierce, R.J., Kune, G.A., Kune, S., Watson, L.F., Field, B., Merenstein, D., Hayes, A. & Irving, L.B. (1989) Dietary and alcohol intake, smoking pattern, occupational risk, and family history in lung cancer patients: Results of a case–control study in males. *Nutr. Cancer*, **12**, 237–248

Pinnock, C.B. & Alderman, C.P. (1992) The potential for teratogenicity of vitamin A and its congeners. *Med. J. Aust.*, **157**, 804–809

Poh-Fitzpatrick, M.B. & Barbera, L.G. (1984) Absence of crystalline retinopathy after long-term therapy with β-carotene. *J. Am. Acad. Dermatol.*, **11**, 111–113

Pollack, J., Campbell, J.M., Potter, S.M. & Erdman, J.W. (1994) Mongolian gerbils (*Meriones unguiculatus*) absorb β-carotene intact from a test meal. *J. Nutr.*, **124**, 869–873

Pool-Zobel, B.L., Bub, A., Muller, H., Wollowski, I. & Rechkemmer, G. (1997) Consumption of vegetables reduces genetic damage in humans: First results of a human intervention trial with carotenoid-rich foods. *Carcinogenesis*, **18**, 1847– 1850

Poor, C.L., Bierer, T.L., Merchen, N.R., Fahey, G.C., Murphy, M. & Erdman, J.W. (1992) Evaluation of the preruminant calf as a model for the study of human carotenoid metabolism. *J. Nutr.*, **122**, 262–268

Poor, C.L., Bierer, T., Merchen, N.R., Fahey, G.C. & Erdman, J.W. (1993) The accumulation of α- and β-carotene in serum and tissues of preruminant calves fed raw and steamed carrot slurries. *J. Nutr.*, **123**, 1296–1304

van Poppel, G., Kok, F.J. & Hermus R.J.J. (1992) Beta-carotene supplementation in smokers reduces the frequency of micronuclei in sputum. *Br. J. Cancer*, **66**, 1164–1168

van Poppel, G., Spanhaak, S. & Ockhuizen, T. (1993) Effect of beta-carotene on immunological indexes in healthy male smokers. *Am. J. clin. Nutr.*, **57**, 402–407

van Poppel, G., Poulsen, H., Loft, S. & Verhagen, H. (1995) No influence of beta carotene on oxidative DNA damage in male smokers. *J. natl Cancer Inst.*, **87**, 310–311

Potischman, N. & Brinton, L.A. (1996) Nutrition and cervical neoplasia. *Cancer Causes Control*, **7**, 113–126

Potischman, N., McCulloch, C.E., Byers, T., Nemoto, T., Stubbe, N., Milch, R., Parker, R., Rasmussen, K.M., Root, M., Graham, S. & Campbell, T.C. (1990) Breast cancer and dietary and plasma concentrations of carotenoids and vitamin A. *Am. J. clin. Nutr.*, **52**, 909–915

Potischman, N., Herrero, R., Brinton, L.A., Reeves, W.C., Stacewicz-Sapuntzakis, M., Jones, C.J., Brenes, M.M., Tenorio, F., de Britton, R.C. & Gaitan, E. (1991a) A case–control study of nutrient status and invasive cervical cancer. *Am. J. Epidemiol.*, **134**, 1347–1355

Potischman, N., McCulloch, C.E., Byers, T., Houghton, L., Nemoto, T., Graham, S. & Campbell, T.C. (1991b) Associations between breast cancer, plasma triglycerides, and cholesterol. *Nutr. Cancer*, **15**, 205–215

Potischman, N., Hoover, R.N., Brinton, L.A., Swanson, C.A., Herrero, R., Tenorio, F., de Britton, R.C., Gaitan, E. & Reeves, W.C. (1994) The relations between cervical cancer and serological markers of nutritional status. *Nutr. Cancer*, **21**, 193–201

Potter, J.D. & McMichael, A.J. (1986) Diet and cancer of the colon and rectum: A case–control study. *J. natl Cancer Inst.*, **76**, 557–569

Prabhala, R.H., Maxey, V., Hicks, M.J. & Watson, R.R. (1989) Enhancement of the expression of activation markers on human peripheral blood mononuclear cells by *in vitro* culture with retinoids and carotenoids. *J. Leukocyte Biol.*, **45**, 249–254

Prabhala, R.H., Garewal, H.S., Hicks, M.J., Sampliner, R.E. & Watson, R.R. (1991) The effects of 13-*cis*-retinoic acid and beta-carotene on cellular immunity in humans. *Cancer*, **67**, 1556–1560

Prasad, K.N. & Kumar, R. (1996) Effect of individual and multiple antioxidant vitamins on growth and morphology of human nontumorigenic and tumorigenic parotid acinar cells in culture. *Nutr. Cancer*, **26**, 11–19

Prince, M.R., Frisoli, J.K., Goetschkes, M.M., Stringham, J.M. & LaMuraglia, G.M. (1991) Rapid serum carotene loading with high-dose β-carotene: Clinical implications. *J. cardiovasc. Pharmacol.*, **17**, 343–347

Princen, H.M.G., van Poppel, G., Vogelezang, C., Buytenhek, R. & Kok, F.J. (1992) Supplementation with vitamin E but not β-carotene *in vivo* protects low density lipoprotein from lipid peroxidation *in vitro*. Effect of cigarette smoking. *Arteriosclerosis Thrombosis*, **12**, 554–562

Pung, A., Rundhaug, J.E., Yoshizawa, C.N. & Bertram, J.S. (1988) β-Carotene and canthaxanthin inhibit chemically- and physically-induced neoplastic transformation in 10T1/2 cells. *Carcinogenesis*, **9**, 1533–1539

Pung, A., Franke, A., Zhang, L.X., Ippendorf, H., Martin, H.D., Sies, H. & Bertram, J.S. (1993) A synthetic carotenoid inhibits carcinogen-induced neoplastic transformation and enhances gap junctional communication. *Carcinogenesis*, **14**, 1001– 1005

Raj, A.S. & Katz, M. (1985) Beta-carotene as an inhibitor of benz[*a*]pyrene and mitomycin induced chromosome breaks in bone marrow of mice. *Can. J. genet. Cytol.*, **27**, 598–602

Ramaswamy, G. & Krishnamoorthy, L. (1996) Serum carotene, vitamin A, and vitamin C levels in breast cancer and cancer of the uterine cervix. *Nutr. Cancer*, **25**, 173–177

Ramaswamy, P.G., Krishnamoorthy, L., Rao, V.R. & Bhargava, M.K. (1990) Vitamin and provitamin A levels in epithelial cancers: A preliminary study. *Nutr. Cancer*, **14**, 273–276

Rao, M.N., Ghosh, P. & Lakshman, M.R. (1997) Purification and partial characterization of a cellular carotenoid-binding protein from ferret liver. *J. biol. Chem.*, **272**, 24455–24460

Rapola, J.M., Virtamo, J., Ripatti, S. Huttunen, J.K., Albanes, D., Taylor, P.R. & Heinonen, O.P. (1997) Randomised trial of tocopherol and β-carotene supplements on incidence of major coronary events in men with previous myocardial infarction. *Lancet*, **349**, 1715–1720

Rautalahti, M., Albanes, D., Haukka, J., Roos, E., Gref, C.-G. & Virtamo, J. (1993) Seasonal variation of serum concentrations of β-carotene and α-tocopherol. *Am. J. clin. Nutr.*, **57**, 551–556

Reaven, P.D., Khouw, A., Beltz, W.F., Parthasarathy, S.M. & Witztum, J.L. (1993) Effect of dietary antioxidant combinations in humans. Protection of LDL by vitamin E but not by β-carotene. *Arteriosclerosis Thrombosis*, **13**, 590–600

Redlich, C.A., Grauer, J.N., van Bennekum, A.M., Clever, S.L., Ponn, R.B. & Blaner, W.S. (1996) Characterization of carotenoid, vitamin A, and α-tocopherol levels in human lung tissue and pulmonary macrophages. *Am. J. respir. crit. Care Med.*, **154**, 1436–1443

Renner, H.W. (1985) Anticlastogenic effect of beta-carotene in Chinese hamsters: Time and dose response with different mutagens. *Mutat. Res.*, **144**, 251–256

Renner, H.W. (1990) In vivo effects of single or combined dietary antimutagens on mutagen-induced chromosomal aberrations. *Mutat. Res.*, **244**, 185–188

Rettura, G., Stratford, F., Levenson, S.M. & Seifter, E. (1982) Prophylactic and therapeutic actions of supplemental beta-carotene in mice inoculated with C3HBA adenocarcinoma cells: Lack of therapeutic action of supplemental ascorbic acid. *J. natl Cancer Inst.*, **69**, 73–77

Ribaya-Mercado, J.D., Holmgren, S.C., Fox, J.G. & Russell, R.M. (1989) Dietary β-carotene absorption and metabolism in ferrets and rats. *J. Nutr.*, **119**, 665–668

Ribaya-Mercado, J.D., Lopez-Miranda, J., Ordovas, J.M., Blanco, M.C., Fox, J.G. & Russell, R.M. (1993) Distribution of β-carotene and vitamin A in lipoprotein fractions of ferret serum. *Ann. N.Y. Acad. Sci.*, **691**, 232–237

Riboli, E., Gonzalez, C.A., Lopez-Abente, G., Errezola, M., Izarzugaza, I., Escolar, A., Nebot, M., Hemon, B. & Agudo, A. (1991) Diet and bladder cancer in Spain: A multicenter case–control study. *Int. J. Cancer*, **49**, 214–219

Richards, G.A., Theron, A.J., van Rensburg, C.E.J., van Rensburg, A.J., van der Merwe, C.A., Kuyl, J.M. & Anderson, R. (1990) Investigation of the effects of oral administration of vitamin E and beta-carotene on the chemiluminescence responses and the frequency of sister chromatid exchanges in circulating leukocytes from cigarette smokers. *Am. Rev. respir. Dis.*, **142**, 648–654

Richardson, S., Gerber, M. & Cenee, S. (1991) The role of fat, animal protein and some vitamin consumption in breast cancer: A case control study in southern France. *Int. J. Cancer*, **48**, 1–9

Riemersma, R.A., Wood, D.A., Macintyre, C.C.A., Elton, R.A., Gey, K.F. & Oliver, M.F. (1991) Risk of angina pectoris and plasma concentrations of vitamins A, C, and E and carotene. *Lancet*, **337**, 1–5

Rimm, E.B., Stampfer, M.J., Ascherio, A., Giovannucci, E., Colditz, G.A. & Willett, W.C. (1993) Vitamin E consumption and the risk of coronary heart disease in men. *New Engl. J. Med.*, **328**, 1450–1456

Ringer, T.V., DeLoof, M.J., Winterrowd, G.E., Francom, S.F., Gaylor, S.K., Ryan, J.A., Sanders, M.E. & Hughes, G.S. (1991) Beta-carotene's effects on serum lipoproteins and immunologic indices in humans. *Am. J. clin. Nutr.*, **53**, 688–694

Risch, H.A., Jain, M., Choi, N.W., Fodor, J.G., Pfeiffer, C.J., Howe, G.R., Harrison, L.W., Craib, K.J. & Miller, A.B. (1985) Dietary factors and the incidence of cancer of the stomach. *Am. J. Epidemiol.*, **122**, 947–959

Risch, H.A., Burch, J.D., Miller, A.B., Hill, G.B., Steele, R. & Howe, G.R. (1988) Dietary factors and the incidence of cancer of the urinary bladder. *Am. J. Epidemiol.*, **127**, 1179–1191

Risch, H.A., Jain, M., Marrett, L.D. & Howe, G.R. (1994) Dietary fat intake and risk of epithelial ovarian cancer. *J. natl Cancer Inst.*, **86**, 1409–1415

Ritenbaugh, C., Peng, Y.M., Aickin, M., Graver, E., Branch, M. & Alberts, D.S. (1996) New carotenoid values for foods improve relationship of food frequency questionnaire intake estimates to plasma values. *Cancer Epidemiol. Biomarkers Prev.*, **5**, 907–912

Rock, C.L. & Swendseid, M.E. (1992) Plasma beta-carotene response in humans after meals supplemented with dietary pectin. *Am. J. clin. Nutr.*, **55**, 96–99

Rock, C.L., Swendseid, M.E., Jacob, R.A. & McKee, R.W. (1992) Plasma carotenoid levels in human subjects fed a low carotenoid diet. *J. Nutr.*, **122**, 96–100

Rock, C.L., Demitrack, M.A., Rosenwald, E.N. & Brown, M.B. (1995) Carotenoids and mentrual cycle phase in young women. *Cancer Epidemiol. Biomarkers Prev.*, **4**, 283–288

Rock, C.L., Flatt, S.W., Wright, F.A., Faerber, S., Newman, V., Kealey, S. & Pierce, J.P. (1997) Responsiveness of carotenoids to a high vegetable diet intervention designed to prevent breast cancer recurrence. *Cancer Epidemiol. Biomarkers Prev.*, **6**, 617–623

Roe, D.A. (1987) Photodegradation of carotenoids in human subjects. *Fed. Proc.*, **46**, 1886–1889

Rohan, T.E., McMichael, A.J. & Baghurst, P.A. (1988) A population-based case–control study of diet and breast cancer in Australia. *Am. J. Epidemiol.*, **128**, 478–489

Rohan, T.E., Howe, G.R., Freidenreich, C.M., Jain, M. & Miller, A.B. (1993) Dietary fibre, vitamins A, C, and E, and risk of breast cancer: A cohort study. *Cancer Causes Control*, **4**, 29–37

Rohan, T.E., Howe, G.R., Burch, J.D. & Jain, M. (1995) Dietary factors and risk of prostate cancer: A case-control study in Ontario, Canada. *Cancer Causes Control*, **6**, 145–154

Roidt, L., White, E., Goodman, G.E., Wahl, P.W., Omenn, G.S., Rollins, B. & Karbeck, J.M. (1988) Association of food frequency questionnaire estimates of vitamin A intake with serum vitamin A levels. *Am. J. Epidemiol.*, **128**, 645–654

Romert, L., Jansson, T., Curvall, M. & Jenssen, D. (1994) Screening for agents inhibiting the mutagenicity of extracts and constituents of tobacco products. *Mutat. Res.*, **322**, 97–110

Rose, B., Mehta, P.P. & Loewenstein, W.R. (1993) Gap-junction protein gene suppresses tumorigenicity. *Carcinogenesis*, **14**, 1073–1075

Ross, R.K., Shimizu, H., Paganini Hill, A., Honda, G. & Henderson, B.E. (1987) Case–control studies of prostate cancer in blacks and whites in southern California. *J. natl Cancer Inst.*, **78**, 869–874

Rossing, M.A., Vaughan, T.L. & McKnight, B. (1989) Diet and pharyngeal cancer. *Int. J. Cancer*, **44**, 593–597

Rybski, J.A., Grogan, T.M., Aickin, M. & Genslerf, H.L. (1991) Reduction of murine cutaneous UVB-induced tumor-infiltrating TG lymphocyes by dietary canthaxanthin. *J. invest. Dermatol.*, **97**, 892–897

Sahyoun, N.R., Jacques, P.F. & Russell, R.M. (1996) Carotenoids, vitamins C and E, and mortality in an elderly population. *Am. J. Epidemiol.*, **144**, 501–511

Saintot, M., Astre, C., Scali, J. & Gerber, M. (1995) Within-subjects seasonal variation and determinants of inter-individual variations of plasma β-carotene. *Int. J. Vit. Nutr. Res.*, **65**, 169-174

Salonen, J.T., Nyyssonen, K., Parviainen, M., Kantola, M., Korpela, H. & Salonen, R. (1993) Low plasma beta-carotene, vitamin E and selenium levels associate with accelerated carotid atherogenesis in hypercholesterolemic eastern Finnish men (Abstract). *Circulation*, **87**, 678

Salvadori, D.M.F., Ribeiro, L.R., Oliveira, M.D.M., Pereira, C.A.B. & Becak, W. (1992a) The protective effect of β-carotene on genotoxicity induced by cyclophosphamide. *Mutat. Res.*, **265**, 237–244

Salvadori, D.M., Ribeiro, L.R., Oliveira, M.D., Pereira, C.A. & Becak, W. (1992b) Beta-carotene as a modulator of chromosomal aberrations induced in mouse bone marrow cells. *Environ. mol. Mutag.*, **20**, 206–210

Salvadori, D.M.F., Ribeiro, L.R. & Natarajan, A.T. (1993) The anticlastogenicity of β-carotene evaluated on human hepatoma cells. *Mutat. Res.*, **303**, 151–156

Salvadori, D.M.F., Ribeiro, L.R. & Natarajan, A.T. (1994) Effect of β-carotene on clastogenic effects of mitomycin C, methyl methanesulphonate and bleomycin in Chinese hamster ovary cells. *Mutagenesis*, **9**, 53–57

Sanders, T.A.B., Haines, A.P., Wormald, R., Wright, L.A. & Obeid, O. (1993) Essential fatty acids, plasma cholesterol, and fat-soluble vitamins in subjects with age-related maculopathy and matched control subjects. *Am. J. clin. Nutr.*, **57**, 428–433

Sanderson, M.J., White, K.L.M., Drake, I.M. & Schorah, C.J. (1997) Vitamin E and carotenoids in gastric biopsies: The relation to plasma concentrations in patients with and without *Helicobacter pylori* gastritis. *Am. J. clin. Nutr.*, **65**, 101–106

Sankaranarayanan, R., Mathew, B., Varghese, C., Sudhakaran, P.R., Menon, V., Jayadeep, A., Nair, M.K., Mathews, C., Mahalingam, T.R., Balaram, P. & Nair, P.P. (1997) Chemoprevention of oral leukoplakia with vitamin A and beta-carotene: An assessment. *Eur. J. Cancer*, **33**, 231–236

Santamaria, L. & Bianchi, A. (1989) Cancer chemoprevention by supplemental carotenoids in animals and humans. *Prev. Med.*, **18**, 603–623

Santamaria, L., Bianchi, A., Arnaboldi, A. & Andreoni, L. (1981) Prevention of the benzo(α)-pyrene photocarcinogenic effect by β-carotene and canthaxanthine. *Med. Biol. Environ.*, **9**, 113–120

Santamaria, L., Bianchi, A., Arnaboldi, A. & Bermond, P. (1983a) Dietary carotenoids block photocarcinogenic enhancement by benzo(a)-pyrene and inhibit its carcinogenesis in the dark. *Experientia*, **39**, 1043–1045

Santamaria, L., Bianchi, A., Arnaboldi, A., Andreoni, L. & Bermond, P. (1983b) Benzo[*a*]pyrene carcinogenicity and its prevention by carotenoids. Relevance in social medicine. In: Meyskens, F.L. & Pradad, K.N., eds, *Modulation and Mediation of Cancer by Vitamins*, Basel, Karger, pp. 81–88

Santamaria, L., Bianchi, A., Arnaboldi, A., Ravetto, C., Bianchi, L., Pizzala, R., Andreoni, L., Santagati, G. & Bermond, P. (1988) Chemoprevention of indirect and direct chemical carcinogenesis by carotenoids as oxygen radical quenchers. *Ann. N.Y. Acad. Sci.*, **534**, 584–596

Santos, M.S., Meydani, S.N., Leka, L., Wu, D., Fotouhi, N., Meydani, M., Hennekens, C.H. & Gaziano, J.M. (1996) Natural killer cell activity in elderly men is enhanced by beta-carotene supplementation. *Am. J. clin. Nutr.*, **64**, 772–777

Santos, M.S., Leka, L.S., Ribaya-Mercado, J.D., Russel, R.M., Meydani, M., Hennekens, C.H., Gaziano, J.M. & Meydani, S.N. (1997) Short- and long-term beta-carotene supplementation do not influence T cell-mediated immunity in healthy elderly persons. *Am. J. clin. Nutr.*, **66**, 917–924

Sarkar, A., Mukherjee, B. & Chatterjee, M. (1994) Inhibitory effect of beta-carotene on chronic 2-acetylamino-fluorene-induced hepatocarcinogenesis in rat: Reflection in hepatic drug metabolism. *Carcinogenesis*, **15**, 1055–1060

Sarkar, A., Mukherjee, B. & Chatterjee, M. (1995a) Inhibition of 3′-methyl-4-dimethyl-aminoazobenzene-induced hepatocarcinogenesis in rat by dietary beta-carotene: Changes in hepatic anti-oxidant defense enzyme levels. *Int. J. Cancer*, **61**, 799–805

Sarkar, A., Bishayee, A. & Chatterjee, M. (1995b) Beta-carotene prevents lipid peroxidation and red blood cell membrane protein damage in experimental hepatocarcinogenesis. *Cancer Biochem. Biophys.*, **15**, 111–125

Schardein, J.L. (1993) *Chemically Induced Birth Defects*, 2nd Ed., New York, Marcel Dekker, pp. 549–555

Schiedt, K. & Liaaen-Jensen, S. (1995) Isolation and analysis. In: Britton, G., Liaaen-Jensen, S. & Pfander, H., eds, *Carotenoids,* Vol. 1A, *Isolation and Analysis,* Basel, Birkhäuser Verlag, pp. 81–108

Schierle, J., Härdi, W., Faccin, N., Bühler, I. & Schüepp, W. (1995) Example 8: Geometrical isomers of β,β-carotene: A rapid, routine method for quantitative determination. In: Britton, G., Liaaen-Jensen, S. & Pfander, H., eds, *Carotenoids,* Vol. 1A, *Isolation and Analysis,* Basel, Birkhäuser Verlag, pp. 265–272

Schmitz, H.H., Poor, C.L., Wellman, R.B. & Erdman, J.W. (1991) Concentrations of selected carotenoids and vitamin A in human liver, kidney and lung tissue. *J. Nutr.,* **121,** 1613–1621

Schober, S.E., Comstock, G.W., Helsing, K.J., Salkeld, R.M., Morris, J.S., Rider, A.A. & Brookmeyer, R. (1987) Serologic precursors of cancer. I. Prediagnostic serum nutrients and colon cancer risk. *Am. J. Epidemiol.,* **126,** 1033–1041

Schüep, W., Hess, D. & Schierle, J. (1995) Example 7: Human plasma: Simultaneous determination of carotenoids, retinol and tocopherols. In: Britton, G., Liaaen-Jensen, S. & Pfander, H., eds, *Carotenoids,* Vol. 1A, *Isolation and Analysis,* Basel, Birkhäuser Verlag, pp. 261–264

Schwartz, J & Shklar, G. (1987) Regression of experimental hamster cancer by beta carotene and algae extracts. *J. oral maxillofac. Surg.,* **45,** 510–515

Schwartz, J. & Shklar, G. (1988) Regression of experimental oral carcinomas by local injection of beta-carotene and canthaxanthin. *Nutr. Cancer,* **11,** 35–40

Schwartz, J.L. & Shklar, G. (1997) Retinoid and carotenoid angiogenesis: A possible explanation for the enhanced oral carcinogenesis. *Nutr. Cancer,* **27,** 192–199

Schwartz, J., Suda, D. & Light, G. (1986) Beta carotene is associated with the regression of hamster buccal pouch carcinoma and the induction of tumor necrosis factor in macrophages. *Biochem. Biophys. Res. Commun.,* **136,** 1130–1135

Schwartz, J., Shklar, G., Reid, S. & Trickler, D. (1988) Prevention of experimental oral cancer by extracts of *Spirulina–Dunaliella* algae. *Nutr. Cancer,* **11,** 127–134

Schwartz, J.L., Sloane, D. & Shklar, G. (1989) Prevention and inhibition of oral cancer in the ham-

ster buccal pouch model associated with carotenoid immune enhancement. *Tumor Biol.,* **10,** 297–309

Schwartz, J.L., Flynn, E. & Shklar, G. (1990) The effect of carotenoids on the antitumor immune response *in vivo* and *in vitro* with hamster and mouse immune effectors. *Ann. N.Y. Acad. Sci.,* **587,** 92–109

Schwartz, J.L., Flynn, E., Trickler, D. & Shklar, G. (1991) Directed lysis of experimental cancer by beta-carotene in liposomes. *Nutr. Cancer,* **16,** 107–124

Schweigert, F.J. & Eisele, W. (1990) Parenteral β-carotene administration to cows: Effect on plasma levels, lipoprotein distribution and secretion in the milk. *Z. Ernährungswiss.,* **29,** 184–191

Schweigert, F.J., Rosival, I., Rambeck, W.A. & Gropp, J. (1995) Plasma transport and tissue distribution of [^{14}-C] β-carotene and [^{3}-H] retinol administered orally to pigs. *Int. J. Vit. Nutr. Res.,* **65,** 95–100

Scott K.J., Thurnham D.I., Hart D.J., Bingham S.A. & Day K. (1996) The correlation between the intake of lutein, lycopene and β-carotene from vegetables and fruits and blood plasma concentrations in a group of women ages 50–65 years in the UK. *Br. J. Nutr.,* **75,** 409–418

Seddon, A.M., Ajani, U.A., Sperduto, R.D., Hiller, R., Blair, N., Burton, T.C., Farber, M.D., Gragoudas, E.S., Haller, J., Miller, D.T., Yannuzzi, L.A. & Willett, W. (1994a) Dietary carotenoids, vitamin A, C, and E, and advanced age-related macular degeneration. *J. Am. med. Assoc.,* **272,** 1413–1420

Seddon, J.M., Christen, W.G., Manson, J.E., LaMotte, F.S., Glynn, R.J., Buring, J.E. & Hennekens, C.H. (1994b) The use of vitamin supplements and the risk of cataract among US male physicians. *Am. J. public Health,* **84,** 788–792

Seifter, E., Rettura, G., Padawer, J. & Levenson, S.M. (1982) Moloney murine sarcoma virus tumors in CBA/J mice: Chemopreventive and chemotherapeutic actions of supplemental beta-carotene. *J. natl Cancer Inst.,* **68,** 835–840

Seifter, E., Rettura, G., Padawer, J., Stratford, F., Goodwin, P. & Levenson, S.M. (1983) Regression of C3HBA mouse tumor due to X-ray therapy combined with supplemental beta-carotene or vitamin A. *J. natl Cancer Inst.,* **71,** 409–417

Seifter, E., Rettura, G., Padawer, J., Stratford, F., Weinzweig, J., Demetriou, A.A. & Levenson, S.M. (1984) Morbidity and mortality reduction by supplemental vitamin A or beta-carotene in CBA mice given total-body gamma-radiation. *J. natl Cancer Inst.*, **73**, 1167–1177

Select Committee of GRAS Substances (1979) *Evaluation of the Health Aspects of Carotene (Beta-Carotene) as a Food Ingredient* (FDA/BF-80/37), Bethesda, Maryland, Life Sciences Research Office, Federation of American Societies for Experimental Biology

Sen, C.K. & Packer, L. (1996) Antioxidant and redox regulation of gene transcription. *FASEB J.*, **10**, 709–720

Shapiro, S.S., Mott, D.J. & Machlin, L.J. (1984) Kinetic characteristics of β-carotene uptake and depletion in rat tissues. *J. Nutr.*, **114**, 1924–1933

Shekelle, R.B., Lepper, M., Liu, S., Maliza, C., Raynor, W.J., Jr, Rossof, A.H., Paul, O., Shryock, A.M. & Stamler, J. (1981) Dietary vitamin A and risk of cancer in the Western Electric study. *Lancet*, **ii**, 1185–1190

Shi, H., Furr, H.C. & Olson, J.A. (1991) Retinoids and carotenoids in the bovine pineal gland. *Brain Res. Bull.*, **26**, 235–239

Shibata, A., Paganini Hill, A., Ross, R.K. & Henderson, B.E. (1992a) Intake of vegetables, fruits, beta-carotene, vitamin C and vitamin supplements and cancer incidence among the elderly: A prospective study. *Br. J. Cancer*, **66**, 673–679

Shibata, A., Paganini Hill, A., Ross, R.K., Yu, M.C. & Henderson, B.E. (1992b) Dietary beta-carotene, cigarette smoking, and lung cancer in men. *Cancer Causes Control*, **3**, 207–214

Shibata, A., Mack, T.M., Paganini Hill, A., Ross, R.K. & Henderson, B.E. (1994) A prospective study of pancreatic cancer in the elderly. *Int. J. Cancer*, **58**, 46–49

Shikany, J.M., Witte, J.S., Henning, S.M., Swendseid, M.E., Bird, C.L., Frankl, H.D., Lee, E.R. & Haile, R.W. (1997) Plasma carotenoids and the prevalence of adenomatous polyps of the distal colon and rectum. *Am. J. Epidemiol.*, **145**, 552–557

Shivapurkar, N., Tang, Z., Frost, A. & Alabaster, O. (1995) Inhibition of progression of aberrant crypt foci and colon tumor development by vitamin E and

beta-carotene in rats on a high-risk diet. *Cancer Lett.*, **91**, 125–132

Shklar, G. & Schwartz, J. (1988) Tumor necrosis factor in experimental cancer regression with alphatocopherol, beta-carotene, canthaxanthin and algae extract. *Eur. J. Cancer clin. Oncol.*, **24**, 839–850

Shklar, G., Schwartz, J., Trickler, D. & Reid, S. (1989) Regression of experimental cancer by oral administration of combined alpha-tocopherol and beta-carotene. *Nutr. Cancer*, **12**, 321–325

Shklar, G., Schwartz, J., Trickler, D. & Cheverie, S.R. (1993) The effectiveness of a mixture of beta-carotene, alpha-tocopherol, glutathione, and ascorbic acid for cancer prevention. *Nutr. Cancer*, **20**, 145–151

Shu, X.O., Gao, Y.T., Yuan, J.M., Ziegler, R.G. & Brinton, L.A. (1989) Dietary factors and epithelial ovarian cancer. *Br. J. Cancer*, **59**, 92–96

Shu, X.O., Zheng, W., Potischman, N., Brinton, L.A., Hatch, M.C., Gao, Y.T. & Fraumeni, J.F. (1993) A population-based case–control study of dietary factors and endometrial cancer in Shanghai, People's Republic of China. *Am. J. Epidemiol.*, **137**, 155–165

Sies, H. & Stahl, W. (1995) Vitamins E and C, β-carotene, and other carotenoids as antioxidants. *Am. J. clin. Nutr.*, **62**, 1315S–1321S

Simic, M.G. (1992) Carotenoid free radicals. *Meth. Enzymol.*, **213**, 444–453

Simpson, K.L. (1990) Use of food composition tables for retinol and provitamin A carotenoid content. *Meth. Enzymol.*, **190**, 237–241

Sivakumar, B. & Parvin, S.G. (1997) Characteristics of carotene cleavage enzyme from rat intestine (Abstract). In: *Abstracts for the 16th International Congress on Nutrition, Montreal, 27 July–1 August 1997*, p. 127

Slattery, M.L., Schuman, K.L., West, D.W., French, T.K. & Robison, L.M. (1989) Nutrient intake and ovarian cancer. *Am. J. Epidemiol.*, **130**, 497–502

Slattery, M.L., Abbott, T.M., Overall, J.C., Jr, Robison, L.M., French, T.K., Jolles, C., Gardner, J.W. & West, D.W. (1990) Dietary vitamins A, C, and E and selenium as risk factors for cervical cancer. *Epidemiology*, **1**, 8–15

Slattery, M.L., Potter, J.D., Coates, A., Ma, K.N., Berry, T.D., Duncan, D.M. & Caan, B.J. (1997) Plant foods and colon cancer: An assessment of specific foods and their related nutrients (United States). *Cancer Causes Control*, **8**, 575–590

Smith, A.H. & Waller, K.D. (1991) Serum beta-carotene in persons with cancer and their immediate families. *Am. J. Epidemiol.*, **133**, 661–671

Smucker, R., Block, G., Coyle, L., Harvin, A. & Kessler, L. (1989) A dietary and risk factor questionnaire and analysis system for personal computers. *Am. J. Epidemiol.*, **129**, 455–459

Snodderly, D.M. (1995) Evidence for protection against age-related macular degeneration by carotenoids and antioxidant vitamins. *Am. J. clin. Nutr.*, **62** (Suppl.), 1448S–1461S

Snodderly, D.M., Russett, M.D., Land, R.I. & Krinsky, N.I. (1990) Plasma carotenoids of monkeys (*Macaca fascicularis* and *Saimiri sciureus*) fed a nonpurified diet. *J. Nutr.*, **120**, 1663–1671

Snodderly, D.M., Handelman, G.J. & Adler, A.J. (1991) Distribution of individual macular pigment carotenoids in the central retina of macaque and squirrel monkeys. *Invest. Ophthalmol. vis. Sci.*, **32**, 268–279

Snodderly, D.M., Shen, B., Land, R.I. & Krinsky, N.I. (1997) Dietary manipulation of plasma carotenoid concentrations of squirrel monkeys (*Saimiri sciureus*). *J. Nutr.*, **127**, 122–129

Som, S., Chatterjee, M. & Banerjee, M. (1984) β-Carotene inhibition of 7,12-dimethyl-benz[*a*]-anthracene-induced transformation of murine mammary cells *in vitro*. *Carcinogenesis*, **5**, 937–940

Speek A.J., Speek-Saichua S. & Schreurs W.H.P. (1988) Total carotenoid and β-carotene content of Thai vegetables and the effect of processing. *Food Chem.*, **27**, 245–257

Sperduto, R.D., Ferris, F.L. & Kurinij, N. (1990) Do we have a nutritional treatment for age-related cataract or macular degeneration? *Arch. Ophthalmol.*, **108**, 1403–1405

Sperduto, R.D., Hu, T.-S., Milton, R.C., Zhao, J.-L., Everett, D.F., Cheng, Q.-F., Blot, W.J., Bing, L., Taylor, P.R., Jun-Yao, L., Dawsey, S. & Guo, W.-D. (1993) The Linxian cataract studies: Two nutrition intervention studies. *Arch. Ophthalmol.*, **111**, 1246–1253

Stacewicz-Sapuntzakis, M., Bowen, P.E., Kikendall, W. & Burgess, M. (1986) Levels of various carotenoids and retinol in serum of middle aged men and women. *Fed. Proc.*, **45**, 592

Stacewicz-Sapuntzakis, M., Bowen, P.E., Kikendall, J.W. & Burgess, M. (1987) Simultaneous determination of serum retinol and various carotenoids: Their distribution in middle-aged men and women. *J. Micronutr. Anal.*, **3**, 27–45

Stähelin, H.B., Gey, K.F., Eichholzer, M., Ludin, E., Bernasconi, F., Thurneysen, J. & Brubacher, G. (1991) Plasma antioxidant vitamins and subsequent cancer mortality in the 12-year follow-up of the Prospective Basel Study. *Am. J. Epidemiol.*, **133**, 766–775

Stahl, W. & Sies, H. (1992) Uptake of lycopene and its geometrical isomers is greater from heat-processed than from unprocessed tomato juice in humans. *J. Nutr.*, **122**, 2161–2166

Stahl, W. & Sies, H. (1996) Lycopene: A biologically important carotenoid for humans? *Arch. Biochem. Biophys.*, **336**, 1–9

Stahl, W., Schwarz, W., Sundquist, A.R. & Sies, H. (1992) *cis–trans* Isomers of lycopene and β-carotene in human serum and tissues. *Arch. Biochem. Biophys.*, **294**, 173–177

Stahl, W., Sundquist, A.R., Hanusch, M., Schwarz, W. & Sies, H. (1993) Separation of β-carotene and lycopene geometric isomers in biological samples. *Clin. Chem.*, **39**, 810–814

Stahl, W., Schwarz, W., von Laar, J. & Sies, H. (1995) all-*trans*-β-Carotene preferentially accumulates in human chylomicrons and very low density lipoproteins compared with the 9-*cis* geometrical isomer. *J. Nutr.*, **125**, 2128–2133

Stahl, W., Nicolai, S., Briviba, K., Hanusch, M., Broszeit, G., Peters, M., Martin, H.-D. & Sies, H. (1997) Biological activities of natural and synthetic carotenoids: Induction of gap junctional communication and singlet oxygen quenching. *Carcinogenesis*, **18**, 89–92

Steering Committee of the Physicians' Health Study Research Group (1988) Preliminary report: Findings from the aspirin component of the ongoing Physicians' Health Study. *New Engl. J. Med.*, **318**, 262–264

Steineck, G., Hagman, U., Gerhardsson, M. & Norell, S.E. (1990) Vitamin A supplements, fried foods, fat and urothelial cancer. A case–referent study in Stockholm in 1985–87. *Int. J. Cancer*, **45**, 1006–1011

Steinel, H.H. & Baker, R.S.U. (1990) Effects of beta-carotene on chemically-induced skin tumours in HRA/Skh hairless mice. *Cancer Lett.*, **51**, 163–168

Steinmetz, K.A, Potter, J.D & Folsom, A.R (1993) Vegetables, fruit, and lung cancer in the Iowa Women's Health Study. *Cancer Res.*, **53**, 536–543

Stich, H.F. & Dunn, B.P. (1986) Relationship between cellular levels of beta-carotene and sensitivity to genotoxic agents. *Int. J. Cancer*, **38**, 713–717

Stich, H.F., Stich, W., Rosin, M.P. & Vallejera, M.O. (1984) Use of the micronucleus test to monitor the effect of vitamin A, beta-carotene and canthaxanthin of the buccal mucosa of betel nut/tobacco chewers. *Int. J. Cancer*, **34**, 745–750

Stich, H.F., Hornby, A.P. & Dunn, B.P. (1985) A pilot beta-carotene intervention trial with Inuits using smokeless tobacco. *Int. J. Cancer*, **36**, 321–327

Stich, H.F., Hornby, A.P. & Dunn, B.P. (1986) Beta-carotene levels in exfoliated mucosa cells of population groups at low and elevated risk for oral cancer. *Int. J. Cancer*, **37**, 389–393

Stich, H.F., Rosin, M.P., Hornby, A.P., Mathew, B., Sankaranarayanan, R. & Nair, M.K. (1988) Remission of oral leukoplakia and micronuclei in tobacco/betel quid chewers treated with beta-carotene and with beta-carotene plus vitamin A. *Int. J. Cancer*, **42**, 195–199

Stich, H.F., Rosin, M.P., Hornby, A.P., Mathew, B., Sankaranarayanan, R. & Nair, M.K. (1990a). Pilot intervention studies with carotenoids. In: Krinsky, N.I., Mathews-Roth, M.M. & Taylor, R.F., eds, *Carotenoids: Chemistry and Biology*, New York, Plenum Press, pp. 313–321

Stich, H.F., Tsang, S.S. & Palcic, B. (1990b) The effect of retinoids, carotenoids and phenolics on chromosomal instability of bovine papillomavirus DNA-carrying cells. *Mutat. Res.*, **241**, 387–393

Stivala, L.A., Savio, M., Cazzalini, O., Pizzala, R., Rehak, L., Bianchi, L., Vannini, V. & Prosperi, E. (1996) Effect of β-carotene on cell cycle progression of human fibroblasts. *Carcinogenesis*, **17**, 2395–2401

Street, D.A., Comstock, G.W., Salkeld, R.M., Schuep, W. & Klag, M.J. (1994) Serum antioxidants and myocardial infarction. Are low levels of carotenoids and alpha-tocopherol risk factors for myocardial infarction? *Circulation*, **90**, 1154–1161

Stryker, W.S., Kaplan, L.A., Stein, E.A., Stampfer, M.J., Sober, A. & Willett, W.C. (1988) The relation of diet, cigarette smoking, and alcohol consumption to plasma beta-carotene and alpha-tocopherol levels. *Am. J. Epidemiol.*, **127**, 283–296

Stryker, W.S., Stampfer, M.J., Stein, E.A., Kaplan, L., Louis, T.A., Sober, A. & Willett, W.C. (1990) Diet, plasma levels of beta-carotene and alpha-tocopherol, and risk of malignant melanoma. *Am. J. Epidemiol.*, **131**, 597–611

Sturgeon, S.R., Ziegler, R.G., Brinton, L.A., Nasca, P.C., Mallin, K. & Gridley, G. (1991) Diet and the risk of vulvar cancer. *Ann. Epidemiol.*, **1**, 427–437

Suda, D., Schwartz, J. & Shklar, G. (1986) Inhibition of experimental oral carcinogenesis by topical beta-carotene. *Carcinogenesis*, **7**, 711–715

Suda, D., Schwartz, J. & Shklar, G. (1987) GGT reduction in beta carotene-inhibition of hamster buccal pouch carcinogenesis. *Eur. J. Cancer clin. Oncol.*, **23**, 43–46

Suzuki, T., Nakashima, M., Ohishi, N. & Yagi, K. (1996) Absorption and isomerization of 9-*cis* β-carotene in rats. *J. clin. Biochem. Nutr.*, **21**, 1–15

Svensson, A. & Vahlquist, A. (1995) Metabolic carotenemia and carotenoderma in a child. *Acta derm. venereol.*, **75**, 70–71

Takagi, S., Kishi, F., Nakajima, K., Kimura, Y. & Nakano, M. (1990) A seasonal variation of carotenoid composition in green leaves and effect of environmental factors on it. *Sci. Rep. Fac. Agr. Okayama Univ.*, **75**, 1–7

Tanaka, T., Morishita, Y., Suzui, M., Kojima, T., Okumura, A. & Mori, H. (1994) Chemoprevention of mouse urinary bladder carcinogenesis by the naturally occurring carotenoid astaxanthin. *Carcinogenesis*, **15**, 15–19

Tanaka, T., Makita, H., Ohnishi, M., Mori, H., Satoh, K. & Hara, A. (1995a) Chemoprevention of rat oral carcinogenesis by naturally occurring xanthophylls, astaxanthin and canthaxanthin. *Cancer Res.*, **55**, 4059–4064

Tanaka, T., Kawamori, T., Ohnishi, M., Makita, H., Satoh, K. & Hara, A. (1995b) Suppression of azoxymethane-induced rat colon carcinogenesis by dietary administration of naturally occurring xanthophylls astaxanthin and canthaxanthin during the postinitiation phase. *Carcinogenesis*, **16**, 2957–2963

Tang, X. & Edenharder, R. (1997) Inhibition of the mutagenicity of 2-nitrofluorene, 3-nitrofluoranthene and 1-nitropyrene by vitamins, porphyrins and related compounds, and vegetable and fruit juices and solvent extracts. *Food Chem. Toxicol.*, **35**, 373–378

Tang, G. & Russell, R.M. (1991) Formation of all-*trans* retinoic acid and 13-*cis*-retinoic acid from all-*trans* retinyl palmitate in humans. *J. Nutr. Biochem.*, **2**, 210–213

Tang, G.-W., Wang, X.-D., Russell, R.M. & Krinsky, N.I. (1991) Characterization of β-apo-13-carotene and β-apo-14′-carotenal as enzymatic products of excentric cleavage of β-carotene. *Biochemistry*, **30**, 9829–9834

Tang, G.-W., Blanco, M.C., Fox, J.G. & Russell, R.M. (1995) Supplementing ferrets with canthaxanthin affects the tissue distribution of canthaxanthin, other carotenoids, vitamin A and vitamin E. *J. Nutr.*, **125**, 1945–1951

Tangney, C.C., Brownei, C. & Wu, S.M. (1991) Impact of menstrual periodicity on serum lipid levels and estimates of dietary intake. *J. Am. Coll. Nutr.*, **10**, 107–113

Tavani, A., Negri, E., Franceschi, S. & La Vecchia, C. (1994) Risk factors for esophageal cancer in lifelong nonsmokers. *Cancer Epidemiol. Biomarkers Prev.*, **3**, 387–392

Tavani, A., Pregnolato, A., Negri, E., Franceschi, S., Serraino, D., Carbone, A. & La Vecchia, C. (1997) Diet and risk of lymphoid neoplasms and soft tissue sarcomas. *Nutr. Cancer*, **27**, 256–260

Taylor, A. (1993) Cataract: Relationship between nutrition and oxidation. *J. Am. Coll. Nutr.*, **12**, 138–146

Taylor, A., Jacques, P.F. & Epstein E.M. (1995) Relations among aging, antioxidant status, and cataract. *Am. J. clin. Nutr.*, **62** (Suppl.), 1439S–1447S

Tee, E.S. & Lim, C.L. (1991) Carotenoids composition and content of Malaysian vegetables and fruits by the AOAC and HPLC methods. *Food Chem.*, **41**, 309–339

Teicher, B.A., Schwartz, J.L., Holden, S.A., Ara, G. & Northey, D. (1994) *In vivo* modulation of several anticancer agents by beta-carotene. *Cancer Chemother Pharmacol.*, **34**, 235–241

Teikari, J.M., Laatikainen, L., Virtamo, J., Haukka, J., Rautalahti, M., Liesto, K. & Heinonen, O.P. (1995) Alpha-tocopherol and beta carotene in age-related macular degeneration, a placebo-controlled clinical trial (Abstract). *Invest. Ophthalmol. vis. Sci.*, **36**, S9

Temple, N.J. & Basu, T.K. (1987) Protective effect of beta-carotene against colon tumors in mice. *J. natl Cancer Inst.*, **78**, 1211–1214

Terao, J. (1989) Antioxidant activity of β-carotene-related carotenoids in solution. *Lipids*, **24**, 659–661

Terwel, L. & van der Hoeven, J.C.M. (1985) Antimutagenic activity of some naturally occurring compounds towards cigarette-smoke condensate and benzo[a]pyrene in the *Salmonella*/-microsome assay. *Mutat. Res.*, **152**, 1–4

Thompson, J.N., Duval, S. & Verdier, P. (1985) Investigation of carotenoids in human blood using high-performance liquid chromatography. *J. Micronutr. Anal.*, **1**, 81–91

Thurnham, D.I. (1990) Anti-oxidant vitamins and cancer prevention. *J. Micronutr. Anal.*, **7**, 279–299

Thurnham, D.I. (1994) Carotenoids: Functions and fallacies. *Proc. Nutr. Soc.*, **53**, 77–87

Thurnham, D.I. & Flora, P.S. (1988) Do higher vitamin A requirements in men explain the difference between the sexes in plasma provitamin A carotenoids and retinol (Abstract). *Proc. Nutr. Soc.*, **47**, 181A

Thurnham, D.I., Smith, E. & Flora, P.S. (1988a) Concurrent liquid-chromatographic assay of retinol, α-tocopherol, β-carotene, α-carotene, lycopene and β-cryptoxanthin in plasma with tocopherol acetate as internal standard. *Clin. Chem.*, **34**, 377–381

Thurnham, D.I., Munoz, N., Lu, J., Wahrendorf, J., Zheng, S., Hambidge, K.M. & Crespi, M. (1988b) Nutritional and haematological status of Chinese farmers: The influence of 13.5 months treatment with riboflavin, retinol and zinc. *Eur. J. clin. Nutr.*, **42**, 647–660

Thurnham, D.I., Singkamani, R., Kaewichit, R. & Wongworapat, K. (1990) Influence of malaria infection on peroxyl-radical trapping capacity in plasma from rural and urban Thai adults. *Br. J. Nutr.*, **64**, 257–271

Thurnham, D.I., Northrop-Clewes, C.A., Paracha, P.I. & McLoone, U.J. (1997) The possible significance of parallel changes in plasma lutein and retinol in Pakistani infants during the summer season. *Br. J. Nutr.*, **78**, 775–784

Toma, S., Benso, S., Albanese, E., Palumbo, R., Cantoni, E., Nicolo, G. & Mangiante, P. (1992) Treatment of oral leukoplakia with beta-carotene. *Oncology*, **49**, 77–81

Tomita, Y., Himeno, K., Nomoto, K., Endo, H. & Hirohata, T. (1987) Augmentation of tumor immunity against syngeneic tumors in mice by beta-carotene. *J. natl Cancer Inst.*, **78**, 679–681

Toniolo, P., Riboli, E., Protta, F., Charrel, M. & Cappa, A.P.M. (1989) Calorie-providing nutrients and risk of breast cancer. *J. natl Cancer Inst.*, **81**, 278–286

Tonucci, L.H., Holden, J.M., Beecher, G., Khachik, F., Davis, C.S. & Mulokozi, G. (1995) Carotenoid content of thermally processed tomato-based food products. *J. Agric. Food Chem.*, **43**, 579–586

Torun, M., Yardim, S., Gonenc, A., Sargin, H., Menevse, A. & Simsek, B. (1995) Serum beta-carotene, vitamin E, vitamin C and malondialdehyde levels in several types of cancer. *J. clin. Pharmacol. Ther.*, **20**, 259–263

Truscott, D.G. (1996) β-Carotene and disease: A suggested pro-oxidant and anti-oxidant mechanism and speculations concerning its role in cigarette smoking. *J. Photochem. Photobiol.*, **35**, 233–235

Trush, M.A. & Kensler, T.W. (1991) An overview of the relationship between oxidative stress and chemical carcinogenesis. *Free Radicals Biol. Med.*, **10**, 201–209

Tsuda H., Uehara, N., Iwahori, Y., Asamoto, M., Iigo. M., Nagao, M., Matsumoto, K., Ito, M. & Hirono, I. (1994) Chemopreventive effects of beta-carotene, alpha-tocopherol and five naturally occurring antioxidants on initiation of hepatocarcinogenesis by 2-amino-3-methylimidzo[4,5-*f*]quinoline in the rat. *Jpn. J. Cancer Res.*, **85**, 1214–1219

Tsugane, S., Kabuto, M., Imai, H., Gey, F., Tgei, Y., Hanaoka, T., Sugano, K. & Watanabe, S. (1993) *Helicobacter pylori,* dietary factors, and atrophic gastritis in five Japanese populations with different gastric cancer mortality. *Cancer Causes Control*, **4**, 297–305

Tsushima, M., Maoka, T., Katsuyama, M., Kozuka, M., Matsuno, T., Tokuda, H., Nishino, H. & Iwashima, A. (1995) Inhibitory effect of natural carotenoids on Epstein-Barr virus activation activity of a tumor promoter in Raji cells. A screening study for anti-tumor promoters. *Biol. Pharm. Bull.*, **18**, 227–233

Tuyns, A.J., Riboli, E., Doornbos, G. & Pequignot, G. (1987a) Diet and esophageal cancer in Calvados (France). *Nutr. Cancer,* **9**, 81–92

Tuyns, A.J., Haelterman, M. & Kaaks, R. (1987b) Colorectal cancer and the intake of nutrients: Oligosaccharides are a risk factor, fats are not. A case–control study in Belgium. *Nutr. Cancer*, **10**, 181–196

Tyurin, V.A., Kagan, V.E., Corongiu, F.P., Day, B.W., Banni, S., Tyurina, Y.Y. & Carta, G. (1997) Peroxidase-catalyzed oxidation of beta-carotene in HL-60 cells and in model systems: Involvement of phenoxyl radicals. *Lipids*, **32**, 131–142

UK Subgroup of the ECP-EURONUT-IM Study Group (1992) Plasma vitamin concentrations in patients with intestinal metaplasia and in controls. *Eur. J. Cancer Prev.*, **1**, 177–186

Umegaki, K., Takeuchi, N., Ikegami, S. & Ichikawa, T. (1994a) Effect of beta-carotene on spontaneous and X-ray-induced chromosomal damage in bone marrow cells of mice. *Nutr. Cancer*, **22**, 277–284

Umegaki, K., Ikegami , S., Inoue, K., Ichikawa, T., Kobayashi, S., Soeno, N. & Tomabechi, K. (1994b) Beta-carotene prevents X-ray induction of micronuclei in human lymphocytes. *Am. J. clin. Nutr.*, **59**, 409–412

US Department of Agriculture (1976–94) *Composition of Foods* (Agriculture Handbooks No. 8-1-8-22), Washington DC, US Government Printing Office

Valsecchi, M.G. (1992) Modelling the relative risk of esophageal cancer in a case–control study. *J. clin. Epidemiol.*, **45**, 347–355 van't Veer, P., Kolb, C.M., Verhoef, P., Kok, F.J., Schouten, E.G., Hermus, R.J.J. & Sturmons, F. (1990) Dietary fiber, beta-carotene and breast cancer: Results from a case–control study. *Int. J Cancer*, **45**, 825–828

van't Veer, P., Strain, J.J., Fernandez-Crehuet, J., Martin, B.C., Thamm, M., Kardinaal, A.F.M., Kohlmeier, L., Huttunen, J.K., Martin-Moreno, J.M. & Kok, F.J. (1996) Tissue antioxidants and post-menopausal breast cancer: The European Community Multicentre Study on Antioxidants, Myocardial Infarction, and Cancer of the Breast (EURAMIC). *Cancer Epidemiol. Biomarkers Prev.*, **5**, 441–447

Vena, J.E., Graham, S., Freudenheim, J., Marshall, J., Zielezny, M., Swanson, M. & Sufrin, G. (1992) Diet in the epidemiology of bladder cancer in western New York. *Nutr. Cancer*, **18**, 255–264

Verhoeven, D.T.H., Assen, N., Goldbohm, R.A., Dorant, E., van't Veer, P., Sturmans, F., Hermus, R.J.J. & van den Brandt, P.A. (1997) Vitamins C and E, retinol, beta carotene and dietary fibre in relation to breast cancer risk: A prospective cohort study. *Br. J. Cancer*, **75**, 149–155

Verreault, R., Chu, J., Mandelson, M. & Shy, K. (1989) A case–control study of diet and invasive cervical cancer. *Int. J. Cancer*, **43**, 1050–1054

de Vet, H.C., Knipschild, P.G., Willebrand, D., Schouten, H.J. & Sturmans, F. (1991) The effect of beta-carotene on the regression and progression of cervical dysplasia: A clinical experiment. *J. clin. Epidemiol.*, **44**, 273–283

Villard, L. & Bates, C.J. (1987) Dietary intake of vitamin A precursors by rural Gambian pregnant and lactating women. *Hum. Nutr. appl. Nutr.*, **41A**, 135–145

Virtanen, S.M., van't Veer, Kok, F., Kardinaal, A.F.M. & Aro, A. for the EURAMIC Study Group (1996) Predictors of adipose tissue carotenoid and retinol levels in nine countries. *Am. J. Epidemiol.*, **144**, 968–979

van Vliet, T., van Schaik, F., van Schoonhoven, J. & Schrijver, J. (1991) Determination of several retinoids, carotenoids and E vitamers by high-performance liquid chromatography. Application to plasma and tissues of rats fed a diet rich in either β-carotene or canthaxanthin. *J. Chromatogr.*, **553**, 179–186

van Vliet, T., van Schaik, F. & van den Berg, H. (1992) Beta-carotene metabolism: The enzymatic cleavage to retinal. *Netherlands J. Nutr.*, **53**, 186–190

van Vliet, T., van Schaik, F., van den Berg, H. & Schreurs, W.H.P. (1993) Effect of vitamin A and β-carotene intake on dioxygenase activity in rat intestine. *Ann. N.Y. Acad. Sci.*, **691**, 220–222

van Vliet, T., van Shaik, F. & van den Berg, H. (1996a) *In vitro* measurement of β-carotene cleavage activity: Methodological considerations and the effects of other carotenoids on β-carotene cleavage. *Int. J. Vit. Nutr. Res.*, **66**, 77–85

van Vliet, T., van Vlissingen, M.F., van Schaik, F. & van den Berg, H. (1996b) β-Carotene absorption and cleavage in rats is affected by the vitamin A concentration of the diet. *J. Nutr.*, **126**, 499–508

Wahlqvist, M.L., Wattanapenpaiboon, N., Macrae, F.A., Lambert, J.R., MacLennan, R., Hsu-Hage, B.H.-H. & Australian Polyp Prevention Investigators (1994) Changes in serum carotenoids in subjects with colorectal adenomas after 24 mo of β-carotene supplementation. *Am. J. clin. Nutr.*, **60**, 936–943

Wald, N.J., Boreham, J., Hayward, J.L. & Bulbrook, R.D. (1984) Plasma retinol, β-carotene and vitamin E levels in relation to the future risk of breast cancer. *Br. J. Cancer*, **49**, 321–324

Wald, N.J., Thompson, S.G., Densem, J.W., Boreham, J. & Bailey, A. (1988) Serum beta-carotene and subsequent risk of cancer: Results from the BUPA Study. *Br. J. Cancer*, **57**, 428–433

Wang, X.-D. (1994) Review: Absorption and metabolism of β-carotene. *J. Am. Coll. Nutr.*, **13**, 314–325

Wang, C.-J., Chou, M.-Y. & Lin, J.-K. (1989) Inhibition of growth and development of the transplantable C-6 glioma cells inoculated in rats by retinoids and carotenoids. *Cancer Lett.*, **48**, 135–142

Wang, C.-J., Shiah, H.-S. & Lin, J.-K. (1991a) Modulatory effect of crocetin on aflatoxin B_1 cytotoxicity and DNA adduct formation in C3H10T1/2 fibroblast cell. *Cancer Lett.*, **56**, 1–10

Wang, C.-J., Shiow, S.J. & Lin, J.K. (1991b) Effects of crocetin on the hepatotoxicity and hepatic DNA binding of aflatoxin B_1 in rats. *Carcinogenesis*, **12**, 459–462

Wang, X.-D., Tang, G.-W., Fox, J.G., Krinsky, N.I. & Russell, R.M. (1991) Enzymic conversion of β-carotene in β-apocarotenals and retinoids by human, monkey, ferret, and rat tissues. *Arch. Biochem. Biophys.*, **285**, 8–16

Wang, X.-D., Krinsky, N.I., Marini, R.P., Tang, G.-W., Yu, J., Hurley, R., Fox, J.G. & Russell, R.M. (1992) Intestinal uptake and lymphatic absorption of β-carotene in ferrets: A model for human β-carotene metabolism. *Am. J. Physiol.*, **263**, G480–G486

Wang, G., Dawsey, S.M., Li, J., Taylor, P.R., Li, B., Blot, W.J., Weinstein, W.M., Liu, F., Lewin, K.J., Wang, H., Wiggett, S., Gail, M.H. & Yang, C.S. (1994) Effects of vitamin/mineral supplementation on the prevalence of histological dysplasia and early cancer of the esophagus and stomach: Results from the general population trial in Linxian, China. *Cancer Epidemiol. Biomarkers Prev.*, **3**, 161–166

Wang, X.-D., Krinsky, N.I., Benotti, P.N. & Russell, R.M. (1994) Biosynthesis of 9-*cis*-retinoic acid from 9-*cis*-β-carotene in human intestinal mucosa *in vitro*. *Arch. Biochem. Biophys.*, **313**, 150–155

Wang, X.-D., Marini, R.P., Hebuterne, X., Fox, J.G., Krinsky, N.I. & Russell, R.M. (1995) Vitamin E enhances the lymphatic transport of β-carotene and its conversion to vitamin A in the ferret. *Gastroenterology*, **108**, 719–726

Wang, C.J., Cheng, T.-C., Liu, J.-Y., Chou, F.-P., Kuo, M.-L. & Lin, J.-K. (1996) Inhibition of protein kinase C and proto-oncogene expression by crocetin in NIH/3T3 cells. *Mol. Carcinog.*, **17**, 235–240

Wang, X.-D., Russell, R.M., Liu, C., Stickel, F., Smith, D.E. & Krinsky, N.I. (1996) β-Oxidation in rabbit liver *in vitro* and in the perfused ferret liver contributes to retinoic acid biosynthesis from β-apocarotenoic acids. *J. biol. Chem.*, **271**, 26490–26498

Wang, X.D., Krinsky, N.I., Chun, L., Peacocke, M., & Russell, R.M. (1997) β-Apo-14′-carotenoic acid trans-activates the response element of retinoic acid receptor 2 gene via its conversion into retinoic acid (Abstract). *FASEB J.*, **11**, A181

Waters, M.D., Brady, A.L., Stack, H.F. & Brockman, H.E. (1990) Antimutagenicity profiles for some model compounds. *Mutat. Res.*, **238**, 57–85

Watson, R.R., Prabhala, R.H., Plezia, P.M. & Alberts, D.S. (1991) Effect of beta-carotene on lymphocyte subpopulations in elderly humans: Evidence for a dose–response relationship [published erratum appears in *Am. J. clin. Nutr.* 1991, **53**, 988]. *Am. J. clin. Nutr.*, **53**, 90–94

Weber, U., Goerz, G., Baseler, H. & Michaelis, L. (1992) Canthaxanthin retinopathy. Follow-up for over 6 years (Abstract). *Klin. Monatsbl. Augenheilkd.*, **201**, 174–177

Weedon, B.C.L. & Moss, G.P. (1995) Structure and nomenclature. In: Britton, G., Lioaec-Jensen, S. & Pfander, H., eds, *Carotenoids*, Vol. 1A, *Isolation and Analysis*, Basel, Birkhäuser Verlag, pp. 27–70

Weiser, H., Riss, G. & Biesalski, H.K. (1993) Uptake and metabolism of β-carotene isomers in rats. *Ann. N.Y. Acad. Sci.*, **691**, 223–225

Weitberg, A.B., Weitzman, S.A., Clark, E.P. & Stossel, T.P. (1985) Effects of antioxidants on antioxidant–induced sister chromatid exchange formation. *J. clin. Invest.*, **75**, 1835–1841

West, D.W., Slattery, M.L., Robison, L.M., Schuman, K.L., Ford, M.H., Mahoney, A.W., Lyon, J.L. & Sorensen, A.W. (1989) Dietary intake and colon cancer: Sex- and anatomic site specific associations. *Am. J. Epidemiol.*, **130**, 883–894

West, D.W., Slattery, M.L., Robison, L.M., French, T.K. & Mahoney, A.W. (1991) Adult dietary intake and prostate cancer risk in Utah: A case–control study with special emphasis on aggressive tumors. *Cancer Causes Control*, **2**, 85–94

West, S., Vitale, S., Hallfrisch, J., Munoz, B., Muller, D., Bressler, S. & Bressler, N.M. (1994) Are antioxidants or supplements protective for age-related macular degeneration? *Arch. Ophthalmol.*, **112**, 222–227

White, W.S., Peck, K.M., Ulman, E.A. & Erdman, J.W. (1993a) The ferret as a model for evaluation of the bioavailability of all-*trans* β-carotene and its isomers. *J. Nutr.*, **123**, 1129–1139

White, W.S., Peck, K.M., Bierer, T.L., Gugger, E.T. & Erdman, J.W. (1993b) Interactions of oral β-carotene and canthaxanthin in ferrets. *J. Nutr.*, **123**, 1405–1413

White, W.S., Stacewicz-Sapuntzakis, M., Erdman, J.W., Jr & Bowen, P.E. (1994) Pharmacokinetics of β-carotene and canthaxanthin after ingestion of individual and combined doses by human subjects. *J. Am. Coll. Nutr.*, **13**, 665–671

Whittemore, A.S., Wu Williams, A.H., Lee, M., Zheng, S., Gallagher, R.P., Jiao, D.A., Zhou, L., Wang, X.H., Chen, K., Jung, D., Teh, C.-Z., Ling, C., Yao, X.J., Paffenbarger, R.S. & Henderson, B.E. (1990) Diet, physical activity, and colorectal cancer among Chinese in North America and China. *J. natl Cancer Inst.*, **82**, 915–926

WHO (1966) *WHO Expert Committee on Biological Standardization, 18th Report* (WHO tech. Rep. Ser. 329), Geneva

WHO (1990) *Canthaxanthin* (Food Addit. Ser. 26), Geneva, pp. 45–73

Whong, W.-Z., Stewart, J., Brockman, H.E. & Ong, T.-M. (1988) Comparative antimutagenicity of chloro-phyllin and five other agents against aflatoxin B_1-induced reversion in*Salmonella typhimurium* strain TA98. *Teratog. Carcinog. Mutag.*, **8**, 215–224

Willett, W.C., Polk, B.F., Underwood, B.A., Stampfer, M.J., Pressel, S., Rosner, B., Taylor, J.O., Schneider, K. & Hames, C.G. (1984) Relation of serum vitamins A and E and carotenoids to the risk of cancer. *New Engl. J. Med.*, **310**, 430–434

Willett, W.C., Sampson, L., Stampfer, M.J., Rosner, B., Bain, C., Witschi, J., Hennekens, C.H. & Speizer, F.E. (1985) Reproducibility and validity of a semiquanti-tative food frequency questionnaire. *Am. J. Epidemiol.*, **122**, 51–65

Witt, E.H., Reznick, A.Z., Viguie, C.A., Starke Reed, P. & Packer, L. (1992) Exercise, oxidative damage and effects of antioxidant manipulation. *J. Nutr.*, **122**, 766–773

Wolterbeek, A.P.M., Schoevers, E.J., Bruyntjes, J.P., Rutten, A.A.J.J.L. & Feron, V.J. (1995a) Benzo[a]-pyrene-induced respiratory tract cancer in hamsters fed a diet rich in beta-carotene. A histomorphologi-cal study. *J. Environ. Pathol. Toxicol. Oncol.*, **14**, 35–43

Wotterbeek, A.P.M., Roggeband, R., van Moorsel, C.J.A., Baan, R.A., Koeman, J.H., Feron, V.J. & Rutten, A.A.J.J.L. (1995b) Vitamin A and β-carotene influence the level of benzo[a]pyrene-induced DNA adducts and DNA-repair activities in hamster tracheal epithe-lium in organ culture. *Cancer Lett.*, **91**, 205–214

Woodall, A.A., Jackson, M.J. & Britton, G. (1997) Carotenoids and protection of phospholipids in solu-tion or in liposomes against oxidation by peroxyl radicals: Relationship between carotenoid structure and protective ability. *Biochim. biophys. Acta*, **1336**, 575–586

Woutersen, R.A. & van Garderen-Hoetmer, A. (1988) Inhibition of dietary fat promoted development of (pre)neoplastic lesions in exocrine pancreas of rats and hamsters by supplemental selenium and beta-carotene. *Cancer Lett.*, **42**, 79–85

Wu, A.H., Henderson, B.E., Pike, M.C. & Yu, M.C. (1985) Smoking and other risk factors for lung cancer in women. *J. natl Cancer Inst.*, **74**, 747–751

WuLeung, W.T., Butrum, R.R. & Chang, F.H. (1972) *Food Composition Table for Use in East Asia*, Rome, United Nations Food and Agriculture Organization

Xu, M.J., Plezia, P.M., Alberts, D.S., Emerson, S.S., Peng, Y.M., Sayers, S.M., Liu, Y., Ritenbaugh, C. & Gensler, H.L. (1992) Reduction in plasma or skin alpha-tocopherol concentration with long-term oral administration of beta-carotene in humans and mice. *J. natl Cancer Inst.*, **84**, 1559–1565

Yamamoto, I., Maruyama, H. & Moriguchi, M. (1994). Effect of beta-carotene, sodium ascorbate and cellulose on 1,2-dimethylhydrazine-induced intesti-nal carcinogenesis in rats. *Cancer Lett.*, **86**, 5–9

Yang, C.S., Sun, Y.-H., Yang, Q., Miller, K.W., Li, G., Zheng, S., Ershow, A.G., Blot ,W.J. & Li, J.-Y. (1984) Vitamin A and other deficiencies in Linxian, a high esophageal cancer incidence area in northern China. *J. natl Cancer Inst.*, **73**, 1449–1453

Yong, L., Forman, M.R., Beecher, G.R., Granbard, B.I., Campbell, W.S., Reichmar, M.E., Taylor, P.R., Lanza, E., Holden, J.M. & Judd, J.T. (1994) Relationship between dietary intake and plasma concentrations of carotenoids in pre-menopausal women: Application of the USDA-NCI carotenoid food composition data-base. *Am. J. clin. Nutr.*, **60**, 223–230

Yong, L.C., Brown, C.C., Schatzkin, A., Dresser, C.M., Slesinski, M.J., Cox, C.S. & Taylor, P.R. (1997) Intake of vitamins E, C, and A and risk of lung cancer. The NHANES I epidemiologic followup study. First National Health and Nutrition Examination Survey. *Am. J. Epidemiol.*, **146**, 231–243

You, W.C., Blot, W.J., Chang, Y.S., Ershow, A.G., Yang, Z.T., An, Q., Henderson, B., Xu, G.W., Fraumeni, J.F., Jr & Wang, T.G. (1988) Diet and high risk of stomach cancer in Shandong, China. *Cancer Res.*, **48**, 3518–3523

You, C.-S., Parker, R.S., Goodman, K.J., Swanson, J.E. & Corso, T.N. (1996) Evidence of *cis–trans* isomerization of 9-*cis*-β-carotene during absorption in humans. *Am. J. clin. Nutr.*, **64**, 177–183

Yu, M.W., Zhang, Y.J., Blaner, W.S. & Santella, R.M. (1994) Influence of vitamins A, C, and E and beta-carotene on aflatoxin B_1 binding to DNA in woodchuck hepatocytes. *Cancer*, **73**, 596–604

Yu, M.W., Chiang, Y.C., Lien, J.P. & Chen, C.J. (1997) Plasma antioxidant vitamins, chronic hepatitis B virus infection and urinary aflatoxin B_1–DNA adducts in healthy males. *Carcinogenesis*, **18**, 1189–1194

Yuan, J.M., Wang, Q.S., Ross, R.K., Henderson, B.E. & Yu, M.C. (1995) Diet and breast cancer in Shanghai and Tianjin, China. *Br. J. Cancer*, **71**, 1353–1358

Yun, T.-K., Kim, S.-H. & Lee, Y.-S. (1995) Trial of a new medium-term model using benzo(a)pyrene induced lung tumor in newborn mice. *Anticancer Res.*, **15**, 839–846

Zaridze, D., Lifanova, Y., Maximovitch, D., Day, N.E. & Duffy, S.W. (1991) Diet, alcohol consumption and reproductive factors in a case–control study of breast cancer in Moscow. *Int. J. Cancer*, **48**, 493–501

Zaridze, D., Evstifeeva, T. & Boyle, P. (1993) Chemoprevention of oral leukoplakia and chronic esophagitis in an area of high incidence of oral and esophageal cancer. *Ann. Epidemiol.*, **3**, 225–234

Zbinden, G. & Studer, A. (1958) [Animal experiments on chronic resistance to β-carotene, lycopene, 7,7′-dihydro-β-carotene and bixin.] *Lebensmitt. Untersuch. Forsch.*, **108**, 113–134 (in German)

Zechmeister, L. (1962) *cis–trans Isomeric Carotenoids, Vitamin A and Arylpolyenes*, Vienna, Springer Verlag

Zeng, S., Furr, H.C. & Olson, J.A. (1992) Metabolism of carotenoid analogs in humans. *Am. J. clin. Nutr.*, **56**, 433–439

Zhang, L.-X., Cooney, R.V. & Bertram, J.S. (1991) Carotenoids enhance gap junctional communication and inhibit lipid peroxidation in C3H 10T1/2 cells: Relationship to their cancer chemopreventive action. *Carcinogenesis*, **12**, 2109–2114

Zhang, L.-X., Cooney, R.V. & Bertram, J.S. (1992) Carotenoids up-regulate *connexin43* gene expression independent of their provitamin A or antioxidant properties. *Cancer Res.*, **52**, 5707–5712

Zhang, L., Blot, W.J., You, W.C., Chang, Y.S., Liu, X.Q., Kneller, R.W., Zhao, L., Liu, W.D., Li, J.Y., Jin, M.L., Xu, G.W., Fraumeni, J.F., Jr & Yang, C.S. (1994) Serum micronutrients in relation to precancerous gastric lesions. *Int. J. Cancer*, **56**, 650–654

Zhang, Y.H., Kramer, T.R., Taylor, P.R., Li, J.Y., Blot, W.J., Brown, C.C., Guo, W., Dawsey, S.M. & Li, B. (1995) Possible immunologic involvement of antioxidants in cancer prevention. *Am. J. clin. Nutr.*, **62**, 1477S–1482S

Zhang, S., Tang, G., Russell, R.M., Mayzel, K.A., Stampfer, M.J., Willett, W.C. & Hunter, D.J. (1997) Measurement of retinoids and carotenoids in breast adipose tissue and a comparison of concentrations in breast cancer cases and control subjects. *Am. J. clin. Nutr.*, **66**, 626–632

Zheng, W., Blot, W.J., Shu, X.O., Diamond, E.L., Gao, Y.T., Ji, B.T. & Fraumeni, J.F. (1992a) Risk factors for oral and pharyngeal cancer in Shanghai, with emphasis on diet. *Cancer Epidemiol. Biomarkers Prev.*, **1**, 441–448

Zheng, W., Blot, W.J., Shu, X.O., Gao, Y.T., Ji, B.T., Ziegler, R.G. & Fraumeni, J.F. (1992b) Diet and other risk factors for laryngeal cancer in Shanghai, China. *Am. J. Epidemiol.*, **136**, 178–191

Zheng, W., Blot, W.J., Diamond, E.L., Norkus, E.P., Spate, V., Morris, J.S. & Comstock, G.W. (1993) Serum micronutrients and the subsequent risk of oral and pharyngeal cancer. *Cancer Res.*, **53**, 795–798

Zheng, W., Sellers, T.A., Doyle, T.J., Kushi, L.H., Potter, J.D. & Folsom, A.R. (1995) Retinol, antioxidant vitamins, and cancers of the upper digestive tract in a prospective cohort study of postmenopausal women. *Am. J. Epidemiol.*, **142**, 955–960

Zhu, D., Caveney, S., Kidder, G.M. & Naus, C.C. (1991) Transfection of C6 glioma cells with connexin 43 cDNA: Analysis of expression, intercellular coupling, and cell proliferation. *Proc. natl Acad. Sci. USA*, **88**, 1883–1887

Ziegler, R.G., Morris, L.E., Blot, W.J., Pottern, L.M., Hoover, R. & Fraumeni, J.F. (1981) Esophageal cancer among black men in Washington, DC. II. Role of nutrition. *J. natl Cancer Inst.*, **67**, 1199–1206

Ziegler, R.G., Brinton, L.A., Hamman, R.F., Lehman, H.F., Levine, R.S., Mallin, K., Norman, S.A., Rosenthal, J.F., Trumble, A.C. & Hoover, R.N. (1990) Diet and the risk of invasive cervical cancer among white women in the United States. *Am. J. Epidemiol.*, **132**, 432–445

Ziegler, R.G., Mayne, S.T. & Swanson, C.A. (1996) Nutrition and lung cancer. *Cancer Causes Control*, **7**, 157–177

Appendix 1

The concept of activity profiles of antimutagens

To facilitate an analysis of data from the open literature on antimutagenicity in short-term tests, we have applied the concept of activity profiles already used successfully for mutagenicity data (Waters *et al.*, 1988, 1990) to antimutagenicity data. The activity profiles display an overview of multi-test and multi-chemical information as an aid to the interpretation of the data. They can be organized in two general ways: for mutagens that have been tested in combination with a given antimutagen or for antimutagens that have been tested in combination with a given mutagen (Waters *et al.*, 1990). The profile presented here is an example of mutagens that have been tested in combination with a single antimutagen and they are arranged alphabetically by the names of the mutagens tested. These plots permit rapid visualization of considerable data and experimental parameters, including the inhibition as well as the enhancement of mutagenic activity. A data listing, arranged in the same order as the profile, is also given to summarize the short-term test used, the doses of mutagens and antimutagens, the response induced by the antimutagens, and the relevant publications.

The antimutagenicity profile graphically shows the doses for both the mutagen and antimutagen and the test response (either inhibition or enhancement) induced by the antimutagen. The resultant profiles are actually two parallel sets of bar graphs (Figure 1). The upper graph displays the mutagen dose and the range of antimutagen doses tested. The lower graph shows either the maximum percent inhibition represented by a bar directed upwards from the origin or the maximum percent enhancement of the genotoxic response, represented by a bar directed downwards. A short bar drawn across the origin on the lower graph indicates that no significant (generally < 20%) difference in the response was detected between the mutagen tested alone or the mutagen tested in combination with the antimutagen. Codes used to represent the short-term tests in the data listings have been reported previously (Waters *et al.*, 1988), and the subset of tests represented in this paper are shown in the Appendix.

In assembling the data base on antimutagens and presumptive anticarcinogens, the literature was surveyed for the availability of antimutagenicity data (Waters *et al.*, 1990), and publications were selected that presented original, quantitative data for any of the genotoxicity assays that are in the scope of the genetic activity profiles (Waters *et al.*, 1988).

The same short-term tests used to identify mutagens and potential carcinogens are being used to identify antimutagens and potential anticarcinogens. The tests are generally those for which standardized protocols have been developed and published. Many of these tests have been evaluated by the USEPA Gene-Tox Program (Waters, 1979; Green and Auletta, 1980; Waters and Auletta, 1981; Auletta *et al.*, 1991) or the National Toxicology Program (Tennant *et al.*, 1987; Ashby and Tennant, 1991) for their performance in detecting known carcinogens and noncarcinogens or known mutagens and nonmutagens (Upton *et al.*, 1984; Waters *et al.*, 1994).

It is not clear at the present time whether antimutagenicity observed in short-term tests is a reliable indicator of anticarcinogenicity since the available data are incomplete. Information on both antimutagenicity and anticarcinogenicity in vivo for a number of chemical classes is required before such a conclusion can be drawn. Clearly, antimutagenicity tests performed *in vitro* will not detect those compounds that act in a carcinogenicity bioassay *in vivo,* for example, to alter the activity of one or more enzyme systems not present *in vitro.* Rather, the in-vitro tests will detect only those compounds that inhibit the metabolism of the carcinogen directly, react directly with the mutagenic species to inactivate them or otherwise show an effect that is demonstrable *in vitro*. Thus, it is essential to confirm putative antimutagenic activity observed in vitro through the use of animal models. Indeed, the interpretation of antimutagenicity data from short-term tests must be subjected to all of the considerations that apply in the interpretation of mutagenicity test results. Moreover, the experimental variable of the antimutagens used must be considered in addition to the variables of the mutagens and short-term tests used. Obvious examples of parameters that must be considered in evaluating results from short-term tests *in vitro* are: (1) the endpoint of the test, (2) the presence or absence of an exogenous metabolic system, (3) the inducer that may have been used in conjunction with the preparation of the metabolic system, (4) the concentration of S9 or other metabolic system used and whether that concentration has been optimized for the mutagen under test, (5) the relative time and order of presentation of the mutagen and the antimutagen to the test system, (6) the concentration ratio of the mutagen relative to the antimutagen, (7) the duration of the treatment period, and (8) the outcome of the test, i.e. inhibition or enhancement of mutagenicity. Similar considerations apply to the evaluation of in vivo tests for antimutagenicity.

References

Ashby, J. & Tennant, R.W. (1991) Definitive relationships among chemical structure, carcinogenicity and mutagenicity for 301 chemicals tested by the US NTP. *Mutat. Res.*, **257**, 229–306

Auletta, A.E., Brown, M., Wassom, J.S. & Cimino, M.C. (1991) Current status of the Gene-Tox program. *Environ. Health Perspectives*, **96**, 33–36

Green, S. & Auletta, A. (1980) Editorial introduction to the reports of 'The Gene-Tox Program': An evaluation of bioassays in *Genetic Toxicology*. *Mutat. Res.*, **76**, 165–168

Tennant, R.W., Margolin, B.H., Shelby, M.D., Zeiger, E., Haseman, J.K., Spalding, J., Caspary, W., Resnick, M., Stasiewicz, S., Anderson, B. & Minor, R. (1987) Prediction of chemical carcinogenicity in rodents from in vitro genetic toxicity assays. *Science*, **236**, 933–941

Upton, A.C., Clayson, D.B., Jansen, J.D., Rosenkranz, H.S. & Williams, G.M. (1984) Report of ICPEMC Task Group 5 on the differentiation between genotoxic and non-genotoxic carcinogens. *Mutat. Res.*, **133**, 1–49

Waters, M.D. (1979) Gene-Tox Program. In: Hsie, A.W., O'Neill, J.P. & McElheny, V.K., eds, *Mammalian Cell Mutagenesis: The Maturation of Test Systems* (Banbury Report 2), Cold Spring Harbor, NY, CSH Press, pp 451–466

Waters, M.D. & Auleta, A. (1981) The GENE-TOX program: Genetic activty evaluation. *J. chem. Inf. Computer Sci.*, **21**, 35–38

Waters, M.D., Stack, H.F., Brady, A.L., Lohman, P.H.M., Haroun, L. & Vainio, H. (1988) Use of computerized data listings and activity profiles of genetic and related effects in the review of 195 compounds. *Mutat. Res.*, **205**, 295–312

Waters, M.D., Brady, A.L., Stack, H.E. & Brockman, H.E. (1990) Antimutagenicity profiles for some model compounds. *Mutat. Res.*, **238**, 57–85

Waters, M.D., Stack, H.F., Jackson, M.A., Bridges, B.A. & Adler, I.-D. (1994) The performance of short-test tests in identifying potential germ cell mutagens: A qualitative and quantitative analysis. *Mutat. Res.*, **341**, 109–131

Figure 1. Schematic diagram of an antimutagenicity profile. Profiles are organized to display either the antimutagenic activity of various antimutagens in combination with a single mutagen or the activity of a single antimutagen with various mutagens. The upper bar graph displays the mutagen concentration and the range of antimutagen concentrations tested. The lower graph shows either the maximum percent inhibition, represented by a bar directed upwards from the origin, or the maximum percent enhancement of the genotoxic response, represented by a bar directed downwards. As illustrated in the lower graph, a bar across the origin indicates that no significant (< 20%) effect was detected (designated as 'negative data' in the text). Test codes are defined in Appendix 2.

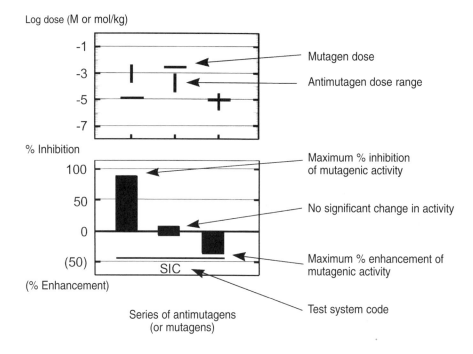

Appendix 2

Definitions of test codes

Test	Definition
AIA	Aneuploidy, animal cells *in vitro*
AIH	Aneuploidy, human cells *in vitro*
BID	Binding (covalent) to DNA *in vitro*
BSD	*Bacillus subtilis rec* strains, differential toxicity
CBA	Chromosomal aberrations, animal bone-marrow cells *in vivo*
CHF	Chromosomal aberrations, human fibroblasts *in vitro*
CHL	Chromosomal aberrations, human lymphocytes *in vitro*
CIC	Chromosomal aberrations, Chinese hamster cells *in vitro*
CVA	Chromosomal aberrations, other animal cells *in vivo*
DIH	DNA strand breaks, cross-links or related damage, human cells *in vitro*
DMX	*Drosophila melanogaster*, sex-linked recessive lethal mutation
ECK	*Escherichia coli* K12, mutation
G9H	Gene mutation *hprt* locus, Chinese hamster V79 cells *in vitro*
GIA	Gene mutation, other animal cells *in vitro*
HMM	Host mediated assay, microbial cells in animal hosts
MVM	Micronucleus formation, mice *in vivo*
SA0	*Salmonella typhimurium* TA100, reverse mutation
SA5	*Salmonella typhimurium* TA1535, reverse mutation
SA7	*Salmonella typhimurium* TA1537, reverse mutation
SA8	*Salmonella typhimurium* TA1538, reverse mutation
SA9	*Salmonella typhimurium* TA98, reverse mutation
SCG	*Saccharomyces cerevisiae*, gene conversion
SHL	Sister chromatid exchange, human lymphocytes *in vitro*
SHT	Sister chromatid exchange, transformed human cells *in vitro*
SIC	Sister chromatid exchange, Chinese hamster cells *in vitro*
SIM	Sister chromatid exchange, mouse cells *in vitro*
SIT	Sister chromatid exchange, transformed cells *in vitro*
SLH	Sister chromatid exchange, human lymphocytes *in vivo*
SPM	Sperm morphology, mouse
TCM	Cell transformation, C3H 10T1/2 mouse cells
URP	Unscheduled DNA synthesis, rat primary hepatocytes *in vitro*

IARC Monographs on the Evaluation of Carcinogenic Risks to Humans
ISSN 0250 9555

Volume 1*
Some Inorganic Substances, Chlorinated Hydrocarbons, Aromatic Amines, N-Nitroso Compounds, and Natural Products
1972; 184 pages; ISBN 92 832 1201 0

Volume 2*
Some Inorganic and Organometallic Compounds
1973; 181 pages; ISBN 92 832 1202 9

Volume 3*
Certain Polycyclic Aromatic Hydrocarbons and Heterocyclic Compounds
1973; 271 pages; ISBN 92 832 1203 7

Volume 4
Some Aromatic Amines, Hydrazine and Related Substances, N-Nitroso Compounds and Miscellaneous Alkylating Agents
1974; 286 pages; ISBN 92 832 1204 5

Volume 5*
Some Organochlorine Pesticides
1974; 241 pages; ISBN 92 832 1205 3

Volume 6*
Sex Hormones
1974; 243 pages; ISBN 92 832 1206 1

Volume 7*
Some Anti-Thyroid and Related Substances, Nitrofurans and Industrial Chemicals
1974; 326 pages; ISBN 92 832 1207 X

Volume 8
Some Aromatic Azo Compounds
1975; 357 pages; ISBN 92 832 1208 8

Volume 9
Some Aziridines, N-, S- and O-Mustards and Selenium
1975; 268 pages; ISBN 92 832 1209 6

Volume 10*
Some Naturally Occurring Substances
1976; 353 pages; ISBN 92 832 1210 X

Volume 11*
Cadmium, Nickel, Some Epoxides, Miscellaneous Industrial Chemicals and General Considerations on Volatile Anaesthetics
1976; 306 pages; ISBN 92 832 1211 8

Volume 12*
Some Carbamates, Thiocarbamates and Carbazides
1976; 282 pages; ISBN 92 832 1212 6

Volume 13
Some Miscellaneous Pharmaceuticals
1977; 255 pages; ISBN 92 832 1213 4

Volume 14*
Asbestos
1977; 106 pages; ISBN 92 832 1214 2

Volume 15*
Some Fumigants, the Herbicides 2,4-D and 2,4,5-T, Chlorinated Dibenzodioxins and Miscellaneous Industrial Chemicals
1977; 354 pages; ISBN 92 832 1215 0

Volume 16
Some Aromatic Amines and Related Nitro Compounds – Hair Dyes, Colouring Agents and Miscellaneous Industrial Chemicals
1978; 400 pages; ISBN 92 832 1216 9

Volume 17
Some N-Nitroso Compounds
1978; 365 pages; ISBN 92 832 1217 7

Volume 18*
Polychlorinated Biphenyls and Polybrominated Biphenyls
1978; 140 pages; ISBN 92 832 1218 5

Volume 19*
Some Monomers, Plastics and Synthetic Elastomers, and Acrolein
1979; 513 pages; ISBN 92 832 1219 3

Volume 20*
Some Halogenated Hydrocarbons
1979; 609 pages; ISBN 92 832 1220 7

Volume 21
Sex Hormones (II)
1979; 583 pages; ISBN 92 832 1521 4

Volume 22
Some Non-Nutritive Sweetening Agents
1980; 208 pages; ISBN 92 832 1522 2

Volume 23*
Some Metals and Metallic Compounds
1980; 438 pages; ISBN 92 832 1523 0

Volume 24
Some Pharmaceutical Drugs
1980; 337 pages; ISBN 92 832 1524 9

Volume 25
Wood, Leather and Some Associated Industries
1981; 412 pages; ISBN 92 832 1525 7

Volume 26
Some Antineoplastic and Immunosuppressive Agents
1981; 411 pages; ISBN 92 832 1526 5

Volume 27
Some Aromatic Amines, Anthraquinones and Nitroso Compounds, and Inorganic Fluorides Used in Drinking Water and Dental Preparations
1982; 341 pages; ISBN 92 832 1527 3

Volume 28
The Rubber Industry
1982; 486 pages; ISBN 92 832 1528 1

Volume 29
Some Industrial Chemicals and Dyestuffs
1982; 416 pages; ISBN 92 832 1529 X

Volume 30
Miscellaneous Pesticides
1983; 424 pages; ISBN 92 832 1530 3

Volume 31*
Some Food Additives, Feed Additives and Naturally Occurring Substances
1983; 314 pages; ISBN 92 832 1531 1

Volume 32*
Polynuclear Aromatic Compounds, Part 1: Chemical, Environmental and Experimental Data
1983; 477 pages; ISBN 92 832 1532 X

Volume 33*
Polynuclear Aromatic Compounds, Part 2: Carbon Blacks, Mineral Oils and Some Nitroarenes
1984; 245 pages; ISBN 92 832 1533 8

Volume 34
Polynuclear Aromatic Compounds, Part 3: Industrial Exposures in Aluminium Production, Coal Gasification, Coke Production, and Iron and Steel Founding
1984; 219 pages; ISBN 92 832 1534 6

Volume 35
Polynuclear Aromatic Compounds: Part 4: Bitumens, Coal-Tars and Derived Products, Shale-Oils and Soots
1985; 271 pages; ISBN 92 832 1535 4

*Out-of-print

Volume 36
**Allyl Compounds, Aldehydes,
Epoxides and Peroxides**
1985; 369 pages; ISBN 92 832 1536 2

Volume 37
**Tobacco Habits Other than Smoking;
Betel-Quid and Areca-Nut Chewing;
and Some Related Nitrosamines**
1985; 291 pages; ISBN 92 832 1537 0

Volume 38
Tobacco Smoking
1986; 421 pages; ISBN 92 832 1538 9

Volume 39
**Some Chemicals Used in Plastics
and Elastomers**
1986; 403 pages; ISBN 92 832 1239 8

Volume 40
**Some Naturally Occurring and Synthetic
Food Components, Furocoumarins
and Ultraviolet Radiation**
1986; 444 pages; ISBN 92 832 1240 1

Volume 41
**Some Halogenated Hydrocarbons
and Pesticide Exposures**
1986; 434 pages; ISBN 92 832 1241 X

Volume 42
Silica and Some Silicates
1987; 289 pages; ISBN 92 832 1242 8

Volume 43
Man-Made Mineral Fibres and Radon
1988; 300 pages; ISBN 92 832 1243 6

Volume 44
Alcohol Drinking
1988; 416 pages; ISBN 92 832 1244 4

Volume 45
**Occupational Exposures in Petroleum
Refining; Crude Oil and Major
Petroleum Fuels**
1989; 322 pages; ISBN 92 832 1245 2

Volume 46
**Diesel and Gasoline Engine Exhausts
and Some Nitroarenes**
1989; 458 pages; ISBN 92 832 1246 0

Volume 47
**Some Organic Solvents, Resin
Monomers and Related Compounds,
Pigments and Occupational Exposures
in Paint Manufacture and Painting**
1989; 535 pages; ISBN 92 832 1247 9

Volume 48
**Some Flame Retardants and Textile
Chemicals, and Exposures in the
Textile Manufacturing Industry**
1990; 345 pages; ISBN: 92 832 1248 7

Volume 49
Chromium, Nickel and Welding
1990; 677 pages; ISBN: 92 832 1249 5

Volume 50
Some Pharmaceutical Drugs
1990; 415 pages; ISBN: 92 832 1259 9

Volume 51
**Coffee, Tea, Mate, Methylxanthines
and Methylglyoxal**
1991; 513 pages; ISBN: 92 832 1251 7

Volume 52
**Chlorinated Drinking-Water;
Chlorination By-products; Some
other Halogenated Compounds;
Cobalt and Cobalt Compounds**
1991; 544 pages; ISBN: 92 832 1252 5

Volume 53
**Occupational Exposures in
Insecticide Application, and Some
Pesticides**
1991; 612 pages; ISBN 92 832 1253 3

Volume 54
**Occupational Exposures to Mists and
Vapours from Strong Inorganic Acids;
and other Industrial Chemicals**
1992; 336 pages; ISBN 92 832 1254 1

Volume 55
Solar and Ultraviolet Radiation
1992; 316 pages; ISBN 92 832 1255 X

Volume 56
**Some Naturally Occurring
Substances: Food Items and
Constituents, Heterocyclic Aromatic
Amines and Mycotoxins**
1993; 600 pages; ISBN 92 832 1256 8

Volume 57
**Occupational Exposures of Hairdressers
and Barbers and Personal Use of
Hair Colourants; Some Hair Dyes,
Cosmetic Colourants, Industrial
Dyestuffs and Aromatic Amines**
1993; 428 pages; ISBN 92 832 1257 6

Volume 58
**Beryllium, Cadmium, Mercury and
Exposures in the Glass
Manufacturing Industry**
1994; 444 pages; ISBN 92 832 1258 4

Volume 59
Hepatitis Viruses
1994; 286 pages; ISBN 92 832 1259 2

Volume 60
Some Industrial Chemicals
1994; 560 pages; ISBN 92 832 1260 6

Volume 61
**Schistosomes, Liver Flukes and
*Helicobacter pylori***
1994; 280 pages; ISBN 92 832 1261 4

Volume 62
Wood Dusts and Formaldehyde
1995; 405 pages; ISBN 92 832 1262 2

Volume 63
**Dry cleaning, Some Chlorinated
Solvents and Other Industrial
Chemicals**
1995; 558 pages; ISBN 92 832 1263 0

Volume 64
Human Papillomaviruses
1995; 409 pages; ISBN 92 832 1264 9

Volume 65
**Printing Processes and Printing Inks,
Carbon Black and Some Nitro
Compounds**
1996; 578 pages; ISBN 92 832 1265 7

Volume 66
Some Pharmaceutical Drugs
1996; 514 pages; ISBN 92 832 1266 5

Volume 67
**Human Immunodeficiency Viruses and
Human T-cell Lymphotropic Viruses**
1996; 424 pages; ISBN 92 832 1267 3

Volume 68
**Silica, Some Silicates, Coal Dust and
para-Aramid Fibrils**
1997; 506 pages; ISBN 92 832 1268 1

Volume 69
**Polychlorinated Dibenzo-para-dioxins
and Polychlorinated Dibenzofurans**
1997; 666 pages; ISBN 92 832 1269 X

Volume 70
**Epstein-Barr Virus and Kaposi's Sarcoma
Herpesvirus/Human Herpesvirus 8**
Publication due May 1998. c. 480 pages;
ISBN 92 832 1270 3

Supplements to Monographs

Supplement No.1*
Chemicals and Industrial Processes
Associated with Cancer in Humans
(Volumes 1 to 20)
1979; 71 pages; ISBN 92 832 1404 8

Supplement No. 2
Long-Term and Short-Term
Screening Assays for Carcinogens: A
Critical Appraisal
1980; 426 pages; ISBN 92 832 1404 8

*Supplement No. 3***
Cross Index of Synonyms and Trade
Names in Volumes 1 to 26
1982; 199 pages; ISBN 92 832 1405 6

*Supplement No.4***
Chemicals, Industrial Processes and
Industries Associated with Cancer in
Humans (Volumes 1 to 29)
1982; 292 pages; ISBN 92 832 1407 2

*Supplement No. 5***
Cross Index of Synonyms and Trade
Names in Volumes 1 to 36
1985; 259 pages; ISBN 92 832 1408 0

Supplement No. 6
Genetic and Related Effects:
An Updating of Selected IARC
Monographs from
Volumes 1 to 42
1987; 729 pages; ISBN 92 832 1409 9

Supplement No. 7
Overall Evaluations of
Carcinogenicity: An Updating
of IARC Monographs
Volumes 1 to 42
1987; 440 pages; ISBN 92 832 1411 0

*Supplement No. 8***
Cross Index of Synonyms
and Trade Names in
Volumes 1 to 46
1989; 346 pages; ISBN 92 832 1417 X

IARC Scientific Publications
ISSN 0300 5085

*No. 1***
Liver Cancer
1971; 176 pages; ISBN 0 19 723000 8

No. 2
Oncogenesis and Herpesviruses
Edited by P.M. Biggs, G. de Thé and
L.N. Payne
1972; 515 pages; ISBN 0 19 723001 6

*No. 3***
N-Nitroso Compounds: Analysis and
Formation
Edited by P. Bogovski, R. Preussman
and E.A. Walker
1972; 140 pages; ISBN 0 19 723002 4

*No. 4***
Transplacental Carcinogenesis
Edited by L. Tomatis and U. Mohr
1973; 181 pages; ISBN 0 19 723003 2

No. 5/6
Pathology of Tumours in Laboratory
Animals. Volume 1: Tumours of the Rat
Edited by V.S. Turusov
1973/1976; 533 pages; ISBN 92 832 1410 2

*No. 7***
Host Environment Interactions in the
Etiology of Cancer in Man
Edited by R. Doll and I. Vodopija
1973; 464 pages; ISBN 0 19 723006 7

*No. 8***
Biological Effects of Asbestos
Edited by P. Bogovski, J.C. Gilson,
V. Timbrell and J.C. Wagner
1973; 346 pages; ISBN 0 19 723007 5

No. 9
N-Nitroso Compounds in the Environment
Edited by P. Bogovski and E.A. Walker
1974; 243 pages; ISBN 0 19 723008 3

*No. 10***
Chemical Carcinogenesis Essays
Edited by R. Montesano and L. Tomatis
1974; 230 pages; ISBN 0 19 723009 1

*No. 11***
Oncogenesis and Herpes-viruses II
Edited by G. de-Thé, M.A. Epstein and
H. zur Hausen
1975; Two volumes, 511 pages and
403 pages; ISBN 0 19 723010 5

No. 12
Screening Tests in Chemical
Carcinogenesis
Edited by R. Montesano, H. Bartsch and
L. Tomatis
1976; 666 pages; ISBN 0 19 723051 2

*No. 13***
Environmental Pollution and
Carcinogenic Risks
Edited by C. Rosenfeld and W. Davis
1975; 441 pages; ISBN 0 19 723012 1

No. 14
Environmental N-Nitroso
Compounds. Analysis and Formation
Edited by E.A. Walker, P. Bogovski and
L. Griciute
1976; 512 pages; ISBN 0 19 723013 X

*No. 15***
Cancer Incidence in Five Continents,
Volume III
Edited by J.A.H. Waterhouse,

C. Muir, P. Correa and J. Powell
1976; 584 pages; ISBN 0 19 723014 8

*No. 16***
Air Pollution and Cancer in Man
Edited by U. Mohr, D. Schmähl and
L. Tomatis
1977; 328 pages; ISBN 0 19 723015 6

*No. 17***
Directory of On-Going Research in
Cancer Epidemiology 1977
Edited by C.S. Muir and G. Wagner
1977; 599 pages; ISBN 92 832 1117 0

*No. 18***
Environmental Carcinogens. Selected
Methods of Analysis. Volume 1: Analysis
of Volatile Nitrosamines in Food
Editor-in-Chief: H. Egan
1978; 212 pages; ISBN 92 932 1118 9

*No. 19***
Environmental Aspects of N-Nitroso
Compounds
Edited by E.A. Walker, M. Castegnaro,
L. Griciute and R.E. Lyle
1978; 561 pages; ISBN 0 19 723018 0

*No. 20***
Nasopharyngeal Carcinoma: Etiology
and Control
Edited by G. de Thé and Y. Ito
1978; 606 pages; ISBN 0 19 723019 9

*No. 21***
Cancer Registration and its
Techniques
Edited by R. MacLennan, C. Muir,
R. Steinitz and A. Winkler
1978; 235 pages; ISBN 0 19 723020 2

*out-of-print

No. 22
Environmental Carcinogens:
Selected Methods of Analysis.
Volume 2: Methods for the
Measurement of Vinyl Chloride in
Poly(vinyl chloride), Air, Water and
Foodstuffs
Editor-in-Chief: H. Egan
1978; 142 pages; ISBN 92 832 1122 7

No. 23*
Pathology of Tumours in Laboratory
Animals.
Volume II: Tumours of the Mouse
Editor-in-Chief: V.S. Turusov
1979; 669 pages; ISBN 0 19 723022 9

No. 24*
Oncogenesis and Herpesviruses III
Edited by G. de-Thé, W. Henle and F. Rapp
1978; Part I: 580 pages, Part II: 512
pages; ISBN 0 19 723023 7

No. 25
Carcinogenic Risk: Strategies for
Intervention
Edited by W. Davis and C. Rosenfeld
1979; 280 pages; ISBN 0 19 723025 3

No. 26*
Directory of On-going Research in
Cancer Epidemiology 1978
Edited by C.S. Muir and G. Wagner
1978; 550 pages; ISBN 0 19 723026 1

No. 27
Molecular and Cellular Aspects of
Carcinogen Screening Tests
Edited by R. Montesano, H. Bartsch and
L. Tomatis
1980; 372 pages; ISBN 0 19 723027 X

No. 28*
Directory of On-going Research in
Cancer Epidemiology 1979
Edited by C.S. Muir and G. Wagner
1979; 672 pages; ISBN 92 832 1128 6

No. 29*
Environmental Carcinogens. Selected
Methods of Analysis. Volume 3: Analysis
of Polycyclic Aromatic Hydrocarbons
in Environmental Samples
Editor-in-Chief: H. Egan
1979; 240 pages; ISBN 0 92 932 1129 4

No. 30*
Biological Effects of Mineral Fibres
Editor-in-Chief: J.C. Wagner
1980; Two volumes, 494 pages &
513 pages; ISBN 0 19 723030 X

No. 31
N-Nitroso Compounds: Analysis,
Formation and Occurrence

Edited by E.A. Walker, L. Griciute,
M. Castegnaro and M. Börzsönyi
1980; 835 pages; ISBN 0 19 723031 8

No. 32
Statistical Methods in Cancer
Research.Volume 1: The Analysis of
Case-control Studies
By N.E. Breslow and N.E. Day
1980; 338 pages; ISBN 92 832 0132 9

No. 33*
Handling Chemical Carcinogens in
the Laboratory
Edited by R. Montesano, H. Bartsch,
E. Boyland, G. Della Porta, L. Fishbein,
R.A. Griesemer, A.B. Swan and L. Tomatis
1979; 32 pages; ISBN 0 19 723033 4

No. 34
Pathology of Tumours in Laboratory
Animals. Volume III: Tumours of the
Hamster
Editor-in-Chief: V.S. Turusov
1982; 461 pages; ISBN 0 19 723034 2

No. 35*
Directory of On-going Research in
Cancer Epidemiology 1980
Edited by C.S. Muir and G. Wagner
1980; 660 pages; ISBN 0 19 723035 0

No. 36
Cancer Mortality by Occupation and
Social Class 1851–1971
Edited by W.P.D. Logan
1982; 253 pages; ISBN 0 19 723036 9

No. 37
Laboratory Decontamination and
Destruction of Aflatoxins B$_1$, B$_2$, G$_1$,
G$_2$ in Laboratory Wastes
Edited by M. Castegnaro, D.C. Hunt,
E.B. Sansone, P.L. Schuller,
M.G. Siriwardana, G.M. Telling,
H.P. van Egmond and E.A. Walker
1980; 56 pages; ISBN 92 832 1137 5

No. 38*
Directory of On-going Research in
Cancer Epidemiology 1981
Edited by C.S. Muir and G. Wagner
1981; 696 pages; ISBN 0 19 723038 5

No. 39
Host Factors in Human Carcinogenesis
Edited by H. Bartsch and B. Armstrong
1982; 583 pages;
ISBN 0 19 723039 3

No. 40
Environmental Carcinogens: Selected
Methods of Analysis. Volume 4: Some
Aromatic Amines and Azo Dyes in the
General and Industrial Environment

Edited by L. Fishbein, M. Castegnaro,
I.K. O'Neill and H. Bartsch
1981; 347 pages; ISBN 0 92 932 1140 5

No. 41*
N-Nitroso Compounds: Occurrence
and Biological Effects
Edited by H. Bartsch, I.K. O'Neill,
M. Castegnaro and M. Okada
1982; 755 pages; ISBN 0 19 723041 5

No. 42*
Cancer Incidence in Five Continents
Volume IV
Edited by J. Waterhouse, C. Muir,
K. Shanmugaratnam and J. Powell
1982; 811 pages; ISBN 0 19 723042 3

No. 43
Laboratory Decontamination and
Destruction of Carcinogens in
Laboratory Wastes: Some
N-Nitrosamines
Edited by M. Castegnaro,
G. Eisenbrand, G. Ellen, L. Keefer,
D. Klein, E.B. Sansone, D. Spincer,
G. Telling and K. Webb
1982; 73 pages; ISBN 92 832 1143 X

No. 44
Environmental Carcinogens: Selected
Methods of Analysis.
Volume 5: Some Mycotoxins
Edited by L. Stoloff, M. Castegnaro,
P. Scott, I.K. O'Neill and H. Bartsch
1983; 455 pages; ISBN 92 932 1144 8

No. 45*
Environmental Carcinogens: Selected
Methods of Analysis.
Volume 6: N-Nitroso Compounds
Edited by R. Preussmann,
I.K. O'Neill, G. Eisenbrand,
B. Spiegelhalder and H. Bartsch
1983; 508 pages; ISBN 92 832 1145 6

No. 46*
Directory of On-going Research in
Cancer Epidemiology 1982
Edited by C.S. Muir and G. Wagner
1982; 722 pages; ISBN 0 19 723046 6

No. 47*
Cancer Incidence in Singapore 1968–1977
Edited by K. Shanmugaratnam,
H.P. Lee and N.E. Day
1983; 171 pages; ISBN 0 19 723047 4

No. 48*
Cancer Incidence in the USSR (2nd
Revised Edition)
Edited by N.P. Napalkov, G.F. Tserkovny,
V.M. Merabishvili, D.M. Parkin,
M. Smans and C.S. Muir
1983; 75 pages; ISBN 0 19 723048 2

*Out-of-print

No. 49
Laboratory Decontamination and Destruction of Carcinogens in Laboratory Wastes: Some Polycyclic Aromatic Hydrocarbons
Edited by M. Castegnaro, G. Grimmer, O. Hutzinger, W. Karcher, H. Kunte, M. Lafontaine, H.C. Van der Plas, E.B. Sansone and S.P. Tucker
1983; 87 pages; ISBN 92 832 1149 9

No. 50*
Directory of On-going Research in Cancer Epidemiology 1983
Edited by C.S. Muir and G. Wagner
1983; 731 pages; ISBN 0 19 723050 4

No. 51
Modulators of Experimental Carcinogenesis
Edited by V. Turusov and R. Montesano
1983; 307 pages; ISBN 0 19 723060 1

No. 52
Second Cancers in Relation to Radiation Treatment for Cervical Cancer: Results of a Cancer Registry Collaboration
Edited by N.E. Day and J.C. Boice, Jr
1984; 207 pages; ISBN 0 19 723052 0

No. 53
Nickel in the Human Environment
Editor-in-Chief: F.W. Sunderman, Jr
1984; 529 pages; ISBN 0 19 723059 8

No. 54
Laboratory Decontamination and Destruction of Carcinogens in Laboratory Wastes: Some Hydrazines
Edited by M. Castegnaro, G. Ellen, M. Lafontaine, H.C. van der Plas, E.B. Sansone and S.P. Tucker
1983; 87 pages; ISBN 92 832 11545

No. 55
Laboratory Decontamination and Destruction of Carcinogens in Laboratory Wastes: Some N-Nitrosamides
Edited by M. Castegnaro, M. Bernard, L.W. van Broekhoven, D. Fine, R. Massey, E.B. Sansone, P.L.R. Smith, B. Spiegelhalder, A. Stacchini, G. Telling and J.J. Vallon
1984; 66 pages; ISBN 92 832 1155 3

No. 56
Models, Mechanisms and Etiology of Tumour Promotion
Edited by M. Börzsönyi, N.E. Day, K. Lapis and H. Yamasaki
1984; 532 pages; ISBN 92 832 1156 1

No. 57*
N-Nitroso Compounds: Occurrence, Biological Effects and Relevance to Human Cancer
Edited by I.K. O'Neill, R.C. von Borstel, C.T. Miller, J. Long and H. Bartsch
1984; 1013 pages; ISBN 92 832 1157 X

No 58
Age-related Factors in Carcinogenesis
Edited by A. Likhachev, V. Anisimov and R. Montesano
1985; 288 pages; ISBN 92 832 1158 8

No. 59
Monitoring Human Exposure to Carcinogenic and Mutagenic Agents
Edited by A. Berlin, M. Draper, K. Hemminki and H. Vainio
1984; 457 pages; ISBN 0 19 723056 3

No. 60
Burkitt's Lymphoma: A Human Cancer Model
Edited by G. Lenoir, G. O'Conor and C.L.M. Olweny
1985; 484 pages; ISBN 0 19 723057 1

No. 61
Laboratory Decontamination and Destruction of Carcinogens in Laboratory Wastes: Some Haloethers
Edited by M. Castegnaro, M. Alvarez, M. Iovu, E.B. Sansone, G.M. Telling and D.T. Williams
1985; 55 pages; ISBN 92 832 11618

No. 62*
Directory of On-going Research in Cancer Epidemiology 1984
Edited by C.S. Muir and G. Wagner
1984; 717 pages; ISBN 0 19 723062 8

No. 63
Virus-associated Cancers in Africa
Edited by A.O. Williams, G.T. O'Conor, G.B. de Thé and C.A. Johnson
1984; 773 pages; ISBN 0 19 723063 6

No. 64
Laboratory Decontamination and Destruction of Carcinogens in Laboratory Wastes: Some Aromatic Amines and 4-Nitrobiphenyl
Edited by M. Castegnaro, J. Barek, J. Dennis, G. Ellen, M. Klibanov, M. Lafontaine, R. Mitchum, P. van Roosmalen, E.B. Sansone, L.A. Sternson and M. Vahl
1985; 84 pages; ISBN: 92 832 1164 2

No. 65
Interpretation of Negative Epidemiological Evidence for Carcinogenicity
Edited by N.J. Wald and R. Doll
1985; 232 pages; ISBN 92 832 1165 0

No. 66
The Role of the Registry in Cancer Control
Edited by D.M. Parkin, G. Wagner and C.S. Muir
1985; 152 pages; ISBN 92 832 0166 3

No. 67
Transformation Assay of Established Cell Lines: Mechanisms and Application
Edited by T. Kakunaga and H. Yamasaki
1985; 225 pages; ISBN 92 832 1167 7

No. 68*
Environmental Carcinogens: Selected Methods of Analysis. Volume 7: Some Volatile Halogenated Hydrocarbons
Edited by L. Fishbein and I.K. O'Neill
1985; 479 pages; ISBN 92 832 1168 5

No. 69*
Directory of On-going Research in Cancer Epidemiology 1985
Edited by C.S. Muir and G. Wagner
1985; 745 pages; ISBN 92 823 1169 3

No. 70
The Role of Cyclic Nucleic Acid Adducts in Carcinogenesis and Mutagenesis
Edited by B. Singer and H. Bartsch
1986; 467 pages; ISBN 92 832 1170 7

No. 71
Environmental Carcinogens: Selected Methods of Analysis. Volume 8: Some Metals: As, Be, Cd, Cr, Ni, Pb, Se, Zn
Edited by I.K. O'Neill, P. Schuller and L. Fishbein
1986; 485 pages; ISBN 92 832 1171 5

No. 72
Atlas of Cancer in Scotland, 1975–1980: Incidence and Epidemiological Perspective
Edited by I. Kemp, P. Boyle, M. Smans and C.S. Muir
1985; 285 pages; ISBN 92 832 1172 3

No. 73
Laboratory Decontamination and Destruction of Carcinogens in Laboratory Wastes: Some Antineoplastic Agents
Edited by M. Castegnaro, J. Adams, M.A. Armour, J. Barek, J. Benvenuto, C. Confalonieri, U. Goff, G. Telling
1985; 163 pages; ISBN 92 832 1173 1

No. 74
Tobacco: A Major International Health Hazard
Edited by D. Zaridze and R. Peto
1986; 324 pages; ISBN 92 832 1174 X

*Out-of-print

No. 75
Cancer Occurrence in Developing Countries
Edited by D.M. Parkin
1986; 339 pages; ISBN 92 832 1175 8

No. 76
Screening for Cancer of the Uterine Cervix
Edited by M. Hakama, A.B. Miller and N.E. Day
1986; 315 pages; ISBN 92 832 1176 6

No. 77
Hexachlorobenzene: Proceedings of an International Symposium
Edited by C.R. Morris and J.R.P. Cabral
1986; 668 pages; ISBN 92 832 1177 4

No. 78
Carcinogenicity of Alkylating Cytostatic Drugs
Edited by D. Schmähl and J.M. Kaldor
1986; 337 pages; ISBN 92 832 1178 2

No. 79
Statistical Methods in Cancer Research. Volume III: The Design and Analysis of Long-term Animal Experiments
By J.J. Gart, D. Krewski, P.N. Lee, R.E. Tarone and J. Wahrendorf
1986; 213 pages; ISBN 92 832 1179 0

No. 80*
Directory of On-going Research in Cancer Epidemiology 1986
Edited by C.S. Muir and G. Wagner
1986; 805 pages; ISBN 92 832 1180 4

No. 81
Environmental Carcinogens: Methods of Analysis and Exposure Measure-ment. Volume 9: Passive Smoking
Edited by I.K. O'Neill, K.D. Brunnemann, B. Dodet and D. Hoffmann
1987; 383 pages; ISBN 92 832 1181 2

No. 82
Statistical Methods in Cancer Research. Volume II: The Design and Analysis of Cohort Studies
By N.E. Breslow and N.E. Day
1987; 404 pages; ISBN 92 832 0182 5

No. 83
Long-term and Short-term Assays for Carcinogens: A Critical Appraisal
Edited by R. Montesano, H. Bartsch, H. Vainio, J. Wilbourn and H. Yamasaki
1986; 575 pages; ISBN 92 832 1183 9

No. 84
The Relevance of N-Nitroso Compounds to Human Cancer: Exposure and Mechanisms
Edited by H. Bartsch, I.K. O'Neill and R. Schulte-Hermann
1987; 671 pages; ISBN 92 832 1184 7

No. 85
Environmental Carcinogens: Methods of Analysis and Exposure Measurement. Volume 10: Benzene and Alkylated Benzenes
Edited by L. Fishbein and I.K. O'Neill
1988; 327 pages; ISBN 92 832 1185 5

No. 86*
Directory of On-going Research in Cancer Epidemiology 1987
Edited by D.M. Parkin and J. Wahrendorf
1987; 685 pages; ISBN: 92 832 1186 3

No. 87*
International Incidence of Childhood Cancer
Edited by D.M. Parkin, C.A. Stiller, C.A. Bieber, G.J. Draper. B. Terracini and J.L. Young
1988; 401 page; ISBN 92 832 1187 1

No. 88*
Cancer Incidence in Five Continents, Volume V
Edited by C. Muir, J. Waterhouse, T. Mack, J. Powell and S. Whelan
1987; 1004 pages; ISBN 92 832 1188 X

No. 89*
Methods for Detecting DNA Damaging Agents in Humans: Applications in Cancer Epidemiology and Prevention
Edited by H. Bartsch, K. Hemminki and I.K. O'Neill
1988; 518 pages; ISBN 92 832 1189 8

No. 90
Non-occupational Exposure to Mineral Fibres
Edited by J. Bignon, J. Peto and R. Saracci
1989; 500 pages; ISBN 92 832 1190 1

No. 91
Trends in Cancer Incidence in Singapore 1968–1982
Edited by H.P. Lee, N.E. Day and K. Shanmugaratnam
1988; 160 pages; ISBN 92 832 1191 X

No. 92
Cell Differentiation, Genes and Cancer
Edited by T. Kakunaga, T. Sugimura, L. Tomatis and H. Yamasaki
1988; 204 pages; ISBN 92 832 1192 8

No. 93*
Directory of On-going Research in Cancer Epidemiology 1988
Edited by M. Coleman and J. Wahrendorf
1988; 662 pages; ISBN 92 832 1193 6

No. 94
Human Papillomavirus and Cervical Cancer
Edited by N. Muñoz, F.X. Bosch and O.M. Jensen
1989; 154 pages; ISBN 92 832 1194 4

No. 95
Cancer Registration: Principles and Methods
Edited by O.M. Jensen, D.M. Parkin, R. MacLennan, C.S. Muir and R. Skeet
1991; 296 pages; ISBN 92 832 1195 2

Registros de cancer: Principios y Métodos
Edited by O.M. Jensen, D.M. Parkin, R. MacLennan, C.S. Muir and R. Skeet
1995; 286 pages; ISBN 92 832 0403 4

Enregistrement des Cancers: Principes et Methodes
Edited by O.M. Jensen, D.M. Parkin, R. MacLennan, C.S. Muir and R. Skeet
1996; 211 pages; ISBN 92 832 0404 2

No. 96
Perinatal and Multigeneration Carcinogenesis
Edited by N.P. Napalkov, J.M. Rice, L. Tomatis and H. Yamasaki
1989; 436 pages; ISBN 92 832 1196 0

No. 97
Occupational Exposure to Silica and Cancer Risk
Edited by L. Simonato, A.C. Fletcher, R. Saracci and T. Thomas
1990; 124 pages; ISBN 92 832 1197 9

No. 98
Cancer Incidence in Jewish Migrants to Israel, 1961-1981
Edited by R. Steinitz, D.M. Parkin, J.L. Young, C.A. Bieber and L. Katz
1989; 320 pages; ISBN 92 832 1198 7

No. 99
Pathology of Tumours in Laboratory Animals, Second Edition, Volume 1, Tumours of the Rat
Edited by V.S. Turusov and U. Mohr
1990; 740 pages; ISBN 92 832 1199 5

*Out-of-print

No. 100
Cancer: Causes, Occurrence and Control
Editor-in-Chief: L. Tomatis
1990; 352 pages; ISBN 92 832 0110 8

No. 101*
Directory of On-going Research in Cancer Epidemiology 1989/90
Edited by M. Coleman and J. Wahrendorf
1989; 828 pages; ISBN 92 832 2101 X

No. 102
Patterns of Cancer in Five Continents
Edited by S.L. Whelan, D.M. Parkin and E. Masuyer
1990; 160 pages; ISBN 92 832 2102 8

No. 103*
Evaluating Effectiveness of Primary Prevention of Cancer
Edited by M. Hakama, V. Beral, J.W. Cullen and D.M. Parkin
1990; 206 pages; ISBN 92 832 2103 6

No. 104
Complex Mixtures and Cancer Risk
Edited by H. Vainio, M. Sorsa and A.J. McMichael
1990; 441 pages; ISBN 92 832 2104 4

No. 105
Relevance to Human Cancer of N-Nitroso Compounds, Tobacco Smoke and Mycotoxins
Edited by I.K. O'Neill, J. Chen and H. Bartsch
1991; 614 pages; ISBN 92 832 2105 2

No. 106
Atlas of Cancer Incidence in the Former German Democratic Republic
Edited by W.H. Mehnert, M. Smans, C.S. Muir, M. Möhner and D. Schön
1992; 384 pages; ISBN 92 832 2106 0

No. 107
Atlas of Cancer Mortality in the European Economic Community
Edited by M. Smans, C. Muir and P. Boyle
1992; 213 pages + 44 coloured maps; ISBN 92 832 2107 9

No. 108
Environmental Carcinogens: Methods of Analysis and Exposure Measurement. Volume 11: Polychlorinated Dioxins and Dibenzofurans
Edited by C. Rappe, H.R. Buser, B. Dodet and I.K. O'Neill
1991; 400 pages; ISBN 92 832 2108 7

No. 109
Environmental Carcinogens: Methods of Analysis and Exposure Measurement. Volume 12: Indoor Air
Edited by B. Seifert, H. van de Wiel, B. Dodet and I.K. O'Neill
1993; 385 pages; ISBN 92 832 2109 5

No. 110*
Directory of On-going Research in Cancer Epidemiology 1991
Edited by M.P. Coleman and J. Wahrendorf
1991; 753 pages; ISBN 92 832 2110 9

No. 111
Pathology of Tumours in Laboratory Animals, Second Edition. Volume 2: Tumours of the Mouse
Edited by V. Turusov and U. Mohr
1994; 800 pages; ISBN 92 832 2111 1

No. 112
Autopsy in Epidemiology and Medical Research
Edited by E. Riboli and M. Delendi
1991; 288 pages; ISBN 92 832 2112 5

No. 113
Laboratory Decontamination and Destruction of Carcinogens in Laboratory Wastes: Some Mycotoxins
Edited by M. Castegnaro, J. Barek, J.M. Frémy, M. Lafontaine, M. Miraglia, E.B. Sansone and G.M. Telling
1991; 63 pages; ISBN 92 832 2113 3

No. 114
Laboratory Decontamination and Destruction of Carcinogens in Laboratory Wastes: Some Polycyclic Heterocyclic Hydrocarbons
Edited by M. Castegnaro, J. Barek, J. Jacob, U. Kirso, M. Lafontaine, E.B. Sansone, G.M. Telling and T. Vu Duc
1991; 50 pages; ISBN 92 832 2114 1

No. 115
Mycotoxins, Endemic Nephropathy and Urinary Tract Tumours
Edited by M. Castegnaro, R. Plestina, G. Dirheimer, I.N. Chernozemsky and H. Bartsch
1991; 340 pages; ISBN 92 832 2115 X

No. 116
Mechanisms of Carcinogenesis in Risk Identification
Edited by H. Vainio, P. Magee, D. McGregor and A.J. McMichael
1992; 615 pages; ISBN 92 832 2116 8

No. 117*
Directory of On-going Research in Cancer Epidemiology 1992
Edited by M. Coleman, E. Demaret and J. Wahrendorf
1992; 773 pages; ISBN 92 832 2117 6

No. 118
Cadmium in the Human Environment: Toxicity and Carcinogenicity
Edited by G.F. Nordberg, R.F.M. Herber and L. Alessio
1992; 470 pages; ISBN 92 832 2118 4

No. 119*
The Epidemiology of Cervical Cancer and Human Papillomavirus
Edited by N. Muñoz, F.X. Bosch, K.V. Shah and A. Meheus
1992; 288 pages; ISBN 92 832 2119 2

No. 120*
Cancer Incidence in Five Continents, Vol. VI
Edited by D.M. Parkin, C.S. Muir, S.L. Whelan, Y.T. Gao, J. Ferlay and J. Powell
1992; 1020 pages; ISBN 92 832 2120 6

No. 121
Time Trends in Cancer Incidence and Mortality
By M. Coleman, J. Estéve, P. Damiecki, A. Arslan and H. Renard
1993; 820 pages; ISBN 92 832 2121 4

No. 122
International Classification of Rodent Tumours. Part I. The Rat
Editor-in-Chief: U. Mohr

Respiratory System
1992; 57 pages; ISBN 92 832 0121 3
US$23

Soft Tissue and Muscoskeletal System
1992; 62 pages; ISBN 92 832 01221

Urinary System
1993; 27 pages; ISBN 92 832 0123 X

Haematopoietic System
1992; 46 pages; ISBN 92 832 0124 8
US$ 23

Integumentary System
1993; 45 pages; ISBN 92 832 0125 6

Endocrine System
1994; 75 pages; ISBN 92 832 0126 4

Central Nervous System: Heart; Eye; Mesothelium
1994; 80 pages; ISBN 92 832 0127 2

*Out-of-print

Male Genital System
1997; 52 pages; ISBN 92 832 0128 0

Female Genital System
1997; 83 pages; ISBN 92 832 0129 9

Digestive System
Publication due May 1997; 109 pages;
ISBN 92 832 0130 2

No. 123
**Cancer in Italian Migrant
Populations**
Edited by M. Geddes, D.M. Parkin,
M. Khlat, D. Balzi and E. Buiatti
1993; 292 pages; ISBN 92 832 2123 0

No. 124
**Postlabelling Methods for the
Detection of DNA Damage**
Edited by D.H. Phillips,
M. Castegnaro and H. Bartsch
1993; 392 pages; ISBN 92 832 2124 9

No. 125
**DNA Adducts: Identification and
Biological Significance**
Edited by K. Hemminki, A. Dipple,
D.E.G. Shuker, F.F. Kadlubar,
D. Segerbäck and H. Bartsch
1994; 478 pages; ISBN 92 832 2125 7

No. 126
**Pathology of Tumours in Laboratory
Animals, Second Edition. Volume 3:
Tumours of the Hamster**
Edited by U. Mohr and V. Turosov
1996; 464 pages; ISBN 92 832 2126 5

No. 127
**Butadiene and Styrene: Assessment
of Health Hazards**
Edited by M. Sorsa, K. Peltonen, H.
Vainio and K. Hemminki
1993; 412 pages; ISBN 92 832 2127 3

No. 128
**Statistical Methods in Cancer
Research. Volume IV. Descriptive
Epidemiology**
By J. Estève, E. Benhamou and L. Raymond
1994; 302 pages; ISBN 92 832 2128 1

No. 129
**Occupational Cancer in Developing
Countries**
Edited by N. Pearce, E. Matos,
H. Vainio, P. Boffetta and M. Kogevinas
1994; 191 pages; ISBN 92 832 2129 X

No. 130*
**Directory of On-going Research in
Cancer Epidemiology 1994**
Edited by R. Sankaranarayanan,
J. Wahrendorf and E. Démaret
1994; 800 pages; ISBN 92 832 2130 3

No. 132
**Survival of Cancer Patients in
Europe: The EUROCARE Study**
Edited by F. Berrino, M. Sant,
A. Verdecchia, R. Capocaccia,
T. Hakulinen and J. Estève
1995; 463 pages; ISBN 92 832 2132 X

No. 134
**Atlas of Cancer Mortality in Central
Europe**
W. Zatonski, J. Estéve, M. Smans,
J. Tyczynski and P. Boyle
1996; 175 pages plus 40 coloured maps;
ISBN 92 832 2134 6

No. 135
**Methods for Investigating Localized
Clustering of Disease**
Edited by F.E. Alexander and P. Boyle
1996; 235 pages; ISBN 92 832 2135 4

No. 136
Chemoprevention in Cancer Control
Edited by M. Hakama, V. Beral,
E. Buiatti, J. Faivre and D.M. Parkin
1996; 160 pages; ISBN 92 832 2136 2

No. 137
**Directory of On-going Research in
Cancer Epidemiology 1996**
Edited by R. Sankaranarayan, J.
Warendorf and E. Démaret
1996; 810 pages; ISBN 92 832 2137 0

No. 138
Social Inequalities and Cancer
Edited by M. Kogevinas, N. Pearce, M.
Susser and P. Boffetta
1997; 412 pages; ISBN 92 832 8138 9

No. 139
Principles of Chemoprevention
Edited by B.W. Stewart, D. McGregor
and P. Kleihues
1996; 358 pages; ISBN 92 832 2139 7

No. 140
**Mechanisms of Fibre
Carcinogenesis**
Edited by A.B. Kane, R. Saracci, P.
Boffetta and J.D. Wilbourn
1996; 135 pages; ISBN 92 832 2140 0

No. 142
**Application of Biomarkers in Cancer
Epidemiology**
Edited by P. Toniolo, P. Boffetta,
D.E.G. Shuker, N. Rothman, B. Hulka
and N. Pearce
1997; 318 pages; ISBN 92 832 2142 7

No. 143
**Cancer Incidence in Five Continentss
Vol VII.**
Edited by D.M. Parkin, S.L. Whelan, J.
Ferlay, L. Raymond & J. Young
1997; 1240 pages; ISBN 92 832 2143 5

No. 144
**International Incidence of Childhood
Cancer, Vol. II**
Edited by D.M. Parkin, E. Kramárová,
C.A. Stiller, J.G.J. Draper, E. Masuyer, J.
Michaelis, J. Neglia and S. Qureshi
Publication due September 1998; c. 500
pages; ISBN 92 832 2144 3

No. 145
**Cancer Survival in Developing
Countries**
Edited by R. Sankaranarayanan, R.J.
Black and D.M. Parkin Publication due
October 1998; c. 250 pages; ISBN 92
832 2145 1

No. 146
**Short- and Medium-term
Carcinogenicity Tests, Mutation
Analysis, and Multistage Models in
Risk Identification**
Publication due September 1998
c. 320 pages; ISBN 92 832 2146 X

*Out-of-print

IARC Technical Reports

No. 1
Cancer in Costa Rica
Edited by R. Sierra, R. Barrantes,
G. Muñoz Leiva, D.M. Parkin,
C.A. Bieber and N. Muñoz Calero
1988; 124 pages;
ISBN 92 832 1412 9

No. 2*
SEARCH: A Computer Package to Assist the Statistical Analysis of Case-Control Studies
Edited by G.J. Macfarlane, P. Boyle and
P. Maisonneuve
1991; 80 pages; ISBN 92 832 1413 7

No. 3
Cancer Registration in the European Economic Community
Edited by M.P. Coleman and E. Démaret
1988; 188 pages; ISBN 92 832 1414 5

No. 4*
Diet, Hormones and Cancer: Methodological Issues for Prospective Studies
Edited by E. Riboli and R. Saracci
1988; 156 pages; ISBN 92 832 1415 3

No. 5*
Cancer in the Philippines
Edited by A.V. Laudico, D. Esteban and
D.M. Parkin
1989; 186 pages; ISBN 92 832 1416 1

No. 6
La genèse du Centre international de recherche sur le cancer
By R. Sohier and A.G.B. Sutherland
1990, 102 pages; ISBN 92 832 1418 8

No. 7
Epidémiologie du cancer dans les pays de langue latine
1990, 292 pages; ISBN 92 832 1419 6

No. 8
Comparative Study of Anti-smoking Legislation in Countries of the European Economic Community
By A. J. Sasco, P. Dalla-Vorgia and
P. Van Der Elst
1992; 82 pages; ISBN: 92 832 1421 8

Etude comparative des Législations de Contrôle du Tabagisme dans les Pays de la Communauté économique européenne
By A. J. Sasco, P. Dalla-Vorgia and
P. Van Der Elst
1995; 82 pages; ISBN 92 832 2402 7

No. 9*
Epidémiologie du cancer dans les pays de langue latine
1991; 346 pages; ISBN 92 832 1423 4

No. 10
Manual for Cancer Registry Personnel
Edited by D. Esteban, S. Whelan,
A. Laudico and D.M. Parkin
1995; 400 pages; ISBN 92 832 1424 2

No. 11
Nitroso Compounds: Biological Mechanisms, Exposures and Cancer Etiology
Edited by I. O'Neill and H. Bartsch
1992; 150 pages; ISBN 92 832 1425 0

No. 12*
Epidémiologie du cancer dans les pays de langue latine
1992; 375 pages; ISBN 92 832 1426 9

No. 13
Health, Solar UV Radiation and Environmental Change
By A. Kricker, B.K. Armstrong,
M.E. Jones and R.C. Burton
1993; 213 pages; ISBN 92 832 1427 7

No. 14*
Epidémiologie du cancer dans les pays de langue latine
1993; 400 pages; ISBN 92 832 1428 5

No. 15
Cancer in the African Population of Bulawayo, Zimbabwe, 1963–1977
By M.E.G. Skinner, D.M. Parkin,
A.P. Vizcaino and A. Ndhlovu
1993; 120 pages; ISBN 92 832 1429 3

No. 16
Cancer in Thailand 1984–1991
By V. Vatanasapt, N. Martin,
H. Sriplung, K. Chindavijak, S. Sontipong,
S. Sriamporn, D.M. Parkin and J. Ferlay
1993; 164 pages; ISBN 92 832 1430 7

No. 18
Intervention Trials for Cancer Prevention
By E. Buiatti
1994; reprinted 1996, 52 pages; ISBN
92 832 1432 3

No. 19
Comparability and Quality Control in Cancer Registration
By D.M. Parkin, V.W. Chen, J. Ferlay,
J. Galceran, H.H. Storm and S.L. Whelan
1994; revised 1996, 110 pages plus
diskette;
ISBN 92 832 1433 1

Comparabilidad y Control de Calidad en los Registros de Cancer
By D.M. Parkin, V.W. Chen, J. Ferlay, J.
Galceran, H.H. Storm and S.L. Whelan
1995; 125 pages + diskette
ISBN 92 832 0402 6

Comparabilité et Contrôle de Qualité dans 'Enriegistrement des Cancers
By D.M. Parkin, V.W. Chen, J. Ferlay, J.
Galceran, H.H. Storm and S.L. Whelan
1996; 123 pages + diskette
ISBN 92 832 0403 5

No. 20
Epidémiologie du cancer dans les pays de langue latine
1994; 346 pages; ISBN 92 832 1434 X

No. 21*
ICD Conversion Programs for Cancer
By J. Ferlay
1994; 24 pages plus diskette;
ISBN 92 832 1435 8

No. 22*
Cancer in Tianjin
By Q.S. Wang, P. Boffetta,
M. Kogevinas and D.M. Parkin
1994; 96 pages; ISBN 92 832 1437 4

No. 23*
An Evaluation Programme for Cancer Preventive Agents
By Bernard W. Stewart
1995; 40 pages; ISBN 92 832 1438 2

No. 24
Peroxisome Proliferation and its Role in Carcinogenesis
1995; 85 pages; ISBN 92 832 1439 0

No. 25
Combined Analysis of Cancer Mortality in Nuclear Workers in Canada, the United Kingdom and the United States of America
By E. Cardis, E.S. Gilbert, L.
Carpenter, G. Howe, I. Kato, J. Fix, L.
Salmon, G. Cowper, B.K. Armstrong,
V. Beral, A. Douglas, S.A. Fry, J. Kaldor,
C. Lavé, P.G. Smith, G. Voelz and
L. Wiggs
1995; 160 pages; ISBN 92 832 1440 4

No. 26
Mortalité par Cancer des Immigrés en France, 1979-1985
By C. Bouchardy, M. Khlat, P. Wanner
and D.M. Parkin
1998; 150 pages; ISBN 92 832 2404 3

No. 27
The risk of Cancer in Three Generations of Young Israelis:
By J. Iscovich and D.M. Parkin
1998; 92pages; ISBN 92 832 1441 2

No. 28
Survey of Cancer Registries in the European Union
By H. Storm, I. Clemmensen and R. Black
1998; c. 40 pages; ISBN 92 832 1442 0

No. 29
International Classification of Childhood Cancer 1996
By E. Kramárová, C.A. Stiller, J. Ferlay, D.M. Parkin, G.J.
Draper, J. Michaelis,
J. Neglia and S. Qureshi
1997; 48 pages + diskette;
ISBN 92 832 1443 9

No. 30
**Cancer Risk from Occupational Exposure to Wood
Dust:** By P. Demer and P. Boffetta
1998; 95 pages; ISBN 92 832 1444 7

No. 31
Histological Groups for Compartive Studies
By D.M. Parkin, K. Shanmugarathnam, L. Sobin, J. Ferlay
and S. Whelan
1998; 67 pages + diskette
ISBN 92 832 1145 US$ 26

No. 32
Automated Data Collection in Cancer Registration
By R.J. Black, L. Simonato and H. Storm
1998; c. 48 pages; ISBN 92 832 1146 3 US$ 26

IARC CancerBases
ISSN 1027 5614

No. 1
EUCAN90: Cancer in the European Union (Electronic
Database with Graphic Display)
By J. Ferlay, R.J. Black, P. Pisani, M.T. Valdivieso and D.M.
Parkin
1996; Computer software on 3.5" IBM diskette + user's
guide (50 pages);
ISBN 92 832 1450 1

No. 2
**CIVII: Electronic Database of Cancer Incidence in Five
Continents**
By J. Ferlay
1997; Computer software on 3.5" IBM diskettes + user's
guide (63 pages);
ISBN 92 832 1449 8

IARC Non-Serial Publications

Alcool et Cancer
By A. Tuyns
1978; 48 pages; US$ 9

**Cancer Morbidity and Causes of Death among
Danish Brewery Workers**
By O.M. Jensen
1980; 143 pages
1SBN 92 832 1403 X; US$ 15

**Directory of Computer Systems Used in Cancer
Registries**
By H.R. Menck and D.M. Parkin
1986; 236 pages; US $10

**Facts and Figures of Cancer in the European
Community**
By J. Estève, A. Kricker, J. Ferlay and D.M. Parkin
1993; 52 pages; ISBN 92 832 1427; US$ 9

An Introduction to Cancer Epidemiology
By I. dos Santos Silva
Publications in English, French and Spanish due
September 1998. US$ 40

**Pathology and Genetics of Tumours of the Nervous
System**
Edited by P. Kleihues and W.K. Cavanee
1997; 255 pages; ISBN 92 832 1148X US$ 85

All IARC Publications are available directly from
**IARCPress, 150 Cours Albert Thomas, F-69372 Lyon cedex 08, France (Fax: +33 4 72 73 83 02;
E-mail:press@iarc.fr).**

**IARC Monographs and Technical Reports are also available from the
World Health Organization Distribution and Sales, CH-1211 Geneva 27 (Fax: +41 22 791 4857)
and from WHO Sales Agents worldwide.**

**IARC Scientific Publications, IARC Handbooks and IARC CancerBases are also available from
Oxford University Press, Walton Street, Oxford, UK OX2 6DP (Fax: +44 1865 267782).**